12/08

THE ENCYCLOPEDIA OF

PHOBIAS, FEARS, AND ANXIETIES

THIRD EDITION

Ronald M. Doctor, Ph.D.
Ada P. Kahn, Ph.D.
and
Christine Adamec

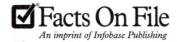

Facts On File
An imprint of Infobase Publishing

The Encyclopedia of Phobias, Fears, and Anxieties, Third Edition

Facts On File, Inc.
An imprint of Infobase Publishing
132 West 31st Street
New York NY 10001

Library of Congress Cataloging-in-Publication Data

Doctor, Ronald M. (Ronald Manual)
The encyclopedia of phobias, fears, and anxieties / Ronald M. Doctor, Ada P. Kahn, and Christine Adamec.—3rd ed.
p. ; cm.
Includes bibliographical references and index.
ISBN-13: 978-0-8160-6453-3 (alk. paper)
ISBN-10: 0-8160-6453-9 (alk. paper)
1. Phobias—Dictionaries. 2. Fear—Dictionaries. 3. Anxiety—Dictionaries. I. Kahn, Ada P. II. Adamec, Christine A., 1949–III. Title. IV. Title: Phobias, fears, and anxieties.
[DNLM: 1. Phobic Disorders—Dictionary—English. 2. Anxiety—Dictionary—English. 3. Fear—Dictionary—English. WM 13 D637e 2008]
RC535.D63 2008
616.85′22003—dc22   2007015217

Facts On File books are available at special discounts when purchased in bulk quantities for businesses, associations, institutions, or sales promotions. Please call our Special Sales Department in New York at (212) 967-8800 or (800) 322-8755.

You can find Facts On File on the World Wide Web at http://www.factsonfile.com

Text design by Cathy Rincon

Printed in the United States of America

VB Hermitage 10 9 8 7 6 5 4 3 2 1

This book is printed on acid-free paper and contains 30% post-consumer recycled content.

CONTENTS

PREFACE

This encyclopedia explores in depth diverse aspects of phobias, fears, and anxieties. Information on these subjects has developed along with our knowledge of other areas of mental health. Just as our understanding of the human psyche is far from complete, so too is our understanding of the origins and management of phobias, fears, and anxieties. This second edition explores additional life areas related to anxieties as well as many complementary approaches.

This book deals with experiences we all have at times but that for some of us become a persistent and sometimes devastating problem. Although we don't fully understand the causes of the problem, or why some people are more susceptible to it than others, we have been more fortunate in treating phobias, fears, and anxieties. Behavioral therapies have been shown to be particularly effective, and self-help techniques are flourishing. Drugs have also been useful, but the biochemical and physiological mechanisms underlying phobias, fears, and anxieties are still only partially understood. It is clear that anxiety and related disorders are much more than a physical or even behavioral response alone. The complex nature of the problem confronts the clinician and researcher at every turn.

In preparing the contents of *The Encyclopedia of Phobias, Fears, and Anxieties,* we were guided by several purposes. First, we wanted to be inclusive rather than restrictive, and thus we were quite liberal in choosing entries. For example, some entries (such as fears of voodoo, magic, etc.) are socio-cultural in emphasis rather than psychological, in order to present a broad perspective. Some entries concern esoteric manifestations of phobias but are included for purposes of depth. Most of the known technical names of specific phobias are defined and described to the extent that information is available from the literature of psychology and psychiatry. Entries range from descriptions of symptoms to explanations of treatments for the disorders, from some concepts of historical interest to some self-help suggestions for phobic individuals.

The Encyclopedia of Phobias, Fears, and Anxieties is intended for both lay readers and health-care professionals. We have tried to use easy-to-understand language without becoming overly simplistic, so that the book can be used by psychologists, social workers, teachers, and family members as well as by individuals who are facing phobias, fears, or anxieties. To give the book an added usefulness for phobic individuals, we have carefully selected some self-tests and self-help suggestions (such as how to relieve a fear of flying). Our suggestions are general, but references are included for more complete and specific self-help approaches in each entry. Professionals will find this a convenient reference guide for short descriptions of concepts they want to explain to patients or clients, and for details they may seek in the course of their own writing, teaching, or counseling. For all who seek information to this field, we hope *The Encyclopedia of Phobias, Fears, and Anxieties* will prove a valuable source of information not otherwise available in one place.

Space limitations have dictated conciseness; to assist readers seeking additional information, we have included in many entries references to relevant books and journal articles. We have also included an extensive bibliography at the end of the book.

Preparing this book has given us a deeper appreciation of humanity's struggle with the elusive force within. We hope that you, too, find it enlightening.

—Ronald Manual Doctor, Ph.D.
Northridge, California
—Ada P. Kahn, Ph.D.
Evanston, Illinois

ACKNOWLEDGMENTS

We appreciate the cooperation of the American Psychiatric Association for permitting reproduction of instructive tables and charts.

We thank many librarians in the reference department of Rush North Shore Medical Center, Skokie, Illinois, and the Skokie Public Library for their ongoing assistance in locating research materials and obtaining data sources through the metropolitan Chicago area North Suburban Inter-library Loan Service, Wheeling, Illinois. Also, we thank librarians in the Division of Library and Information Management, American Medical Association, Chicago; the Northwestern University Medical Library, Chicago; the library of the Institute for Psychoanalysis, Chicago; the Oviatt Library, California State University, Northridge, California; the Wellcome Institute for the Study of the History of Medicine, London; and the library at the Maudsley Hospital, University of London, for their assistance.

We thank Jennifer Welbourne, Rebecca Burkhardt, and Michelle Pellegrino for their assistance with research.

—Ronald M. Doctor, Ph.D.
Northridge, California
—Ada P. Kahn, Ph.D.
Evanston, Illinois

INTRODUCTION: A HISTORICAL OVERVIEW OF PHOBIAS

Phobias are common in the United States and throughout the world. An estimated 19.2 million adults over age 18 in the United States, or 9 percent of the population, have experienced specific phobic reactions at some time in their lives. Phobic objects, people, or situations are extremely variable, ranging from fear of large ferocious dogs, a phobia many people can understand, to other phobias that most people find baffling, such as fear of gravity, fear of developing a fever, or fear of strangers. In addition, about 15 million adults (6.8 percent of the population) in any given year suffer from social phobia, in which they avoid or feel anxious about interacting with others. About 1.8 million people (less than 1 percent of the adult population) have agoraphobia that is not associated with panic disorder. Agoraphobia is often characterized by individuals' fear of leaving their homes or safe areas, lest something dire occur to them.

Whatever the phobia, the individual's life is often dominated by this intense fear, both at work (if the phobic person *can* work) and at home, and it often makes life extremely difficult for both the phobic person and family members. For example, the agoraphobic parent cannot attend parent-teacher meetings or travel comfortably with their family. The social phobic shuns social gatherings, even those honoring a beloved spouse, and may have difficulty writing checks in public. The individual with a specific phobia goes to great lengths

to avoid the feared object. Avoidance is a critical marker for labeling a behavior as phobic.

Most phobics know that their extreme fears are irrational and may even seem silly, yet they continue to be transfixed by them, trapped and unable to escape from them. However, today psychotherapy and medications can often ease the way for the phobic person, greatly enhancing his or her life, at last largely freeing them from the emotional bonds that have held them captive.

Phobias are different from fears, in both their intensity and their importance in the person's life. Many experts have debated why people develop phobias. Some experts believe that phobias are hardwired into the brain as evolutionary rudiments (called *prepared fears*), while others believe they stem from unresolved conflicts in childhood or traumas. In some cases, the origin of a phobia cannot be determined, even by a skilled therapist. Talented therapists, though, should be able to provide considerable relief to most people suffering from phobias, even when they cannot ascertain the initial source of the phobia.

This introduction covers key theories about the origins of the term *phobia*, describes the difference between fears and phobias, and discusses some general theories about why phobias develop, as well as offering some newer theories that have been advanced to explain phobias. In addition, a historical overview on views about phobias and phobics from the past to the present is also provided.

The Use of the Term *Phobia*

According to author Paul Errara, M.D., in his article on the historical aspects of the concept of phobia, the word *phobia* itself is derived from the Greek word for flight, terror, and strangulation. Phobos was a Greek god who caused panic and fear among the enemies of those who worshipped him. However, for the most part, the term *phobia* did not appear in common usage until the 19th century.

In the latter half of the 19th century, the word *phobia* was used in the same sense that it is used today, meaning an intense fear out of proportion to the apparent stimulus. These fears cannot be explained or reasoned away, and phobic individuals avoid the feared situations wherever and whenever possible.

With the proliferation of many different names that were given to various phobias (mainly by psychoanalytic theorists), confusion increased. Naming phobias ultimately led to the idea that each phobia had its own root cause and individual treatment. However, phobias share certain features. Early on, theorists were aware of the strikingly unreasonable quality of the fears, of their chronic nature, and their fluctuating intensity.

As understanding of how the mind works advanced during the 19th century, and particularly in its latter part, phobias were described increasingly in psychiatric literature. The term agoraphobia was introduced in 1872, in Otto Westphal's (1824–1902) classic paper describing three agoraphobic cases (all of whom were male):

> . . . impossibility of walking through certain streets or squares or possibility of so doing only with resultant dread of anxiety . . . no loss of consciousness . . . vertigo was excluded by all patients
>
> . . . no hallucinations nor delusions to cause the strange fear . . . agony was much increased at those hours when the particular streets dreaded were deserted and the shops closed. The subjects experienced great comfort from the companionship of men or even an inanimate object, such as a vehicle or a cane. The use of beer or wine also allowed the patient to pass through the feared locality

with comparative comfort. One man even sought, without immoral motives, the companionship of a prostitute as far as his own door . . . some localities are more difficult of access than others; the patient walking far in order not to traverse them . . .

> Strange to say, in one instance, the open country was less feared than sparsely housed streets in town. Case three also had a dislike to crossing a certain bridge. He feared he would fall into the water
>
> . . . In two cases the onset of the disease had been sudden; in the third the fear had been gradually increasing for a number of years. In two of the cases there was no hereditary predisposition to mental or nervous disease; in the third case a sister was epileptic and ancestors had had some peculiar seizures.

Westphal labeled his patients as having *agoraphobia* because their state was characterized principally by a dread or *phobia* that occurred in the streets or in public places, like the *agora* (the Greek word for "market"). He commented that for agoraphobics, the thought of the feared situation frequently was as distressing as the actual situation itself. (This is still a valid observation.) Writers in France, England, and Germany commented on Westphal's paper and contributed information of their own to the increasing body of literature about this syndrome. Within the next century, researchers and therapists recognized that the fear of fear was a central concept in agoraphobia.

In 1895, Henry Maudsley (1835–1918), British psychiatrist and author, included all phobias under the heading *melancholia* and advised against the trend of giving a special name to each variety of phobic situation, as many phobias often were noticed together or successively in the same individual.

Phobias versus Fears

Many people do not like snakes or spiders. Some people, however, have irrationally excessive fears and may exhibit a marked reaction to even a drawing or the mere *thought* of snakes and spiders (or another feared object). Any reminders of the feared item will increase the heart rate of the phobic person, as well as their blood pressure and hormone levels. (Secretions of hormones such as cortisol will spike during times of a real or perceived threat.)

The primary difference between a normal fear that is shared by many people and a chronic phobia is that a phobia is irrational and impedes the individual's daily life. When the fear becomes overwhelming, persistent, and enveloping and impedes an individual from normal functioning, it is considered a phobia.

Some fears and phobias stem from modern-day issues such as the fear of terrorism, which, if taken to extremes, could develop into irrational avoidance. Other fears are more individual, such as a fear of caves, which may be based on claustrophobia or caused by a distressing experience of being lost or trapped in a cave for many hours.

The intensity and chronicity of a phobia are far greater than the reaction of simple fear. According to authors Aaron Beck, M.D., and Gary Emery in their book, *Anxiety Disorders and Phobias: A Cognitive Perspective,* "One of the key qualities that makes a fear into a phobia is the magnification of the amount of risk in a feared situation and the degree of harm that will come from being in that situation. Because of the greater hazard the phobic person imputes to situation or object, he experiences much greater anxiety than the non-phobic individual in the fear situation, as well as a greater desire to avoid it."

Traumatic Experiences

Some phobias evolve from traumatic experience, often occurring in childhood. A child who was bitten by a dog may fear all dogs even though the experience is suppressed or forgotten. Someone who was trapped in an elevator and frightened may develop a fear of elevators and even a generalized fear of small enclosed spaces (claustrophobia). Adults abused as children may associate some objects to their childhood abuse; for example, a child who was injured by an iron thrown by her mother avoided irons as an adult.

A Multiplicity of Phobias

Beck and Emery describe what they call "spreading phobias," or phobias that have evolved beyond the original feared object to other items that are somehow linked with the initial phobia: "For example, a laborer was struck by a truck while painting a white line on a road and subsequently developed a phobia of working on the road. The phobia then spread to a fear of riding a motorcycle or bicycle on a road."

Many phobic individuals suffer from more than one phobia. Beck and Emery described a doctor who feared flying, sitting in a large audience, speaking before large groups, and going to parties. A therapist found the underlying common factor of each of these phobias by asking the doctor what he thought could occur in each of these situations. He discovered that the doctor felt he could lose control and harm someone or humiliate himself. "He was afraid of traveling in an airplane because he feared he would go berserk, lose control of himself, or strike out at other passengers. At public gatherings, he feared he would jump up, wave his arms, and shout obscenities at the audience. He had a recurring fantasy of sitting in the second row at a concert and completely disrupting the performance by vomiting over the person seated in front of him, or of stepping on people's feet as he left his seat. He feared he would distract the entire audience from the music. . . . His fear of speaking at professional meetings was related to a fear of demolishing someone else's theory. His anxiety at cocktail parties was related to the thought that he might spill a drink and also by the thought that he might impulsively tell people that they were stupid."

Avoidance: The Common Reaction to Phobias

Many phobic people are able to avoid the things that they fear, unless they are ubiquitous. Those who fear social contact find it difficult to avoid people altogether unless they become recluses, while those who fear snakes can generally avoid them. It is when an individual, for whatever reason, is compelled to encounter and then *remain* with the object of the phobia, such as when the phobic person reacts by freezing rather than taking flight, which is the most stressful time.

Fear as an Engrained Evolutionary Response

Many experts believe that there are some basic fears that may be hardwired into the human brain as an autonomic internal protection against dangerous creatures or other experiences. Some examples are the fears of lightning, thunder, darkness, blood, spiders, snakes, high places, angry people, and storms, as well as the infant's fear of strangers that manifests at about the same time that the baby starts to crawl.

Many experts believe that humans have experienced and displayed their responses to certain primordial fears from before prerecorded history to the present day, and that such fears may have been largely adaptive in times long past. For example, it is likely that the ancient cave dweller was extremely fearful of snakes, spiders, and many other real threats, just as many people today continue to shrink from such creatures—even though they rarely represent a threat to modern individuals. Some evidence for engrained fears comes from the fact that 85 percent of the people who are terrified of snakes have never seen a live snake.

According to Isaac M. Marks and Randolph M. Nesse in an article in *Ethology and Sociology,* "Factors that have shaped anxiety-regulation mechanisms can explain prepotent and prepared tendencies to associate anxiety more quickly with certain cues than with others. These tendencies lead to excess fear of largely archaic dangers, like snakes, and too little fear of new threats, like cars." This point is important to emphasize, because modern individuals are far more at risk from death or injury from a car crash than from a tiny household spider or a harmless garden snake.

In a 1998 article in the *British Journal of Medical Psychology* on considering emotional disorders from an evolutionary perspective, Randolph Nesse pointed out that some clinical states of anxiety are actually adaptive in some situations. Animal phobia is a useful response when an individual is confronted with dangerous animals, while social phobia is an adaptive response when there is a valid threat to an individual's reputation or status. Agoraphobia is adaptive as well when a person faces an environment that includes dangerous predators, while hypochondria is adaptive when perceived health threats are valid.

Despite the apparent evolutionary aspect of fears and phobias, which may have become maladaptive reactions in a 21st-century world, today there are many available treatments for individuals suffering from debilitating phobias. The ancient cave dweller could not seek out a therapist who was an expert in exposure therapy, nor could he talk it out with a cognitive behavior psychotherapist or take an antianxiety medication to ease his suffering. These options—and a variety of other means to resolve phobias, fears, and anxieties—are now available and even commonplace in the 21st century.

The Element of Disgust and Boundary Transgressions in Phobias

Some authors have discussed phobias in terms of two key elements: disgust and the fear of being touched and thus contaminated by the feared object. These elements are almost always present among those with phobias of natural items. In their article on disgust and phobias in a 2006 article in *Body & Society,* Mick Smith and Joyce Davidson say that many phobic individuals whose phobias are related to natural items (such as insects, snakes, cats, or even some foods) are concerned with actively avoiding the object specifically because the elements of disgust and the fear of being touched by the feared object are so intense. Even when the phobic individual has never been touched by the feared object, he or she fears that such a touch would be intolerable. In addition, the feared object represents a lack of order and is experienced as a direct threat to the individual's personal boundaries. Say the authors, "Such intrusions might be thought threatening, not because they pose a physical danger (evolutionary naturalism), nor because they are associated with the polluting effects of human bodily waste (psychoanalytic naturalism), but because they are indicative of nature itself transgressing the very basis of the symbolic order on which modern society and self-identity are founded."

The authors described one spider phobic who could not enter or stay in a room unless she repeatedly checked for spiders. Yet, unlike nonphobics who would either kill the spider or leave, the spider phobic would be transfixed if she actually did see a spider. "An escape route would have been planned but probably not taken advantage of, as she freezes and experiences a desperate need to keep the spider within her view. Her fear of leaving the room and losing sight of the spider may be indicative of a reluctance to surrender the very limited amount of control she has over the situation, in the form of knowledge of the feared object's location."

In one case, a patient feared onions. If the onion was not peeled, she was not fearful, but, if any layers were removed, she could not bear to look at or be in contact with the onion, in part because of her fear that she might accidentally ingest the onion, which she found disgusting.

Looking Back in History at Phobias

It is instructive to consider a brief historical overview of phobias to provide a backdrop of understanding how humans have evolved from the past to the present day.

Early Events

Throughout history, phobic reactions have been noted by authors and other individuals. Hippocrates (460–377 B.C.E.) may have been one of the first authors to describe morbid fears when he wrote about a highly phobic individual who seemed to fear heights, precipices, and flute music:

> He would not go near a precipice, or over a bridge or beside even the shallowest ditch, and yet he could walk in the ditch itself. When he used to begin drinking, the girl flute-player would frighten him; as soon as he heard the first note of the flute at a banquet, he would be beset by terror. He used to say he could scarcely contain himself when night fell; but during the day (when there were people about him) he would hear this instrument without feeling any emotion.

Phobias and Superstitions

Historically, much fearful behavior was attributed to superstitious beliefs in witchcraft, demonology, and evil spirits. Indeed, Robert Burton characterized the changes that took place during the 17th century when he wrote, "Tis a common practice of some men to go first to a witch, then to a physician; if one cannot, the other shall; if they cannot bend Heaven, they will try Hell."

John Bunyan (1628–88), English preacher, writer, and author of *The Pilgrim's Progress*, noted his own fear of bells ringing and church steeples:

> Now, you must know, that before this I had taken much delight in ringing, but my conscience beginning to be tender, I thought such practice was but vain, and therefore forced myself to leave it, yet my mind hankered; wherefore I should go to the steeple house, and look on it, though I durst not ring. But I thought this did not become religion yet I forced myself, and would look on still; but quickly after, I stand under a main beam, that lay overthwart the steeple, from side to side, thinking there I might stand sure, but then I should think again, Should the bell fall with a swing, it might first hit the wall, and then rebounding upon me, might kill me for all this beam. This made me stand in the steeple door; and now, thought I, I am safe enough; for if a bell should then fall, I can slip out behind these thick walls, and so be preserved not withstanding.
>
> So, after this, I would yet to go see them ring, but would not go farther than the steeple door; but then it came into my head, How, if the steeple itself should fall? And this thought, it may fall for aught I know, when I stood and looked on, did continually so shake my mind, that I durst not stand at the steeple door any longer, but was forced to flee, for fear the steeple should fall upon my head.

Bunyan demonstrated a common feature of phobias: their tendency to spread. At first, he feared just the straight fall of the bell, then its bouncing course, and finally the complete crashing destruction of the whole steeple.

Botanist François Boissier de Sauvages (1706–67) created a systematic listing of his medical observations, and he termed what are now known as phobias as either hysterical vertigo or hypochondriacal vertigo. He thought that these symptoms stemmed from a problem with the retina of the eye that caused an increased sensitivity. He described a woman who became dizzy every time she entered an empty church; however, if she entered a church full of parishioners, she experienced no dizziness.

In 1789, Benjamin Rush (1745–1813), American physician, author, and signer of the Declaration of Independence, published an article in which he offered his definition of phobia: "I shall define phobia to be a fear of an imaginary evil, or an undue fear of a real one." He then listed 18 species of fear named according to the object of excessive fear or aversion, such as dirt or rats.

Samuel Johnson (1709–84), English author, critic, and lexicographer, indicated that he suffered from a fear of death and crowded places when he asked to be excused from jury duty because he came "very near fainting . . . in all crowded places."

In the 18th century, the French surgeon A. Le Camus (1722–72) described what we now call phobias in his book *Des Aversions*. Le Camus labeled phobias as *aversions* that he believed were related to the various senses, seeing, hearing, touching, tasting, or smelling. Le Camus described King James I of England as overwhelmed with terror at the very sight of an unsheathed sword. Le Camus described other individuals who fled from the smell of apples or upon seeing a mouse or observing the presence of cream.

During the late 18th–early 19th century, imaginative naming was in vogue, perhaps in an emulation of Linnaeus (1707–78), the Swedish botanist and originator of the system of biologic taxonomic classification and nomenclature. For several decades, many types of phobias were described and named. Many names are still in use and can be found in this encyclopedia.

Sigmund Freud and Phobias

Sigmund Freud's writing and theorizing at the end of the 19th century contributed to an increased interest in both the causes and the treatment of anxieties and phobias. In 1895, Freud wrote *Obsessions and Phobias: Their Psychical Mechanism and Their Aetiology*. In this paper, he distinguished obsessions from phobias by suggesting that in the case of phobias, the patient's emotional state was always one of morbid anxiety, while in the case of obsessions, other emotional states such as doubt or anger could also occur at the same time.

In 1905, Freud wrote about a case that came to be known as "Little Hans," a five-year-old boy who was afraid of horses falling. Dr. Freud's analysis emphasized "infantile sexuality," and the Oedipal complex in which Hans repressed fear of his father's anger toward him for his attraction to his mother. The concept of expressed conflict for phobia became the psychoanalytic interpretation.

The symbolism always concerned an unacceptable aggressive or sexual impulse, regardless of the individual's own personality or previous experiences. Freud arrived at this analysis through correspondence with Hans's father and never actually saw the boy.

Freud classified phobia as an anxiety neurosis or a form of hysteria, and his original idea was that the phobia was an unconscious attempt by the individual to deal with anxiety by substitution and by displacement of anxieties that are foreign to the ego. Freud suggested that phobias related to objects had unconscious symbolic meanings and that they represented regressions to earlier infantile fears and anxieties, usually centered around Oedipal conflicts. (An Oedipal conflict is a child's attraction to the parent of the opposite sex, a conflict which is naturally resolved by healthy individuals.)

To Freud, the object that was feared always symbolized some form of sexual anxiety, and every phobia, therefore, was invested with some element of sexual anxiety. He believed a phobia was a symbolic expression of repressed feelings and the punishment linked to them in the unconscious. Freud distinguished between common phobias, such as of snakes and death, as well as between specific phobias of circumstances (such as going outside) that do not inspire fear in normal individuals.

Beyond Dr. Freud

Many psychotherapists have built upon Freud's ideas, accepting some of them, modifying others, and also adding new understanding to the mechanisms of anxiety, fears, phobias, obsessive-compulsive behavior, and depression among those who suffer from these problems. For example, most descriptions of patients with obsessive-compulsive disorder include some discussion of phobias. The converse is also true, and some modern authorities (e.g., Chambless and Goldstein) believe that phobias are closely related to obsessive-compulsive disorders and in fact are operationally and dynamically similar to them.

In 1876, French psychiatrist Legrand du Saulle (1830–86) referred to a phobia that he called "peur des espaces" (fear of spaces). According to author David Trotter, an English professor at Cambridge University, in his 2004 article on agoraphobia in

Victorian Literature and Culture: "Legrand was keen to emphasize the syndrome's ubiquity; panic might strike anywhere, on bridges and ferries, as well as in city streets and squares. He characterized the onset of an attack as a hesitation at a boundary: the transition between street and square, the edge of a pavement, an upstairs window overlooking a limitless expanse. Here, the sufferer, unable either to advance or to retreat, begins to tremble, or shiver, or breaks out in a sweat."

In some circumstances the phobia is not present. Trotter wrote of a patient who was a cavalry officer who could not cross open spaces while in civilian clothing, yet once he was arrayed in soldierly garb, he trotted across them with ease on horseback.

In the late 19th century, psychiatrists referred to a fear of contamination as *mysophobia*. Other experts believed that mysophobia could connect itself to objects, such as the woman who has a fear of tallow or any objects that contained tallow.

In 1890, philosopher and psychologist William James (1842–1910) wrote of "pathological fears" and "certain peculiarities in the expression of ordinary fear" in *The Principles of Psychology*. James believed that agoraphobia was a survival strategy in long past years, but was not useful in more modern times.

In 1903, Pierre Janet (1859–1947), a French psychologist, classified neurotic disorders into two major divisions. To him, hysteria denoted disturbances in sensation, movement, and consciousness; these are still considered characteristic symptoms of that syndrome. Psychasthenia, on the other hand, included most of the neurotic phenomena, such as phobias, anxiety, obsessions, and depression.

One of Janet's patients is of historical interest because, a quarter of a century before Janet presented him to his students, the patient had been examined by Legrand du Saulle when he was studying the problem of agoraphobia. Janet wrote:

> He was about 25, when there started what he himself called "the trouble with spaces." He was crossing the Place de la Concorde (alone, it should be noted) when he felt a strange sensation of dread. His breathing became rapid and he felt as if he were suffocating; his heart was beating violently and his legs were limp, as if half-paralyzed. He could go neither forwards nor backwards, and he had to exert a tremendous effort, bathed in sweat, to reach the other side of the square. From the time of that first episode on, he took a great dislike to the Place de la Concorde and decided that he would not risk going there again alone. However, a short while after the same sensation of anxiety recurred on the Invalides Bridge, and then in a street, which though it was narrow, seemed long and was quite steep.

Although the patient had regained temporary relief of his symptoms while he was under Legrand du Saulle's care, according to Janet:

> His illness was not cured and continued to develop slowly. The anxiety he would experience whenever he had to venture out into a place that was at all open was so severe that it became impossible for him to control it, and he was no longer able to cross any square. Some dozen years ago he had to escort a young girl to her house. As long as he was with her everything was all right, but when she had left him, he was unable to go back home. Five hours later, noticing that though it was getting dark and was raining, he had not yet returned, his wife became alarmed and went out in search of him. She found him ashen and shivering with cold on the edge of the Place des Invalides, which he had been completely unable to cross.

After this unpleasant experience, the patient was not allowed to go out alone, which was exactly what he wanted, since his attacks could thus be controlled. Whenever he came to a village square, he would begin to tremble and breathe heavily and develop tics. He repeated the phrase: "Mama, Rata, bibi, bitaquo. I'm going to die." His wife had to hold him tightly by his arm and then he would calm down and cross the square without further incident. His wife had to accompany him absolutely everywhere, even when he went to the toilet.

In 1913, Emil Kraepelin (1856–1926), a German psychiatrist, included a chapter on irrepressible ideas and irresistible fears in his textbook. He regarded personality factors as by-products of a diseased brain or a faulty metabolism. Genetic defects were believed to be the cause of mental illness at that time. Later these organic interpretations were largely overturned by others who took a more psychodynamic approach, although, as evidenced by the massive research effort directed to the use of medications, biological views still predominate.

The Development of Theories and Therapies for Phobias

Developments in the latter half of the 20th century and into the 21st have led to an increased knowledge about anxiety and phobic disorders as well as new directions in treating them. The treatment of choice, in most therapy settings, is a focus on helping people cope with phobic reactions. In many therapeutic settings, therapists use an integrated perspective to treat phobic people.

While each perspective offers value, none explains all the phenomena that various individuals experience. While some psychiatrists suggest that phobias are maintained by unconscious conflicts that remain in the unconscious mind, other psychotherapists focus instead on the avoided behavior and thoughts of the individual, such as the catastrophic misinterpretation of danger.

Some experts have suggested that phobias are derived from conditioned emotional experiences, and that the phobic object may have been part of a traumatic situation. On this basis, any object has an equal potential to become a phobic stimulus. Some say that certain phobic responses may be learned though imitating the reactions of others, or vicarious learning. Another theory is that phobic reactions are learned by the positive consequences that follow (for example, soothing attention from a parent of a school-phobic child). This type of learning is called "operant conditioning." O. Hobart Mowrer, author and psychologist (1907–82), proposed a "two-factor" theory in which conditioned anxiety was maintained by avoidance behavior (operant) that served to reduce this anxiety and therefore reinforced it.

Those who take a biological perspective suggest that a biological function may contribute to anxieties, phobias, panic attacks, and obsessive-compulsive behaviors. All organisms may have been prepared by evolutionary history to acquire fears of certain things more than others, such as snakes, spiders, and the dark.

Today, millions of people have some form of anxiety disorder, including a phobia. Anxiety is currently described as a cluster of symptoms that does not imply any theory of causation. While psychoanalysis has been used as a treatment for anxiety disorders, in many cases, understanding the source of the anxiety does not necessarily resolve it or the unwanted behaviors. As a result, many experts question the effectiveness of psychoanalysis.

Behavior Therapy

In the late 1950s and early 1960s, the system of behavior therapy was developed. The shift to behavioral therapies for phobias is probably mostly attributable to the work of Joseph Wolpe (1915–97) and his classic work on reciprocal inhibition, *Psychotherapy by Reciprocal Inhibition* (1959). Early behavioral researchers speculated that they could be effective by looking at an individual's symptoms, working with them directly, and systematically desensitizing them from the effect of these symptoms by gradual exposure to them. Through a wide variety of behavior-therapy techniques, thousands of individuals have learned to cope with or be free of their anxiety.

Theories of behavioral therapy suggest that a phobia is a learned response and therefore the response can also be *un*learned. Behavioral therapists use techniques that involve gradual exposure of the individual to whatever is feared. Exposure may take place in real life or may occur in the person's imagination. For example, a person with a fear of heights may imagine himself on a higher and higher hill without anxiety or may be taken to progressively higher hills; it is the gradualness of the exposure that is the important factor.

It is now understood that phobic and obsessive-compulsive disorders are two very different conditions, although they both have anxiety as a common underlying symptom. Also, psycho-physiological measures in the study of anxiety disorders have been expanded, making it possible now to distinguish certain groups of phobias that have clinical correlates. Thus, in addition to talking therapy, current therapy may now include periodic examinations of cardiovascular, pulmonary, endocrine, or neurological changes, as well as pharmacologic aspects.

Exposure Therapy

There are various types of exposure therapy that seek to decrease the intensity of a phobia or extinguish it altogether. Exposure therapy may be gradual or intense, depending on the therapist and the particular means and goals. Individuals may be exposed to photographs or computer images of the feared item, slowly increasing their confidence until they can face the actual feared thing. Other experts support a more rapid form of exposure/desensitization known as *flooding.*

Other Therapies

Some phobic individuals have found relief from their debilitating symptoms through hypnotherapy, while others have learned ways to deal with their phobias by joining self-help groups or participating in group therapy with fellow phobics. Hypnotherapy has yet to prove its lasting positive, therapeutic effects.

Often issues related to feeling stupid and crazy need to be dealt with, since the family of the phobic person may have expressed annoyance and irritation at the irrational behavior and may have mistakenly assumed that the phobic person could simply "get over it" if he or she tried hard enough. A very promising approach to anxiety treatment involves the use of Eye Movement Desensitization and Reprocessing (EMDR), in which imagined exposure coupled with eye movements help "process" the traumatic roots of the fear.

Medications

Antianxiety medications such as benzodiazepines may be used with phobic individuals, in conjunction with therapy. Antidepressants may also be helpful to some, as either adjunctive therapies to benzodiazepines or by themselves. Often the first antianxiety medication that is used provides relief, although, in some cases, the physician must try a variety of medications before the individual obtains respite. Medications alone are insufficient to combat active phobias. Instead, a combination

EXAMPLES OF PHOBIAS

Creatures in nature

Apiphobia; melisophobia: bees
Arachnophobia: spiders
Batrachophobia: frogs
Entomophobia: insects
Equinophobia: horses
Icthyphobia: fish
Musephobia; murophobia: mice
Ophidiophobia: snakes
Ornithophobia: birds
Zoophobia: animals

Natural phenomena

Acluphobia; nyctophobia: night, darkness
Acrophobia; hysophobia: heights
Anemophobia: wind
Astraphobia: lightning
Brontophobia; keraunophobia: thunder
Ombrophobia: rain
Potomophobia: rivers
Siderophobia: stars

Blood/Injury/Illness

Algophobia; odynophobia: pain
Belonephobia: needles
Dermatophobia: skin lesions
Hematophobia; homophobia: blood
Pyrexeophobia; febriphobia: fever
Molysmophobia; mysophobia: contamination
Traumatophobia: injury

Social

Aphephobia; haptephobia: being touched
Catagelophobia: ridicule
Ereuthophobia: blushing
Graphophobia; scriptophobia: writing
Kakorrhaphiophobia: failure
Scopophobia: being looked at
Xenophobia: strangers

Miscellaneous

Ballisophobia: missiles
Barophobia: gravity
Claustrophobia: confinement
Dementophobia: insanity
Erythrophobia: the color red
Harpaxophobia: robbers
Levophobia: objects to the left
Trichopathophobia; trichophobia: hair

of psychotherapy and medication is often the optimal treatment for phobic individuals.

Research Continues to Provide New Information

State-of-the-art technology in medical and pharmacological research is used as a diagnostic and therapeutic tool. The advent of relatively safe, appropriate drugs to relieve anxieties has enabled many individuals to work effectively with therapists or by themselves to overcome phobias, anxieties, panic disorders, and obsessive-compulsive behaviors.

Interaction between psychotherapy and biology is increasingly better understood. Researchers now believe that, coupled with medical, scientific, and technological advances, the future treatment of phobic individuals will lean toward self-help. (Many self-help techniques and self-help groups have developed in recent years.)

One example of techniques that are used to treat phobias is body awareness, which many phobic individuals learn through the use of biofeedback. With such techniques, individuals—particularly those who have panic attacks—learn concrete, rapid tools for relaxation and objective ways to validate their relaxation skills if they doubt their ability to relax. Further, individuals learn to develop increased self-confidence and to control the power of stress.

Therapy for phobias, in most cases, concentrates on helping the individual focus on the present, switching from internal thoughts to imagining sensations, and training the phobic person to face fears realistically, become more assertive, express anger when appropriate, and use anxiety constructively.

Conclusion

Millions of people in the United States are extremely unhappy because they are trapped in unhealthy phobias. The fears of spiders, snakes, and "things that go bump in the night" are likely to remain as long as humans continue to exist, with some individuals becoming phobic toward such objects and others who remain normally frightened. New phobias may develop, such as an excessive concern over terrorist attacks beyond the genuine threat to most individuals.

Mental health professionals are constantly learning new techniques to assist phobic individuals and will continue to discover new therapies and methods to ease the anguish for phobic individuals in the United States and other countries around the globe.

Beck, Aaron T., M.D., and Gary Emery, *Anxiety Disorders and Phobias: A Cognitive Perspective* (New York: Basic Books, 2005).

Chambless, Dianne L., and Alan J. Goldstein, *Agoraphobia: Multiple Perspective on Theory and Treatment* (New York: John Wiley and Sons, 1982).

Errara, Paul, "Some Historical Aspects of the Concept, Phobia." *The Psychiatric Quarterly,* April 1962, pp. 325–336.

Lewis, Aubrey, "A Note on Classifying Phobia." *Psychological Medicine* 6, 1976, pp. 21–22.

Marks, Isaac M., *Fears, Phobias and Rituals* (New York: Oxford University Press, 1987).

———, "The Classification of Phobic Disorders." *British Journal of Psychiatry* 116, 1970, pp. 377–386.

———, and Randolph M. Nesse, "Fear and Fitness: An Evolutionary Analysis of Anxiety Disorders." *Ethology and Sociobiology* 15, 1994, pp. 247–261.

Nesse, Randolph, "Emotional Disorders in Evolutionary Perspective." *British Journal of Medical Psychology* 71, 1998, pp. 397–415.

Smith, Mick, and Joyce Davidson, "'It Makes My Skin Crawl . . .': The Embodiment of Disgust in Phobias of 'Nature.'" *Body & Society* 12, no. 1, 2006, pp. 43–67.

Trotter, David, "The Invention of Agoraphobia." In *Victorian Literature and Culture,* 2004, pp. 463–474.

ENTRIES A to Z

abandonment, fear of Fear of the loss of the presence of someone or a group that is extremely important to the individual, as well as the love and protection they provide. Even the threat (real or imagined) of abandonment can cause severe stress. Some children develop a fear of abandonment because their parents threaten to send them away as a disciplinary measure. Sometimes children fear that one or both parents will neglect or desert them, and, in some cases, this is a valid fear. Often, children are removed from homes and placed with relatives or in foster care.

Many adults also have a general fear of abandonment. Adults fear abandonment when there is a risk of losing a loved one on whom they are dependent, whether from divorce, death, illness, or some other cause. Another form of the fear of abandonment is the fear of loss of status or of having power taken away. Studies of individuals with AGORAPHOBIA indicate that they develop a greater degree of dependency directly related to the fear of abandonment.

Fear of abandonment is a state of anticipation of undesirable events in the future. Many people live their lives around this anticipatory fear.

See also AGING, FEAR OF; ALONE, FEAR OF BEING; CHILDHOOD FEARS; RETIREMENT, FEAR OF.

ablutophobia Fear of washing or bathing. The term also relates to an incessant preoccupation with washing or bathing. Individuals who have OBSESSIVE-COMPULSIVE DISORDER may be preoccupied with frequent handwashing or alternately with an obsession against washing or bathing. Manifestations of this fear include avoidance (long periods without washing), excessive anxiety when contemplating washing or when actually attempting to wash, and anxiety and dread when seeing others wash.

See also BATHING, FEAR OF.

Campbell, Robert Jean, M.D., *Psychiatric Dictionary* (New York: Oxford University Press, 1981).

abortion Abortion is the interruption or loss of any pregnancy before the fetus is capable of living. Considering and undergoing an abortion leads to sources of anxiety for many women. For example, some mourn the loss of their fetus while others, years later, fantasize about how old the lost child would have been. Women who have anxiety surrounding an abortion may undergo mental health counseling before and after the procedure. The subject of abortion is also a source of anxiety for the fathers-to-be, who may share in the decision-making process regarding continuation of the pregnancy.

The term *abortion* usually refers to induced or intentional termination of a pregnancy, while *spontaneous abortion*, the natural loss of a pregnancy, is usually referred to as a *miscarriage.*

Throughout history, many women have coped with the anxieties of self-abortion and tried innumerable abortifacients without success, and indeed, in many cases, requiring emergency medical care and incurring permanent injury. Such items have included concentrated soap solutions, ingestion of quinine pills, or castor oil or other strong laxatives. These methods can be dangerous to a woman's physical health and not necessarily effective as abortifacients.

Women who find themselves with an unwanted pregnancy should seek counseling to determine their options and help relieve the stresses of the situation.

Selecting the Safest Method

To minimize anxieties and fears, a woman should seek information and counseling before seeking an abortion. Once the decision is made, women should have a medical examination before undergoing an abortion to become aware of a possible cardiac condition or bleeding disorder. In the United States, Planned Parenthood, with offices in many large cities, can provide information on clinics and services. Local health departments can provide names of services that meet acceptable health standards. Women may feel less stressed and more confident if they have a recommendation from a trusted physician, or from a member of a local hospital gynecology staff.

See also PREGNANCY, FEAR OF.

abreaction   Emotional release resulting from remembering a painful experience that has been forgotten or repressed because it was consciously painful. In some cases, the process of abreaction helps an individual gain insight into the roots of a phobia or an anxiety reaction. The therapeutic effect of abreaction is through discharge of the painful emotions, relief from them, and probably some DESENSITIZATION to the emotional expression itself. Sigmund Freud's colleague Eugene Bleuler noted the therapeutic effects of catharsis with his client Anna O.

See also CATHARSIS.

abstraction anxiety   See MATHEMATICS ANXIETY; NUMBERS, FEAR OF.

acarophobia   Fear of small objects, such as INSECTS, worms, mites, and nonliving items such as PINS AND NEEDLES.

See also WORMS, FEAR OF; NEEDLES, FEAR OF; SMALL OBJECTS.

acceptance   A favorable attitude on the part of the therapist toward the phobic or anxious individual under treatment. The therapist conveys an implicit respect and regard for each client as an individual, without necessarily implying either approval of behavior or an emotional attachment toward the client. Acceptance has been defined as "valuing or prizing all aspects of the client including the parts that are hateful to himself or appear wrong in the eyes of

society." The term acceptance is used interchangeably with UNCONDITIONAL POSITIVE REGARD by client-centered therapists. It is a nonjudgmental condition that is seen as a necessary quality in any therapy.

See also CLIENT-CENTERED PSYCHOTHERAPY.

accidents, fear of   Fear of accidents is known as dystychiphobia. Those who fear having accidents fear behaving in any way that might result in injury to themselves or to other persons, or in damage to property or the environment. Accident phobics associate certain factors with accidents and tend to avoid them. The situations they might avoid include risky jobs, atmospheric conditions, a tiring work schedule, and equipment failure. They also are fearful of personal factors such as inattention, errors of perception, risk-taking, and decision making. Fear of accidents is related to a fear of decision-making and a fear of errors. Some people who fear accidents also fear injury to themselves.

See also DECISIONS, FEAR OF; ERROR, FEAR OF; INJURY, FEAR OF.

accommodation   A term that describes how a therapist adapts language and specific techniques to the characteristics of the individual patient. Accommodation enhances trust and rapport and therefore helps promote change for the individual or family.

See also FAMILY THERAPY; PSYCHOTHERAPY.

Minuchin, S., *Families and Family Therapy* (London: Tavistock, 1974).

acculturation, fear of   Acculturation is a process associated with increased anxieties and fears. In situations where there are linguistic or cultural communication barriers or an individual's expectations are not congruent with what takes place, anxieties can be heightened. As reported in an editorial in *Canadian Family Physician* (vol. 41, October 1995) the anxieties of the immigration experience are compounded particularly for individuals whose future residency status is in question.

There may be behavioral changes, such as increasing alcohol and tobacco consumption following immigration. When different family members become accustomed to the new culture at different rates, conflicts can arise between the generations, adding to the overall anxiety.

Increasingly, physicians are seeing immigrant patients from ethnic backgrounds that do not use the Western medical model. Some of these patients see Western medicine as one of many healing systems. Cultural expectations can cause anxieties for both physicians and patients. For example, some East Indian women cannot allow pelvic examination by male physicians, even those from their own culture. Because such examination can be construed as grounds for divorce, the relatively simple procedure of a physical examination becomes both a cultural and a medical issue.

Practitioners of biomedicine should address the clinical issues surrounding folk beliefs and behaviors in a culturally sensitive manner, according to an article in *The Journal of the American Medical Association* (March 1, 1994). Lee M. Pachter, D.O., associate director of inpatient pediatrics, St. Francis Hospital and Medical Center, Hartford, Connecticut, wrote: "A culturally sensitive health care system is one that is not only accessible, but also respects the beliefs, attitudes and cultural lifestyles of its patients. It is a system that is flexible and acknowledges that health and illness are in large part molded by variables such as ethnic values, cultural orientation, religious beliefs, and linguistic considerations."

Dr. Pachter explained that most medical folk beliefs and practices are not harmful and do not interfere with biomedical therapy. Under these circumstances, the clinician should not attempt to dissuade the patient from these beliefs, but instead educate him or her as to the importance of the biomedical therapy in addition to the patient-held belief. However, any ethnomedical practice that has the potential for serious negative outcome needs to be discouraged, but this must be done in a sensitive and respectful way. Replacing dangerous practices with alternatives that fit into the patient's ethnocultural belief system are often met with acceptance.

Reducing Anxieties Involved in Interactions between Physicians and Patients

Pachter recommended three strategies for physicians treating ethnic populations.

- Become aware of the commonly held folk medical beliefs and behaviors of the patient's community.
- Assess the likelihood of a particular patient or family acting on these beliefs during a specific illness episode.
- Arrive at a way to successfully negotiate between the two belief systems.

Following a study conducted in Canada, researchers drew up a list of recommendations to reduce anxieties on the part of the physician as well as the patient.

- Be aware of your own cultural biases.
- Determine whether language will be an issue during office visits.
- Develop an office guide for immigrant patients including typical questions asked during an examination, needs for disrobing and types of examinations and testing procedures and their importance.
- Prepare a list of local agencies that are available to help with multicultural issues.
- Train the nurse or receptionist to explain the preliminary aspects of routine examination procedures.
- Encourage patients to share their culture and lifestyle with you. Explain that you are not trying to pry into their lives but need the information for accurate diagnoses and appropriate therapy.
- Ask before going ahead with any procedures. By seeking permission and explaining the procedures the mystery is removed and patients become partners in the activity rather than objects of scrutiny. Compliance improves with understanding.
- Take advantage of opportunities for cross-cultural learning in group discussions with other professionals from different cultural backgrounds.

See also ACCULTURATION, FEAR OF; COMPLEMENTARY THERAPIES; CROSS-CULTURAL INFLUENCES; MIGRATION; PERSONAL SPACE.

Cave, Andrew et al., "Physicians and immigrant patients." *Canadian Family Physician* 41, October 1995, pp. 1,685–1,690.

Pachter, Lee M., "Physicians should not ignore folk medicine beliefs and remedies" *The Journal of the American Medical Association* (March 1, 1994).

acerophobia (acerbophobia) Fear of sourness. The word is derived from the Latin *accer,* meaning "sharp, sour." Such fears would lead to avoidance of acerbic foods or other products.

See also SMELLS, FEAR OF; SOURNESS, FEAR OF; TASTES, FEAR OF.

acetycholine See LITHIUM CARBONATE.

achluophobia Fear of the dark (also known as NYCTOPHOBIA). Manifestations of this fear include not going out at night, increased anxiety as dusk approaches, not wanting to look out at the darkness (for example, closing shades in order to avoid looking out), avoidance of looking into dark rooms, and having light available constantly. Freud quoted a child who was afraid of the dark as saying, "If someone talks, it gets lighter," implying that darkness is associated with loneliness and separation.

See also DARKNESS, FEAR OF; NIGHT, FEAR OF.

acid dew, fear of Fear of acid dew is a contemporary fear in technologic societies. Acid dew is a side effect of AIR POLLUTION and is formed when dewdrops absorb chemicals expelled in automobile exhaust or smoke from coal-burning factories. Some people fear the dew because of suspected or unknown health effects and because they feel helpless with regard to avoiding or controlling the presence of the noxious substances in their environment.

See also ACID RAIN, FEAR OF.

acid rain, fear of Fear of acid rain is a late 20th-century fear brought about by high industrialization and AIR POLLUTION in many parts of the world. People fear acid rain because they fear the unknown health consequences of breathing the polluted air that results after rain falls. They fear a lack of control over their environment and feel forced to breathe the polluted air.

See also ACID DEW, FEAR OF.

acousticophobia A morbid fear of noise. Also spelled akousticophobia. This may also be a fear of sounds or particular sounds.

See also PHONOPHOBIA; NOISE, FEAR OF.

acquired immunodeficiency syndrome (AIDS)/ human immunodeficiency virus (HIV) The acquired immunodeficiency syndrome is one of the most feared, complicated, and devastating diseases ever identified. It is caused by the human immunodeficiency virus, which is most frequently contracted through unprotected sexual acts and transmitted through the lining of the vagina, vulva, penis, rectum, or mouth during sex. Another route of transmission is through shared needles used by injection drug abusers. Pediatric AIDS can be contracted by a newborn from an infected mother, although treatment during pregnancy greatly reduces the risk of the newborn's infection with HIV. AIDS is the final stage of the illness caused by HIV. As of this writing, there is no cure for HIV or AIDS.

According to the Centers for Disease Control and Prevention (CDC), HIV harms the CD4 positive T cells, which are an important part of the immune system. The normal CD4 cell count in a person with a healthy immune system ranges from 500 to 1,800 per cubic millimeter of blood. AIDS is definitively diagnosed when the CD4 cell count falls below 200. AIDS is also diagnosed if the patient has tested positive for HIV and has developed infections common to patients with AIDS, such as *Pneumocystis carinii pneumonia* (PCP) or tuberculosis.

An estimated 1 million people in the United States had HIV/AIDS in 2004. The incidence of AIDS peaked in the United States in 1993 at 80,000 new cases. In 2004, about 42,500 new cases of AIDS were reported.

As can be seen from the table, the numbers of people diagnosed with AIDS each year in the United States has *increased* from 39,513 people in 2000 to 42,514 in 2004; however, the number of people who are dying from the disease has declined, due

ESTIMATED NUMBERS OF AIDS DIAGNOSES, DEATHS, AND PERSONS LIVING WITH AIDS, 2000–2004

	2000	2001	2002	2003	2004
AIDS diagnoses	39,513	39,206	40,267	41,831	42,514
AIDS deaths	17,139	17,611	17,544	17,849	15,798
Persons living with AIDS	320,177	341,773	364,496	388,477	415,193

Source: Centers for Disease Control and Prevention, "A Glance at the HIV/AIDS Epidemic" Department of Health and Human Services, (April 2006). Downloaded May 11, 2006 from http://www.cdc.gov/hiv/resources/factsheets/At-A-Glance.htm.

to new medical therapies. In 2001, 17,611 people died from AIDS, but in 2004, the death rate had declined to 15,798 people.

Testing for HIV in individuals who may be at risk is extremely important. According to Jeffrey L. Greenwald, M.D., and his colleagues in their 2006 article for *Current Infectious Disease Reports,* many patients fail to get tested until the later stages of infection and as many as half of patients with HIV infection are diagnosed with AIDS a year later because of the lateness of their diagnosis.

Worldwide, according to the Joint United Nations Programme on HIV/AIDS, about 40 million people had HIV in 2006, and 25 million people had died of AIDS up to that time. According to a 2006 report from the General Assembly of the United Nations, in considering individuals infected globally with HIV, women represent half of all those who are infected. The infection rate among women is even higher in Africa: 60 percent.

An estimated one of every 20 children in sub-Saharan Africa has become orphaned because the parents have died of AIDS. AIDS is also the leading global cause of premature death among men and women ages 15–59 years.

Historical Background

The first cases of immune system failure were recognized in 1981 among gay men, blood infusion recipients, and injecting drug users of illegal drugs, when physicians noticed a pattern of people in groups who were diagnosed with rare diseases, such as *Pneumocystitis carinii.* In 1982, the disease which caused the failure of the immune system received its name, *acquired immune deficiency syndrome* (AIDS). Scientists at that time also identified the key routes of transmission as through contaminated blood, sexual intercourse, and mother-to-child infection in newborn babies.

In 1983, the lymphadenpathy-associated virus (LAV) was isolated in France by Dr. Luc Montagnier. This virus was later to be known as the human immunodeficiency virus (HIV).

In 1984, Dr. Robert Gallo, an American physician, identified HIV as the cause of AIDS.

During the mid-1980s, many people with AIDS discovered their illness for the first time in an emergency room when an AIDS-defining condition was diagnosed. Before 1986, HIV testing was not generally available except to a few people enrolled in research studies. Then some laws began to change, and, for example, states began requiring pregnant women and newborn infants to be tested for the virus, so that they could obtain medical treatment for their newborn or yet-to-be-born infants.

In the 1980s, there was a very high level of concern and fear surrounding both HIV and AIDS, and many people in the general public wrongly believed that the disease could be caught in much the same way as the common cold. When some individuals were identified as being infected with HIV or having developed AIDS, they were often ostracized because of this fear of contagion. Some children who were HIV-positive were harassed out of public schools because of their infection status. When their parents tried to educate parents and other individuals that only an exchange of body fluids could infect other children, they were not believed. Many people feared that their children would contract HIV from a mere association with infected children and nothing anyone said assuaged this fear.

In the 1990s, as education about HIV and AIDS began to take effect, most people began to realize that HIV was generally not a threat to children, nor was it a threat to adults unless they engaged in risky behaviors. The virus could only be contracted through specific routes, such as unprotected sexual acts and injected drug use, as well as from an infected mother to her child if she did not take medical precautions.

Transmission of HIV/AIDS

In the United States, according to the Centers for Disease Control and Prevention (CDC), about 65 percent of males (28,143 males) diagnosed with HIV/AIDS in 2004 contracted the virus through male-to-male sexual contact. Sixteen percent of males contracted the virus through heterosexual contact, and 14 percent were infected through illicit intravenous drug use. Male-to-male sexual contact and injection drug use together were the causes of infection in 5 percent of the male cases. In 1 percent of the cases of males diagnosed in 2004, the method of transmission was unknown.

Among the 10,410 females diagnosed with HIV/AIDS in 2004, most infected females (78 percent) contracted the virus through heterosexual contact, while 20 percent were infected as a result of injected drug use. It is unknown how females obtained the virus in 2 percent of the cases.

Anxieties About HIV/AIDS

People who fear contracting HIV/AIDS may reduce their sexual contacts, have less interest in sexual activity, have sexual difficulties, stop participating in activities with others, feel depressed or anxious for no obvious reason, and have sleeplessness, nightmares, or loss of appetite. They may feel guilty for their past behaviors.

Fears almost always refer to the possibility of unpleasant future events. In this case, the prospect of an early and often painful death will evoke fear. Bodily changes, the prospect of loss of function, and loss of economic success and security are scary. An emotionally generous, compassionate, and supportive community is essential to a meaningful and less fearful life with AIDS.

Some experts believe that a *generational forgetting* has occurred with regard to AIDS and that an insufficient level of fear exists in the 21st century among some people. Some individuals no longer believe that risky behaviors can lead to infection with HIV and thus they may be more likely to engage in risky behaviors.

Reactions to Diagnosis. Individuals may experience grief, heartbreak, and uncertainty when they learn that they have contracted HIV or that they have full-blown AIDS. They may be anxious about their impending losses, including the loss of their health, the loss of the freedom to live each day without the threat of sudden illness, and the loss of freedom to make plans for the future. Individuals may experience these feelings of loss long before any actual physical symptoms begin.

In the early stages of the virus, the infected person may wonder how long it will take to become ill, whether they will experience pain, what treatments will be available, who will take care of them, and how they can maintain hope in the face of such great uncertainty.

Anger is often a major reaction to the discovery that one is HIV positive. According to experts, the anger may be directed at possible sources of infection, past sexual partners, or needle-sharing friends, or it may be directed at oneself for not having been responsible for past behavior. However, anger can also contribute to the "fighting spirit" that some people with AIDS acknowledge as a source of their continued psychological and physical survival.

Relationship with Health Care Professionals. The primary doctor-patient relationship can provide constancy and comfort, as well as uncertainty. For people with HIV/AIDS, the association with a caring physician may constitute one of the patient's most enduring and emotionally intimate connections. Experts suggest that a successful relationship with the doctor can mean shared expectations, good communication, and satisfaction about their collaboration at all stages of illness up to and including the patient's death, should that occur.

Physicians and patients currently have considerably different attitudes about their prospects of health and survival after diagnosis than in earlier years. Before 1987, many patients were told that they had only six months to a year to live after diagnosis. In the 21st century, a diagnosis of HIV no longer means an imminent demise.

Family and Friends: Disclosure and Support. For people who discover that they are HIV positive, there is usually no urgency about disclosure (except to sexual or needle-sharing partners). However, if one is hospitalized for infections that are often associated with AIDS, family and friends frequently discover or guess the problem. Disclosure is usually a highly charged topic.

When family members and friends learn about an individual's HIV status, they may react with varying degrees of acceptance. Many people do not know *how* they should act or what they should say. Some people may avoid the infected person, while others become overly solicitous. Unsuspecting parents may feel guilt and anger. Most relatives and friends need time to adjust to the news. Family and friends are understandably upset, sad, angry, and distraught when they learn that a loved one has HIV. However, it is important for friends to express reassurance that the relationship to the HIV-infected person will remain close.

Confidentiality is an important issue. One who is close enough to the infected individual to be informed of his or her HIV status should not betray that trust and should not gossip with mutual friends.

During acute illness, after hospital discharge, or when the illness becomes chronic, the question of providing practical assistance arises. People with AIDS may truly need help, yet they may be resistant at acknowledging or accepting this need. Friends can be most helpful by making it clear that they are not "taking over" but instead they wish to do whatever the ill person indicates is important. Friends can let it be known that they are available for specific tasks, such as providing transportation to the physician's office, cooking, or delivering some meals.

Symptoms and Diagnostic Path

Patients infected with HIV may have no symptoms for years; however, eventually as the infection progresses to the final stage of AIDS, they become ill frequently and have a much slower recovery than normal from common infections and viruses. Some symptoms may occur within about one or two months after exposure to HIV, including tiredness, headache, and fever. (These symptoms may occur with many other illnesses as well.)

Individuals who may be at risk for having contracted HIV (because of recent sexual contacts with individuals who are infected or who are considered at risk for infection with HIV for other reasons) should request testing. In addition, intravenous users of illicit drugs who share needles are also at high risk and should be tested.

Symptoms that may occur from months to years before the onset of AIDS may include

- rapid weight loss
- recurring fevers and profuse night sweats
- frequent oral or vaginal yeast infections
- profound lack of energy
- persistent skin rashes
- swollen lymph glands in the armpits, groin, or neck
- short-term memory loss

In addition, some individuals who are HIV positive develop sores in the mouth, genitals, and anus. Children with HIV may have slow growth and frequent illnesses.

If the patient with HIV is undiagnosed and untreated, multiple illnesses can cause the condition to deteriorate to the level of AIDS. Opportunistic infections, uncommon in healthy people, may develop in a person weakened by HIV/AIDS, such as infection with Pneumocystis carinii pneumonia, Mycobacterium avium complex, Cytomegalovirus, tuberculosis, toxoplasmosis, cryptosporidiosis, hepatitis C, and the human papilloma virus (HPV).

Opportunistic infections may cause the following symptoms in individuals with HIV/AIDs:

- breathing problems
- problems with the mouth such as white spots (thrush), sores, dryness, loose teeth, and trouble swallowing
- weight loss
- vision loss
- severe headaches
- skin rashes or itching
- fever for longer than 2 days
- diarrhea
- extreme fatigue
- confusion and forgetfulness

Individuals with AIDS are at risk for some forms of cancer, such as cancers of the immune system (lymphomas), cervical cancer, and Kaposi's sarcoma, which presents with spots in the skin or mouth.

Testing for the virus. The presence of HIV is diagnosed with testing, such as with the enzyme immune assay (EIA) test, and results are available within one to two weeks. False positives do occur, although they are rare. If the initial test is positive, it is confirmed with a second test such as the Western Blot test. There are also rapid HIV tests that are licensed for use in the United States, and these tests can provide results in 20 minutes. If the rapid HIV test is positive, a further confirming test should be given. As of this writing, there are four rapid HIV tests that have been approved by the FDA, including the OraQuick Advance Rapid HIV1/2 Antibody Test, the Reveal G2 Rapid HIV-1 Antibody Test, the Uni-Gold Recombigen HIV Test, and the Multisport HIV-1/HIV-2 Rapid test.

Home self-tests for HIV are available. A home test requires a finger prick of blood collected on a special card, which is then sent to a laboratory. Such tests can be purchased at pharmacies. As of this writing, only the Home Access test is approved by the Food and Drug Administration (FDA).

Individuals who test positive for HIV should be tested for other sexually transmitted diseases, since they have an increased risk for such diseases. Patients should also be tested for tuberculosis and hepatitis, since the risk is increased for infection with these diseases as well.

Patients with HIV/AIDS will need to be followed carefully by their physicians.

Treatment Options and Outlook

Highly active antiretroviral therapy (HAART), a customized combination of different medications, is the mainstay treatment for many patients with HIV/AIDS, and there are a variety of individual medications that may be prescribed. Doctors individualize treatment, and they take into account the patient's level of the virus, the CD4 lymphocyte count, and any clinical symptoms.

There are some side effects to HAART; for example, HAART has been reported to be linked to increased cholesterol levels as well as to an abnormal blood sugar (glucose) metabolism. Also, because they often feel significantly better, some patients wrongly believe that they are cured and, as a result, stop taking their medication. This is a very

unwise course because without their medication their immune system will no longer be protected, and the patient will become sicker.

Risk Factors and Preventive Measures

Males who engage in unprotected sex with other males have an increased risk for contracting HIV, as are those who use shared needles to inject drugs. Individuals who engage in unprotected heterosexual sex with others at risk for HIV are themselves at risk for contracting HIV.

African Americans who contract HIV have an increased risk for death from AIDS compared to other races or ethnicities, although the reason for this is unknown. One theory is that the virus is not identified until a later stage in African Americans, when it is more difficult to treat.

Sex workers and other individuals who engage in unprotected sex with multiple partners have an increased risk for contracting HIV.

Newborn infants whose mothers are infected with HIV have a 25 percent risk for contracting the virus; however, if pregnant women are treated with antiretroviral medication, the risks diminish considerably.

See also DISEASE, FEAR OF; EPIDEMIC ANXIETY; ILLNESS PHOBIA; MASS HYSTERIA; PLAGUE, FEAR OF THE; PSYCHOSEXUAL ANXIETIES; SEXUALLY TRANSMITTED DISEASES, FEAR OF.

Centers for Disease Control and Prevention, "Basic Statistics." Available online. URL: http://www.cdc.gov/hiv/topics/surveillance/basic.htm. Downloaded May 11, 2006.

Greenwald, Jeffrey L., M.D., et al., "A Rapid Review of Rapid HIV Antibody Tests." *Current Infectious Disease Reports* 8, 2006, pp. 125–131.

Joint United Nations Programme on HIV/AIDS, 25 Years of AIDS, 2006. Available online. URL: http://data.unaids.org/pub/FactSheet/2006/20060428_FS_25years ofAIDS_en.pdf. Downloaded May 19, 2006.

United Nations General Assembly, Declaration of Commitment on HIV/AIDS: Five Years Later. Report of the Secretary General. March 26, 2006. Available online. URL: http:data.unaids.org/pub/Report/2006/20060324_SGReport_GA-A60737_en.pdf. Downloaded May 19, 2006.

acrophobia A fear of heights, also known as hypsophobia. This is one of the commonest phobias in the general population. According to a study by Agras, about .4 percent of the population has a phobia to heights, and only about 2 percent of those seek treatment. Treatment commonly involves EXPOSURE THERAPY, in which graded exposure to heights is made while in a state of relative relaxation. For example, a person might start exposure with looking out the second-floor window until relaxation or comfort is achieved and then move on to third and subsequent floors in the same manner. In severe cases, a therapist or trained support person may be necessary.

Individuals who have acrophobia fear being on high floors of buildings or on the tops of hills or mountains. They usually feel anxious approaching the edge of precipices such as BRIDGES, rooftops, stairwells, railings, and overlooks. They usually fear FALLING and being injured. Some feel and fear an uncontrollable urge to jump. They may have fantasies and physical sensations of falling even when on firm ground.

Fear of ELEVATORS, ESCALATORS, balconies, and stairways are related to a fear of heights, as is sometimes a fear of FLYING or FALLING. In severe cases, the individual cannot even stand on the lower steps of a ladder without experiencing some anxiety. Often fear of driving on freeways or highways has an acrophobic component in that these roadways are frequently elevated.

In psychoanalysis, fear of falling from high places sometimes represents fear of punishment for forbidden wishes or impulses.

See also HEIGHTS, FEAR OF.

ACTH (adrenocorticotrophic hormone) A substance secreted by the pituitary gland to control release of steroid hormones from the adrenal cortex. STRESS leads to simultaneous release into the circulation of both ACTH and beta-endorphin, a type of amino acid. ACTH is also known as corticotropin.

See also ENDORPHIN.

active analytic technique A psychotherapeutic approach that differs from the classical or expectant technique of PSYCHOANALYSIS. Active techniques are aimed at modifying the troublesome responses of ANXIETIES, PHOBIAS, and OBSESSIONS in individuals. Active techniques encourage reenactment of events that may have led to development of the habits or phobias that the individual seeks to change. This approach, which stems from psychoanalytic therapies, predates and foreshadowed the behavioral techniques that are more commonly used in treating anxiety today. Names associated with this technique are Sandor Ferenczi, Wilhelm Stekel, Franz Alexander, and Thomas French.

acupressure Sometimes referred to as ACUPUNCTURE without needles, acupressure embraces the same concepts of energy flow and point stimulation as the original science but uses the pressure of the therapist's fingers for point stimulation. Acupressure is used by many people for relief of physical symptoms as well as anxieties. Acupressure is thought to combine the science of acupuncture with the power of the healing touch and has been most widely used for pain control.

In Oriental medicine, acupressure is helpful in conditions where the body's energy balance has been upset by a variety of physical and/or emotional stresses. Because it is an extremely gentle technique, acupressure is sometimes used by individuals who are fearful of needles.

See also ACUPUNCTURE; COMPLEMENTARY THERAPIES; SHIATSU.

acupuncture A technique used to relieve anxieties as well as pain for many people. It has been used for thousands of years as a component of Chinese medicine. It is based on the theories about the body's "vital energy" (*chi*), which is said to circulate through "meridians" along the surfaces of the body. The ancient theory holds that illness and disease result from imbalances in vital energy, which can be remedied when therapy is applied to "acupuncture points" located along the meridians. The goal of acupuncture is to rebalance the flow of energy, promoting health and preventing future imbalance. The points are believed to have certain electrical properties, which, when stimulated, can alter chemical neurotransmitters in the body and bring about a healing response. Practitioners of acupuncture insert hair-thin stainless steel needles into body surfaces at acupuncture points.

In addition to reduction of anxieties and relaxation, many people have used acupuncture for many conditions, including osteoporosis, asthma, back pain, painful menstrual cycles and migraine headaches.

Increasing Acceptance of Acupuncturists

In the mid-1990s, acupuncture was permitted in all 50 states. In some states, only physicians are permitted to practice acupuncture, while other states allow the procedure to be performed by lay acupuncturists under medical supervision or by unsupervised lay persons. In the United States, an estimated 3,000 medical doctors and osteopaths have studied acupuncture and use it in practice, up from 500 a decade before. Additionally, some 7,000 nonphysicians use acupuncture for a wide array of problems, sometimes in conjunction with massage, herbal therapies, and other traditional Eastern techniques.

In 1990, the U.S. secretary of education recognized the National Accreditation Commission for Schools and College of Acupuncture and Oriental Medicine as an accrediting agency. However, the Food and Drug Administration considers acupuncture needles to be "investigational" devices and has not approved the use of acupuncture for any disease treatment. In the early 1990s, the U.S. Food and Drug Administration estimated that 9 million to 12 million acupuncture treatments are performed annually in the United States. In the mid-1990s, nearly 100 private insurers and Medicaid programs in some states covered acupuncture for some conditions.

Choosing an Acupuncturist

Individuals choosing a therapist to perform acupuncture should be examined by their physician first. Some conditions are beyond the scope of acupuncture treatment and demand immediate medical attention. Discuss your expectations with the acupuncturist. Ask how long until you can expect to see a change in your condition. Be suspicious of promises of a quick cure, especially if you have had

your problem for some time. If you don't see progress after six to eight treatments, reevaluate your choice of treatment and the practitioner.

Check the credentials of the acupuncturist you are considering. Ask whether he or she is certified by the National Commission for the Certification of Acupuncturists. Discuss the costs of the procedure. Depending on the area of the country, and whether or not the acupuncturist is a physician, fees vary. Usually the first visit is considerably higher than subsequent visits.

Weigh the risks of acupuncture. There have been reports of serious complications attributed to acupuncture needles. However, most acupuncturists use sterile, disposable needles that come in a sealed package.

See also ACUPRESSURE; ADDICTIONS, FEAR OF; COMPLEMENTARY THERAPIES.

Campbell, A., "A doctor's view of acupuncture: Traditional Chinese theories are unnecessary." *Complementary Therapies in Medicine* 6, 1998, pp. 152–155.

Helms, Joseph M., "An Overview of Medical Acupuncture." *Alternative Therapies* 4, no. 3, May 1998, pp. 35–45.

James, R., "There is more to acupuncture than the weekend course," *Complementary Therapies in Medicine* 6, 1998, pp. 203–207.

Martyn, Peter, "Acupuncture Successful in Treating Addictions," *The Toronto Star,* September 10, 1995.

addiction, fear of Fear of the development of a physical and psychological dependence on a chemical substance. Alcohol, tobacco, CAFFEINE, narcotics, as well as some sedatives that may have been prescribed by physicians for the treatment of anxiety, can produce addiction in individuals who are prone to addictive behaviors. Most people are not fearful of a caffeine addiction, but many are fearful of using drugs such as narcotics, BARBITURATES, and BENZODIAZEPINES because of a fear of possible addiction to these drugs. It *is* possible to develop an addiction to these substances, which is why they are all scheduled drugs under the Controlled Substances Act, and why physicians have special guidelines that they must follow with most of these drugs.

Some individuals in moderate to severe pain are afraid to take pain medications lest they become addicted; however, studies have shown that few patients with pain who are under competent medical care will develop addictions unless they have a history of substance abuse. Instead, individuals who abuse prescription medications that they obtain from others in an illicit manner are far more likely to develop addiction, in part because they use higher than normal dosages and also because they use the drugs to obtain a euphoria rather than to control pain.

Some physicians are fearful of causing addiction in patients and, as a result, may undertreat pain, particularly among the elderly. Some studies have shown that elderly cancer patients have been undertreated for pain. Since most narcotics are inexpensive, and thus, cost is not a factor, it is likely that the undertreating physicians were concerned about possible addiction should they prescribe narcotics.

Addiction is a physiological condition, but it also has important psychological and social consequences, such as individuals centering their lives around the use of the addictive substance and a willingness to go to great lengths to obtain the drug. Some individuals who fear becoming addicted worry that they may become so totally involved in their addiction that they might neglect or harm other people. Others fear the loss of control that is implied by addiction.

When individuals are addicted to alcohol and/or drugs, they may become neglectful of their children and their jobs and may even become guilty of acts of CHILD ABUSE. The abuse of some drugs can incite aggression in otherwise nonaggressive individuals, for example, anabolic steroids, COCAINE, or METH-AMPHETAMINE.

Some individuals have a psychological but not a physical dependence on some types of medications, such as antianxiety medications. Even after discontinuing a medication, such patients may continue to carry the drug around with them, because the mere possession of the drug is comforting, whereas its absence would be distressing. As long as they have the drug in their physical possession, they know that it is available if they believe that they need it.

It is clear that a number of people with anxiety disorders will use drugs and alcohol to avoid the anxiety experience. Estimates are, for example, that almost one-third of alcoholics have an active anxiety disorder that is masked by the alcohol use.

See also ALCOHOL, FEAR OF; ANXIETIES; SEDATIVES, FEAR OF.

Gwinnell, Esther, M.D., and Christine Adamec, *The Encyclopedia of Addictions and Addictive Behaviors.* (New York: Facts On File, Inc., 2005).

adenosine   A naturally occurring chemical in most living cells. Adenosine is a source of energy in metabolic activities at the cellular level, is also associated with nerve impulse transmissions, and may be involved in causing some anxiety disorders.

See also BIOLOGICAL BASIS FOR ANXIETY.

adenylate cyclase   An enzyme-linked chemical secreted by the body that affects HORMONE functions.

adjustment   Change or accommodation by which the individual can adapt himself to the immediate environment. For example, a phobic individual may make adjustments in his route to work so that he will not encounter a fearful situation along the way, such as a bridge, tunnel, or overpass. An agoraphobic may arrange to have a trusted friend or relative go with him or her to necessary appointments.

See also BRIDGES, FEAR OF.

adolescent depression   See DEPRESSION, ADOLESCENT.

adolescent suicide   See SUICIDE, ADOLESCENT.

adoption   The legal assumption of all parental rights and obligations to a child not born to an individual, and which rights and responsibilities are conferred by a court. Adoptive parents may be stepparents, relatives, or nonrelatives.

Both the decision whether to adopt and acting on that decision cause multiple anxieties. Many individuals who adopt children are infertile, and, before they choose to adopt, they must give up the hope of having a biological child. This is very difficult for most people. Many infertile individuals have endured the anguish of waiting for the results of a variety of tests and treatments in their attempts to achieve a pregnancy. Once it has been established that there is no treatment that will help or that treatments have been ineffectual, the decision to adopt and all the pressures surrounding that decision must be faced.

If they decide to adopt, many prospective parents are consumed with anxiety of the unknown, such as the fear that they will not be able to adopt a child or the fear that the birth parents may change their minds, and, of course, the possibility of eventual emotional or health problems with the adopted child. However, according to *The Encyclopedia of Adoption* and other sources, few birth parents change their minds about adoption after a baby is placed with the adoptive family, and the majority of decision reversals occurs before the placement of the child with an adoptive family. Some highly publicized stories of adoption losses by the media have misled the public into believing that adoption is riskier than it usually is.

Adoptive couples today have far more choices to make than, for example, in the 1980s which may also cause more anxieties. There are a variety of adoption channels, such as a private or public agency (public agencies primarily place children in foster care). Families may also choose to arrange their own adoption, seeking out the assistance of an attorney or adoption agency only after they have located a pregnant woman in the United States who is interested in placing her child for adoption when it is born.

The prospective parents must decide whether to adopt a child from the United States or from another country. In addition, some prospective parents consider open adoptions, in which birth parents and adoptive parents know each other's identities and may maintain contact through the years as the child grows up. (Very few international adoptions are open adoptions.)

Another source of anxiety is the home study, a process in which the prospective parents are evaluated as to their fitness to be parents. They must have an approved home study before they can adopt a child. The prospective parents must undergo the scrutiny of a social worker as well as have physical examinations to confirm that they are healthy enough to raise a child. Their financial resources

are reviewed to verify that they have sufficient income to raise a child. The agency also runs other checks, such as a police check to rule out any criminal convictions and a check of the state child abuse registry to confirm that the individuals seeking to adopt have not abused any children in the past. If a single person wishes to adopt a child, he or she will also undergo scrutiny, including questions about who would care for the child if the adult became incapacitated. Only a small part of the home study, despite its name, is a visit to the home to determine if it is a safe place to raise a child.

If the family is adopting a child from another country, in most cases, they must travel there, which is an anxiety-inducing process for many people, particularly those who have never traveled outside the United States. The prospective parents must also be fingerprinted and obtain a passport. There is a great deal of paperwork that must be accomplished with an international adoption, although a good agency will provide some assistance.

Once approved, prospective parents often worry about how long it will take to adopt their child or even if they will ever receive a child. However, most prospective adoptive parents report that it is the evaluation and approval process which is most difficult.

Once a child is placed with the family, the adoption may not be finalized for about six months, depending on state law. The family may be fearful that some unknown event will somehow subvert the adoption process, although as mentioned, such an occurrence rarely happens.

Once the adoption is finalized, the family is equal under the law to parents to whom a child was born. If the child was born in the United States, the original birth certificate will be altered, inserting the names of the adoptive parents as the parents. In most states, the original birth certificate is sealed. If the child was born in another country, the adoptive parents often receive a birth certificate from that country. However, some parents choose to re-adopt the child in a state court, so that they can obtain a U.S. birth certificate that includes the adoptive parents' names as the parents on the new birth certificate.

For adoptive parents, even after finalization, other anxiety-producing events lie ahead: such as knowing how and when to tell children they are adopted; dealing with the anxiety that this information may bring to them at various stages of their lives; and recognizing the possibility that when they are older, adult children may wish to locate their birth parents. Most adoption experts report that children should learn about their adoption from their adoptive parents, usually before they begin attending kindergarten. Simple explanations are best at first, and more detailed explanations should follow later, at the child's level of understanding.

Studies have shown that most adopted children grow up to be healthy adults. Those with the greatest risk for problems in adolescence and adulthood are children adopted as older children or children who have been sexually abused in the past. However, there are no guarantees with adoption (as with having a child born to the family), and a healthy baby may grow up to become a troubled adult.

See also COMMUNICATION; PARENTING.

Adamec, Christine, and Laurie C. Miller, M.D., *The Encyclopedia of Adoption,* 3rd ed. (New York: Facts On File, Inc., 2006).

adrenaline   A hormone secreted by the central, or medullary, portion of the adrenal glands that produces an increase in heart rate, a rise in blood pressure, and a contraction of abdominal blood vessels (often leading to "butterflies"). Anxiety and panic are the subjective reactions to these changes. These sympathetic changes can be reversed by activation of the parasympathetic system.

See also EPINEPHRINE; NEUROTRANSMITTERS; NORADRENERGIC SYSTEM.

adrenergic blocking agents   Substances that inhibit certain responses to adrenergic, or adrenalinelike (energizing), nerve activity. The term adrenergic blocking agents (ABA) is also applied to drugs that block the action of the neurotransmitters epinephrine and norepinephrine. Ergot alkaloids were first discovered to alter responses to sympathetic nerve stimulation. ABAs are selective in action and are classed as alpha ABAs (alpha blockers or alpha-receptor blocking agents) and beta ABAs (or beta blockers or beta-receptor block-

ing agents), depending which types of adrenergic receptors they affect. Medications for anxiety may involve both alpha-receptor blockers and beta blockers, although the beta blockers are used primarily for performance anxiety such as public speaking or test taking.

See also ADRENERGIC DRUGS; ADRENERGIC SYSTEM.

adrenergic drugs   Substances that stimulate activity of adrenaline (epinephrine) or mimic its functions. Adrenergic drugs produce stimulation of the central nervous system, thereby increasing anxiety. ADs are part of a group of sympathomimetic amines that includes ephedrine, amphetamines, and isoproterenol. Adrenergic agents are produced naturally in plants and animals but can also be developed synthetically.

See also ADRENERGIC BLOCKING AGENTS; ADRENERGIC SYSTEM; DRUGS.

adrenergic system   The part of the AUTONOMIC NERVOUS SYSTEM that is influenced by adrenergic drugs, which stimulate the activity of epinephrine or mimic the functions of epinephrine.

See also ADRENERGIC BLOCKING AGENTS; ADRENERGIC DRUGS.

adultery   Adultery refers to sexual intercourse between a married individual and another person who is not the legal spouse; adultery is also known as extramarital sex. Historically, in many countries, adultery has been considered a taboo and major (and sometimes the only) ground for divorce. In the United States, adultery is a source of anxiety within marriages and in many cases, contributes to DEPRESSION in one or both partners in the marriage.

Adultery and extramarital affairs carry the strong threat of acquiring a SEXUALLY TRANSMITTED DISEASE. Even when participants in an affair try to keep it a secret, it can produce anxieties, conflict and guilt feelings on the part of one involved in the affair and emotions ranging from anger to depression in the other partner left behind.

See also LIVE-IN; MARRIAGE, FEAR OF.

advantage by illness The benefit or relative satisfaction a sick person gains from being ill. Freud differentiated between primary and secondary advantages, or gains, by illness. In primary advantage, the psychic mechanism is preserved because inaction and withdrawal lower ANXIETY levels and avoid the emergence of possibly destructive impulses. In secondary advantage, the individual consciously or unconsciously perceives an environmental gain, such as sympathy and attention from family members, removal of responsibilities or possible failure, and avoidance of frightening situations. Some phobic individuals (especially agoraphobics) experience some advantage to having a phobia, which may cause resistance to therapy.

See also AGORAPHOBIA; PHOBIA; SECONDARY GAIN.

adverse drug reactions Physical or mental reactions that occur after taking a prescribed or over-the-counter drug or herbal remedy. How particular individuals react to drugs depends on many factors, including their genetic susceptibility, general health, history of allergies, attitude in taking the drugs, medical history, tolerance to bodily changes, and other drugs or foods that the individual has consumed within the same timeframe.

An example of an adverse drug reaction is the extremely high blood pressure that may result from the combination of taking a drug in the category known as MONOAMINE OXIDASE (MAO) INHIBITORS when it is also consumed with wines, cheeses, or other foods that contain TYRAMINES. Individuals who consume alcohol and prescription drugs may experience adverse drug reactions.

Adverse drug reactions may range from mild stomachaches, headaches, or skin rashes to heart attacks, seizures, and even death. A mental reaction could include feelings of anxiety or confusion or HALLUCINATIONS. Anyone who receives a prescription for any drug as part of therapy to help deal with a phobia or anxiety should ask the physician about possible adverse reactions.

Individuals should follow any restrictions on their prescribed medication labels and should also carefully read the labels of all over-the-counter drugs as well. If individuals wish to use herbal remedies, they should check with their physician first to ensure that these remedies are not dangerous to them because of other medications that they take. For example, the combination of vitamin E and warfarin (Coumadin) can lead to dangerous internal bleeding.

People with anxiety disorders are often conditioned to react to bodily sensations that are unusual. Drug side effects can trigger anxiety in people afraid of their bodily sensations.

aelurophobia See CATS, FEAR OF.

aeroacrophobia Fear of open, high spaces. Aeroacrophobia includes fear of being at great heights, such as in an airplane. This should be differentiated from airsickness, which is a vertigo-type disturbance.

See also FLYING, FEAR OF; VERTIGO, FEAR OF.

aeronausiphobia Fear of airplanes; fear of vomiting due to airsickness.

See also FLYING, FEAR OF.

aerophagia Fear of swallowing air.

See also AIR, FEAR OF.

aerophobia A fear of air, drafts, gases, or airborne noxious influences. Also known as air phobia. Sometimes this term is used as a label for the fear of flying.

See also AIR, FEAR OF; FLYING, FEAR OF; WIND, FEAR OF.

affective disorders Affective disorders are classified in the *DIAGNOSTIC AND STATISTICAL MANUAL OF MENTAL DISORDERS*, fourth edition, as MOOD DISORDERS and are often associated with anxiety. Affective disorders are so named because they involve changes in affect, a term that is roughly equivalent to emotion, or mood. In this group of disorders, the individual experiences mood disturbances that are intense enough to warrant professional attention. An individual who has an affective, or mood, disorder may have feelings of extreme sadness or intense, unrealistic elation with the disturbances in mood not due to any other physical or mental disorder. Some mood disorders have been thought to be related to ANXIETY. For example, AGORAPHOBIA is sometimes associated with DEPRESSION. The depression may be a reaction to the demoralization that accompanies the phobic's feelings of incompetence, ineffectualness, and loss of self-respect. Some agoraphobics may feel disappointed and hopeless about themselves and aware of their fearful dependency on their spouses or significant others. However, as phobics gain more mastery over their problems during the course of treatment, the depression that accompanies agoraphobia usually improves.

Mood disorders differ from thought disorders; schizophrenic and paranoid disorders are predominantly disturbances of thought, although individuals who have those disorders may also have some distortion of affect. A disorder of the thought processes is not a common feature in affective disorders; however, if the disorder reaches extreme intensity, there may be a change in thought pattern, but the change in thought will be somewhat appropriate to the extremes of emotion that the person is experiencing.

Affective disorders have been known throughout history. There are descriptions of mood disorders in the early writings of the Egyptians, Greeks, Hebrews, and Chinese. There are descriptions in the works of Shakespeare, Dostoyevski, Poe, and Hemingway. Many historical figures have suffered from recurrent depression, including Moses, Rousseau, Dostoyevski, Queen Victoria, Lincoln, Tchaikovsky, and Freud.

Symptoms and Diagnostic Path

BIPOLAR DISORDER and depressive disorders sometimes occur according to a seasonal pattern, with a regular cyclic relationship between the onset of the mood episodes and particular 60-day periods of the year.

A mood syndrome (depressive or manic) is a group of associated symptoms that occur together for a short duration. For example, major depressive syndrome is defined as a depressed mood or loss of interest of at least two weeks' duration, accompanied by several associated symptoms, such as weight loss and difficulty concentrating.

A mood episode (major depressive, manic, or hypomanic) is a mood syndrome not due to a known organic factor and not part of a nonmood psychotic disorder such as schizophrenia or delusional disorder. A mood disorder is diagnosed by the pattern of mood episodes. For example, the psychiatric diagnosis of major depression is made when there have been one or more major depressive episodes without a history of a manic or unequivocal hypomanic episode.

Manic Episodes. Individuals who have manic episodes have distinct periods during which the predominant mood is either elevated, expansive, or irritable. They may have inflated self-esteem, decreased need for sleep, accelerated and loud speech, flight of ideas, distractibility, grandiose delusions, or flamboyancy. The disturbance may cause marked impairment in their working or social activities or relationships; an episode may require hospitalization to prevent harm to themselves or others. They may experience rapid shifts of mood, with sudden changes to anger or depression.

The mean age for the onset of manic episodes is in the early twenties, but many new cases appear after age 50.

Hypomanic Episodes. These are mood disturbances not severe enough to cause marked impairment in social or work activities or to require hospital care.

Major Depressive Episodes. Individuals who experience a major depressive episode have either depressed mood (in children or adolescents, irritable mood) or loss of interest or pleasure in all, or almost all, activities for at least two weeks. Their symptoms are persistent in that they occur for most of the day, nearly every day, during at least a two-week period. Associated symptoms may include appetite disturbance, change in weight, sleep disturbance, decreased energy, feelings of worthlessness or excessive or inappropriate guilt, difficulty concentrating, restlessness, such as an inability to sit still, pacing, hand-wringing, pulling or rubbing of hair, and recurrent thoughts of death or of attempting suicide. The average age of onset of depressive episodes is in the late 20s, but a major depressive episode may begin at any age. They are more common among women than among men.

Bipolar Disorders.   Bipolar disorders (episodes of mania and depression) are equally common in males and females. Bipolar disorder seems to occur at much higher rates in first-degree biologic relatives of people with bipolar disorder than in the general population.

Cyclothymia.   This is a condition in which there are numerous periods of hypomanic episodes and numerous periods of depressed mood or loss of interest or pleasure that is not severe enough to meet the criteria for a major depressive episode.

Dysthymia.   This is a history of a depressed mood for at least two years that is not severe enough to meet the criteria for a major depressive episode.

Causes of Affective Disorders.   Many factors contribute to mood disorders. The major causative categories are biological, psychosocial, and sociocultural. There seems to be a hereditary predisposition because the incidence of mood disorders is higher among relatives of individuals with clinically diagnosed affective disorders than in the general population. There was considerable research during the 1970s and 1980s to explore the view that depression and manic episodes both may arise from disruptions in the delicate balance of the levels of the brain chemicals called biogenic amines. Biogenic amines serve as neural transmitters or modulators that regulate the movement of nerve impulses across the synapses from one neuron to the next. Two such amines involved in affective disorders are norepinephrine and 5-hydroxytryptamine (serotonin). Some drugs are known to have antidepressant properties, and they biochemically increase the concentrations of one or the other (or both) of these transmitters.

Psychosocial and biochemical factors may work together to cause affective disorders. For example, stress has been considered as a possible precipitating factor in many cases. Stress may also affect the biochemical balance in the brain, at least in predisposed persons. Mild depressions frequently follow significant life stresses, such as the death of a family member. Many other life events may precipitate changes in mood, especially those involving lowered self-esteem, thwarted goals, physical disease or abnormality, or ideas of deterioration or death.

Some individuals may have personality characteristics that predispose them to affective disorders, such as negative views of themselves, of the world, and of the future. A stressful life event for these individuals simply activates previously dormant negative thoughts. Generally, individuals who become manic are ambitious, outgoing, energetic, care what others think about them, and are sociable before their episodes and after remission. On the other hand, depressive individuals appear to be more obsessive, anxious, and self-deprecatory. They often have rigid consciences and are prone to feelings of guilt and self-blame.

Depressed individuals tend to interact with others differently from the way manics do. For example, some manic individuals do not want to rely on others and try to establish a social role in which they can dominate others. On the other hand, depressed individuals take on a role of dependency and look to others to provide support and care; this is also the case with agoraphobics.

According to many researchers, feelings of helplessness and a loss of hope are central to depressive reactions. In severe depression, "learned helplessness" may occur when the individual sees no way to cope with his or her situation and gives up trying.

Treatment Options and Outlook

Mood disorders are treated with behavior therapy as well as drugs. Some behavioral approaches, known as cognitive and cognitive-behavioral therapies, involve efforts to correct the individual's thoughts and beliefs (implicit and explicit) that underlie the depressed state. Therapy includes attention to unusual stressors and unfavorable life situations, and observing recurrences of depression.

Medical intervention includes the use of antidepressant, tranquilizing, and antianxiety drugs. Lithium carbonate, a simple mineral salt, is used to control manic episodes and is also used in some cases of depression where the underlying disorder is basically bipolar. Lithium therapy is often effective in preventing cycling between manic and depressive episodes.

Death Rates.   The death rate for depressed individuals seems to be about twice as high as that for the general population because of the higher incidence of suicide. Manic individuals also have a high risk of death because of accidents (with or without alcohol as a contributing factor), neglect of proper precautions to safeguard health, or physical exhaustion.

See also ALCOHOLISM; ANTIDEPRESSANTS; ANXIO-LYTICS; DEPRESSION, ADOLESCENT; BIPOLAR DISORDER; ENDOGENOUS DEPRESSION; EXOGENOUS DEPRESSION; SEASONAL AFFECTIVE DISORDER; SUICIDE, FEAR OF; TRANQUILIZERS.

American Psychiatric Association, *Diagnostic and Statistical Manual of Mental Disorders,* 4th ed. (Washington, DC: American Psychiatric Association, 1994).

age distribution of fears, phobias, and anxiety

During their first few weeks of life, infants exhibit fear responses. Sudden, loud noises or loss of support typically result in fearful reactions such as crying and stiffening of the body. The number of stimuli to which a child responds with fear increases as the child gets older. During the second half of the first year, and through the second year, fear of strangers is fairly common. After the first two years, fear of animals shows an increasing incidence from around age three and by four or five comprises the largest category of children's fears. After age four or five, animal fears tend to decline. New fears involve more intangible or abstract objects or situations, such as fear of imaginary creatures, monsters, and the dark. Fear of creatures usually declines steadily and becomes negligible after 10 or 11 years for most children. Fears associated with school and social life then become more prominent.

As many as 40 percent of CHILDHOOD FEARS persist into adulthood. In a significant epidemiological study by Stuart Agras et al. in 1969, three different patterns of specific fears occurred over a broad age range. The greatest number of specific fears and phobias was during childhood, usually peaking before age 10. Another cluster of fears, including fears of doctors and medical procedures such as injections, showed a peak occurrence at about age 20. Then there was a rapid decline in prevalence during the adolescent and early adult years. By the sixth decade, the same fears were negligible. Fears of death, injury, illness, separation, and crowds showed a steady increase in prevalence up to age 60, and then also declined. Another pattern, involving fears of ANIMALS, SNAKES, HEIGHTS, STORMS, ENCLOSED SPACES and social situations, showed an increasing prevalence up to age 20 and then declined gradually, suggesting that these fears tend to persist much longer than the others. Stuart Agras, a Stanford University psychiatrist, suggests that this constellation of fears had survival value to primitive man and therefore are relatively universal reactions.

In 1975, Isaac Marks, a British psychiatrist affiliated with the Maudsley Hospital, London University, and Michael Gelder, a British psychiatrist at the University of Oxford, reported that more severe fears, phobias, and anxiety states also show age-related patterns. For specific phobias involving heights and storms, they reported an average age of onset of about 22.7 years. Social phobias and extreme shyness had a mean onset of 18.9 years, and the average age for the onset of agoraphobia was 23.9 years of age. The latter percentage corresponds closely to age of onset for agoraphobia of 24 years found by Ronald M. Doctor, Ph.D., professor of psychology, California State University, Northridge, California.

See also SHYNESS; SOCIAL PHOBIA.

Doctor, Ronald M., "Major Results of a Large Scale Survey of Agoraphobics," In R. DuPont, *Phobia: Comprehensive Summary of Modern Treatment* (New York: Brunner/Mazel, 1982), pp. 203–214.

Marks, Isaac, *Fears and Phobias* (London: Heinemann Medical, 1969).

Scarr, S., and P. Salapatek, "Patterns of Fear Development in Infancy," *Merrill Palmar Quarterly* 16, 1970, pp. 53–90.

aggression A general term for a variety of hurtful or destructive behaviors that appear outside the range of what is socially and culturally acceptable. Anxiety is often the outcome to the victim of aggressive acts. Fear of violence, aggression, or even confrontation are common triggers of anxiety.

Aggression includes extreme self-assertiveness, social dominance to the point of producing resentment in others, and a tendency toward hostility. Individuals who show aggression may do so for many reasons, including frustration, as a compensatory mechanism for low SELF-ESTEEM, lack of affection, hormonal changes, or illness. Aggression may be motivated by fears, anger, over-competitiveness, or directed toward harming or defeating others.

An individual with an aggressive personality may behave unpredictably at times. For example, such an individual may start arguments inappropriately with friends or members of the family and harangue them angrily. The individual may write letters of an angry nature to government officials or others with whom he or she has some quarrel.

The opposite of aggression is passivity. The term *passive aggression* relates to behavior which seems to be compliant but where "errors, mistakes, or accidents" for which no direct responsibility is assumed results in difficulties or harm to others. Patterns of behaviors such as making "mistakes" that harm others are considered "passive aggressive".

See also PASSIVE-AGGRESSIVE PERSONALITY DISORDER.

aging, fear of   Fear of aging is known as gerontophobia. Many people fear aging, which is a normal process throughout life. In older individuals, aging involves some characteristic patterns of late life changes that can be distinguished from diseases and social adversities. Fear of aging is based on fears of being alone, of being without resources, and of being incapable of caring for oneself both intellectually and physically.

agitation   Excessive movement, usually nonpurposeful, that is associated with or is symptomatic of tension or anxiety. Examples of agitation are wringing of the hands, pacing, and inability to sit still.

See also ANXIETIES; SYMPTOM.

agoraphobia   Agoraphobia is the most common phobic disorder for which people seek treatment. It is also the most disabling. Although the *Diagnostic and Statistical Manual of Mental Disorders*, fourth edition (American Psychiatric Association, 1994) focuses on agoraphobia with panic disorders, cases of agoraphobia without panic as a precursor have

also been reported. Often these cases begin in the teenage years and manifest overtly or symptomatically in the mid-twenties.

Estimates are that about 8–10 percent of the population experience occasional unexpected panic attacks. Some 50 percent of people who experience panic attacks could develop agoraphobia if left untreated. Only about 1–3 percent of people with panic experience fears of future attacks.

Stress is a major precipitant of panic attacks but there may be a biological contribution that leads to increased vulnerability. Through classical conditioning, situations where panic has occurred quickly become conditioned to anxiety, and, as a means of coping, avoidance becomes the first line of defense. Medicine is often used to treat panic attacks, but it is much less effective in treating agoraphobia. Behavioral techniques of exposure are highly effective with agoraphobia. There is evidence that dependency is associated with the development of

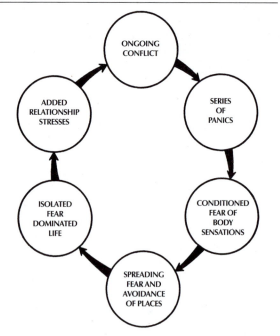

THE CYCLE OF AGORAPHOBIA

Reprinted by permission, from *Overcoming Agoraphobia*, by Dr. Alan Goldstein and Berry Stainback (New York: Viking Penguin, 1987).

MAIN EFFECTS OF AGORAPHOBIA ON SUBJECTS' LIVES

112 Men	%	818 Women	%
Unable to work	42	Social restrictions	29
Lack of social contacts	29	Personal psychological effect	23
Personal psychological effect	11	Marital disharmony	14
Marital disharmony	9	Unable to work	14
Travel restrictions	4	Travel restrictions	11
Guilt about children	2	Guilt about children	6

Reproduced from *Fears, Phobias, and Rituals: An Interdisciplinary Perspective,* by I. M. Marks (copyright © 1987 Oxford University Press; reproduced by permission).

agoraphobia, with many showing separation anxiety and school phobia in childhood.

Current evidence indicates that people who develop agoraphobia also tend to catastrophize about body sensations (which have taken on conditioned anxiety reactions) and come to interpret these sensations as onset of panic. This, of course, leads to panic and intense anxiety and perpetuates the cycle of fear reactions. Underlying this cycle may be a reduced sense of self-efficacy, or belief in the ability to help oneself.

A central component of agoraphobia is fear of fear itself. The agoraphobic syndrome is a complex phobic disorder that usually occurs in adults. The major features are a variable combination of characteristic fears and the avoidance of public places, such as streets, stores, public transportation, crowds, and tunnels.

Agoraphobia is well known in many languages. For example, in German, it is *platzangst;* in French, *peur des espaces* or *horreur du vide.* The English term is derived from the Greek root "agora," meaning the place of assembly, the marketplace. The original definition meant fear of going out into open spaces such as streets or isolated areas. Now the term agoraphobia is applied to many disabling fears, usually involving a group of fears centering around distance from a safe place. Consequently, agoraphobics commonly fear going away from home, going into the street, into stores, occupying center seats in churches, theaters, or public transportation, crowded places, large rooms where many people are gathered, or being far from help.

Although agoraphobia has been recognized as far back as Hippocrates' time, until the latter half of the 20th century, the term agoraphobia and the agoraphobic syndrome were not well defined. Individuals who were afraid to go out were considered unusual or peculiar. Some received sympathy, some received ridicule. Even today, many agoraphobics conceal their disorder for long periods, especially if they work outside the home. Sometimes only family members and close associates are aware of the individual's problem.

Historical Background

In 1871, Alexander Karl Otto Westphal (1863–1941), a German neurologist, coined the term agoraphobia, because the most striking symptom of the condition was anxiety that appeared when a phobic individual walked across open spaces or through empty streets. He described this as the "impossibility of walking through certain streets or squares, or possibility of so doing only with resultant dread of anxiety."

The previous year, Moritz Benedikt (1825–1920), an Austrian physician, described the condition but suggested that the central feature was dizziness rather than anxiety. He suggested the name *Platzschwindel,* which meant "dizziness in public places." Although the term is no longer used, many individuals still report some of the same symptoms, including palpitations, trembling, sweating, nausea, pressure in the chest, headaches, breathlessness, and blushing. Some individuals have anticipatory anxiety and fear of dying. Some fear that they may attract unwanted attention.

In 1871, Westphal observed that anxiety in agoraphobia is based on ideas (cognitive factors) and not brought about by stimuli in the environment.

SYMPTOMS AND WORST FEARS DURING A PANIC, AS LISTED BY 100 PATIENTS WITH AGORAPHOBIA (IN ENGLAND)

Symptoms	%	Worst Fears	Listed as First Fear (%)	Listed as Second Fear (%)
Nervous and tense	93	Death	13	20
Dizzy or faint	83	Fainting/collapsing	38	16
Agitated	80	Heart attack	4	4
Palpitations	74	Becoming mentally ill	6	1
Weak legs	73	Causing a scene	6	7
Trembling/shaking	72	Inability to get home/to place of safety	6	26
Feeling totally unable to cope	66	Losing control (e.g., becoming hysterical)	7	9
Stomach churning	65	Other personal illness	10	7
Sweating/perspiring	65			
Shortness of breath	59			
Confused	58			
Things not quite real	57			
Loss of control	52			
Tightness/pressure in the head	43			
Difficulty with eyes (blurred vision, etc.)	36			
Feeling of becoming paralyzed	19			

Reproduced from *Fears, Phobias, and Rituals: An Interdisciplinary Perspective,* by I. M. Marks (copyright © 1987 Oxford University Press; reproduced by permission).

In 1885, a clinical description of a female agoraphobic patient appeared in the literature with a comment that the condition was uncommon among women. Interestingly, all five of Westphal's original agoraphobic patients were men! Now, however, the condition is much more common among women than men. Current estimates are that approximately 80 percent to 85 percent of the agoraphobics who seek treatment are women.

In 1912, American psychologist Morton Prince (1854–1929) wrote that such phobias "occur in people of all types and characteristics, amongst the normally self-reliant as well as amongst the timid."

Symptoms and Diagnostic Path

Agoraphobia usually begins with a panic experience followed by extreme sensitivity to bodily sensations, self-judgment, helplessness, and social anxiety. Social fears, fear of embarrassment, or fear of sensations may lead to avoidance of critical situations and thus avoidance of the frightening feelings.

Most agoraphobia begins in early adulthood, between the ages of 18 and 35, with 24 years as an average age, but many individuals do not seek treatment until about 10 years after its onset. In this regard, agoraphobia differs from most simple phobias, which originate during childhood. Agoraphobia rarely occurs in children. However, it may be that childhood anxieties, such as school phobia, fear of the dark or of leaving parents, or night terrors, might sensitize someone to later agoraphobia; both problems may reflect a generally fearful disposition.

Some people who have agoraphobia can pinpoint the overt onset of their disability to some incident or situation. Typical examples that have been reported to therapists are a sudden bereavement, losing a baby at birth, the emotional and physical strain of a difficult pregnancy, or a state of acute shock following major surgery and a period of isolation or incapacity.

The death of a parent or spouse is a major crisis for most individuals. For an agoraphobic, however, such an event, or the threat of it, may lead to panic attacks. The same is true when college or a job transfer threatens to separate the agoraphobic from an emotional-support figure.

In many individuals, however, the agoraphobia is not triggered by a major life event. For example, some report relatively insignificant incidents at the onset of their agoraphobia, such as a minor fall on a slippery street, or being startled outdoors in the dark by a lamppost or dog. Many individuals do not recall any single stressful event preceding their first agoraphobic panic attack. However, these attacks usually do occur while the individual is under some nonacute stress, such as marital conflict, the illness of a child, engagement, marriage, pregnancy, bereavement, or physical illness.

Many individuals report that their agoraphobia began suddenly with an unexpected, spontaneous panic attack (usually lasting from two to 10 minutes) during a situation that they later came to fear and avoid. Some say the panic occurred while crossing the street, at a bus stop, or while in a crowded store.

One Australian study reported that more agoraphobia begins in summer weather than in the colder months. It may be that agoraphobic individuals become unusually anxious when they notice physical changes such as sweating and increased heart and breathing rates, which occur in everyone during hot weather.

Agoraphobia may develop within a few hours or over several years after a precursory stage of vague, intermittent anxiety. After the first anxiety attack, some individuals experience anxiety only when they return to the same or similar surroundings.

RATING OF PANIC PROVOCATION BY AGORAPHOBICS*

Activity	Panic-Provoking	No Problem
Driving freeways	42.6%	29.4%
Airplanes	38.8	17.7
Closed-in places	24.5	17.1
Heights	23.1	17.9
Audiences	22.0	20.2
Department store	20.4	27.4
Crowds	18.1	15.2
Bridges	14.8	39.3
Supermarket lines	11.2	34.9
Parties	10.8	34.7
Being alone	10.8	50.8
Elevators	10.0	37.2
Restaurants	09.6	36.1
Unfamiliar places	07.9	20.9

*N = 477
Adapted from S. L. Williams, "On the Nature and Measurement of Agoraphobia," *Progress in Behavior Modification* 19, 1985, pp. 109–144.

LOCATIONS OF FIRST PANIC ATTACKS*

Location	Percentage
Auto	15%
At work	9%
Home	8%
Public places	8%
Restaurant	8%
School	7%
Away from home	7%
Store	6%
Bridge	4%
Public transportation	4%
Street	4%

*Locations in which first panic attack occurred and percent of agoraphobics with first panic in these locations.
Ronald M. Doctor. In R. L. DuPont (ed.), *Phobia: Comprehensive Summary of Modern Treatment* (New York: Brunner-Mazel, 1982).

For most, the fear generalizes to other situations that also elicit fear.

Once the phobic reaction happens a few times, a type of learning called *conditioning* occurs, and the reaction tends to happen more frequently in certain places. Conditioning is the process by which the fearful reactions become associated with particular things or places.

The feeling of panic in agoraphobia, like other panics, cannot be controlled easily. Some people who experience panic attacks may be predisposed (due to personality, social learning history, or perhaps genetic factors) to develop agoraphobia while others who have panic attacks do not. Usually agoraphobia becomes chronic, but it may fluctuate, depending on responses to minor occurrences in the environment. An individual may have periods of relative freedom from the disorder, sometimes with complete remissions of the fears. Research shows, however, that over time, without treatment, the agoraphobia will worsen. Agoraphobia often develops in anxious, shy people. Some agoraphobics tend to be indecisive, have little initiative, feel guilty, and are self-demeaning, believing they should be able to get out of their situation themselves. They may become increasingly withdrawn into their restricted life. There is some evidence that dependency and perfectionism are associated with a subgroup of people who develop agoraphobia. There is also substantial clinical evidence that emotional suppression is strongly associated with the development of agoraphobia.

One theory about the cause of agoraphobia is that experience in certain individuals' learning process conditioned them to regard the world as a dangerous place. Many agoraphobics have had at least one agoraphobic parent, and many have had at least one parent who is somewhat fearful. In some cases, they received mixed messages from their parents; while they were encouraged to achieve, they were not well prepared to deal with the world, either because they were overprotected, taught that home is the only safe place, or underprotected, having to take on too much responsibility at an early age.

When agoraphobics seek treatment, they are often in a constant state of alertness, have a passive and dependent attitude, and show a tendency toward sexual inhibition. Typically, the agoraphobic admits to being generally anxious and often expresses feelings of helplessness and discouragement. However, many agoraphobics were formerly active, sociable, outgoing persons. Some agoraphobics abuse alcohol and drugs, and researchers are beginning to uncover the extent of such abuse. Some current estimates place 30 percent of alcoholics as having a primary anxiety disorder that leads to the chronic use of alcohol.

General Symptoms. A common characteristic of agoraphobia is a history of panic attacks in which the individual experiences symptoms of extreme excitement, distortion of perceptions, and an overwhelming sense of imminent catastrophe, loss of control, or fear of public humiliation. A fear of the fear then develops in which the individual begins experiencing anxiety in anticipation of panic reaction. The result is avoidance of the feared situation.

Situations that bring on anxiety in agoraphobia have common themes involving distance from home or other safe places, crowds, and confinement. Crowds and confinement bring on these anxieties because the individual often feels trapped and cannot leave easily, for example, in a waiting line for a bus or train, or in a crowded department store.

Still other agoraphobics are afraid to be home alone or to be outside alone. They require constant companionship. Casual observers sometimes feel the agoraphobic is lazy and shirking routine responsibility, but this is not true. Most individuals who are agoraphobic fear that they will lose control over their own reactions and that their fear may lead to a panic attack. Some are afraid of fainting, having a heart attack, dying among strangers, screaming, attacking someone, or otherwise attracting unwanted attention and causing embarrassment.

Agoraphobic people avoid specific fear-provoking situations in different ways. Most tend to avoid places that might trigger their phobia. Some phobic individuals feel better with someone they trust and may habitually depend on having a companion when they go out because a reassuring person can make a frightening situation seem safer. Some agoraphobics feel better in a public place just knowing there is a policeman or doctor nearby. Generally, stimulation (physical, emotional, perceptual) will trigger anxiety, so agoraphobic individuals generally avoid such situations as crowds, noisy places, traffic, bright lights, and movement.

Symptoms include general anxiety, spontaneous panic attacks, and occasional depersonalization. DEPERSONALIZATION is a change in the perception or experience of the self so that the feeling of one's own reality is temporarily lost. This is manifested in a sense of self-estrangement or unreality, which may include the feeling that one's extremities have changed in size, or a sense of perceiving oneself from a distance (usually from above). Depersonalization occurs in the absence of any mental disorder when an individual is experiencing overwhelming anxiety, stress, or fatigue. Experiences of depersonalization, in and of themselves, are common (nearly 50 percent of adults report having had a depersonalization experience).

For some individuals, anxiety in agoraphobia may be aggravated by certain predictable situations, such as arguments between marital partners and general STRESS. For some, the anxiety is nearly always relieved somewhat in the presence of a trusted companion. Some individuals relieve their anxiety by having with them a dog or an inanimate object such as an umbrella or shopping cart (SOTERIA).

Some agoraphobics develop ways to live more comfortably with their disorder. For example, those who go to movie theaters or churches may be less frightened if they sit in an aisle seat so that they can make a fast exit if they experience a panic attack. Having a cell phone available is another comfort.

In severe cases, individuals may also have panic attacks, depression, feelings of depersonalization, obsessions, and other symptoms. Historically, other terms that were used to describe agoraphobic symptoms include anxiety hysteria, locomotor anxiety, street fear, phobic-anxiety-depersonalization syndrome, anxiety syndromes, phobic-anxious states, pseudoneurotic schizophrenia, and nonspecific insecurity fears.

Many agoraphobics have episodes of depression. The first episode may occur within weeks or months of the first panic attack. Individuals complain of feeling "blue," having crying spells, feeling hopeless or irritable, with a lack of interest in work and difficulty in sleeping. Agoraphobia is often aggravated during a depressive episode. The increased anxiety may make individuals less motivated to work hard at tasks (such as going out) that they previously did with difficulty.

Some agoraphobics are also claustrophobic. Usually claustrophobia is present before the agoraphobia develops. The common factor between the two phobias is that escape is blocked, at least temporarily. Some people fear confinement in a barber or beautician's chair, or a dentist's chair; some fear taking a bath in the nude. Some individuals who

FREQUENCY OF SYMPTOMS OTHER THAN PHOBIAS IN AGORAPHOBICS COMPARED WITH HEALTHY CONTROLS*

	Agoraphobics	Healthy
General anxiety	80%	17%
Depression	30	3
Obsessional symptoms	10	3
Depersonalization	37	13
Loss of libido	53	3

*N = 30 in each group
Modified from Buglass, Clarke, Henderson, Kreitman, and Presley (1977), using their numbers for symptoms "clearly present," in A. M. Mathews, M. G. Gelder, and D. W. Johnston, *Agoraphobia: Nature and Treatment* (New York: Guilford Press, 1981).

are phobic about bridges fear them because long, narrow bridges with open sides high above a river offer no way out except to cross. Others fear tunnels and elevators for similar reasons.

Many agoraphobics develop some sexual dysfunctions due to anxiety and depression. Dr. Isaac Marks reported in 1969 that inability to achieve orgasm is not uncommon in agoraphobic women. Some agoraphobic men complain of general impotence or premature ejaculation. Anxiety from any cause reduces capacity for sexual enjoyment, and panic attacks and background tension are features of agoraphobia. Many women report that generalized anxiety and panic in agoraphobia tend to be worse just prior to and during menstruation.

Symptoms of the phobic anxiety in agoraphobia may include the many physical sensations that accompany other anxiety states, such as dry mouth, sweating, rapid heartbeat, hyperventilation, faintness, and dizziness.

The mental sensations an agoraphobic experiences include a fear of losing control and behaving in a disinhibited way, of having a heart attack because of the rapid heart action, of fainting if the anxiety becomes too intense, and of being surrounded by unsympathetic onlookers. Following is a table indicating the thoughts (cognitions) of some agoraphobics.

Panic Attacks. Panic attacks are specific periods of the sudden onset of intense apprehension, fearfulness, or terror, often associated with feelings of impending doom. During panic attacks there are symptoms such as difficulty in breathing (hyperventilation), palpitations, chest pain or discomfort,

PERCENTAGE OF AGORAPHOBIC PEOPLE REPORTING CERTAIN SITUATIONS THAT RELIEVE ANXIETY

Situation	%
Being accompanied by spouse	85
Sitting near the door in a hall or restaurant	76
Focusing my mind on something else	63
Taking dog, baby carriage, etc.	62
Being accompanied by a friend	60
Talking problems over with my doctor	62
Talking problems over with a friend	62
"Talking sense to myself"	52

Reprinted with permission from Andrew M. Mathews, Michael G. Gelder and Derek W. Johnston's *Agoraphobia: Nature and Treatment* (New York: Guilford Press, 1981).

COGNITIONS IN AGORAPHOBIA

	First Fear	Second Fear
Fainting/collapsing	37.9%	15.8%
Death	13.2%	19.7%
Other personal illness	10.4%	9.7%
Losing control (e.g., becoming hysterical)	7.4%	6.7%
Causing a scene	6.2%	25.8%
Inability to get home to place of safety	5.9%	8.5%
Becoming mentally ill	5.8%	7.0%
Heart attack	4.1%	4.0%
Other	8.9%	3.0%

From Mathews, Gelder, and Johnston's *Agoraphobia: Nature and Treatment* (New York: Guilford Press, 1981).

choking or smothering sensations, and the fear of going crazy or losing control. For diagnostic purposes, the panic "syndrome" is characterized by three panic attacks within a two-week span of time. Panic syndrome leads to agoraphobia in many individuals.

Obsessions. Some agoraphobics may develop obsessional thinking about certain situations, objects, or places where the fear reaction might occur. Obsessions are recurrent, persistent ideas, thoughts, images, or impulses that are not experienced as voluntarily produced but rather as ideas that invade consciousness. Obsessional or worried thinking is difficult to control, often gravely distorts or exaggerates reality, and is the source of much anticipatory anxiety. Compulsive (superstitious) behavior may develop in an attempt to reduce obsessional thoughts and the anxiety that results from them. Some agoraphobics often have obsessive symptoms, such as ritual checking or thoughts of harming others by strangling, stabbing, or other means. They may avoid being alone with their own infants because they fear harming them. Some agoraphobics fear that they might jump from heights or in front of an oncoming train. Obsessional behavior is usually present *before* an individual develops agoraphobia.

Effects on Social Functioning and Marriage. When individuals tend to avoid situations that provoke fear, their lives become restricted to varying extents. For example, they give up visiting homes of friends, shopping, and accompanying their children to school. They become fearful even when anticipating these situations. Some individuals report that their anticipatory fear is worse than the fear they actually experience in the situation.

Many agoraphobics become socially disabled because they cannot travel to work, visit friends, or shop. They may refuse invitations and often make excuses for not going out. Various adjustments are necessary to compensate for the phobic's lack of participation in family life and activities outside the home.

At the time they come for treatment, most agoraphobics are married. In most research projects involving agoraphobics, spouses are fairly well adjusted and integrated individuals. In some cases, therapists use the Maudsley Marital Questionnaire to assess the individual's perception of his or her marriage before and after treatment. Questions relate to categories of marital and sexual adjustment, orgasmic frequency, work and social adjustment, and "warmth" items. When agoraphobia improves with treatment, marriages usually remain stable or improve.

Agoraphobia may strain a marriage because the phobic person may ask the spouse to take over any chores that require going out, such as shopping, picking up children, and doing errands, and because spouses often must fulfill social obligations without the companionship of their mates. Spouses are additionally stressed by having to be "on call" in case anxiety attacks occur that require communication or a trip home to soothe the agoraphobic. Thus a couple that may have been happy may be driven apart by the disorder, with each blaming the other for a lack of understanding. The husband may think that the wife is not trying to overcome her phobic feelings, and the agoraphobic wife may think that her husband does not understand her suffering. The wife may become so preoccupied with fighting her daily terrors that she focuses little attention on their marital relationship and her husband's needs. However, in cases where the agoraphobic has an understanding, patient, and loving spouse, this support can be an asset in overcoming the agoraphobic condition. The spouse can attend training sessions with the therapist, attend group therapy sessions, and act as the "understanding companion" when the agoraphobic is ready to venture out.

Agoraphobia and Alcoholism.   Alcohol plays a significant role in the lives of many agoraphobics. As Hippocrates wrote in his *Aphorisms,* "Wine drunk with an equal quantity of water puts away anxiety and terrors."

In the early 1970s, J. A. Mullaney and C. J. Trippett described "a treatable complication of the phobic-anxiety syndrome: i.e., addiction to various habituating sedatives such as barbiturates, nonbarbiturate sedatives, minor tranquilizers and alcohol." These addictions were viewed as attempts to self-medicate for chronic anticipatory anxiety, believed to develop in response to panic attacks. Alcohol is effective in relieving chronic anticipatory anxiety, and agoraphobics may escalate to alcoholism in a mistaken attempt to prevent panic, for which it is not effective. In fact, alcohol may even exacerbate panic by contributing to a feeling of loss of control and to strange body sensations. Some agoraphobic men say that drinking helps to calm them before they venture out into public and that they avoid social situations where alcohol is not served. Likewise, some agoraphobic men say that drinking helps them to drive, as well as to be able to go to school or hold a job.

Use of alcohol to cope with panic or to overcome withdrawal due to anxiety not only increases the risk of alcoholism but may interfere with effective treatment of the agoraphobia, since central nervous system depressants reduce the efficacy of exposure treatment.

While the hypothesis that alcohol is used as self-medication or a tension reducer is complex and controversial, many researchers agree that alcohol is functionally related to agoraphobia through its capacity to relieve symptoms associated with the phobic syndrome. In one study (Mullaney and Trippet, 1979, noted in Bibb, 1986), the mean age of onset for agoraphobia among inpatient alcoholics preceded that for alcohol abuse. This led to speculation that the alcoholism might result from self-medication for a preexisting phobic disorder. In a later study, however, no consistent order of onsets was found.

In a 1986 study at the American University, Washington, D.C., (Bibb, 1986), findings indicated that outpatient agoraphobics are at clear risk for alcoholism. The research indicated that about 10 percent of agoraphobic patients were alcoholic, with men both somewhat more likely to be alcoholic and more likely to engage in severe pathological drinking. These findings probably underestimate the true extent of alcohol abuse in this population, however, because subjects selected from outpatient treatment settings tend to be healthier and more motivated than the wider agoraphobic population. Additionally, self-reports of alcoholism probably provide a conservative estimate due to alcoholic denial, as well as problems identifying alcoholics in remission. Many agoraphobics with a history of alcohol abuse consider themselves recovered, but such individuals may be particularly vulnerable to relapse, since they believe that alcohol helps them cope with anxiety and panic.

In the 1986 study, the use of alcohol to self-medicate for phobic discomfort was reported by 91 percent of those with a history of alcoholism and 43 percent of those without such a history, suggesting that it may be a common practice among agoraphobics. Of the individuals who later became alcoholic, 33 percent reported that their earliest use of alcohol was mostly for control of phobic symptoms, indicating that a pattern of alcohol use for phobic control may lead to alcoholism for a substantial minority of individuals. Based on these findings, it appears that self-medication with alcohol for dysphoria associated with the phobic syndrome may represent enduring and intentional patterns.

Alcohol-abusing agoraphobics may differ from their nonalcoholic peers in several ways. Histories of disturbed childhoods are common both for agoraphobics and alcoholics, and such histories are important in determining the causes of combined alcoholism and agoraphobia. Disturbed childhoods of alcoholic agoraphobics frequently include familial alcoholism and depression. Also, children whose early attachments to caretakers are characterized by lack of consistent support as well as by frightening and dangerous interactions may fail to learn a sense of trust and security, and they may be particularly vulnerable to later psychopathology, such as panic attacks and agoraphobia; alcoholism may be one mode of coping for such individuals.

Depression is also frequently evident in the clinical pictures of both agoraphobia and alcoholism, and it appears to be linked to panic attacks.

Agoraphobics who have alcohol-abuse problems may also be more socially anxious than their nonalcoholic peers. High rates of social phobia have been noted among inpatient alcoholics, and major depression has been found to increase both the likelihood and intensity of agoraphobia and social anxieties. According to the American University study, alcoholic agoraphobics are more phobic and anxious on a variety of measures than their nonalcoholic counterparts. More social phobia among outpatient agoraphobics with a history of alcoholism is consistent with previous reports of high rates of social phobia, as well as agoraphobia, among inpatient alcoholics. Also, alcoholic agoraphobics are more avoidant of feared situations when accompanied, not when alone. Their social anxiety and relative failure to benefit from companionship is consistent with their more disordered and abusive childhoods. Children raised in the belief that caretakers are undependable and perhaps frightening may be less likely as adults to believe that companionship in the face of danger is beneficial. They may learn to mistrust or fear social contacts, and perhaps to respond to fearful situations with catastrophic thinking or extreme anticipation of physical or psychosocial trauma.

The prevalence of alcohol abuse among agoraphobic individuals and its relationship to the development and course of the agoraphobic syndrome are still unclear, but it appears that there may be definite relationships.

Biological Basis for Agoraphobia. Many autonomic and biochemical changes occur during agoraphobic attacks; these changes may be similar to those experienced during anxiety, depression, and sudden fright. Spontaneous panics are accompanied by physical changes including increased heart rate and elevated blood pressure.

Temporary aggravation of fear may be caused by stimulants such as caffeine and yohimbine, by inhalation of carbon dioxide, infusion of sodium lactate or isoproterenol, or by hyperventilation, heat, and physical or mental effort. This may reflect a general tendency of anxious people to overreact to certain autonomic sensations produced in these various ways. The dexamethasone suppression test (used to diagnose major depression) is generally normal, and mitral valve prolapse (MVP) is not especially frequent among agoraphobics.

Some researchers hold the view that panic attacks associated with agoraphobia may be associated with hypoglycemia or mitral valve prolapse (MVP), a usually benign condition more common in women than in men, in which a defect in the shape of a mitral heart valve may cause a sudden rapid, irregular heartbeat. Some studies have shown a higher incidence of these conditions among agoraphobics, but current evidence indicates that while hypoglycemia (which is clinically quite rare) and mitral valve prolapse can produce body sensations that the individual reacts to with anxiety, they cannot cause agoraphobia, and treatment for these conditions does not cure agoraphobia. Likewise, there is *no* evidence that agoraphobia is caused by or linked to an inner-ear disorder.

In some treatment centers, as part of a diagnostic workup, agoraphobic patients are given a sodium-lactate challenge test. Individuals who have panic disorder have attacks when they are injected with sodium lactate, a substance found in everyone's body that affects the acidity of the blood. Such individuals may have a sensitivity to this or some other substance that triggers neurotransmitters in the brain to set off panic. Sodium lactate is produced by muscles during exercise. Some individuals get panic attacks when they exercise; this condition was once known as "effort syndrome." About eighty percent of those who suffer panic attacks will experience one in reaction to intravenous infusion of sodium lactate; nonpanic sufferers do not feel anything more than tingling or fatigue.

More recent studies have indicated that once a lactate-reactive person completes a behavioral treatment, their reactivity is no longer present. This would suggest that lactate reactivity is a state factor in the individual dependent on the presence of anxiety rather than a causative factor in phobic disorders.

See also LOCUS CERULEUS; NEUROTRANSMITTERS.

Treatment Options and Outlook

Treatment of agoraphobia is more complicated than treatment of simple phobias, because panic attacks themselves are at the root of the disorder (see table on p. 28).

There are many treatments for agoraphobia. Often several are combined. Most treatments are exposure-based; that is, the major component involves exposing the agoraphobic to situations that are frightening and commonly avoided, in order to demonstrate that there is no actual danger. Treatment may include direct exposure, such as having the individual walk or drive away from a safe place or a safe person, or to enter a crowded shopping center, in a structured way. Indirect exposure is also used; this may involve use of films with fear-arousing cues. Systematic desensitization is included in this category, as this procedure is characterized by exposure (either in imagination or *in vivo*) to the least reactive elements of a situation or object until the anxiety response no longer occurs. Then the next less reactive element or item is presented, and so on until the individual can be exposed to the most critical aspect without a strong anxiety response. Another imaginal procedure for anxiety treatment involves flooding, or continuous presentation of the most reactive elements of a situation until anxiety reduction occurs.

Behavior therapy may involve educating individuals about their reactions to anxiety-producing situations, explaining the physiology and genetics involved (where applicable) and teaching breathing exercises that help correct hyperventilation. Three to six months of behavior therapy is effective in many cases, and supportive and behavioral techniques often reduce the anxiety level.

In recent years, exposure behavioral therapy has been used increasingly to treat agoraphobics. This is also known as *in vivo* therapy, meaning that it uses real-life exposure to the threat. It is thought that facing the fearful situation with appropriate reinforcement can help the individual undo the learned fear. Some therapists develop a "contract" with the phobic individual and set up specific goals for each week, such as walking one block from home, then two and three, taking a bus, and progressing after each session. Many therapists accompany the phobic individuals as they venture forth into public places, particularly in the early stages of treatment. In some cases, therapists train spouses or family members to accompany the phobic individual. Structured group therapy with defined goals and social-skill training for agoraphobics and their families is helpful.

Socially anxious agoraphobic individuals may benefit from assertion training while they partici-

pate in a therapy program. They may gradually expose themselves to social situations of increasing difficulty after successfully performing social skills during the assertion training sessions.

Psychotherapy can help agoraphobics resolve past conflicts that may have contributed to their condition. Before investigating the causes of the problem, however, the therapist usually tries to relieve symptoms with behavioral therapies. Drug therapy may be used at the same time. By itself, psychotherapy does not seem to be an adequate way to treat agoraphobia.

Drug therapy is sometimes useful for agoraphobics, particularly those who have panic attacks, and it enhances the results of exposure-based treatments for many individuals, at least initially. Ideally, drugs should be used for three to six months and then discontinued once the individual has some control over bodily sensations. In some individuals, attacks never recur, although in others they return months or years later. If they do, a second course of drug treatment is often successful. The treatment of choice today for agoraphobia involves use of behavioral exposure therapy and judicious use of medication, with the latter withdrawn as progress is made in behavioral therapy.

Drugs used in the treatment of panic attacks associated with agoraphobia include the tricyclic antidepressants and the monamine-oxidase inhibitors (MAOIs) (which are also used to treat severe depression), and alprazolam (Xanax), an antianxiety drug. Research at the National Institutes of Mental Health indicates that drugs such as tricyclic antidepressants are successful in reducing panic attacks. Some antianxiety agents, such as Valium, Xanax, and Librium, reduce anticipatory fear but can lead to abuse as individuals take increasing doses to prevent panic attacks.

Self-help is useful for many agoraphobics. Some support groups encourage agoraphobics to go out together and offer one another mutual support. In this way, individuals share common experiences, learn coping tips, and have an additional social outlet. Some agoraphobics get together for outings, help take children to and from school, arrange programs, and retrain themselves out of their phobias. Since recovery from agoraphobia is a long-term process, self-help groups can provide valuable support during this process.

Involvement of spouses and family members in treatment, researchers say, produces more continuing improvement with better results than treatment involving the agoraphobic alone. The reason for greater improvement lies in motivation for continued "practice" in facing feared situations both between sessions and after treatment has ended. Home-based treatment, where patients proceed at their own pace within a structured treatment program, produce fewer dropouts than the more intensive, prolonged exposure or pharmacological treatments, but suffer from lack of necessary support.

Research. Agoraphobia is one of the phobias most actively studied by researchers and clinicians. Researchers believe that developing improved treatments for agoraphobia will be based on better definition of the agoraphobic phenomenon, and on improved measurement of treatment effects.

To assess agoraphobic conditions, researchers have devised many tests, most of which are behavioral in nature. Such tests include STANDARDIZED BEHAVIORAL AVOIDANCE TESTS (SBATs), Individualized Behavioral Tests (IBATs), the Fear Questionnaire, the Mobility Inventory for Agoraphobics, Phobic Avoidance Hierarchy Ratings, Agoraphobia Severity Ratings, Agoraphobia Cognitions Questionnaire, Body Sensations Questionnaire, Self-Monitoring Activities Form, Self-Monitoring of Anxiety Form, and the Anxiety Sensitivity Index.

Researchers are also trying to clarify the relationship of agoraphobic behavior to depression, obsessions and compulsions, and depersonalization. One measure to assess these areas is the Beck Depression Inventory, devised in 1961 to assess changes in the level of depression as a function of agoraphobia treatment. The BDI contains 21 groups of state-

KIND OF HELP AND EFFECTS

	Psychiatrist	Psychologist	Counselor	Medical Doctor	Other	F	df	P
Whom did you see?	36.6% (149)	22.3% (90)	9% (28)	22% (89)	8.9% (36)	15.42	4/399	.001
How long?								
1 mo. = 1	4.4%	7.3%	25.0%	20.7%	14.3%			
1–3 mo. = 2	7.7%	32.7%	16.7%	10.3%	28.6%			
4–6 mo. = 3	8.8%	12.7%	25.0%	3.4%	7.1%			
7–12 mo. = 4	6.6%	9.1%	8.3%	0	14.3%			
12+ mo. = 5	72.5%	38.2%	25.0%	65.5%	35.7%			
x =	4.35	3.38	2.92	3.79	3.29	6.14	4/198	.01
Results on phobias								
much better = 1	6.3%	5.6%	11.5%	2.6%	17.9%			
slightly better = 2	18.7%	19.7%	30.8%	9.1%	21.4%			
none = 3	64.8%	63.4%	53.8%	83.1%	60.7%			
negative = 4	10.2%	9.9%	3.8%	5.2%	0			
x =	2.79	2.79	2.50	2.92	2.43	4.22	4/326	.01
Results on non-phobias								
insight = 1	19.4%	16.1%	9.5%	3.3%	19.2%			
awareness = 2	16.3%	21.4%	33.3%	10.0%	15.4%			
skills = 3	2.0%	5.4%	4.8%	07.7%				
none = 4	53.1%	42.9%	47.6%	78.3%	53.8%			
negative = 5	9.2%	14.3%	4.8%	8.3%	3.8%			
x =	3.16	3.18	3.05	3.78	3.08	3.43	4/257	.01

R. M. Doctor, "Major Results of a Large-scale Survey of Agoraphobics," in DuPont's (ed.) *Phobia: A Comprehensive Survey of Modern Treatments* (New York: Bruner/Mazel, 1982).

ments representing different levels of severity of depression. Another test is the Middlesex Hospital Questionnaire, devised in 1968. This 48-item questionnaire allows assessment of psychopathological features common to many agoraphobics.

Researchers suggest that adequate assessment of agoraphobia should include physiological measures, because agoraphobics often complain about the physiological concomitants of an anxiety reaction: palpitations, sweating, muscular tension, gastrointestinal upset, and labored breathing. Routine physiological recording has become more important since the early 1980s, when panic attacks were recognized as the central feature of the agoraphobic syndrome.

See also ADDICTION, FEAR OF; ALCOHOLISM; ANTI-DEPRESSANTS; ANXIETY; ANXIETY DISORDERS; BEHAVIOR THERAPY; CLAUSTROPHOBIA; CONDITIONING; CONTEXTUAL THERAPY; DEPRESSION; FLOODING; INDIVIDUALIZED BEHAVIOR AVOIDANCE TESTS [IBATS]; MAUDSLEY MARITAL QUESTIONNAIRE; PANIC; PHOBIA; PHOBIC DISORDERS; PSYCHOTHERAPY.

American Psychiatric Association, *Diagnostic and Statistical Manual of Mental Disorders*. 4th ed. (Washington, DC: American Psychiatric Association, 1994).

Barlow, D. H., and Maria T. Waddell, "Agoraphobia," in *Clinical Handbook of Psychological Disorders*. Edited by D. H. Barlow (New York: Guilford Press, 1985).

Bibb, James L., and Dianne L. Chambless, "Alcohol Use and Abuse Among Diagnosed Agoraphobics," *Beh. Res. Ther.* 24, no. 1 (1986): pp. 49–58.

Doctor, R. M., "Major Results of a Large-scale Survey of Agoraphobics," in DuPont (ed.), *Phobia* (New York: Brunner/Mazel, 1982).

Fishman, Scott M., and David V. Sheehan, "Anxiety and Panic: Their Cause and Treatment," *Psychology Today,* April 1985.

Frampton, Muriel, *Agoraphobia: Coping with the World Outside* (Wellingstorough, Northamptonshire: Turnstone Press, 1984).

Himadi, William G. et al., "Assessment of Agoraphobic-II, Measurement of Clinical Change," *Beh. Res. Ther.* 24, no. 2, 1986, pp. 321–332.

Marks, Isaac M., *Fears, Phobias and Rituals* (New York: Oxford University Press, 1987).

———, "Agoraphobia Syndrome (Phobic State Anxiety)" *Arch. Gen. Psychiat.* December 1970.

———, *Fears and Phobias* (New York: Academic Press, 1969).

Mathews, Andrew M. et al., *Agoraphobia: Nature and Treatment* (New York: Guilford Press, 1981).

Mavissakalian, M., and D. Barlow, *Phobia: Psychology and Pharmacologic Treatment* (New York: Guilford Press, 1981).

Mullaney, J. A., and C. J. Trippett, "Alcohol Dependence and Phobias: Clinical Description and Relevance," *Brit. J. Psychiat.* 135, 1979, pp. 565–573.

Thyer, Bruce A., "Alcohol Abuse among Clinically Anxious Patients," *Behav. Res. Ther.* 24, no. 3, 1986, pp. 357–359.

agraphobia Fear of sexual abuse.
See also SEXUAL ABUSE; SEXUAL FEARS.

agrizoophobia Fear of wild animals.
See also ANIMALS, FEAR OF WILD.

agyiophobia Fear of being in a street. Fear of streets is also known as dromophobia. This fear is related to agoraphobia and topophobia, or fear of specific places.
See also AGORAPHOBIA; LANDSCAPES.

aibohphobia Fear of palindromes.

aichmophobia Fear of pointed objects, such as knives, nails, and forks. The word is derived from the Greek term *aichme,* which means "spear, point." Psychoanalytically, an aichmophobic will avoid these objects because they arouse threatening impulses to use them against others. Symptoms of this phobia may lead to unusual eating habits, such as eating alone or without silverware, or to the selection of an occupation in which the phobic individual will not encounter dangerous implements or their symbolic equivalents.
See also BEING TOUCHED, FEAR OF; KNIVES, FEAR OF; POINTS, FEAR OF.

aichurophobia Fear of points or pointed objects.
See also POINTS, FEAR OF.

AIDS, fear of See ACQUIRED IMMUNODEFICIENCY SYNDROME.

ailurophobia See CATS, FEAR OF.

air, fear of Air fear, or anemophobia, is the fear of wind or strong drafts. Some individuals have these fears when the weather changes (for example, when dark clouds appear) or at places where they can hear the wind. This fear may be related to a fear of motion, a fear of thunderstorms, a fear of whirlpools, or a fear of waves.

See also CYCLONES, FEAR OF; WAVES, FEAR OF; WIND, FEAR OF.

airplane phobia See FLYING, FEAR OF.

air pollution, fear of Many people fear air pollution because of its negative health effects. Some individuals who have a fear of contamination, or fear of illness, also fear air pollution. This is not an unreasonable fear, however, because prolonged exposure to polluted air has caused headaches, nausea, and possibly cancer, and it aggravates lung conditions. Air pollution causes anxieties because many individuals fear the known as well as unsuspected effects of air pollution.

See also ACID DEW, FEAR OF; ACID RAIN, FEAR OF; CONTAMINATION, FEAR OF; POLLUTION, FEAR OF.

airsickness, fear of Fear of airsickness (aeronausiphobia) includes fears of NAUSEA, VOMITING, and DIZZINESS while on an airplane. Individuals who fear vomiting, or seeing others vomit, may also fear being airsick themselves or seeing others afflicted. Some social phobics who fear being seen while vomiting or looking ill also fear becoming airsick. Some who fear FLYING do so out of a fear of becoming airsick. Like seasickness, airsickness is caused by unaccustomed MOTION that overstimulates the semicircular canals, the center for the sense of balance in the inner ear. Airsickness is more likely to happen in turbulent air when the plane rises and drops abruptly. Individuals prone to airsickness can help themselves by choosing a seat between the wings, reclining in the seat with their head still and their eyes either closed or fixed on the ceiling rather than looking out.

See also MOTION, FEAR OF; FLYING, FEAR OF.

albuminurophobia Fear of kidney disease.

See also DISEASE PHOBIA; KIDNEY DISEASE, FEAR OF.

alcohol, fear of The concern that alcohol could take over one's life in a harmful way, often much as a parent, sibling, or other key relative was severely affected by ALCOHOLISM. Individuals with little personal identity, low self-esteem, or feelings of helplessness and dependence might have exaggerated fears of becoming alcoholic due to their personal qualities and feelings of having no control of their lives.

See also AGORAPHOBIA; HANGOVER; HEADACHES.

alcoholism A physiological and psychological dependence on alcohol. According to the Substance Abuse and Mental Health Services Administration, about 3.5 percent of the population in the United States ages 12 and older is dependent on alcohol, or about 8 million people in 2006. Many people who are alcohol-dependent also abuse other drugs, such as MARIJUANA or prescription medications.

Some fearful and anxious people become dependent on alcohol to provide relief from their symptoms. Because alcohol exerts both mental and physical effects, it becomes a major part of the dependent person's life. Many agoraphobics become alcoholics as a way of coping with their fears. Some agoraphobic individuals do not leave their homes at all, so it is fairly easy for them to conceal their alcoholism. (They can have alcohol delivered to their homes.) There is emerging evidence that over 30 percent of alcoholics are actually anxiety- or panic-ridden people who use alcohol for its anxiety-relief properties. They may prefer alcohol to the use of antianxiety medications.

Studies by Petrakis et al. reported in *Alcohol Research & Health* have shown that people who are dependent on alcohol have nearly a five times greater risk of having GENERALIZED ANXIETY DISORDER than those who are not alcoholics. They also have more than twice the risk of having POST-TRAUMATIC STRESS DISORDER. Individuals who are alcoholics have an above-average risk for the development of DEPRESSION and BIPOLAR DISORDER. It is believed by some experts that alcoholism may trigger psychiatric disorders in some individuals, while others believe individuals with psychiatric disorders use alcohol as a means of self-medication. There are arguments for both cases and it is impossible to generalize to the entire population of individuals with alcoholism.

According to the American Psychiatric Association's *DIAGNOSTIC AND STATISTICAL MANUAL OF MENTAL DISORDERS* (FOURTH EDITION), as many as 90 percent of adults in the United States have had some experience with alcohol and a substantial number (60 percent of males and 30 percent of females) have had one or more alcohol-related adverse life events, such as driving after consuming too much alcohol or missing school or work due to a hangover.

Historical Background

The term *alcoholism* was coined by Swedish scientist Magnus Huss in 1852, when he identified a condition involving abuse of alcohol and labeled it *alkoholismus chronicus.* However, references to the problem of alcoholism are also found in the earlier works of Benjamin Rush, an 18th-century American physician, considered the "father of American psychiatry," as well as even further back in time, to the Roman philosopher Seneca. In 1956, the American Medical Association and the American Bar Association officially recognized alcoholism as a "disease," an action that affected the legal status of alcoholics, alcoholism-related state and federal laws, program financing, insurance coverage, and hospital admissions.

How Alcohol Affects the Body

Contrary to popular belief, alcohol is a depressant and not a stimulant. The effects of alcohol are felt most noticeably in the central nervous system. As sensitivity is reduced in the nervous system, the higher functions of the brain are dulled, which may lead to impulsive actions, loud speech, and lack of physical control. The drinker's face may turn red or pale. While drinking, the alcoholic often loses any sense of guilt or embarrassment, gains more self-confidence, and loses inhibitions as the alcohol deadens the normal restraining influences of the brain. Large quantities of alcohol will impair physical reflexes, coordination, and mental acuteness.

The long-term use of alcohol can lead to many severe health problems, such as major damage to the liver (requiring liver transplant), and an increased risk for the development of some forms of cancer (colorectal cancer, esophageal cancer, and stomach cancer). In addition, the alcoholic has an increased risk of developing pancreatitis, dementia, and heart disease.

Alcoholics Anonymous and Self-Help

Founded in 1935, Alcoholics Anonymous is an international organization devoted to maintaining the sobriety of its members and helping them control the compulsive urge to drink by offering them support, fellowship, and understanding. The program includes the individual's admission that he or she cannot control their drinking, the sharing of experiences, problems and concerns at meetings, and the willingness to help others who are in need of support.

At the core of the program is the desire to stop drinking. Members follow a 12-step program, which stresses faith, disavowal of personal responsibility, passivity in the hands of God or a higher power, the confession of past and current wrongdoing to those who were harmed, and other required actions.

Symptoms and Diagnostic Path

The National Institute on Alcohol Abuse and Alcoholism says that alcoholism is characterized by an individual who exhibits three or more of the following indicators:

- a tolerance to alcohol (which means that more alcohol is needed than in the past in order to achieve intoxication)

- withdrawal symptoms if alcohol is not consumed (such as shakiness, nausea, sweating, and other physical symptoms)

- the use of alcohol in a greater quantity than was intended

- the persistent desire to cut back or control use
- a significant amount of time that is spent on obtaining, using, or recovering from the use of alcohol
- neglect of an individual's normal social, occupational, or recreational tasks
- drinking that occurs to avoid withdrawal symptoms
- continued use of alcohol despite physical and psychological problems

Stages of Alcoholism. In the first phase of dependence on alcohol, the heavy social drinker may feel no effects from alcohol. In the second phase, the drinker experiences memory lapses relating to events that happen during drinking episodes. In the third phase, there is lack of control over alcohol and the drinker cannot be certain of discontinuing drinking by choice. The final phase begins with long binges of intoxication, and there are observable mental or physical complications.

Behavioral symptoms may include hiding bottles, aggressive or grandiose behavior, irritability, jealousy, or uncontrolled anger, frequent change of jobs, repeated promises to self and others to give up drinking, and neglect of proper eating habits and personal appearance. Physical symptoms may include unsteadiness, confusion, poor memory, nausea, vomiting, shaking, weakness in the legs and hands, irregular pulse, and redness and enlarged capillaries in the face.

Treatment Options and Outlook
Medical help for alcohol dependence includes detoxification, or assistance in overcoming withdrawal symptoms, and psychological, social, and physical treatments. Treatment may be received in an inpatient facility or an outpatient clinic.

Medications such as disulfiram (Antabuse), an aversive medication, are also often used by many treatment centers after the individual is alcohol free, to enable him or her to stay off alcohol. If the individual who takes disulfiram consumes any amount of alcohol, even a minor amount that is included in food, he or she will become extremely nauseous and vomit copiously. Even the alcohol in cologne or shaving lotion may cause vomiting in some individuals taking disulfiram.

Other medications used to treat alcoholism, and which help to manage the craving for alcohol, are naltrexone (ReVia) and acamprosate (Campral). These drugs have been proven successful in many individuals with alcoholism. However, it is best to combine medication therapy with psychotherapy.

Group psychotherapy is often employed to treat individuals with alcoholism, using a variety of techniques. Individual psychotherapy is also often used. Therapists for alcohol-dependent persons may be psychiatrists, psychologists, or social workers. Social treatments involve family members in the treatment process. Many alcohol-dependent people benefit from an active involvement in groups such as Alcoholics Anonymous.

Risk Factors and Prevention
Many studies have shown that there is a genetic risk for the development of alcoholism, although not all children of alcoholics develop the disorder. In addition, the children of alcoholics who drink may have been affected by environmental factors, i.e., viewing their parents' drinking. However, studies of adopted children have shown that the biological children of alcoholics have a greater risk for developing alcoholism than others, even when they are reared by nonalcoholic adoptive parents to whom they have no genetic relationship.

The only means of prevention of alcoholism is to avoid drinking altogether or to drink in moderation. Many experts believe, however, that individuals with a predisposition to alcoholism cannot drink in moderation.

See also ADDICTION, FEAR OF; AGORAPHOBIA; CODEPENDENCY; CONTROL; EMPLOYEE ASSISTANCE PROGRAMS.

Gwinnell, Esther, M.D., and Christine Adamec, *The Encyclopedia of Drug Abuse.* (New York: Facts On File, Inc., 2008).

Miller, Laurie, M.D., and Christine Adamec, *The Encyclopedia of Adoption.* (New York: Facts On File, Inc., 2006).

Petrakis, Ismene L., M.D., et al., "Comorbidity of Alcoholism and Psychiatric Disorders," *Alcohol Research & Health* 26, no. 2, 2002, pp. 81–89.

alektorophobia   Fear of chickens. This fear may be related to a fear of feathers, of winged creatures, or of flying animals or birds.

See also ANIMALS, FEAR OF; BIRDS, FEAR OF; CHICKENS, FEAR OF; FLYING THINGS, FEAR OF.

Alexander technique A technique to properly move one's body for relief of anxieties and stress and to promote well-being and health. Practitioners of the technique learn to increase conscious awareness of how they use their bodies. The technique was developed by Frederick Mathias Alexander (1869–1955), a Shakespearean actor.

Teachers of the Alexander technique work with individuals to develop mindful involvement so that they learn to move, sit, stand, and walk in new ways to prevent imbalances caused by automatic habits. The technique teaches that the misuse of the body begins in the brain, where thoughts of carrying out an activity cause an unconscious interference with the reflex mechanism by which the thought is translated into action. Interferences are a learned behavior that people pick up unconsciously and then becomes automatic.

The first step is to break the connection between a habitual activity and the thought of carrying the activity out. A new system of movement can be introduced. For example, after years of slumping in front of the computer, our faulty kinesthetic awareness signals the brain that all is correct. Customary behaviors feel right even if they are inefficient or out of balance.

The technique promotes an understanding that a few brief periods of horizontal rest allow a respite from the stresses of the day; overused, fatigued muscles are soothed; and the natural curves of the spine balance their forces.

Recommendations for following the Alexander technique call for lying down in the "position of mechanical advantage" at least once a day for 20 minutes, preferably in the middle of the day. Musicians are advised to fit the "lie-down" time into their practice schedule and to lie down five minutes for every half-hour of practice time. Individuals who do physical fitness training are advised to lie down before the workout to help prevent injury to fatigued muscles.

How to Practice the Technique

Find a quiet place on the floor or large flat table, not a bed. Use a small pile of paperback books to rest your head on. Start by sitting with your legs extended in front of you; they can be bent, but do not cross them. Keep your arms in your lap or relaxed by your sides.

Lean forward over your legs, thinking of the crown of your head extending out over your feet. When you feel that your lower back has lengthened, let your head release forward from the top of your neck and begin to roll back to lie down. Your hips will go down first, then your back, then your shoulders and head; rest your head on the books. The books under your head should be high enough to fill the space made by the natural curve in your neck.

Let your weight settle into the floor. Bring your arms up so that your elbows are pointing away from your sides and your hands are resting on your lower ribs. Keep your hands relaxed with fingers extended.

Bring your legs up one at a time so that your knee points toward the ceiling and your foot is flat on the floor. Keep your legs about shoulder-width apart and your feet as close to your buttocks as is comfortable. After you bring your legs up, you may wish to push the pile of books under your head back a little. They should not be touching your neck.

Allow your body weight to settle into the floor. Notice where you are holding onto the muscles of your body and think about letting them release. Keep your breathing easy and regular. During the 20 minutes, let your mind occasionally return to your feelings of tension and relaxation.

After 20 minutes, get up by rolling your head to the side, followed by your shoulders, then hips and legs. Bring yourself onto hands and knees and slowly bring yourself to standing.

See also BODY THERAPIES; COMPLEMENTARY THERAPIES.

Kahn, Ada P., *The Encyclopedia of Stress and Stress-related Disorders,* 2nd ed. (New York: Facts On File, 2006).

algophobia Fear of pain.
See also PAIN, FEAR OF.

allergies Uncomfortable and sometimes seriously threatening bodily reactions to stimuli, such as airborne substances (pollen or dust), foods (egg yolks or chocolate), or bee stings. Fearful situations can heighten the body's sensitivity and produce allergic reactions that vary greatly between people. Some respond with stomach problems, some with rashes, and others with respiratory disorders such as asthma. Commonly, allergic reactions can trigger anxiety. For example, the asthmatic may become frightened about repeated attacks during which he has trouble breathing. Those who have skin rashes can become so embarrassed, sensitive, and anxious about their appearance that their normal social functioning is impaired during attacks. When allergic disorders are treated medically, some related ANXIETIES usually disappear. Allergic sensitivity heightens the intensity of anxiety.

Allergies are sources of anxieties for many people because symptoms of allergies may make them uncomfortable, sometimes unpredictably. Allergies can lead to anxieties for many reasons. Some allergies limit many people's participation in certain activities, such as hiking in forests, or partaking of certain foods. Some people must curtail their social activities during periods when their allergy symptoms are severe.

According to the American Academy of Allergy and Immunology, 41 million Americans (one in six) have asthma and allergies. Of those, 22.4 million have hay fever and 10 million are affected by eczema, urticaria (hives), angioedema (swelling), and allergic reactions to food, medications, and insect stings. Many people are allergic to insect stings; insect stings account for at least 50 deaths a year.

Symptoms and Diagnostic Path

The most common type of allergy, known as allergic rhinitis, affects the upper respiratory tract. Sufferers of this type of allergy often complain of coldlike symptoms, such as runny eyes, drippy noses, coughing, and congestion. Since allergic rhinitis is often caused by pollen, molds, and spores, it is primarily a seasonal affliction, striking in spring and fall.

Asthma is an allergy that affects the lungs and afflicts some 10 million Americans. Sufferers complain of "attacks," in which the chest tightens and breathing becomes extremely difficult. Some people gasp and fear that they might die at any moment. Asthma causes anxiety for those around the sufferer. Asthma may be caused by a wide variety of allergens, including house dust, certain foods, and feathers. Effective prescription medications are available for asthma.

Many people mistake allergies for other problems and seek medical help only after consistent bouts. Prescription medications are available to relieve allergies.

Treatment Options and Outlook

Most allergies begin during childhood, some 80 percent before the age of 15 years. The first step is to identify the allergen and then to remove the allergen from the person's environment if possible, or take the person away from the allergen. Sometimes a change of climate works, but it may result in other allergies. Some hay fever sufferers have moved to the opposite end of the country only to find new allergens waiting there.

Air conditioners and filters help persons allergic to pollen. A change in occupation or the use of a face mask on the job can help others. Use of hypoallergenic cosmetics (preparations that are compounded without the most common allergens) helps many people.

Seeking the help of a physician who specializes in allergies (allergist) is a wise decision for people who think they have an allergy from an unknown cause. For some individuals, skin tests may be recommended. A minute amount of various materials is exposed to the skin to see which one causes a reaction. Efforts are then made, wherever possible, to eliminate or reduce contact with that allergen.

Though apparently not a direct cause, anxieties and emotional stress can trigger allergic attacks. If you are prone to allergies, it is likely that you will have less trouble with them if you can reduce the anxieties and tension in your life. The allergic person needs some assurance that he or she can live a fairly normal life. If one cannot eliminate his or her allergy, he or she can usually learn how to live with it, sometimes with the use of relaxation techniques and mental imagery.

See also ASTHMA; COMPLEMENTARY THERAPIES; MENTAL IMAGERY; POISON, FEAR OF; RELAXATION.

Kahn, Ada P., *Stress A–Z: A Sourcebook for Facing Everyday Challenges.* (New York: Facts On File, 1998).

alliumphobia Fear of garlic.

See also GARLIC, FEAR OF.

allodoxaphobia Fear of opinions. This may relate to hearing or learning opinions of others or fearing one's own opinions. This fear may also be related to a fear of criticism.

See also CRITICISM, FEAR OF; OPINIONS, FEAR OF OTHERS'.

alone, fear of being Fear of being alone is known as phobophobia and eremophobia. Fear of being alone sometimes relates to AGORAPHOBIA. Another term for the dread of solitude used by American physician and author Benjamin Rush (1745–1813) was "solo phobia." "This distemper is peculiar to persons of vacant minds, and guilty consciences. Such people cannot bear to be alone, especially if the horror of sickness is added to the pain of attempting to think, or to the terror of thinking."*

See also AGING, FEAR OF.

*Runes, D. D., *The Selected Writings of Benjamin Rush* (New York: The Philosophical Library, 1947).

alpha adrenergic blockers See ADRENERGIC BLOCK-ING AGENTS; ADRENERGIC DRUGS.

alpha adrenergic function See ADRENERGIC SYSTEM.

alprazolam The generic name for a pharmaceutical marketed as Xanax. It is in a class of drugs known as benzodiazepine compounds with anti-anxiety and sedative-hypnotic actions. It is efficacious in treating agoraphobia and panic disorders and is also used to treat generalized anxiety disorder. Studies suggest that alprazolam also has antidepressant activity.

Drowsiness is the most common side effect reported. Caution should be observed when other drugs possessing sedative actions are given with alprazolam. Physical and psychological dependence is likely when larger than usual doses are prescribed

or therapy is prolonged. As with all benzodiazepines, treatment should be terminated by gradually reducing the dose.

alternative therapies See COMPLEMENTARY THERAPIES.

altophobia See HEIGHTS, FEAR OF.

Alzheimer's disease A progressive, irreversible disease that is primarily experienced by senior citizens, although younger individuals may also develop an early onset of the disease. Alzheimer's disease is also known as *senile dementia of the Alzheimer's type* (SDAT), and it is the most common form of dementia. It should be noted that the majority of older individuals over age 65 do *not* suffer from dementia, although the risk for dementia increases steadily with aging.

Many people fear developing the disease as they age, particularly when their own parents or other close relatives suffered from Alzheimer's disease. These individuals may also cope with the anxieties of providing care to a person with Alzheimer's as they wonder if they too will suffer from the disease. In fact, most people with Alzheimer's (70 percent) are cared for at home by family members.

Patients who are told that they have Alzheimer's are often distressed. It is frightening for patients in the early stages of Alzheimer's to discover that they have the disease. Sufferers with early Alzheimer's disease are often anxious and fearful and many of them altogether deny that they have the disease.

Alzheimer's disease was originally named in 1906 by Alois Alzheimer (1864–1915) after diagnosing a patient, Auguste D. Subsequent to an autopsy, Dr. Alzheimer discovered that the patient's brain cells were very different from normal brain cells. He also found tangles of a plaquelike substance, which were not seen in the normal brain. Auguste D. was 51 years old at the time of her death and she had an early onset of the disease.

Although there is no known cure for Alzheimer's disease, there are many ongoing research projects underway worldwide. In the United States, this research is at least in part being conducted in anticipation of large numbers of older Baby Boomers (born 1946–1964) entering their retirement years. It will be expensive and difficult to care for greater numbers of patients with Alzheimer's.

According to the National Institute of Neurological Disorders and Stroke, an estimated 6.8 million people in the United States have some form of dementia, and of these, about 4 million people (59 percent) have Alzheimer's disease. Other forms of dementia include vascular dementia, the second most common cause of dementia, which represents nearly 20 percent of all dementias. Frontotemporal dementia (FTD), a disorder of the frontal lobe that is characterized by the degeneration of nerve cells, accounts for 2–10 percent of all cases of dementia. Other forms of dementia comprise the balance of cases.

The causes of Alzheimer's disease are controversial and hotly debated by many researchers and other experts. Some experts believe that the disease is primarily caused by excessive plaques in the brain, while others believe that an excessive production of brain proteins may lead to the disease. Genetic factors also play a clear role and individuals whose parents have Alzheimer's disease have an increased risk for the disease themselves, although it is no certainty that the disease will develop.

Symptoms and Diagnostic Path

The symptoms of Alzheimer's disease vary from person to person. However, they generally include the following:

- a gradual loss of memory, particularly for recent events
- dwindling powers of judgment, reasoning, and understanding
- disorientation
- personality changes
- an inability to perform normal activities of daily living
- difficulty in learning
- loss of language skills
- general intellectual deterioration.

The dementia of Alzheimer's disease is progressive, degenerative, and irreversible, and, eventually, patients with the disease become totally incapable of caring for themselves. Alzheimer's disease is a major cause for admission to long-term care facilities and nursing homes.

The symptoms of Alzheimer's should not be confused with age-associated memory impairment (AAMI), a term that health care professionals use to describe minor memory difficulties that come with age. For example, a person with minor memory difficulties may forget that he or she has an appointment at 4 P.M. A person with Alzheimer's disease may be puzzled by the purpose of the watch on their wrist.

Ruling Out Other Disorders.   Before a diagnosis of Alzheimer's disease is made, a physician should rule out other possible contributing conditions to memory loss in the patient, such as a potentially reversible DEPRESSION, or adverse drug reactions,

COMPARING NORMAL MEMORY FAILURES WITH FAILURES OF ALZHEIMER'S DISEASE	
Person with Normal Memory Failure	**Person with Alzheimer's Memory Failure**
Forgets the time of an appointment.	Forgets how to tell time.
Forgets to read an article someone recommends.	Forgets how to read.
Has minor difficulty driving to a new address and gets lost briefly.	Has major difficulty finding a new address. Forgets how to get home. Forgets how to drive.
Forgets the name of a celebrity or politician.	Forgets the names of common household objects, such as an apple or a chair. Does not recognize family members or know their names.
Pays a few bills late.	Stops paying bills.
Forgets what was eaten for lunch.	Forgets to eat lunch; is unable to prepare lunch.

as well as Parkinson's disease, any major metabolic changes, head trauma, chronic alcoholism, nutritional or vitamin deficiencies, head injuries, and stroke.

Alzheimer's Was Often Misdiagnosed in the Past. Before technologically sophisticated testing procedures became generally available, many sufferers of Alzheimer's were misdiagnosed and consequently mistreated. For example, screen star Rita Hayworth was misdiagnosed with alcoholic dementia in the 1970s. She was later diagnosed as suffering from Alzheimer's disease, from which she died in 1987. Her career ended when she could no longer remember her lines.

Former president Ronald Reagan's diagnosis of Alzheimer's disease was made public by Reagan himself in 1994. This announcement allowed many people to admit to others that they or their relatives had the disease; before this time, it was often considered a shameful and embarrassing subject.

Making the Diagnosis. Alzheimer's disease in the later stages can be diagnosed by most physicians. However, in the earlier stages of the disease, a neurologist is usually the specialist who diagnoses the disease. Often screening devices such as the Mini-Mental State Examination (MMSE) are used to help physicians determine patients' abilities with speaking and writing. Doctors may also ask patients to perform simple tasks, such as drawing the face of a clock and showing where the clock hands would go if it were 5:00. Testing using paper and pencil can help the physician determine whether Alzheimer's is present.

The Use of Brain Scans. Brain scans can be used to rule out strokes, tumors, and other disorders that can cause memory problems similar to those of Alzheimer's disease. In addition, cortical atrophy is present in brain scans in some forms of dementia such as Alzheimer's. The most commonly used brain scans are computed tomography (CT) scans and magnetic resonance imaging (MRI) scans. These scans can show brain atrophy as well as damage to the brain from small strokes. An electroencephalogram (EEG) may be used to detect dementia in patients with moderately severe to severe Alzheimer's disease. This test measures brain waves and patients with Alzheimer's disease will have abnormal brain patterns.

Laboratory Tests. Physicians also usually use laboratory tests to rule other possible diseases out, such as infections or thyroid disease. A complete blood count (CBC) is commonly used to check for infection, and a thyroid-stimulating hormone (TSH) test is used to check for thyroid function. Physicians will usually check the blood glucose levels for diabetes and test the urine for infection.

The Stages of Alzheimer's Disease. According to *The Encyclopedia of Senior Health and Well-Being,* the following are some symptoms of the presence of Alzheimer's disease in the early (mild), moderate, and severe stages of the disease.

Early Stage

- personality changes, such as agitation, anxiety, and depression
- frequent and unexplained mood swings
- changes in the ability to carry on a simple conversation
- temporary confusion while still in one's own neighborhood
- difficulty handling daily tasks that were easy in the past

Moderate Stage

- inability to recognize family members or friends
- combative or aggressive behavior
- a reluctance to engage in any conversations that require more than a one- or two-word answer
- confusion with tasks such as bathing and toileting
- poor personal hygiene, such as wearing stained clothes day after day and failing to bathe or shower regularly
- extreme resistance to any changes in the daily routine

Severe Stage

- speech that is slow or cannot be understood at all
- incontinence of bladder and bowels
- paranoia or extreme suspiciousness
- rages for no reason
- trouble with simple tasks that is unrelated to any physical disabilities

- wandering about the house at night and being sleepy in the daytime (also known as "sundowning")
- difficulty in speaking or in understanding what is said by others (aphasia)

Treatment Options and Outlook

Family members or professional caregivers can use behavior modification to encourage patients with Alzheimer's to continue desired behaviors and to ignore inappropriate behaviors. Some patients in the early stage of the disease can learn to use note-taking or computer recall devices to help them with their memory problems.

In the early stages, many people with Alzheimer's can remain at home if they have patient and educated caregivers. Support groups may also be helpful to many caregivers of Alzheimer's patients. However, in the moderate to severe stages of the disease, few family members can provide the extreme level of care that the patient needs and often the patient must go to a nursing home or other long-term facility.

Medications May Help. Medications are often used to treat patients with Alzheimer's. Although they are no cure, they may allay further deterioration for a period of time. Donepezil hydrochloride (Aricept) is often used with patients who have Alzheimer's disease, and it has been approved for mild to moderate Alzheimer's as well as for the severe dementia that is associated with Alzheimer's disease. Other drugs which are used to treat the disease are rivastigamine (Exelon), tacrine (Cognex), galantamine (Reminyl), and memantine (Namenda). Other drugs may also be used to improve the patient's behavior and mood, such as antidepressants, anticonvulsants, and sedatives. These drugs are used to treat any existing depression (antidepressants), seizures (anticonvulsant), and sleep disorders (sedatives), which often accompany Alzheimer's disease.

In the past, antipsychotic medications were frequently used to treat patients with Alzheimer's as well as other forms of dementia, particularly in nursing homes; however, research has shown that such drugs do not improve the condition. In addition, antipsychotic medications have been associated with an increased risk of death in patients with Alzheimer's. In most cases, however, the deaths were caused by infections or heart disease.

Risk Factors and Prevention

More women than men are affected by Alzheimer's, and about 68 percent of patients with Alzheimer's are female. However, this may be because women statistically outlive men and, with increased age, comes an increased risk for the development of Alzheimer's disease. In fact, age is a primary risk factor for Alzheimer's and the number of people with Alzheimer's doubles every five years after the age of 65 years. Almost half of individuals age 85 years and older have Alzheimer's disease.

Race is another factor and most people diagnosed with Alzheimer's (85 percent) are white. A large percentage of patients with Alzheimer's are in poor health (about two-thirds) with diseases such as diabetes, hypertension, arthritis, and heart disease.

Some genes appear to increase the risk for the development of Alzheimer's; for example, about 40 percent of people with Alzheimer's have a gene that produces apolipoprotein E (ApoE), and those who inherit these genes may develop Alzheimer's, although further research is needed to clarify the genetic risks.

The risk increases further with genetic loading; for example, studies have shown that the risk for developing Alzheimer's disease is 11 percent if neither parent had the disease. The risk increases to 36 percent when one parent has the disease. The risk further increases to 54 percent if both parents have the disease. In the case of identical twins, if one twin has Alzheimer's, the risk for the other twin is 40–50 percent.

DIABETES is a risk factor for Alzheimer's and individuals with diabetes should work to maintain as normal a blood sugar as possible. Some studies have shown that individuals with tightly controlled diabetes have performed better on cognitive tests than individuals with poorly controlled diabetes.

Some studies have linked high levels of blood cholesterol to an increased risk for the development of Alzheimer's disease, and individuals with high cholesterol levels who have not developed Alzheimer's are advised to work to normalize their blood cholesterol to decrease the risk for Alzheimer's.

Untreated hypertension has been shown to be another risk factor for the development of Alzheimer's disease, and, in one study in Europe, individuals over age 60 who received medications for their high blood pressure had a 55 percent lower risk of developing dementia, including both Alzheimer's disease and vascular dementia.

The progression of Alzheimer's disease, once it has begun, cannot be slowed down, but if it is identified in the early stages, many patients can show visible improvement. Because of its devastating and intractable deterioration of functioning, people develop anticipatory fears about possibly having the beginnings of this disorder.

See also DEPRESSION; SUPPORT GROUPS.

Bren, Linda, "Alzheimer's: Searching for a Cure." U.S. Food and Drug Administration. Available online. URL: http://www.fda.gov/fdac/features/2003/403_alz.html. Downloaded December 2, 2006.

Kandel, Joseph, M.D., and Christine Adamec, *The Encyclopedia of Senior Health and Well-Being* (New York: Facts On File, 2003).

amathophobia   See DUST, FEAR OF.

amaxophobia   Fear of being in a vehicle.

See also AUTOMOBILES, FEAR OF; CLAUSTROPHOBIA; TRAINS, FEAR OF; VEHICLES, FEAR OF.

ambivalence   The simultaneous existence of two sometimes contradictory feelings, attitudes, values, goals, or directions. The term was introduced by Eugen Bleuler, a Swiss psychiatrist (1857–1939), to denote the simultaneous occurrence of two antagonistic emotions, such as hatred and love toward the same person, or inclination and disinclination toward the same activity or goal. For example, some individuals have feelings of ambivalence toward parents who dole out love and affection as well as punishment. Some individuals are ambivalent about work, marriage, and other major life issues. Ambivalence is common in PHOBIAS, including AGORAPHOBIA, as there is often a simultaneous approach–avoidance attitude toward potentially fearful situations.

ambulophobia   Fear of walking or riding in vehicles.

amitriptyline   An antidepressant drug known as a tricyclic compound (one of two major classes of antidepressant drugs). It is a popular antidepressant that has a moderate to marked SEDATIVE action. Because the sedative effect of amitriptyline interacts additively with the sedative effect of ALCOHOL, alcohol consumption should be avoided by individuals taking amitriptyline, particularly if they drive a car or work in a hazardous occupation. Amitriptyline compounds are also used to treat HEADACHES associated with depression that are the result of nonorganic causes. Amitriptyline also is known by the trade names Endep, Elavil, Amitid, Domical, Lentizol, Triptafen, and Triptizol.

See also ADVERSE DRUG REACTIONS; ANTIDEPRESSANTS; DEPRESSION; DRUGS; TRICYCLIC ANTIDEPRESSANTS.

amnesia, fear of   Fear of having amnesia is known as amnesiophobia. Amnesia is an inability to recall past experiences, or the loss of memory. There are two basic types of amnesia that people fear. One is anterograde amnesia, or an inability to form new memories, in which the individual either does not consolidate what is perceived into permanent memory storage or cannot retrieve recent memories from storage. The other is retrograde amnesia, which is a loss of the memory of events that occurred before the memory disturbance began. Episodic amnesia refers to a particular event or period in one's life that is forgotten. The episode may have been a significant one that may have led to the development of one or more phobias or anxieties. The fear of amnesia is now commonly related to the development of ALZHEIMER'S DISEASE.

See also REPRESSION.

amnesiophobia   Fear of having amnesia.

See also AMNESIA, FEAR OF.

amphetamines Amphetamines, popularly referred to as "speed," include dextroamphetamines, methamphetamines, and methylphenidates. Amphetamines are sometimes prescribed for DEPRESSION and to give the user a sense of well-being and increased alertness. In some cases, they may relieve anxiety symptoms. They are sometimes abused by individuals who have depression and anxiety, and they should be prescribed only for a limited time and for a specific purpose. All drugs in this group are associated with dependence, and all can produce one or more organic mental disorders, intoxication, delirium, delusional syndrome, or withdrawal syndrome. These drugs also act as appetite suppressants. Because of the possibility of patients' developing dependency on amphetamines, many physicians have stopped prescribing them.

See also ADVERSE DRUG REACTIONS; APPETITE SUPPRESSANTS; DRUGS.

amulets Some individuals who fear witchcraft wear amulets, such as stones, bones, nails, rings, or other objects. Wearers believe that the amulets offer them protection and comfort when facing anxiety about feared situations. Some amulets may have special significance, such as objects found at a significant place of burial or under certain astrological configurations.

See also MAGIC, FEAR OF; WITCHES AND WITCHCRAFT, FEAR OF.

amychophobia Fear of being scratched. Often such fears are associated with avoidance of ANIMALS, particularly cats, dogs, puppies, and kittens. In many cases the fear is irrational and exaggerated; however, for individuals who have severe allergic reactions to animal scratches, animal hair, or fleas, the fear is quite appropriate.

See also ANIMALS, FEAR OF; SCRATCHED, FEAR OF BEING.

amygdala The small, almond-shaped brain structure on both sides of the brain that regulates emotional reactions to perceptions. The amygdala is also the controller of the fear response. Only one inch long, the amygdala is associated with a range of mental conditions from normalcy to post-traumatic stress responses.

The amygdala has become the focal point of numerous research projects. Research involving the amygdala dates from the 1940s, when scientists viewed amygdala lesions in rhesus monkeys. Improved techniques, such as using the neurotoxin, ibotenic acid, to make precise lesions, as well as advanced imaging such as magnetic resonance imaging (MRI) and POSITRON EMISSION TOMOGRAPHY (PET) are partly responsible for a renewed interest in the amygdala.

Researchers are exploring how the amygdala might affect people who suffer from mood disorders, such as BIPOLAR DISORDER, or depression, which runs in families. Such people may have an abnormal increase in blood flow and glucose metabolism. Furthermore, the amygdala occupies a central role in anxiety disorders and post-traumatic stress disorders in that it tends to overreact to conditioned stimuli associated with previous traumatic experience (such as traumatic events, panic attacks, and so on). Shrinkage has been noted in chronic trauma states, but recovery of size occurs with successful treatments.

anablepophobia See HIGH PLACES, FEAR OF LOOKING UP AT.

analgesia Also known as analgia. This is an insensitivity to pain, which may be due to an organic disorder or to psychological factors, while other senses remain intact. Some degree of analgesia can be induced by distraction, such as by light or sound. Analgesia may also occur in hysterical disorders and schizophrenia. Muscle tension associated with ANXIETY can restrict sensitivity to physical sensations.

A second meaning of analgesia is pain relief from medications. Pain-alleviating drugs are referred to as analgesics or analgesic drugs. Analgesics were commonly prescribed for anxiety before the advent of modern tranquilizers. Psychic factors are involved in the experience of pain, including expectations, emotions, and thoughts. When tranquilizers and neuroleptics are used to alleviate pain, mental elements may be more affected than physical elements. Analgesics may induce slight drowsiness. Some analgesics contain narcotics, which may produce drug ADDICTION or dependence. Examples are opium alkaloids, morphine, codeine, and heroin. The morphine antagonists nalorphine and pentazocine are analgesics but are not addictive.

See also PAIN.

O'Brien, Robert and Sidney Cohen, *The Encyclopedia of Drug Abuse* (New York: Facts On File, 1984).

anal stage The second stage of psychosexual development during which libidinal energies are derived from anal activity. The child focuses on the pleasurable feelings of retaining and expelling the feces; this usually occurs during the second year of life. Some phobic reactions and phobias (such as contamination and germ fears, fear of lack of resources such as money, and obsessive-compulsive disorder) relate back to this stage in the individual's development, according to psychoanalytic theory.

See also DEVELOPMENTAL STAGES; OBSESSIVE-COMPULSIVE DISORDERS; PSYCHOANALYSIS.

analysand The individual undergoing psychoanalysis for a phobia or any other reason.

See also PSYCHOANALYSIS.

analysis See PSYCHOANALYSIS.

analysis, fractional A brief therapy method (focused, short-term therapy based on psychoanalytic theory) introduced by Franz Alexander (1891–1964), a Hungarian-American psychoanalyst and pioneer in brief analytic therapy. In fractional analysis, PSYCHOTHERAPY is suspended for prearranged intervals while the individual works through insights already attained, including those related to ANXIETIES and PHOBIAS.

See also BRIEF PSYCHOTHERAPY.

analyst Along with the term psychoanalyst, usually refers to therapists who follow routines

of psychoanalysis as outlined by Sigmund Freud (1856–1939). Analysts who follow concepts of Carl Jung (1875–1963) are called analytical psychologists. Those who use the concepts of Adolf Meyer (1866–1950) are psychobiologists. Those who follow Alfred Adler (1870–1937) are individual psychologists. All these types of analysts try to help individuals with anxieties and phobias.

See also PSYCHOLOGY; PSYCHOANALYSIS.

anamnesis A process by which the individual recalls past events and the feelings associated with them. The word literally means "not forgetting." The term applies to the lengthy process of retrospective investigation into an individual's past prior to diagnosis in long-term treatments for ANXIETY and other disorders.

See also MEDICAL MODEL; MEMORIES.

anaphylaxis, psychic Reactivation of earlier symptoms by an event similar to the one that initially produced the symptoms, such as anxieties or phobias. The initial event may be the sensitizing agent, and the later event the activating agent. For example, the early event may have been a near-drowning and the later event an incident that happens near water, with the result that the individual fears water.

androgens See HORMONES.

androphobia See MEN, FEAR OF; SEXUAL FEARS.

anemophobia See AIR, FEAR OF.

anger An intense and basic emotional state in which one feels a high level of displeasure, frustration, and stress. The spectrum of anger may range from slight irritation to explosive hostility. Anger is a source of energy that is discharged on others, objects, or oneself. Anger and anxiety are incompatible; anger is often used to counteract anxiety.

Physiological changes occur when one feels angry. For example, anger increases the heart rate, blood pressure, and flow of ADRENALINE. Suppressed anger, or hostility, may result in HIGH BLOOD PRESSURE, skin rashes, and HEADACHES and is thought to be the primary cause of heart disease in the Type A personality.

Most people at times are caught between two attitudes with regard to anger. There is the psychological and medical opinion that suppressed anger is physically and psychologically damaging. There are social pressures which at different levels label angry behavior destructive, illegal, or unsophisticated. Further limiting expression of anger is the feeling that such behavior may bring regrets later.

Adults who express anger directly with physical violence or verbal abuse usually do so because they model their behavior on others in their environment or because there seems to be a reward for violent behavior. In American frontier society, for example, violent behavior was common and usually considered to be admirable. Since in most situations it is unacceptable to express anger directly, many people react by becoming sulky or indifferent, or adopting a superior, patronizing attitude toward the person or situation that angered them.

Anger may be helpful and constructive. The exercise that an individual chooses to use to work off anger may do him or her good in other ways. Releasing an angry feeling sometimes brings with it a sense of pleasure. Assertiveness training is a common technique for expressing oneself constructively.

Among athletes, anger can have a harmful effect on athletic performance. Anger drains energy and diverts attention from what must be done at the moment. However, professional athletes are trained to recover quickly from events that arouse anger. In some cases, anger may make a player more forceful and positive.

An individual who expresses anxieties and angry feelings extremely might be given three goals: first, to identify the feelings of anger; secondly to use constructive release of the energy of anger through assertiveness or appropriate physical expression; and third, to identify thought and thought processes that lead to anger. For example, to identify feelings of anger, one might keep a diary of angry feelings and learn to recognize anger before losing control.

The individual will learn to take responsibility for his or her own emotions and stop blaming others for arousing the anger. In learning to use constructive release of the energy of anger, the individual may benefit from assertiveness training and learn to express anger verbally to the appropriate source. Assertive techniques will help the individual increase his feelings of self-esteem, demonstrate internal control over behavior, and harness energy generated by the anger in a nondestructive manner.

Anger can be tied to anxiety in that some people feel anxious whenever they start to get angry and get distracted into anxiety, never really learning to express their feelings through appropriate assertive behavior.

Also, individuals can learn to use energy through physical activity that involves the large muscles, such as running, walking, or playing a racket sport. Other techniques that are helpful in controlling stress and anger are COMPLEMENTARY THERAPIES such as BIOFEEDBACK, GUIDED IMAGERY, and MEDITATION.

It is common to feel angry after the death of a loved one. The anger may be directed toward the deceased for having left the living person alone. Or, the anger may be directed toward the medical care system for not having been able to cure a disease or mend a body after an accident. In the case of accidents, often there is anger at a drunk driver or a person who has taken drugs and committed a crime, or the drug dealer who sold the drugs taken by the perpetrator of the loved one's death. Anger is a normal part of the cycle of the grief reaction. However, prolonged anger that leads to depression may indicate a need to consult a mental health professional.

See also AGGRESSION; ANXIETY; BIOFEEDBACK; COMPLEMENTARY THERAPIES; DEPRESSION; GUIDED IMAGERY; GRIEF; HOSTILITY; REACTION AND GRIEF RESOLUTION.

Kahn, Ada P., *The Encyclopedia of Stress and Stress-related Disorders*, 2nd ed. (New York: Facts On File, 2006).

angina pectoris   A specific type of discomfort in the chest. Angina pectoris is not a sharp pain, but rather a sensation of pressure, squeezing, or tightness. It usually starts in the center of the chest under the breastbone (sternum) and radiates to the throat area. Angina generally results from the muscle fibers of the heart not getting enough blood through the coronary arteries to nourish them. This condition, known as myocardial ischemia, is associated with coronary heart disease and is usually the result of the narrowing of blood vessels by atherosclerosis, or hardening of the arteries. It may also be related to heart failure, other heart conditions, blood deficiency diseases such as anemia, or low blood pressure.

Angina symptoms appear when an individual exerts himself, and the discomfort disappears when he rests. Attacks usually last for only two or three minutes, but if they are triggered by ANXIETY or other emotional tension and the individual cannot relax, they may last ten minutes or more. The first time an individual has uncomplicated angina pectoris, he may fear that he is having a fatal HEART ATTACK. He may become extremely anxious and even have a PANIC ATTACK, which will aggravate his chest pains. He should be reassured that he has little to fear if he rests both physically and mentally.

See also CHOKING, FEAR OF; HEART ATTACK, FEAR OF; HEART ATTACK, ANXIETY FOLLOWING; NARROWNESS, FEAR OF.

anginophobia Fear of ANGINA PECTORIS or related heart problems.

See also CHOKING, FEAR OF; HEART ATTACK, FEAR OF; HEART ATTACK, ANXIETY FOLLOWING; NARROWNESS, FEAR OF.

Anglophobia Fear of England, the English language, and things relating to the English culture.

angst Loosely, anxiety. Angst is a major concept of the existentialist approach to psychology, which tries to understand the essence of human existence by emphasizing basic human values such as love, free will, and self-awareness. The word "angst" is derived from the German term meaning "fear, anxiety, anguish." American psychoanalyst Rollo May (1909–94) described angst as "the inward state of my becoming aware that my existence can become lost, that I can lose myself and my world, that I can

become nothing." Anxiety strikes at the center of an individual's existence, whereas FEAR, in contrast, is a threat to the periphery of physical survival.

See also EXISTENTIAL.

anhedonia A term that refers to an ongoing lack of emotional responsiveness and pleasure in life events; an inability to experience pleasure. A quality commonly found in SCHIZOPHRENIA, anhedonia is contrasted with an excitable personality that might become anxious.

animals, fear of The fear of animals in general is known as zoophobia. Many individuals fear animals in general, as well as fearing wild animals (agrizoophobia) or particular animals such as SNAKES (ophidiophobia), CATS (ailurophobia), DOGS (cynophobia), INSECTS (acarophobia), MICE (musophobia), or SPIDERS (arachnophobia). Animal phobias are often acquired by children through vicarious modeling; for example, by seeing an animal in the context of a frightening situation, such as a dog attacking a person in a movie or on the street; by having a traumatic experience, such as being bitten, or by generalization (for example, an existing fear of dogs that is generalized to a fear of cats).

Animal phobias usually develop early in life, around age four, and rarely occur after age seven or eight. However, if an individual experiences a traumatic event that is related to animals later in life, such as being attacked by a dog, a lasting fear may develop even during adulthood. Most animal phobics are female.

Nearly all children show some fear of one animal or another at some time. Many such fears are overlooked because they cause only mild disturbance. Sometimes these fears disappear spontaneously or are outgrown without any disturbing recurrence. It is only when a child's fear of certain animals radically disturbs his or her normal functioning that therapy becomes necessary; for example, when an individual is fearful of leaving home because of the *possibility* of seeing a dog (or another feared animal) outside the home.

The most common animal phobias are fears of dogs, cats, snakes, worms, spiders, birds, mice, fish, and frogs. While animal fears are prevalent in the general population, fewer people who fear animals seek treatment than do people who have social fears or AGORAPHOBIA, because the fear of animals, usually considered a specific phobia, does not usually disrupt life to the extent that some other phobias do.

In *Totem and Taboo*, Sigmund Freud suggested why many children may fear animals. The relation of the child to animals, he said, has much in common with that of primitive man. The child does not show any trace of the pride that moves adults to recognize a dividing line between his own nature and that of all other animals. The child unhesitatingly attributes full equality to animals and, in fact, may feel more closely related to animals than to the mysterious adult.

Sometimes, however, there is a curious disturbance in this understanding between child and animal. The child suddenly begins to fear a certain type of animal and to protect himself against seeing or touching any member of this species. The result is a clinical picture of an animal phobia. The phobia is usually expressed toward animals in which the child has until then shown the liveliest interest, and it has nothing to do with the particular animal itself. Sometimes animals known to the child only in picture books and fairy stories may become objects of the inordinate anxiety manifested in the phobia.

Psychoanalytically, animals are sometimes considered to represent unconsciously feared parents (for example, a horse might symbolize the father, a bear the mother) or repressed impulses (for example, snakes as phallic symbols).

Freud had also suggested that the essential feature of animal phobia is the displacement of the child's fear from a person who is important in his emotional life onto some animal selected by the child according to individual circumstances. Thus the animal becomes a substitute for the feared person. Moreover, because love, as well as feelings of hate toward the feared object, is transferred in this displacement, the relationship to the feared animal is an ambivalent one.

In this model, the animal phobia has a great advantage to the patient over the original fear, because with appropriate behavior, the phobia permits avoidance of fear and anxiety. While the child succeeds in staying away from the feared animal, he or she is free from anxiety. The fear reappears only when the child leaves the protected domain and enters the danger zone of the dreaded animal.

Unlike Freudian analysts, however, behavioral psychologists emphasize the *learned* nature of animal fears, either through direct-traumatic exposure (classical conditioning) or vicariously by observation, via films, television, newspapers, and stories about animals. Traumatic conditioning is relatively less common (e.g., only about 5 percent of snake phobics have ever had contact with a snake, or even seen one), but many dog, bird, insect, cat, and common animal phobias begin with a traumatic or frightening experience involving one of these animals.

Vicarious conditioning, a far more common means of acquiring a phobia, occurs when the individual observes another person (often a parent) react to a situation, animal, or person with anxiety. One such experience can be enough to instill a permanent fear if identification with the model is strong and the modeling reaction is intense. Viewers of films such as *Jaws* or *The Birds* perhaps can understand how such learning can take place.

Prior to adolescence, there are few gender differences relating to animal phobias. However after adolescence, animal phobias are more prevalent among females.

There is evidence that some animal phobias (such as the fear of snakes) may have an innate component and may perhaps be a vestige of a survival mechanism that kept small children away from dangerous animals for their own safety. These are called *prepared fears.*

See also AMBIVALENCE; CHILDHOOD ANXIETIES, FEARS AND PHOBIAS; SPECIFIC PHOBIAS; SYMBOLISM.

Freud, Sigmund, *Totem and Taboo* (London: Routledge & Kegan Paul, 1950).

animals, fear of wild   Fear of wild animals is known as agrizoophobia.
See also ANIMALS, FEAR OF.

animism   The belief, stemming from primitive times, that inanimate objects possess a soul, consciousness, and will. Some individuals attribute various life characteristics to things they fear, such as mountains, TREES, RIVERS, stones, etc. Because of this belief, some individuals become fearful of inanimate objects. For example, young children may believe that the SUN is alive because it produces light or that a vacuum cleaner eats because it sucks up items from the floor. Because of such beliefs, children as well as adults may become phobic about certain objects and perpetuate their fears to their own children.

See also CHILDHOOD ANXIETIES, FEARS, AND PHOBIAS; FAIRY TALES.

ankylophobia See IMMOBILITY OF A JOINT, FEAR OF.

Anna O. (1859–1936) The first case in psychoanalysis. Anna O. was treated by Breuer and written about by Breuer and Freud in their work, *Studies in Hysteria* (1893–95). The patient's real name was Bertha Pappenheim. She was a pioneer social worker and feminist who became well known for her work with the sick and poor and later traveled extensively, including to the Henry Street Settlement in New York City. At age 21, after sitting at the bedside of her ailing father for months, Bertha was diagnosed as having a malady then called "hysteria." Her symptoms included inability to eat, hallucinations of snakes and death's heads, limb paralysis, and multiple personalities; she attempted suicide. Breuer used a technique to help her that may have been hypnosis or autohypnosis. Later, as she began to talk about memories from the past, her emotional expression had the effect of CATHARSIS, or of inducing relief from her anxieties. Her squinting eyes relaxed, and she and Breuer surmised that her eyes became frozen in that position because she was crying when she tried to see a clock to tell her ailing father the time. Her inability to drink came from having seen a dog drinking out of a glass, which apparently disgusted her. After she relived a traumatic time during her father's last illness, her paralyzed arm became useful again. She later spent some time in sanatoriums and became addicted to morphine, which had been prescribed for her as a sedative. She never married and dedicated her life to improving conditions for women and children.

See also HYPNOSIS.

anniversary reaction Feelings of anxiety or other symptoms that arise at the time of the anniversary of a painful event such as a divorce or the death of a family member or close friend. Recalling and reliving difficult events may trigger anxieties. Some individuals experience bad dreams or minor illnesses on the anniversary of a painful event. Anniversary reactions are often common when an individual has experienced a traumatic event.

See also ANXIETY DISORDERS; GRIEF REACTION AND GRIEF RESOLUTION; POST-TRAUMATIC STRESS DISORDER.

anorexia nervosa See EATING DISORDERS.

anorgasmia (anorgasmy) Inability to achieve orgasm or the absence of the orgasmic phase in the sexual reaction cycle. Some women fear sexual intercourse because of anorgasmia. Anorgasmia may be caused by fears about sexual intercourse, incompatible sexual attitudes in the partners, anatomical and neurophysiological defects, fear of painful intercourse, and sociocultural conditioning.

See also FRIGIDITY; SEXUAL FEARS; SEX THERAPY.

anthophobia Fear of flowers.

See also FLOWERS, FEAR OF.

anthropophobia Fear of people or human society.

See also PEOPLE, FEAR OF.

antianxiety drugs Drugs used to reduce anxiety and tension; they are known also as minor tranquilizers. Antianxiety drugs are used by individuals during times of stress and in treatment of stress-related physical disorders under the supervision of a physician.

See also ANXIETY.

antibiotics Drugs used to treat infectious diseases by destroying pathogenic or noxious microorganisms. Antibiotics are generally not effective in treating viral diseases. The best-known antibiotics are penicillin and streptomycin. Antibiotics are produced by or derived from living cells, such as molds, yeasts, or bacteria, or are manufactured as synthetic chemicals with effects similar to natural antibiotics. Some antibiotics act by interfering with the ability of bacteria to reproduce; others disrupt the pathogen's normal life functions.

Since the discovery that ribonucleic acid (RNA) has effects on learning and retention, antibiotics have been of interest to psychologists. In experiments, some antibiotics seem to block long-term memory with no effect on short-term memory. Some phobias may have origins in long-term memories. Just how antibiotics influence retention is not yet clear.

See also DRUGS, FEAR OF NEW.

anticholinergics Substances that block or interfere with the acetycholine transmission of impulses in the parasympathetic nervous system. The parasympathetic nervous system actively produces relaxation, calmness, digestion, and sleep.

The best-known natural substances with anticholinergic effects are atropine (used as a drug to dilate the eyes) and scopolamine (a plant substance used with morphine to induce sleep). Some antidepressants and antipsychotic drugs have anticholinergic properties; anticholinergic effects sometimes include unpleasant side effects, such as extreme dryness of the mouth. Many synthetic anticholinergics are used to treat nervous-system disorders such as Parkinson's disease.

See also AGORAPHOBIA; ANTIDEPRESSANTS; DEPRESSION; DRUGS, FEAR OF NEW; DRY MOUTH.

anticonvulsives Substances that prevent convulsions or limit their frequency or severity. In high doses, TRANQUILIZERS and hypnotic drugs may act as anticonvulsants. Anticonvulsives are also known as antiepileptics. Many anticonvulsives are central nervous system depressants and also reduce the incidence of anxiety symptoms.

See also DRUGS, FEAR OF NEW.

antidepressants Medications used to treat DEPRESSION and anxiety. There are several major categories of drugs used to treat depression, including tricyclic antidepressants (TCAs), selective serotonin reuptake inhibitors (SSRIs), serotonin norephinephrine inhibitors (SNRIs), and monoamine oxidase inhibitors (MAOIs). BUPROPION (Wellbutrin) is an atypical depression medication that is approved by the Food and Drug Administration (FDA) to treat depression. If the individual has BIPOLAR DISORDER, he or she may be treated with lithium, which may relieve some of the depression of bipolar disorder, although lithium is categorized as a mood stabilizer.

It is important to understand that in the early treatment for depression, patients who are severely depressed are at risk for SUICIDE and any indications of suicide, such as talking about a wish for death or a plan to commit suicide, should be reported immediately to the person's physician and/or family members who can then act to help the individual.

Antidepressants are available only by prescription, and because they suppress rather than cure depressive symptoms, they are usually prescribed in conjunction with some type of psychotherapy. Commonly, antidepressant medications take up to two to three weeks to have a full effect (although side effects may begin immediately). The time elapsing before the drug becomes therapeutic varies with the drug. Antidepressants may have to be taken regularly for months or even years, if their gains are to persist. Relapse often occurs upon stopping the drug.

Unlike antianxiety drugs, antidepressants generally do not interfere with exposure therapies. Individuals with phobias or rituals are urged to carry out self-exposure treatment in addition to taking their medication.

Antidepressants are often useful in the treatment of panic disorders and seem to have an inhibitory effect on panic. However, antidepressants are generally not used to treat anxiety by itself or AGORAPHOBIA.

How Antidepressants Work

Because most drugs that are used to treat depression either mimic certain neurotransmitters (biochemicals that allow brain cells to communicate with one another) or they alter their activity, a general hypothesis is that a decrease in the activity or concentration of these neurotransmitters occurs during depression. Unfortunately, neurotransmitters cannot be measured directly. Two of the major neurotransmitters involved appear to be norepinephrine and serotonin. When they work, antidepressants alter the function of neurotransmitters such that the person is less depressed or not depressed.

The precise pharmacologic mechanisms of antidepressant drugs, as well as the balances of neurotransmitters in individuals exhibiting depression, are still debated. As newer, more specific antidepressants are developed, our understanding of antidepressants and depression continues to evolve.

It is important to remember, however, that there are no tests to measure levels of serotonin in the body in spite of the fact that people often talk about antidepressants as correcting a "chemical imbalance."

Tricyclic Antidepressants

Tricyclic antidepressants were often used in the past to treat depression and are still used in many cases. They are referred to as *tricyclic* antidepressants because the chemical diagrams for these drugs resemble three rings connected together. In the late 1940s, imipramine (a tricyclic with the brand name of Tofranil) was first synthesized in the lab. Since then, tricyclics have been heavily tested and frequently used as antidepressants. Other examples of tricyclics are desipramine (Norpramin) and amitriptyline (Elavil).

Tricyclics may elevate mood and improve appetite and sleep patterns in depressed individuals. The effect might more accurately be described as a reduction of depression as opposed to a euphoric stimulation. However, when tricyclics are given to a nondepressed person, they do not elevate their mood; instead, the effects are likely to be feelings of unhappiness and an apparent increase in anxiety.

Tricyclic antidepressants are relatively safe and well tolerated. The primary side effects are sedation and weight gain. Their antidepressant effects, however, often take several weeks to appear, for reasons not yet well understood. Other side effects include dry mouth, blurring of vision, headache, urinary hesitation, and constipation. Excessive sweating is also a common side effect. Drowsiness and dizziness, as well as vertigo, weakness, rapid heart rate, and reduced blood pressure upon standing upright are likely to occur early on but usually disappear within the first several weeks. Tricyclics should be used cautiously in people with heart problems.

Unfortunately, no clinical signs or aspects of a person's medical history indicate which tricyclic antidepressant (or any other type of antidepressant) is likely to be the best for an individual patient. Some depressed individuals may respond remarkably well to one tricyclic antidepressant, but not respond at all to another tricyclic. Due to the time lag of several weeks before any beneficial effects show up, the physician must try first one drug, and then, if positive results are not achieved, prescribe another tricyclic for several weeks. Such waiting and uncertainty may cause some anxiety and frustration for both the individual and the physician.

Use of tricyclics in agoraphobia. When used in the treatment of agoraphobia with panic attacks, tricyclic antidepressants have been shown to cause moderate or marked improvement in the reduction of panic attacks in about 25 percent of those who can tolerate the drug.

Use of tricyclics in obsessive-compulsive disorders. In patients who have obsessive-compulsive disorders, including ritualistic or ruminative (persistently pondering problems) behaviors, the tricyclic drug clomipramine (Anafranil) has been reported to be effective. Clomipramine effectively reduces most symptoms in at least 20 percent of those who can tolerate the drug, according to a National Institute of Mental Health report.

Drug interactions. It is considered good judgment to avoid combining tricyclic antidepressants with MAOIs. Although very rare, a severe interaction between the two drugs can occur, and, in extreme cases, convulsions, seizures, and coma may result. A more commonly occurring drug interaction involves the combination of tricyclics and alcohol or other depressants. Tricyclic antidepressants increase the effects of these substances.

Selective Serotonin Reuptake Inhibitors (SSRIs)

Many physicians prescribe selective serotonin reuptake inhibitors (SSRIs) to treat depression. These drugs inhibit the reuptake of serotonin, thereby allowing for an elevation of mood, and they are highly effective in many individuals. There are many different types of SSRIs, including fluoxetine (Prozac), citalopram (Celexa), fluvoxamine (Luvox), escitalopram (Lexapro), paroxetine (Paxil), and sertraline (Zoloft).

Note that SSRIs should *never* be combined with an MAO inhibitor, because this combination could lead to excessive and dangerously high levels of serotonin. An individual taking an MAO inhibitor should have been off the drug for at least 14 days before starting to use an SSRI antidepressant.

Depending on the particular SSRI, some side effects may include decreased sexual desire in both men and women as well as insomnia. When first taking the drug, some patients may experience increased anxiety and agitation. Rarely, these drugs may induce mania. In addition, in rare cases, SSRIs may cause hyponatremia (below-normal blood levels of sodium).

Serotonin and Norepinephrine Reuptake Inhibitors (SNRIs)

The newest class of antidepressants available in the United States as of this writing is the serotonin and norepinephrine reuptake inhibitor (SNRI). This type of drug blocks the reuptake of both serotonin and norepinephrine, allowing for an enhanced mood state. In addition, they also boost the level of dopamine. Some examples of SNRIs are venlafaxine (Effexor) and duloxetine (Cymbalta). Some research indicates that SNRIs may be useful in treating anxiety as well as depression. Venlafaxine is FDA-approved for the treatment of GENERALIZED ANXIETY DISORDER and SOCIAL PHOBIA, as well as depression. Some physicians use venlafaxine to treat panic disorder and POST-TRAUMATIC STRESS DISORDER.

These drugs may take from two to four weeks before the full antidepressant effect is experienced. SNRIs may be sedating. Higher doses may cause headaches, nervousness and sexual dysfunction. These effects may abate with time.

SNRIs should not be taken with MAO inhibitors. Individuals who decide to stop taking SNRIs should taper off the drug to avoid withdrawal effects, such as nausea and vomiting and headaches.

Other Antidepressants

Some antidepressants do not fit into the category of tricyclics, SSRIs, SNRIs, or MAO inhibitors. A key example of this category is bupropion (Wellbutrin), which is called an atypical antidepressant and is sometimes used to treat ATTENTION-DEFICIT/HYPERACTIVITY DISORDER. Bupropion is also used to treat nicotine addiction (Zyban). This drug should not be used in patients with seizure disorders.

Another medication, mirtazapine (Remeron) is an alpha 2 antagonist that is approved by the FDA for the treatment of depression. It is also used to treat panic disorder, generalized anxiety disorder, and post-traumatic stress disorder.

Monoamine Oxidase Inhibitors (MAOIs)

MAO inhibitors (or MAOIs) are primarily used for people who do not respond adequately to all other forms of antidepressants. They are generally considered less effective than other antidepressants and due to a wider range of potential and often unpredictable complications, their use is limited. However, MAOIs may be recommended for depression, generalized anxiety, and phobic disorders. They are also used to help individuals who have PANIC ATTACKS. Some examples of MAO inhibitors are isocarboxazid (Marplan), phenelzine (Nardil), tranylcypromine (Parnate), and selegiline (Eldepryl).

The discovery of MAOIs' antidepressant effects first occurred by chance. Quite unexpectedly, tuberculosis patients being given the antituberculosis drug iproniazid experienced an elevation of mood. Further testing with related drugs led to the widespread use of MAOIs as antidepressants.

Patients taking MAOIs must avoid the following foods altogether:

- aged cheese in any form (cottage and cream cheese are permitted.)
- yogurt
- Marmite, Bovril, and similar concentrated yeast or *meat* extracts (beware of drinks and stews made with these products), baked products raised with yeast are allowed
- pickled herring
- liver
- alcohol in more than social (i.e., moderate) amounts. (Limit to one glass of beer, wine, or sherry). Avoid Chianti wines altogether.

- broad bean pods (limas, fava, Chinese, English, etc.) and banana skins
- canned figs
- food that is not fresh (or prepared from frozen or newly opened canned food). Take special care to avoid pickled, fermented, smoked, or aged meat, fish, poultry, game, or variety meats (organ meats and offal).
- caffeine in large amounts (such as caffeine in cola drinks)
- chocolate in large amounts
- any food that has given unpleasant symptoms previously

Due to the potential hazards in combining tricyclics and MAOIs, when a tricyclic antidepressant is tried and discontinued because of its ineffectiveness, a gap of several days is recommended before the MAOI is tried. In the reverse case, where the MAOI inhibitor is ineffective and is to be replaced by a tricyclic, a period of two weeks between medications is recommended.

Lithium

For reasons not well understood, lithium is effective in countering both depression and mania and preventing future episodes. It acts without causing sedation, but as with antidepressants, it requires a period of use before its actions take effect. Lithium's side effects may rule it out for use as an antidepressant; for example, lithium commonly causes a significant weight gain as well as sedation. Its toxic effects may include nausea and vomiting, muscular weakness, and confusion.

Some drugs, such as ibuprofen and diuretics, can increase the concentration of lithium in the bloodstream and should be used with caution. Other drugs may interact with lithium to lower or increase its concentration in the blood, and individuals taking lithium should be thoroughly informed by their physicians of possible drug interactions.

Antidepressants have been empirically shown to be moderately effective, but work best when combined with a program of cognitive behavioral therapy and exercise.

Exercise

One of the most commonly effective interventions to depression is exercise. Exercise is usually not of interest to the depressed person yet it has been shown to reduce depression and anxiety consistently. A good therapeutic program should involve exercise and possible medications as a supplement.

See also AGORAPHOBIA; ANXIOLYTICS; BENZODIAZEPINES; ADVERSE DRUG REACTIONS; SEDATIVES.

Stahl, Stephen M., *Essential Psychopharmacology: The Prescriber's Guide*. (Cambridge: Cambridge University Press, 2005).

antihistamines A class of drugs used primarily to counteract the effects of histamine, one of the body chemicals involved in allergic reactions. While they are primarily used for conditions other than ANXIETY, antihistamines also have an antianxiety-sedative effect. The two drugs in this group most likely to be used to treat anxiety are diphenhydramine (brand names: Benadryl, Allerdryl, BayDryl) and hydroxyzine (Atarax, Vistaril, BayRox, Durrax, Neucalm, Orgatrax). Unlike the BENZODIAZEPINES, these drugs do not carry risks of tolerance, habituation, and dependency. This feature may be important for some individuals. However, antihistamines are somewhat less well tolerated than the benzodiazepines and are therefore not as widely used for anxiety.

See also ALLERGIC DISORDERS.

antimanic drug Also known as a mood stabilizer. Antimanic drugs generally refer to medications that are used to alleviate the symptoms of mania and hypomania, as seen in BIPOLAR DISORDER and cyclothymic conditions. Lithium is commonly used for this purpose. Valproate (Depakote, Depakene, Depakote ER) is also used to treat bipolar disorder. Some individuals avoid lithium because it can cause an extensive weight gain not seen with other medications. Some phobic individuals also suffer from bipolar disorder or dysthymic disorders and take antimanic drugs.

See also ANTIDEPRESSANTS.

antipsychotic drugs   A group of drugs that are used to reduce psychotic symptoms such as HALLUCINATIONS and DELUSIONS in individuals who have SCHIZOPHRENIA and who commonly experience such symptoms. Antipsychotic drugs are sometimes prescribed initially in the severe acute mania attacks of BIPOLAR DISORDER. Although LITHIUM is the drug of choice for treating mania, it has a delayed effect, whereas antipsychotic drugs take effect fairly quickly. Antipsychotic drugs are also known as "major tranquilizers" because many antipsychotics are heavily sedating; however, there are many variations in individual response. Common antipsychotics used in the past were haloperidol (Haldol) and chlorpromazine (Thorazine). These drugs are used less frequently today because of the heavy sedation they cause and irreversible long-term side effects that may occur, such as TARDIVE DYSKINESIA.

Antipsychotic drugs are believed to work on receptors in the brain to influence emotional behavior. These actions may influence their antipsychotic effects and may account for a number of ADVERSE DRUG REACTIONS if the antipsychotic is combined with other medications, illegal drugs, or alcohol. It is generally believed that the antipsychotic drugs are not appropriate for use with anxiety reactions in the absence of severe psychotic symptoms.

Newer atypical antipsychotics are far more effective at treating psychosis than drugs used in the past which caused severe side effects, such as extreme weight gain and excessive sedation. Some examples of the newer antipsychotics used to treat schizophrenia and bipolar disorder are aripiprazole (Abilify) and risperidone (Risperdal). They are also used for problems with impulse control and behavioral disturbances in children and adolescents as well as those with dementia.

These drugs block neurochemicals that may be responsible for psychotic symptoms. Risperidone may increase the risk for the development of diabetes and may also cause sedation and weight gain. Aripiprazole may be sedating. It is not believed to cause diabetes but monitoring is recommended.

See also CLOZAPINE; DRUGS.

antlophobia   Fear of floods.
See also FLOOD, FEAR OF.

ants, fear of   Fear of ants is known as myrmecophobia. Individuals who fear ants may also fear other tiny insects. Some individuals who have fears of dirt or contamination may also fear the presence of ants near food or in kitchens. Some who have OBSESSIVE-COMPULSIVE DISORDER may continually wash kitchen counters and the inside of their refrigerators as a RITUAL to assure themselves that no ants or other sources of contamination are present.

See also CONTAMINATION, FEAR OF; DIRT, FEAR OF.

anuptaphobia   Fear of staying single.
See also SINGLE, FEAR OF STAYING.

anxiety   The word anxiety derives from a Greek root meaning "to press tight" or "to strangle." The Latin word *anxius* and its derivatives imply narrowness and constriction, usually with discomfort, particularly in early derivations, in the throat area. Those words denote distress, disquiet, and sadness rather than the uncertainty and fear denoted by the contemporary English word anxious.

Anxiety is an unpleasant feeling of generalized fear and apprehension, often of unknown origin, accompanied by physiological symptoms. This feeling may be triggered by the anticipation of danger, either from thoughts (internal) or from one's environment (external).

Anxiety and fear have similarities and differences. Fear is sometimes defined as a response to a consciously recognized and usually external threat. In a general way, fear is a response to a clear and present danger, whereas anxiety is a response to a situation, object, or person that the individual has come to fear through learning and experience. Anxiety, as noted by the existentialist philosopher Søren Kierkegaard, is the full experience of fear in the absence of a known threat. In both fear and anxiety, however, the body mobilizes itself to meet the threat, and certain physiological phenomena occur. Muscles become tense, breathing is faster, the heart beats more rapidly, and there may be sweating or diarrhea. There may be shakiness, increased breathing and heart rate, and acute sensitivity to environmental stimuli (for example, an intense startle reaction). Some individuals may focus their anxiety on an object, situation, or activity about which they are phobic. For others, general or unknown stimuli may trigger anxiety. This is known as free-floating anxiety. Some individuals may experience a sudden onset of anxiety and notice physical symptoms such as gastrointestinal upset, weakness, or faintness as precursors to a panic attack. Phobic anxiety is the anxiety that occurs only in contact with a particular situation or object.

Anxiety and Depression

While anxiety is not among the criteria by which depressive illness is diagnosed and distinguished from other disorders, anxiety is recognized as a major feature in many cases of depressive illness. The diagnosis of anxiety or depression is difficult in some cases, because symptoms of both disorders often coexist. Many individuals who have anxieties also show some of the symptoms of major depression, including:

Sleep disturbance, such as insomnia or hypersomnia

Eating disturbance—either loss of appetite or increased eating behavior

Loss of capacity for pleasure in usually pleasurable activities; loss of motivation

A slowing of thought, speech and movement, or agitation and an increase in movement and speed of speech

Difficulty in concentration, memory, or decision making

Thoughts of self-reproach, guilt, or profound unworthiness

Profound loss of energy

Hopelessness, often leading to suicidal thoughts or impulses

Hypochondriasis

When an individual focuses anxiety on physical signs or symptoms and is preoccupied with an unfounded fear or belief that he or she has a disease, that situation is a type of anxiety called hypochondriasis.

Freudian views. Freud made the term anxiety, or angst, popular in the psychiatric literature of his time. In his theory of personality, he viewed anxiety as a danger signal alerting the ego to impending threat. Depending on the source of threat, he proposed three types of anxiety: reality anxiety, neurotic anxiety, and moral anxiety. Freud called anxiety resulting from the perception of threat from the external environment REALITY ANXIETY, or FEAR, as a response to an actual threat. He called anxiety resulting from a source of threat generated from unconscious id impulses NEUROTIC ANXIETY, which could take on different forms of intensities resulting in phobias or panic reactions. Freud's third type of anxiety was called "moral anxiety," resulting from unconscious conflicts between the id impulses and the superego, or the conscience. He interpreted moral anxiety as shame or guilt, which is also capable of producing panic and intense anxiety responses.

See also ANXIETY ATTACK, ANXIETY DISORDERS; ANXIETY HIERARCHY; BASIC ANXIETY; CHILDHOOD FEARS; DEPRESSION; AFFECTIVE DISORDERS; PANIC ATTACK; PSYCHOSEXUAL ANXIETY; RESPONSE PROPERTIES; STATE ANXIETY; STIMULUS PROPERTIES; TRAIT ANXIETY.

Bromberg, W., *The Mind of Man: A History of Psychotherapy and Psychoanalysis.* (New York: Harper & Row, 1959).

Fawcett, Jan, and Howard M. Kravitz, "Anxiety Syndromes and Their Relationship to Depressive Illness," *Journal of Clinical Psychiatry* 44 (August 1983).

Jones, E., *The Life and Works of Sigmund Freud* (Garden City, NY: Doubleday, 1961).

Kleinknecht, Ronald A., *The Anxious Self* (New York: Human Sciences Press, 1986).

Marks, Isaac M., *Fears, Phobias and Rituals* (New York: Oxford University Press, 1987).

Price, R. H., *Abnormal Behavior: Perspective in Conflict* (New York: Holt, Rinehart & Winston, 1978).

Stone, Evelyn M., ed., *American Psychiatric Glossary* (Washington, DC: American Psychiatric Press, 1988).

anxiety, ancient Symptoms of anxiety have been mentioned in literature since antiquity. Both the Old and New Testaments contain references to fears, as does the Bhagavad-Gita, a sacred Hindu text. Hippocrates mentioned several instances of fears, phobias, and anxieties.

See also BIBLE.

anxiety, basic A term for a feeling of loneliness and helplessness toward a potentially hostile world.

The term was coined by Karen Horney (1885–1952), a German-born American psychiatrist. Basic anxiety originates in disturbed relationships between parents and children and from social and cultural factors. Hence this concept of basic anxiety differs from Sigmund Freud's concept of anxiety as resulting predominantly from sexual urges and hostility.

See also ANXIETY.

anxiety, cognitive vs. somatic The symptoms of anxiety fall into two categories: cognitive or somatic. Cognitive symptoms of anxiety display themselves as thoughts in the anxious person's mind. Ideas of impending doom are reported as though a horrible event is at hand but the source cannot be pinpointed. Other examples are racing thoughts, inability to concentrate, and runaway imaginations. The only real measure of cognitive anxiety is through self-report. Somatic anxiety is easily measured by a second party. Common symptoms of somatic anxiety are increased heart rate, respiration, and blood pressure; sweating; and muscle tension particularly in the forehead. Perspiration is measured by the Galvanic Skin Response Test (GSR) which measures electroconductivity of the skin.

See also ANXIETY; GALVANIC SKIN RESPONSE.

anxiety, performance See PERFORMANCE ANXIETY.

anxiety, postcoronary bypass See POSTCORONARY BYPASS ANXIETY.

anxiety, psychosexual See PSYCHOSEXUAL ANXIETIES.

anxiety, self-reported Therapists use various ways to evaluate an individual's anxiety. Self-report is one technique. This is often done with a questionnaire.

anxiety, separation See SCHOOL PHOBIA; SEPARATION ANXIETY.

anxiety, signal See SIGNAL ANXIETY.

anxiety and pain See PAIN AND ANXIETY.

anxiety attack The sudden onset of acute anxiety, sometimes starting with pounding of the heart, difficulty in breathing, excessive perspiration, and dizziness. Anxiety attacks always begin in response to a stimulus which may be a bodily sensation, something seen or heard, a thought, or imagining any of these stimuli. Anxiety attacks are triggered by different stimuli for each individual, and each individual will show a different response to an anxiety attack. However, in most cases the main response systems at work are the cognitive (thought processes), autonomic, and muscular. In some individuals, an anxiety attack develops into a full-scale panic attack, in which one experiences unbearable tension, fear of suffocation, or a feeling that he or she may die or that some unnameable disaster is going to occur.

See also ANXIETY; ANXIETY DISORDERS; ANXIETY HIERARCHY; PANIC ATTACK.

anxiety disorders A group of disorders in which anxiety is either the predominant characteristic or it is experienced when the individual confronts a dreaded object or situation or resists obsessions or compulsions. Until 1980, anxiety was considered a one-dimensional condition. Then mental health professionals realized that there are several categories of specific symptom clusters, with unique causes, treatments, and outlooks for improvement for each type of anxiety disorder.

According to the National Institute of Mental Health (NIMH), 40 million adults ages 18 and older in the United States suffer from one or more anxiety disorders in any given year. Anxiety disorders last more than six months and they may worsen if they go untreated. Some individuals with anxiety disorders develop problems with substance abuse or dependence. Nearly half (45 percent) of individuals with one anxiety disorder also suffer from another form of anxiety disorder.

ANXIETY-RELATED CONDITIONS

Disorder	Clinical History	Clinical Examination	Features
Phobia	Specific fear of object	Behavioral observation useful	Can precipitate fear by talking about specific phobia
Hyperventilation syndrome		Precipitated by hyperventilation and relieved by increased CO_2	May represent secondary complication of anxiety attacks
Posttraumatic neurosis	Recurrent dreams, nightmares, and day recollections Specific precipitating event More constant and unremitting Secondary alcoholism and drugs	Mixed features of depression Reluctance to discuss traumatic events	Diagnostic interviews with sodium amytal or hypnosis Treatment with antidepressant helpful
Chronic anxiety state	Chronic, unremitting, and often with no precipitating event Usually no discrete anxiety attacks	Mixed features of depression Obsessive ruminations	Anxiety neurosis may evolve into chronic anxiety state
Early schizophrenia	Typical age of onset Family history Reports of weird experiences	Thought disorders Delusions, hallucinations	Favorable response to neuroleptic drugs
Mania	Previous episode of affective illness Family history	Euphoria or irritability paramount Flight of ideas Grandiosity	Atypical forms of mania may resemble anxiety attack Favorable response to lithium
Agitated depression	Depressive symptomatology paramount Biological signs of depression	Poverty of ideas Delusions of sin, poverty, nihilism, and bizarre somatic complaints	Favorable response to antidepressants or ECT
Hyperthyroidism	Intolerance to heat Profound weakness	Palpable thyroid Exopthalmos	May also respond to propranolol
Cardiac arrhythmias	Often precipitated by caffeine or nicotine	Pulse rate reflects arrhythmia or PAT	EKG corroboration
Angina	Characteristic pain distribution and duration		EKG corroboration. Relief by nitroglycerine
Mitral valve prolapse syndrome	Symptoms referable to cardiovascular system but also mimics classic anxiety attacks	Extrasystolies, tachycardia Midsystolic click	Prolapse of mitral valve during systole Diagnostic echocardiogram shows abnormal mitral valve movement

(Table continues)

ANXIETY-RELATED CONDITIONS *(continued)*

Disorder	Clinical History	Clinical Examination	Features
Hypoparathyroidism	Often previous thyroid operation	Chvostek and Taussig signs Hyperreflexia	Decrease of serum calcium Poor response to anti-anxiety agents
Pheochromocytoma	Episodic or sustained	Marked elevations in blood pressure, flushing Severe headaches	Increased urinary catecholamines Induced by phentolamine and relieved by mecholyl
Insulinoma (hypoglycemia)	Faintness, nausea Seizures		Low blood sugar during attack Abnormal glucose tolerance
Carcinoid syndrome	Itching Flushing of skin	Skin blotches	Increased 5-HIAA in urine
Acute intermittent porphyria	Acute intermittent attacks of colicky abdominal pain Positive family history Personality change	Sinus tachycardia Decreased deep tendon reflexes Occasional cranial nerve involvement Reddish urine	Increased urinary porphobilinogens
Stimulant drugs	Drug use	Paranoid ideation or delusions	Drugs in urine
Caffeinism	Ingestion of large amounts of coffee, tea, etc.		Panic attacks
Hypnotic-sedative drug withdrawal	Ingestion of barbiturates, alcohol, or related agents	Postural hypotension Clouding of consciousness Transient hallucinations	Heightened tolerance to pentobarbital test dose
Presenile dementia	Older onset with other cognitive and behavioral disturbances	Memory and abstraction deficits Emotional lability Little insight into illness	Other features of dementia
Cerebral neoplasm	Unremitting headache vague neurological complaints	Increased intracranial pressure and papilledema Soft or specific neurological signs	
Auras of migraine, temporal lobe lesions, or grand mal epilepsy	Precede headache, amnesic period, altered mental states or seizures No sustained anxiety between attacks Characteristic clinical history for migraine or epilepsy		May be induced by hyperventilation or special provocative procedures EEG changes with temporal lobe or grand mal epilepsy

Following are several of the major categories described in the *DIAGNOSTIC AND STATISTICAL MANUAL OF MENTAL DISORDERS, FOURTH EDITION:*

- GENERALIZED ANXIETY DISORDER
- phobias: specific phobia (formerly simple phobia), social phobia
- AGORAPHOBIA
- PANIC DISORDER
- OBSESSIVE-COMPULSIVE DISORDER
- POST-TRAUMATIC STRESS DISORDER

Primary care physicians have indicated that anxiety disorders are among the most common mental health problems seen in their practice. Yet in primary care settings, anxiety disorders often are underrecognized because anxious individuals frequently present with physical symptoms rather than psychological concerns. Individuals suffering from anxiety disorders are often apprehensive and they are worried, ruminative, and expecting something very bad to happen to themselves or loved ones in the future. They often feel on edge, impatient, and irritable and are easily distracted. Some individuals have anxiety symptoms that are so severe that they are almost totally disabled.

Prevalence of Anxiety Disorders in the United States

The most common form of anxiety disorder is specific phobia and according to the NIMH, about 19.2 million American adults, or about 8.7 percent of individuals 18 and older, have some type of specific phobia in any given year. Often these phobias have their onset in childhood and the median age of onset is age seven.

Social phobia is a problem for an estimated 15 million Americans, and women and men are equally likely to suffer from this disorder. Social phobias generally begin in late childhood or early adolescence. There may be only one particular social situation that elicits anxiety in an individual or, in the case of many people with social phobias, they may feel anxiety in several social situations.

Post-traumatic stress disorder (PTSD) is the next most common form of anxiety disorder and 7.7 million American adults in any given year, or about 3.5 percent of adults 18 and older, suffer from PTSD. PTSD can occur at any age, but the median age of onset is 23 years. It is believed that 30 percent of returning Vietnam veterans suffered from PTSD, and estimates are that an equivalent percentage of the many servicepeople serving in Iraq will return with PTSD. PTSD may also develop in individuals who have been sexually assaulted or terrorized or who have experienced severe accidents, domestic violence, or natural disasters.

Generalized anxiety disorder (GAD) is the next most common form of anxiety disorder, and according to the NIMH, about 6.8 million American adults ages 18 and older, or 3.1 percent of adults 18 and older, suffer from GAD, and this form of anxiety disorder is about twice as common in females as in males. The median age of onset for GAD is 31 years old. GAD is characterized by chronic worry and moderate anxiety as a result.

Fourth in the prevalence of anxiety disorders is panic disorder and about 6 million American adults (2.7 percent of adults ages 18 and older) have panic disorder. Panic disorder is about twice as common among women than men. The median age of onset is 24 years. About a third of those with panic disorder will develop agoraphobia, a disorder in which the person fears being away from a safe place or being trapped (such as being trapped in a left-turn lane). Some people with agoraphobia become housebound, their fear is so intense.

Obsessive-compulsive disorder (OCD) is the least common form of anxiety disorder in the United States, and 2.2 million adults ages 18 and older, or about 1 percent of adults, suffer from OCD. In most cases, the first symptoms occur in childhood or adolescence, but the median age of onset is 19 years.

Types of Anxiety Disorders

Each type of anxiety disorder has its own symptoms, signs, and treatment.

Phobias. People who suffer from phobias feel terror, dread, or panic when confronted with the feared object, situation, or activity. Many have such an overwhelming desire to avoid the source of the fear that it interferes with their jobs, family life, and social relationships. For example, they may lose their job because they fear traveling or eating in front of others. Some become fearful of leaving their homes, and they live hermitlike existences with their window shades pulled down, afraid of light or darkness, insects or birds. They may also fear being assaulted.

Within the category of phobias are specific phobias, social phobias (also known as social anxiety disorder), and agoraphobia. Specific phobias are fears of specific objects or situations; examples of such phobias are the fear of snakes, the fear of flying, or the fear of closed spaces.

Social phobias are fears of situations in which the individual can be watched by others, such as public speaking, or in which individual behavior might prove embarrassing, such as eating in public, using public restrooms, or signing their name in public. Some experts report that genetic factors may be involved with social phobia, so that if a parent or other close relative has the disorder, others in the family are more likely to suffer as well.

Individuals with social phobia often have depression and other forms of anxiety disorders, and substance abuse is a problem among those who medicate themselves with alcohol or drugs. Social phobia is treated with psychotherapy and with medications such as selective serotonin reuptake inhibitors (SSRIs), like fluoxetine (Prozac), sertraline (Zoloft), or citalopram (Celexa). Antianxiety drugs, also known as benzodiazepines, are also used to treat social phobia; for example, clonazepam (Klonopin) is commonly used for social phobia. In addition, beta blockers such as propranolol (Inderal) are sometimes used to treat social phobia.

Agoraphobia, the fear of being away from a safe place, being in a public place, being in a place with no escape, such as a train or plane, or being alone, is the most disabling because sufferers can become housebound. Early treatment is the most effective solution and includes exposure therapies and medications.

Panic Disorder. Individuals who have panic disorder have intense, overwhelming terror and feelings of doom for no apparent reason. These attacks are known as *panic attacks.* Some people suffer from one or two panic attacks but do not develop panic disorder, which is a condition of chronic panic attacks.

Often people suffering a panic attack for the first time rush to the hospital emergency room, convinced they are having a heart attack because their heart is racing and they may experience chest pain. They may also experience chills and/or nausea. Panic attacks are usually brief and peak within about 10 minutes, although some attacks last longer.

When it is determined that a patient's heart is normal, the physician may suggest that panic disorder is the problem. Sufferers cannot predict when the attacks will occur, although certain situations such as driving a car can become associated with them if it was in those situations that the first attack occurred.

People with panic disorder may develop depression and substance abuse. Some experts estimate that about one-third of those with ALCOHOLISM have a panic disorder. Panic disorder is considered highly treatable with cognitive-behavioral therapy and medications. Medications such as lorazepam (Ativan) are used to treat panic disorder, as is alprazolam (Xanax).

Generalized Anxiety Disorder Individuals with GAD are constantly tense and worried, even though most know their worries are irrational and unwarranted. Such individuals may worry constantly about their own health or the health of others or they may worry about money (when finances are not a problem), work, or other issues. Individuals with GAD often have problems with insomnia and may have physical symptoms such as fatigue, muscle pain, nausea, irritability, a frequent need to use the bathroom, breathlessness, etc.

Individuals with GAD are at risk for depression, other anxiety disorders, and substance abuse. GAD is treated with cognitive behavioral therapy and antidepressant medications such as venlafaxine (Effexor), a serotonin norepinephrine reuptake inhibitor (SNRI). Antianxiety medications such as clonazepam (Klonopin) are used to treat GAD, as is alprazolam (Xanax).

Obsessive-Compulsive Disorders Some individuals attempt to cope with their anxiety by associating it with obsessions, which are defined as repeated, unwanted thoughts, or with compulsive behaviors, which are defined as rituals that may spin out of control. Individuals who suffer from obsessive disorders do not automatically have compulsive behaviors. However, most people who have compulsive, ritualistic behaviors also suffer from obsessions. Obsessions

SELF-REPORT OF RESPONSES TO ANXIETY

This self-test suggests 39 different responses you may have as reactions to anxiety. To determine your individualized and specific pattern, imagine that you are in a situation that causes you anxiety. Write a number from 0 to 5 (depending on how frequently you experience that particular effect) in the spaces after the question. If there are two sets of spaces, write the same number in both spaces. (The "A" column refers to autonomic arousal symptoms, "M" to muscular tension, and "C" to cognitive responses.) Column totals reflect relative contributions of these sources of anxiety.

> 0 = Never have this reaction
> 1 = Almost never have it
> 2 = Seldom have it
> 3 = Occasionally have it
> 4 = Frequently have it
> 5 = Almost always have it

	A	M	C
1. I tap my feet or fingers.		—	
2. My stomach flutters or *feels full*.	—		
3. I stammer or stutter.		—	—
4. I clench my teeth or grind them.		—	
5. I kick my foot or bounce it.		—	
6. I bite my nails.			—
7. I pick at things (lint, hair, etc.).			—
8. I feel nausea.	—	—	
9. I have tightness in my chest or feel like a strap is tight across my chest.		—	
10. My hand or head shakes or trembles.		—	
11. My hands feel cold.	—		
12. My hands sweat.	—		
13. My heart beats fast and noticeably.	—		
14. I feel distant from my surroundings.			—
15. I continually have the same or many thoughts running through my head.			—
16. I move awkwardly, bump into things, or drop things.		—	—
17. It is difficult to concentrate.			—
18. I must be aware of everything around me to keep control.			—
19. My head or jaws ache.		—	
20. My head aches with a pounding either behind my eyes or on one side of my head.	—		
21. My forehead aches or the back of my head aches with a kind of pulling ache.		—	
22. The muscles running from my shoulder blades across my shoulders to my neck ache on one side or both sides.		—	
23. My face flushes.	—		
24. I get dizzy.	—	—	
25. I want to be very close to someone.			—
26. I tend to have lapses of awareness.			—
27. I feel like I want to smash something.		—	
28. I have to go to the toilet often.	—		
29. I have difficulty eating or holding down food.	—		
30. My calves, thighs, or feet get tense.		—	
31. I breathe rapidly and shallowly.	—		
32. I have to check things again and again.			—

(Table continues)

SELF-REPORT OF RESPONSES TO ANXIETY *(continued)*

	A	M	C
33. I keep forgetting things.			—
34. I want to retreat and sleep, safe at home.			—
35. I busy myself putting everything in order.			—
36. I have to eat and eat.	—		
37. I produce gas (burp or other).	—		
38. My mouth gets dry.	—		
39. I worry about many things.			—

This scale has no norms. However, there is a maximum score of 70 for each item (14 items; five is the top score for each item). "A" refers to autonomic arousal symptoms; "M" to muscular tension, and "C" to cognitive responses. Generally, total scores above 100 are anxiety reactive. One of the most important factors is the relative values among the three categories. These tell the examiner and testee which system responds the most to stimulation and consequently which type of relaxation intervention would be best suited to the individual. "A" responders do best with a breathing technique. "M" reponders do best with muscle relaxation, such as progressive relaxation. "C" responders do best with mental relaxation, such as meditation, thought stopping, and other techniques.

(chronic worries) increase anxiety and compulsions (chronic rituals) decrease it, building a vicious cycle. Men and women develop OCD about equally.

Individuals who have OCD have involuntary, recurrent, and persistent thoughts or impulses that are distasteful to them. They may have thoughts of violence or of becoming infected by shaking hands with others. These thoughts can be momentary or they may be long-lasting. Generally, individuals with OCD are divided into "checkers" (people who constantly check something) and "washers" (people who wash themselves, often their hands, to excess). However, some people with OCD fall outside these distinctions; for example, they may constantly count things or feel a need to touch items.

The most common obsessions are those that focus on hurting others or on violating socially acceptable behavioral standards, such as cursing in public or making inappropriate sexual advances to others. Individuals with OCD may also focus on religious or philosophical issues that the individual never resolves. Fears of being contaminated inadvertently are common. In this case, washing serves as a means of coping with these thoughts.

Individuals who have compulsions go through repeated, involuntary ritualistic behaviors that are believed to prevent or produce an unrelated future event. Some people with this disorder also suffer from a complementary obsession, as in the case of worries over infection and the resultant behavior of compulsive hand-washing.

Cleaning is an example of a compulsive ritual. If the individual comes in contact with any dirt, he or she may spend hours washing, even to the point that the hands bleed. Hand-washing affects more women than men. Another example of a compulsive ritual is repetitious behavior, such as saying a loved one's name several times every time that person's name comes up in conversation. Compulsives also may check and recheck that their doors are really locked or that electric switches, ovens, and water taps are turned off. Others will retrace a route that they have driven to check that they did not hit a pedestrian or cause an accident without knowing it. More men than women are affected by the checking compulsion.

Obsessive-compulsive disorders are generally chronic and cause moderate to severe disability in their victims. OCD may be accompanied by eating disorders, depression, and other forms of anxiety disorders.

Treatment for OCD generally involves medication such as imipramine (Tofranil) or clomipramine (Anafranil). Exposure therapy is also used, in which individuals are trained to deal with situations that cause them anxiety and to learn to cope without relying on these rituals/compulsions. Drugs usually have little effect in controlling or eliminating problematic reactions.

Post-traumatic Stress Disorder Post-traumatic stress disorder can occur in anyone who has survived a life-threatening physical or mental trauma, such as a physical or sexual assault in childhood or adulthood. The individual with PTSD may be the victim or the trauma may have occurred to a loved one. Individuals with PTSD often also have depression and substance abuse issues and other forms of anxiety disorders.

People with PTSD avoid situations that remind them of the traumatic event. They often become irritable and some become violent, while others become emotionally numb. Despite their wish to avoid thinking about the traumatic event, individuals with PTSD often find themselves fixated on thinking about it. They may have flashbacks in which they feel as if they are experiencing the trauma in the same way as when it actually occurred. A person with a flashback may believe that he or she is actually reexperiencing the trauma. The individual also experiences chronic arousal which causes sleep disturbance, lack of concentration, and anxiety.

Medications can help reduce intense symptoms so that the individual can make better use of behavior therapy or other psychotherapy techniques. Medications such as SSRIs are often used to treat PTSD. In addition to behavioral modification techniques and medication, psychotherapy can be an important component of treatment.

See .EYE MOVEMENT DESENSITIZATION AND REPROCESSING; SOMATIZATION.

See also RESPONSE PROPERTIES; STATE ANXIETY; TRAIT ANXIETY; STIMULUS PROPERTIES.

American Psychiatric Association, *Diagnostic and Statistical Manual of Mental Disorders-Text Revision, 4th ed.* Washington, DC: American Psychiatric Association, 2000.

Marks, Isaac, *Fears, Phobias, and Rituals: Anxiety and Their Disorders* (New York: Oxford University Press, 1987).

National Institute of Mental Health, "The Numbers Count: Mental Disorders in America." Available online. URL: http://www.nimh.nih.gov/publicat/numbers.cfm. Downloaded November 14, 2006.

Anxiety Disorders Interview Schedule (ADIS)

This is a structured interview designed to provide a detailed functional analysis of the anxiety disorder and an accurate diagnosis. The ADIS and the revised version of the ADIS (ADIS-R) were developed from content analysis of clinical interviews with anxiety disorder patients. Questions are branched so that a "yes" or "no" answer will have particular follow-up questions. The interviewer using the ADIS-R (revised) can acquire a reliable set of information on the client for diagnostic purposes, determination of severity, and effective intervention.

The ADIS was developed by Peter DiNardo, David Barlow, Jerome Cerny, Bonnie Vermilyea, James Vermilyea, William Himadi, and Maria Waddell.

anxiety disorders of childhood A group of disorders in which anxiety is the central feature. They include:

Separation Anxiety

Separation anxiety is excessive worry about separation from significant others, such as fears that harm will befall parents or the child and nightmares involving separation themes. School phobia is sometimes considered a form of separation anxiety.

Avoidant Disorders

Avoidant disorders include extreme shyness that prevents interacting with other children and persistent retreat from contact with strangers.

Overanxious Disorder

Overanxious disorder is persistent worrying about the future or humiliations that happened in the past, excessive need for reassurance, and many unfounded physical complaints.

See also CHILDHOOD ANXIETIES, FEARS AND PHOBIAS.

anxiety drugs Also known as antianxiety medications or anxiolytic drugs. Some individuals who have anxieties, fears, and phobias are advised by their physicians to take anxiety drugs, starting with a low dose. It is better if these medications are prescribed in combination with some form of psychotherapy or exposure treatment. When they are effective, antianxiety medications often make the individual more receptive to the *talking therapy* and *exposure therapy* that are used in many forms of psychotherapy and may be particularly receptive to exposure therapy, which is effective in counteracting many forms of phobias.

One widely used class of drugs is the BENZODIAZEPINES. Examples are DIAZEPAM (Valium), ALPRAZOLAM (Xanax), lorazepam (Ativan), and oxazepam (Serax). Benzodiazepines are used to help individuals over a temporary circumstance that brings on anxiety. They are usually less helpful for chronic anxiety, and there is some risk for drug dependence with these medications. These drugs do not improve (on a lasting basis) problems with phobias or compulsive rituals (exposure therapy is the recommended treatment). High doses of benzodiazepines may interfere with exposure therapy if the medication is taken up to four hours before or during exposure sessions.

Sometimes, ANTIDEPRESSANTS are used as anxiety drugs. Many people with anxiety disorders also suffer from DEPRESSION, and these medications can be very helpful to some individuals. Unlike benzodiazepines, high doses of antidepressants do not interfere with exposure therapy. There is evidence, however, that once the anxiety problems and limitations are dealt with the depressive mood abates.

Although not specifically referred to as anxiety drugs, BETA BLOCKERS are another group of drugs that are sometimes used to reduce some of the physical features of anxiety, such as a rapid heartbeat and heart palpitations. These drugs are particularly effective in public speaking situations and with other forms of social anxiety.

See also MONOAMINE OXIDASE INHIBITORS; OBSESSIVE-COMPULSIVE DISORDER; PERFORMANCE ANXIETY; PHOBIAS, RITUALS; WITHDRAWAL EFFECTS OF ADDICTIVE SUBSTANCES.

anxiety hierarchy   A list of anxiety-producing stimuli, ranked from least frightening to most, for use in systematic desensitization and exposure therapies. The ranking is usually done by using SUD units, and the hierarchy relates to a specific stimulus situation, such as riding elevators, making left turns, insects, and so on.

See also BEHAVIOR THERAPY; EXPOSURE THERAPY; SYSTEMATIC DESENSITIZATION.

anxiety hysteria   An obsolete diagnostic term for what is now generally called phobia, phobic disorders, or somataform disorder.

See also PHOBIA.

anxiety neurosis   An obsolete term for ANXIETY DISORDER, no longer used in psychiatric diagnosis or literature.

Anxiety Sensitivity Index (ASI)   The Anxiety Sensitivity Index was developed by Steven Reiss, Department of Psychology, University of Illinois at Chicago, during the late 1980s as a self-report measure of fear or sensitivity to anxiety. The authors claim the ASI has factor and construct validity and behavioral validity. While people who have anxiety disorders score significantly higher on this scale than non-anxiety-prone individuals, those who have AGORAPHOBIA and POST-TRAUMATIC STRESS DISORDERS tend to score even higher (indicating a greater sensitivity to the body sensations of anxiety).

anxiogenic   A term denoting drugs, substances, or activities that tend to raise anxiety levels. For example, in studies of panic disorder with or without agoraphobia, anxiety has been raised by CAFFEINE, yohimbine, sodium lactate or isoproterenol infusion, carbon dioxide inhalation, HYPERVENTILATION, and exercise. Certain stimuli, such as the sight of a dog (if one is phobic about dogs) or looking down from the top of a tall building (if one has a phobia of heights) may be anxiogenic.

See also LACTATE-INDUCED ANXIETY.

anxiolytics   Drugs that are used to combat anxiety or used as minor tranquilizers.

See also ANTIDEPRESSANTS; ANXIETY DRUGS; BENZODIAZEPINES.

anything, fear of   Fear of anything or everything is known as panphobia, panophobia, pantophobia, and pamphobia. When an individual fears anything or everything, the condition may be an anxiety disorder rather than a true phobia.

See also ANXIETY, BASIC; ANXIETY DISORDERS; ANXIETY HIERARCHY.

apeirophobia Fear of infinity.

See also INFINITY, FEAR OF.

aphenphobia Fear of being touched, or of physical contact.

See also BEING TOUCHED, FEAR OF.

apiphobia or apiophobia See BEES, FEAR OF.

apocalypse, fear of Fear of the apocalypse, or end of the world, has always been a part of mankind's anxieties. Primitive man was frightened by natural disasters such as earthquakes, volcanic eruptions, and hurricanes. This sense of change and danger in the natural order may have given him the fear that all life could come to an end at any time. Many early religious rituals and observances were aimed at the preservation of order in nature, with the implication that the balance could tip in the other direction very easily. Some civilizations, including the Aztecs, Hindus, Buddhists, and Greeks, developed beliefs that divided time into a series of ages, with either possible or certain destruction at the end of these ages. Common to several apocalyptic philosophies is the theme of man's deterioration into immoral, disorganized, destructive behavior at the point just preceding the earth's destruction. Like other religions, the Judeo-Christian tradition contains notions of past destruction. The Old Testament chronicles the rebirth of civilization in the story of Noah and the flood; several books of the New Testament include a prediction of the end of the world and the second coming of Jesus Christ. It was a strong belief in Europe that the world would end in the year 1,000.

Contemporary religious groups deemphasize the fear of the end of the world and the anticipation of the rebirth of a new order, but writers and filmmakers during the latter part of the 20th century picked up on the theme. Novels such as Walter M. Miller Jr.'s *A Canticle for Leibowitz* and Walker Percy's *Love in the Ruins* and films such as *Dr. Strangelove, Planet of the Apes,* and *Road Warrior* reflect fears about the end of the world, or at least a cataclysmic finish to civilization as we know it. If artistic expression is a genuine reflection of 20th- and 21st-century fears and anxieties, man is afraid that he is his own worst enemy.

Cavendish, Richard, ed., "End of the World." In *Man, Myth and Magic* (New York: Marshall Cavendish, 1983).

approach-avoidance conflict The conflict that arises when an individual experiences two competing drives simultaneously. Such unresolved conflicts may result in neuroses, such as anxieties and phobias. The term approach-avoidance conflict was developed in the 1950s by Neil Miller, a renowned learning theorist, who together with J. Dollard attempted to translate psychoanalytic theory into learning-theory terms that might be better researchable. The approach-avoidance conflict assumes that each factor has different strengths, or gradients, and that resulting behavior will be decided by the gradient that is stronger at a given time.

See also NEUROSIS.

approximation conditioning See OPERANT CONDITIONING.

aquaphobia See WATER, FEAR OF.

arachibutyrophobia A fear that peanut butter will stick to the roof of one's mouth.

See also PEANUT BUTTER, FEAR OF.

arachnophobia (arachnephobia) See SPIDERS, FEAR OF.

arches, fear of Some individuals may be frightened of arches because the structures may appear less stable and more likely to collapse than angular structures. Arches may also be associated with an aversion to other curved or rounded shapes. The fear may relate to a fear of landscapes in which arches appear.

See also LANDSCAPES, FEAR OF.

arithmophobia   See NUMBERS, FEAR OF.

aromatherapy   The art and science of using essential oils from plants and flowers to reduce anxieties and enhance health. Practitioners of aromatherapy blend essential oils from around the world based on one's current physical, bioenergetic, and emotional condition and apply them with a specialized massage technique focusing on the nervous and lymphatic system. Aromatherapy massage has been used to treat conditions such as job anxieties, muscle soreness, acne, varicose veins, allergies, and emotional conditions.

The art of aromatherapy is fairly new in the United States, but has been used for centuries elsewhere in the world, particularly Egypt and Greece. During World War I, Dr. Jean Valnet, a Parisian physician, used essential oils to treat injured soldiers. He also influenced Marguerite Maury, a biochemist, who developed a special way to apply the penetrating oils with massage.

Finding a Practitioner of Aromatherapy

There is no national organization overseeing training standards in this field. Techniques vary from practitioner to practitioner. Many therapists are employed in spas in larger cities or resort areas. If you are seeking this therapy, look for someone who is a licensed, certified massage practitioner and who can show proof of training in the use of essential oils.

See also COMPLEMENTARY THERAPIES.

arrhenophobia   Fear of men. The fear of women is called gynophobia, while the fear of men is also known as androphobia.

See also MEN, FEAR OF.

arrhythmia   An abnormal heart rhythm, usually detected by an electrocardiogram. When some individuals hear this diagnosis, they become anxious and find it a source of fear. It may or may not be of potential significance, and understanding its significance can relieve subsequent anxieties. Arrhythmias can be caused by several factors, such as coronary artery disease, heart valve problems, or hyperthyroidism. Individuals with this diagnosis should question their physician carefully about possible lifestyle changes they should make as well as the possible need for medication.

See also BIOFEEDBACK; BREATHING; HEART ATTACK, ANXIETY FOLLOWING AND OR, FEAR OF; HIGH BLOOD PRESSURE, FEAR OF; RELAXATION; TYPE A BEHAVIOR PATTERN.

arsonphobia   Fear of fire.

See also FIRE, FEAR OF.

arthritis   A painful, debilitating chronic condition that has been diagnosed by physicians in nearly 43 million American adults. It is also believed that 23 million adults with joint symptoms have not yet been diagnosed. Arthritis is the leading cause of disability in the United States. There are many different forms, including osteoarthritis (the most common form), rheumatoid arthritis, gout, fibromyalgia, and lupus.

Arthritis can cause considerable anxiety and distress because of its effects on the lives of those who are afflicted. About 16 million adults say that arthritis limits their usual activities and 8 million adults say that they have work limitations because of arthritis. At least 80,000 children in the United States have some form of arthritis, and some experts believe the number may be as high as 285,000 children. The percentage of adults with arthritis varies from an estimated low of 18 percent in Hawaii to a high of 37 percent in West Virginia. Arthritis affects individuals of all races and ethnicities. The body and joint pain and discomfort caused by arthritic conditions can cause and/or exacerbate anxiety and the vulnerability to develop anxiety.

According to the Centers for Disease Control and Prevention (CDC), there are more than 100 different rheumatic diseases and conditions that affect the joints, and all of these are collectively called arthritis. A diagnosis of any form of arthritis triggers many accompanying fears and anxieties in the individual, who wonders how their life will be changed and impaired and what they can do to prevent the disease from escalating. They may recall elderly relatives who were severely disabled from arthritis and fear that they too will suffer similar consequences. Fortunately, although there are no cures for arthritis, there are many effective treatments and lifestyle changes that individuals can make to decrease the pain and limit the disability of the disease.

Osteoarthritis, sometimes called *degenerative joint disease,* is the most common form of arthritis and affects an estimated 21 million people in the United States. It typically affects older adults and is caused by wear and tear on the joints, particularly in the joints of the hands, knees, feet, hips, and back. Osteoarthritis usually appears after the age of 40 and may become progressively worse as the individual ages.

Rheumatoid arthritis is the most severe form of arthritis and is caused by the body's immune system attacking the joints and surrounding tissues, often leading to severe deformity of the shoulders, elbows, hands, wrists, feet, and ankles. An estimated 2 million people in the United States have rheumatoid arthritis.

Gout is another common form of arthritis, causing severe swelling and extreme pain, often in the toe or ankle but can be present in any joint. It is caused by the deposit of uric acid crystals. In general, men are more likely to suffer from gout than women, but postmenopausal women are at risk for the development of gout.

Systematic lupus erythematosus (SLE) often known simply as *lupus,* is another form of arthritis in which the immune system produces antibodies to cells and causes widespread tissue damage and inflammation. It can cause damage not only to the joints but also to the kidneys, skin, heart, lungs, blood vessels, and brain. The causes of lupus are unknown but may be linked to environmental, genetic, and hormonal factors. The disease is characterized by flare-ups and remissions.

FIBROMYALGIA is a form of arthritis that causes widespread pain throughout the body, with chronic muscle pain and fatigue. Many patients with fibromyalgia have difficulty sleeping. Severe fatigue is another common indicator of fibromyalgia. The causes of fibromyalgia are unknown but it is believed that genetics play a role and emotional stress may be a factor as well. The inability to function caused by fibromyalgia can produce worry and anxiety.

Symptoms and Diagnostic Path

Depending on the form of arthritis, patients may have pain and swelling and the inflammation may be visible, although it is not always apparent upon a visual inspection. X-rays and sometimes imaging studies such as magnetic resonance imaging (MRI) will help determine if there are any fractures or serious tissue damage.

Blood tests such as for erythrocyte sedimentation rate (ESR) are given to test for possible rheumatoid arthritis or lupus. Physicians may also test for rheumatoid factor (RF) to help with diagnosis, and some may use a test for c-reactive protein, a test that measures inflammation as well.

Gout is often readily diagnosed by the red inflammation and acute pain of the affected area.

Fibromyalgia is diagnosed by the presence of tender points in specific areas of the body as well as by the presence of sleep difficulties and widespread pain.

Treatment Options and Outlook

Many pharmacological and other approaches are available for treating individuals who have arthritis, and the treatment depends on the type of arthritis. However, many patients with arthritis suffer from anxiety and depression. Often antidepressants are prescribed to help ease depression as well as the arthritis pain. Many over-the-counter topical remedies are available for all forms of arthritis.

Osteoarthritis treatment. Nonsteroidal anti-inflammatory drugs (NSAIDs) are often used to treat osteoarthritis. Physical therapy helps some patients, as do prescribed topical transdermal applications of lidocaine (Lidoderm). Some patients receive epidural injections of cortisone to relieve their pain for weeks, months, or longer. Heat and cold therapy as well as massage therapy may be helpful. Surgery is an option for some patients with severe osteoarthritis, who may need the replacement of a joint, particularly the knee. A newer treatment is the injection of a preparation that lubricates the knee joint, and two options are available, including Hyalgan and Synvisc.

Some patients find relief with transcutaneous electrical nerve stimulation (TENS), applied to the painful area.

Increasingly, researchers are trying COMPLEMENTARY THERAPIES, either in conjunction with prescription medication or as sole therapies. Some patients with osteoarthritis have reported relief with ACUPUNCTURE.

Rheumatoid arthritis treatment. With rheumatoid arthritis, NSAIDs are often used, as are corticosteroids. Disease-modifying antirheumatic drugs (DMARDs) may be prescribed to limit joint damage, including hydroxychloroquine (Plaquenil), minocycline (Dynacin, Minocin), methotrexate (Rheumatrex), and other drugs. In addition, medications that inhibit tumor necrosis factor, an element that is present in rheumatoid arthritis, have been developed for patients to use as a self-injection under the skin. Some examples of such drugs include etanercept (Enbrel), infliximab (Remicade), and adalimumab (Humira).

Anakinra (Kinaret) is a newer drug that is used when other medications have not helped rheumatoid arthritis. It blocks the protein that promotes inflammation, which exists in excessive quantities in people with rheumatoid arthritis. Anakinra is administered under the skin. Many other drugs are in development as of this writing.

Gout treatment. Colchicine is used to treat flare-ups of gout. If an individual has frequent bouts of gout, he or she may be placed on allupurinol, a preventive medication. The individual is advised to stay off the affected joint until symptoms remit. Usually the symptoms abate within days.

Fibromyalgia treatment. Fibromyalgia is treated with NSAIDs, massage therapy, and topical creams. Trigger injections of corticosteroids sometimes provide relief. If the pain is severe, narcotics are sometimes used on a temporary basis. Chronic pain may be treated with antidepressants, such as SEROTONIN NOREPINEPHRINE REUPTAKE INHIBITORS (SNRIs). Duloxetine (Cymbalta) is used for this purpose although not specifically approved by the FDA. Acupuncture may provide some relief.

Lupus treatment. Lupus is treated on a symptomatic basis, depending on which part of the body and which symptoms the patient suffers from.

General treatments for patients with arthritis. As a result of early research in PSYCHONEUROIMMUNOLOGY, a few behavioral programs to treat arthritis have been developed. One activity is exercise. The chief benefit of exercise is it moves the blood flow to the affected joints and keeps them flexible. Arthritic individuals may be advised to do stretching exercises to keep their joints moving smoothly and to do strengthening exercises to maintain muscle tone. Walking and nonweight-bearing exercises such as swimming are also helpful.

Some physicians suggest relaxation tapes for patients with arthritis. The logic behind these tapes is that if the mind is distracted by mental exercise, it is less likely to feel the arthritis pain. Additionally, some researchers believe that the relaxation response increases the body's production of endorphins, which are natural painkillers.

Other researchers have used BIOFEEDBACK to train people to relax. In one study, one group of arthritics had biofeedback training; the other had a standard physical therapy program. The group using biofeedback and relaxation felt better; additionally, their ESR blood test measuring the disease's activity showed that their immune systems held stable against the disease or the disease had somewhat abated.

In one study of 63 patients with rheumatoid arthritis, the subjects received training in meditation, which they practiced six hours a week. The control group did not use meditation. After two months the psychological distress of the patients was decreased by 30 percent in the meditation group and by 10 percent in the control group. In addition, after six months, nonspecific inflammation *decreased* by 35 percent in the meditation group, compared to a 11 percent *increase* in the control group. As a result, meditation can provide pain relief.

Psychotherapy may also be helpful for many patients with chronic arthritis. Many psychological forces seem to have a role in autoimmune diseases. Psychotherapy can help arthritis patients understand the possible emotional factors that may be associated with their symptoms and realize that emotional stress can exacerbate their pain. In conjunction with psychotherapy, or by themselves, techniques such as relaxation exercises, meditation, and biofeedback can be helpful to patients with all forms of arthritis.

Risk Factors and Preventive Measures

Individuals with a family history of osteoarthritis or rheumatoid arthritis are at risk for the development of these diseases, and there appears to be a genetic risk for lupus and fibromyalgia as well. Individuals who have been in car accidents have an increased risk for the development of fibromyalgia.

Joint injuries increase the risk of the development of arthritis in that joint.

Age is a risk factor for the development of most forms of arthritis, and a large number of elderly people suffer from osteoarthritis or another type of arthritis.

For individuals with osteoarthritis and rheumatoid arthritis, the best preventive measure is to avoid obesity, which can place additional strain on already overburdened and inflamed arthritis joints.

With the exception of gout, women are more likely to suffer from arthritis than men and, according to the CDC, women account for 60 percent of all arthritis cases.

Individuals who engage in sports or occupations that require repetitive motions are at risk for the development of osteoarthritis.

In general, moderate exercise can reduce the risk for all forms of arthritis and can also improve existing arthritis, although the individual should be careful not to overdo exercise. Walking and swimming are considered good exercise for patients with arthritis.

See also AUTOIMMUNE DISEASES; CHRONIC ILLNESS; GUIDED IMAGERY; IMMUNE SYSTEM; MEDITATION; PAIN; RELAXATION.

Rados, Carol, "Helpful Treatments Keep People with Arthritis Moving," *FDA Consumer Magazine* (March–April 2005). Available online. URL: http://www.fda.gov/fdac/features/2005/2O5pain.html. Downloaded June 16, 2006.

assertiveness training A behavior-therapy technique in which individuals learn how to responsi-

bly express both positive and negative feelings with other people and with a minimum of passivity, aggression, or guilt. Assertiveness training is helpful in treating some agoraphobics, social phobics, speech phobias, and individuals with other phobias, since it focuses on emotional expression that is incompatible with anxiety.

See also AGORAPHOBIA; BEHAVIOR THERAPY.

asthenophobia Fear of fainting, or weakness.

See also FAINTING, FEAR OF; WEAKNESS, FEAR OF.

asthma A lung disease that makes breathing difficult. Because it is a chronic inflammatory lung disease characterized by recurrent breathing problems, it is a source of anxiety to the sufferer as well as his or her family. People with asthma have recurrent attacks or flareups of breathlessness, accompanied by wheezing. Asthma varies from one person to another. Some people have mild to moderate symptoms while others have severe symptoms that can be life threatening. Even in the same individual, asthma attacks can vary in severity from day to day. Often, medical intervention is required, adding to the stress and anxiety produced by this condition.

In many individuals, attacks begin in childhood and tend to become less severe in adulthood; however, asthma attacks can begin at any age. For many people, attacks are brought on by STRESS or ANXIETY. Asthma symptoms are a major cause of lost time from school and work and sleep disturbances.

Symptoms and Diagnostic Path

During a severe attack, breathing becomes increasingly difficult, causing sweating, rapid heart beat, and an increasingly high arousal level. The individual may be unable to speak, cannot lie down or sleep, breathes rapidly, and wheezes loudly. The individual may fear dying and those watching and trying to help the sufferer may add to the overall anxiety level. Asthma may get worse at night because chemical changes in the body narrow airways; there may be delayed allergic reactions, and the airways become cooled.

Asthma may be *extrinsic,* in which an allergy (usually to something inhaled) triggers an attack, or *intrinsic,* in which there seems to be no apparent external cause. Intrinsic asthma tends to develop later in life than extrinsic asthma.

About 10 million Americans have asthma. Of these, about 3 million are children under the age of 18. Asthma affects women and men equally. The reported number of cases of asthma is increasing, but the death rate for asthma in the United States is still one of the lowest in the world.

Understanding Asthma. Contrary to a popular notion, asthma is not a psychosomatic illness. It is a real disease and not a sign of an emotional disturbance. Understanding the physiology involved in asthma can help one manage the disease, reduce the stress it brings, and improve quality of life. In healthy lungs, air moves easily in and out of the airways. During an asthma attack, several things occur:

- *Inflammation narrows the airways.* Inflammation is redness and swelling that occurs in response to a "trigger." (A trigger is something that sets off an asthma episode.) When the airways swell, there is less room for air to get through. Inflammation remains after the attack, increasing the risk of future attacks.

- *Muscle spasms occur.* The airways are ringed by smooth muscles. During an asthma episode, these muscle squeeze the airways, narrowing them further.

- *Mucus production increases.* In some cases, the airways become clogged with thick, sticky mucus. This makes it even harder to move air in and out of the lungs.

Many people get warning signs from hours or days before an attack. Signs may include tiredness, a change in breathing, coughing, change in mucus color, trouble sleeping, itching of the chin or throat, sneezing, headache, dark circles under the eyes, and moodiness.

What Triggers an Asthma Attack. Triggers vary from person to person, and many people with asthma have more than one. Common triggers include:

- *Excitement or stressful situations.* Emotional factors themselves do not cause asthma. However, laughing, crying, yelling may bring on symptoms.

- *Airborne allergens.* An allergen is a substance that causes an allergic response. Common airborne allergens include pollen, dust mites, mold, and animal dander.

- *Common irritants.* These include cigarette smoke (as well as secondhand smoke), smoke from other sources, such as candles, burning leaves or wood-burning stoves, aerosol sprays and other chemicals, and strong odors.

- *Exercise.* Exercise is a trigger for many people; however, most people with asthma can lead active lives and participate in sports. There are steps one can take to reduce the risk of problems.

- *Respiratory infections.* Respiratory infections can be particularly troublesome for children who tend to get more colds than adults.

Asthma is sometimes difficult to diagnose because many of its symptoms resemble emphysema, bronchitis, and lower respiratory infections. For some individuals, the only symptom is a chronic cough, especially at night, or coughing or wheezing occurring only with exercise. Diagnosis is made using a combination of medical history, thorough physical examination, and certain laboratory tests.

Treatment Options and Outlook

Asthma cannot be cured but it can be controlled with proper treatment. With current drug therapies, people who suffer repeated attacks can learn to manage episodes. Quality of life need not be impaired, as demonstrated by successes of athletes and others who have had asthma. There are two main groups of medications. One is anti-inflammatory medications. These can help prevent asthma attacks by reducing swelling. Anti-inflammatory medications include corticosteroids (usually inhaled), cromolyn, and nedocromil. Inhaled steroids are absorbed primarily by the lungs. That means little gets into the bloodstream, lowering the risk of side effects. The second group is the bronchodilators. These medications can open airways during asthma attacks. They include beta2 agonists and theophylline. Asthma sufferers should have a bronchodilator handy.

An asthma sufferer should follow his/her health care provider's instructions for when to take the medication and how much to take. If one has an anti-inflammatory medication, it should be taken regularly, even when feeling fine.

Exercise can improve lung power and wellness. However, before embarking on an exercise program, an asthma sufferer should talk with his/her health care provider. If exercise is a trigger for asthma, warming up before exercising in cold air is necessary. One should wear a scarf or mask over the nose and the mouth. Stick to a safe level of exercise. Follow one's health care provider's directions for taking extra medication before exercising.

Research Under Way. Research on asthma is under way at the National Institutes of Health and is conducted and supported by two units, the National Heart, Lung and Blood Institute (NHLBI) and the National Institute of Allergy and Infectious Diseases. Projects supported by these agencies focus on identifying basic abnormalities that cause asthma, on developing better drug treatments and emergency measures, and on educating people with asthma to help themselves more effectively. Projects supported by the NHLBI involve educational programs to reduce disability from asthma and train patients in asthma self-management techniques while under medical supervision.

Meanwhile, individuals who have asthma have particular concerns about stress, as many become depressed due to their chronically recurring condition and especially anxious during asthma attacks. In cases of children who have asthma, family counseling is often useful for all concerned.

See also ALLERGIES; CHRONIC ILLNESS; DEPRESSION; GUIDED IMAGERY; MEDITATION; STRESS.

astraphobia (astrapophobia)   Fear of lightning; also known as keraunophobia.

See also LIGHTNING, FEAR OF.

astrology, fear of   Some individuals fear their lives are affected by the positions of various planets, stars, or constellations. They consult astrologers who plot their horoscopes, relating the time of birth to the present positions of specific celestial bodies. Astrologers counsel their clients about the advisability of certain actions. While many individuals become fearful and anxious about what they find in their horoscopes, many others follow horoscopes with confidence. The attraction to astrology, as well as the fears aroused by it, probably evolved from ancient fears about the stars and planets and outside or external forces acting on them. (The term "lunacy" was coined by Paracelsus to denote astal influence on sanity.) In an attempt to understand these celestial bodies, astronomers gave names of humans or gods to various constellations of stars and added an anthropomorphic feature to the skies. Some discoveries about sun spots, the influence of the moon on the tides, and eclipses, added to the notion that the earth and its inhabitants might be influenced by the stars and planets. Early forms of medicine were heavily influenced by astrology and numerology. Various religious views added more mystification, and early astronomers gained importance because they were the only individuals who could intercede between man and the heavens to predict the future and advise man about how to avoid fearful predictions.

See also MAGIC, FEAR OF.

ataraxy   Absence of anxiety or confusion; untroubled calmness. Drugs to produce a state of ataraxy are commonly called tranquilizers.

See also ANXIETY; TRANQUILIZERS.

ataxiophobia or ataxophobia   Fear of disorder.

See also DISORDER, FEAR OF.

atelophobia   Fear of imperfection.

See also IMPERFECTION, FEAR OF.

atenolol   A beta-blocking drug that has been used in treating some cases of social phobia, social anxieties, and fear of flying.

See also ANTIDEPRESSANTS; BETA-BLOCKERS; CLASSIFICATION OF PHOBIAS; SOCIAL PHOBIAS.

atephobia   Fear of ruins.

See also RUINS, FEAR OF.

attachment theory   A theory that conceptualizes the ability of human beings to develop strong affectional or object bonds in childhood that manifest in the same way in adulthood. The theory was proposed by British psychiatrist John Bowlby. Attachment theory or object relations theory also refers to many forms of distress and disturbance that can result from unwilling separation. These include anxieties, anger, and depression.

See also ANXIETY; BIRTH TRAUMA; DEPRESSION; SCHOOL PHOBIA; SEPARATION ANXIETY.

attention-deficit/hyperactivity disorder (ADHD)
A persistent pattern of inattention and/or hyperactivity-impulsivity that is more frequent and severe than is typically observed in individuals at a comparable level of development. Children are more frequently diagnosed with ADHD than adolescents and adults, but the disorder may be present at any life stage. In the past, it was commonly believed that children somehow outgrew ADHD in adolescence, but this belief has been debunked. It was also commonly believed that only boys could develop ADHD. However, most experts agree that girls and women may also have ADHD, although females are far more likely to exhibit inattentive behavior than hyperactive behavior.

The symptoms of ADHD are often a source of anxiety to children and adolescents with the disorder, as well as to their parents and teachers. Individuals of all ages who have ADHD may regard themselves as stupid, lazy, or incompetent, largely because this is what they have heard from others. In addition, ADHD in children often sets the stage for adult anxiety, particularly generalized anxiety disorder (GAD), in which worry about the future and one's performance predominate.

Some individuals who are diagnosed with ADHD as adults feel anxious and perhaps stigmatized or troubled by the diagnosis, while others experience relief that their lifelong symptoms of distractibility and inattentiveness have a cause and a name, as well as a treatment.

To make the diagnosis of ADHD, according to the DIAGNOSTIC AND STATISTICAL MANUAL OF MENTAL DISORDERS, FOURTH EDITION, Text Revision (DSM-IV-TR), some hyperactive-impulsive or inattentive symptoms that cause impairment must have been present before age seven, although many individuals are diagnosed after their symptoms have been present for years. Additionally, there must be clear evidence of an interference with developmentally appropriate social, academic, or occupational functioning, and the disorder cannot be better accounted for by another mental disorder, such as an anxiety disorder, dissociative disorder, or a personality disorder.

According to the DSM, there are three primary types of ADHD, including the predominantly inattentive type, the predominantly hyperactive type, and the combined type. ADHD affects about 5–7 percent of the school-age population. According to the National Institute of Mental Health (NIMH), about 4 percent of the adult population ages 18–44 has ADHD.

Symptoms and Diagnostic Path

The symptoms and diagnostic path are somewhat different with children and adolescents than with adults. For example, adults are much less likely to behave in a hyperactive manner, and mostly exhibit inattentiveness.

Symptoms and diagnosis in children and adolescents.   Often ADHD is noticed before the child is age five, particularly when they exhibit overactive, impulsive, and hyperactive behavior. Children who are inattentive may constantly daydream or seem to be in their own world and are startled or sidetracked by others around them. Impulsive children act without thinking, while hyperactive children have great difficulty sitting still. All children may exhibit some elements of inattentiveness, impulsivity, and hyperactivity, but, when they have ADHD, their behavior is extreme and frequent and impairs their performance at school and their social relationships with their family and others.

ADHD is not always diagnosed in those who have the disorder, particularly among children and adolescents who are primarily inattentive. As a result, young people with undiagnosed ADHD often develop very negative attitudes toward school and patterns of school failure. Often this failure could have been avoided with prompt diagnosis and treatment. Even with treatment, however, some individuals with ADHD develop behavioral problems in later life.

Some individuals with ADHD develop substance use disorders; a four-year study by psychiatrist Joseph Biederman and his colleagues demonstrated that untreated adolescents with ADHD have a significantly greater risk for developing substance use disorders than adolescents who had been treated with stimulants.

It is important to note that ADHD exists as a separate entity from other disorders, such as conduct disorder. The essential feature of conduct disorder is a persistent conduct pattern in which the rights of others and age-appropriate societal norms or rules are violated. This pattern often leads to a diagnosis of sociopath as an adult. While both ADHD and conduct disorder may occur in the same individual, it is not assumed that one is a necessary predictor of the other. Making the distinction between disorders has important implications for outcome. Mental health professionals treating individuals with ADHD generally agree that individualized management, on a case-by-case method, is most effective.

The diagnosis of a child or adolescent is based on a description of the child's behavior obtained from parents and teachers, as well as by observation of behavior in the office of the mental health professional. Questions for the child are directed toward features of hyperactivity, impulsiveness, and lack of attention. Such children are often restless, particularly while the physician talks with parents. Rating scales are often used to help diagnose ADHD, such as the Conners' Rating Scales for parents, teachers, and adolescents, the Copeland Symptom Checklist for Children and Adolescents, or the Child Behavior Checklist.

To determine whether the child has an associated disorder, such as a learning disorder or mild mental retardation, psychological tests are always useful.

Symptoms and diagnosis in adults. Many adults discover that they are likely to have ADHD when their own children are diagnosed with the disorder. Others read or hear about ADHD and suspect that they may have the disorder, based on frequent job changes, severe relationship difficulties, and other issues that may occur to the untreated adult with ADHD.

According to the *DSM*, the adult should have exhibited symptoms of ADHD before the age of 7 years, although some experts dispute this age cutoff as arbitrary. To diagnose ADHD in an adult, mental health professionals may use self-rating scales such as the Adult ADHD Self-Report Scale (ASRS) Symptom Checklist, the Barkley Current Symptoms Scale, the Brown Attention Deficit Disorder (ADD) Rating Scale for Adults, or the Copeland Symptom Checklist for Adult ADHD. The Wender Utah Rating Scale is used to retrospectively diagnose adults, by asking the adult questions about childhood behaviors. Some physicians ask their patients to obtain report cards from their former elementary and middle school, so that teacher comments can be viewed for possible indications of ADHD in childhood and adolescence.

The behavior of adults is also observed, for signs of inattentiveness, impulsivity, or hyperactivity. ADHD can be difficult to diagnose because many adults with ADHD also have depression and/or anxiety disorders. In general, most adults with ADHD can sit without constantly jumping up, although they may exhibit signs of hyperactivity such as constantly wiggling legs or squirming about in their seats. They may have difficulty remaining on one subject and may slip from one topic to another topic and yet another topic, with no seeming relationship between any of these topics.

It should be pointed out that extremely intelligent children often exhibit signs of inattentive behavior in the classroom due to boredom, thus a differential diagnosis is essential.

Treatment Options and Outlook

Individualized managed care, on a case-by-case method, is the most effective approach in treating ADHD. Successful treatment of children and adolescents depends on multimodal therapy involving parents, teachers, and mental health professionals. Adults with ADHD often benefit from both medication and therapy. Some adults with ADHD benefit from *coaching,* a specialized form of mentoring that is provided by a person experienced in working with adults with ADHD.

In an effort to reduce stress levels when ADHD is diagnosed, the mental health professional usually explains the nature of ADHD, trying to reduce feelings of guilt and blame in the family and at the same time improve the individual's self-esteem. When there are disorders of family dynamics or a learning disorder underlying the symptoms, these issues must be addressed as well. In the case of a child with ADHD, often other health and educational professionals, such as psychologists, special education specialists, or social workers may become involved.

Behavior modification and cognitive therapy are used in some cases of ADHD.

Methylphenidate (Ritalin) is the most commonly prescribed medication for children with ADHD in the United States, followed by other stimulants, such as amphetamines. There are short-acting forms of these drugs which last about three to four hours and also extended-release forms that last as long as 12 hours. A child on stimulant medication should be evaluated by the prescribing physician with some regularity.

Adolescents who are prescribed stimulants are at risk for misusing or selling their drugs, particularly if they have conduct disorder or a substance use disorder. A 2006 study in the *Journal of the American Academy of Child & Adolescent Psychiatry* divided adolescent and young adult subjects into one group with ADHD whose subjects primarily took stimulants and one group without ADHD who took psychiatric medications, including some stimulants. The researchers found that 11 percent of the ADHD group said that they had sold their medication to others, while no one in the non-ADHD group reported such a diversion of their medications. Additionally, 22 percent of the ADHD group said that they had misused their own medication, versus 5 percent of the non-ADHD group.

The researchers discovered that all of the stimulant drugs that were either misused or diverted to others were immediate-release stimulants. They also found that 80 percent of the individuals who reported having diverted or misused their drugs had either conduct disorder or a substance use disorder. As a result, the researchers recommended that extended-release medications or a non-stimulant drug, such as atomoxetine (Strattera), should be used to treat individuals in these populations who had ADHD. Atomoxetine is specifically approved by the Food and Drug Administration (FDA) for the treatment of ADHD in children and adolescents.

Adults may also be treated with stimulants, while some are treated with antidepressants which have proven effective in treating ADHD. BUPROPION (Wellbutrin) has been demonstrated as helpful for many people with ADHD, although it is not specifically approved by the FDA for the treatment of ADHD.

Both children and adults with ADHD often have other disorders, such as depression or an anxiety disorder, and they need medication and therapy for these conditions as well.

Risk Factors and Preventive Measures

Children, adolescents, and adults whose parents and/or siblings have been diagnosed or are likely to have ADHD have an increased risk for ADHD themselves, since there is a familial link to the disorder. Furthermore, a considerable amount of evidence shows that ADHD symptoms often occur during treatment or the outgoing stages of treatment of traumatized children who struggle with the arousal caused by trauma (See POST-TRAUMATIC STRESS DISORDER.) Differential diagnosis and a thorough life history assessment are important diagnostic information sources.

There are no known preventive measures to take against the possible development of ADHD.

American Psychiatric Association, *Diagnostic and Statistical Manual of Mental Disorders. Fourth Edition. Text Revision (DSM-IV-TR).* Washington, DC: American Psychiatric Association, 2000.

Biederman, J., et al., "Is ADHD a Risk Factor for Psychoactive Substance Use Disorders: Findings from a Four-Year Prospective Follow-up Study," *Journal of the American Academy of Child & Adolescent Psychiatry* 36, no. 1 (1997): 21–29.

Wilens, T. E., et al., "Characteristics of Adolescents and Young Adults with ADHD Who Divert or Misuse their Prescribed Medications," *Journal of the American Academy of Child & Adolescent Psychiatry* 45, no. 4 (2005): 408–414.

attitude, fear   See FEAR.

attribution theory   A theory regarding the individual's perception of the causes of his or her phobias and anxieties. People assign causes for certain types of behavior and seek information to support their theories. Such attributions have important behavioral consequences, since a significant part of the meaning attached to a situation or behavior is the cause to which it is attributed.

atychiphobia Fear of failure.
See also FAILURE, FEAR OF.

aulophobia Fear of seeing, handling, or playing a flute or similar wind instrument. To the psychoanalyst, the flute may serve as a phallic symbol and thus may be related to sexual fears.
See also FLUTE; PHALLIC SYMBOL; SEXUAL FEARS; SYMBOLISM.

aura A signal of an impending migraine headache or epileptic convulsion. The word aura comes from the Greek word for "breeze." An aura may include a feeling of dizziness, nausea, or visions of colored lights. Migraine sufferers' experiences of auras are highly individualized. For example, one may feel numbness or hear strange sounds, while another may be aware of strange tastes or odors. Some individuals become anxious when the aura heralding an attack begins. However, with therapy, an individual can learn to cope with the impending attack and try to abort it with appropriate medication and relaxation.
See also HEADACHES.

aurophobia Fear of gold.
See also GOLD, FEAR OF.

auroraphobia Fear of the auroral lights.

authority, fear of Many individuals fear authority. Some fear authority because the individual loses autonomy and feels dominated. Others fear authority when it loses its sense of legitimacy and becomes associated with coercion. Authority figures or groups within the family or government are feared when they are out of touch with the needs of their subordinates. A power structure that is opposed to social needs generally produces fear rather than cooperation and respect. A clash between two authority figures (e.g., two parents) is also disruptive and disturbing.
See also BUREAUCRACY, FEAR OF.

autodysomophobia A fear or delusion that the individual himself has a vile or repugnant odor. This phobia, often combined with automysophobia, or a fear of being dirty, is often associated with obsessive-compulsive disorder and may consequently result in excessive washing or an avoidance of social situations.
See also BODY ODOR, FEAR OF; DELUSIONS; DIRTY, FEAR OF BEING; OBSESSIVE-COMPULSIVE DISORDER; ODORS, FEAR OF.

autogenic training A form of psychotherapy that uses both body and mind to treat anxieties and other mental problems. Autogenic training, which originated in Germany in the early 20th century, is a self-help as well as therapeutic technique, involving a variety of breathing and relaxation exercises and exploration of the subconscious, with or without the help of a therapist. The system was developed by Johannes Schultz and was based on earlier work done by German neuropathologist Oskar Vogt.
See also RELAXATION THERAPY.

Schultz, J., and W. Luthe, *Autogenic Training: A Psychophysiological Approach in Psychotherapy* (New York: Grune & Stratton, 1959).

autohypnosis A form of self-hypnosis sometimes used with anxiety reactions to promote relaxation on cue in fearful situations. In general, autohypnosis by itself will not significantly relieve anxiety responses. It can, however, be used as a supplement to behavioral therapy to make images more vivid and to heighten one's ability to concentrate.

autoimmune disease A diverse group of disorders in which the immune system mistakes parts of its own body for the enemy, causing symptoms that can lead to anxieties and fears and symptoms of debilitating and long-term disease.

The main characteristic of these disorders is inflammation, varying from the merely irritating to the potentially deadly, as in diabetes. For example, in Type I diabetes, the immune system has damaged the body's insulin-producing capabilities.

Resulting autoimmune diseases can be either systemwide or specific to a particular body part. Rheumatoid arthritis and systemic lupus erythematosus are also autoimmune diseases.

See also ARTHRITIS; COMPLEMENTARY THERAPIES; DIABETES, FEAR OF; IMMUNE SYSTEM; MIND/BODY CONNECTIONS; PSYCHO-NEUROIMMUNOLOGY.

automation   The transition to automated production systems in the workplace where machines do the repetitive manual elements of the work process. As a result of automation, workers may be displaced or left with mainly supervisory functions. Either of these situations can lead to anxieties and fears regarding future employment.

Most industries, particularly manufacturing, have experienced displacement of workers as a result of automation of their production lines. Today, offices have been automated as well. It is estimated that office workers spend as much as 90 percent of their time at computers. The advent of computers has also meant automation of the delivery of services. A good example is the automatic bank teller, which not only cashes checks and deposits money but can provide those services 24 hours a day.

The introduction of automation is generally considered a positive step if the worker is assisted by the machine but maintains some CONTROL over its services. However, if operator skills and knowledge are taken over by the machine, the resulting monotony, lack of control, and social isolation may result in anxieties and stress.

Even when automation requires high skill from process operators, the monitoring of machines can become monotonous. Skills are used only during a small percentage of the work hours, and mechanical breakdowns can mean loss of work already completed. All of these elements have been shown to constitute sources of anxiety at both the psychological and physiological level and stress reactions.

See also AUTONOMY; BOREDOM, FEAR OF; CONTROL.

automobiles, fear of   Fear of automobiles is known as motorphobia and ochophobia.

See also DRIVING A CAR, FEAR OF.

automysophobia   Fear of being dirty.

See also DIRTY, FEAR OF BEING.

autonomic nervous system   The part of the nervous system that regulates involuntary functions and activates endocrine glands, smooth muscle, breathing, and heart muscle. The autonomic nervous system (ANS) is involved in the physiological changes that are part of expression and emotion; anxiety reactions are primarily those of the ANS. Increases in heart rate, perspiration on the face and palms of the hands, muscle tension, dry mouth, and queasy stomach result from activation of the ANS.

The part of the ANS known as the sympathetic nervous system (SNS) prepares the body for meeting emergencies and to deal with threats to one's well-being. SNS changes include increased respiration, increased heartbeat, perspiration, and muscle tension. When an event is judged as threatening, neural impulses are sent to the adrenal gland (the adrenal medulla), which in turn releases the hormones epinephrine (also known as adrenaline) and norepinephrine (noradrenaline) into the bloodstream, where they are circulated to various organ systems that they stimulate. The physical changes one perceives when anxious or frightened are partly a result of these hormones stimulating organs activated by the SNS.

Another branch of the ANS, called the parasympathetic nervous system (PNS), conserves energy and is activated when the individual moves toward calm, quiet, and relaxed states. The PNS helps to slow heart rate, reduce blood pressure, and facilitate digestion. In cases of extreme fright or shock and for some individuals who are fearful of blood or injury, there is a strong PNS response, which results in lowered blood pressure, dizziness, or fainting.

See also BLOOD PRESSURE; DIZZINESS; FAINTING.

EFFECTS OF AUTONOMIC NERVOUS SYSTEM ON BODILY SYSTEMS

Organ System	Sympathetic Branch	Parasympathetic Branch
Eyes/pupils	Dilates	Constricts
Heart rate	Increases Decreases	
Bronchia/Lungs	Dilates	Constricts
Salivary glands	Reduces saliva (thick)	Increases saliva (watery)
Stomach	Inhibits function	Stimulates function
Adrenal Medulla	Secretes epinephrine and norepinephrine	No effect
Sweat glands (hands and feet)	Increases sweating	No effect
Blood flow	Increases to skeletal muscles	No effect

autonomic side effect   Disturbance of the autonomic nervous system. This effect may be a result of the use of antipsychotic and antianxiety drugs. The autonomic side effects include higher or lower blood pressure, blurred vision, nasal congestion, dryness of the mouth, dizziness, seizures, psychotic symptoms, depression, and reduced sexual drive.

See also ADVERSE DRUG REACTION; AUTONOMIC NERVOUS SYSTEM.

autonomy   A feeling of being in CONTROL associated with attitudes of independence and freedom that may take many forms. An individual may express autonomy by making simple decisions for oneself. When one loses a sense of autonomy, one may experience anxieties, lose self-esteem, and become frustrated. In developing a sense of autonomy, peer groups play an important role. Children with good peer relationships generally acquire good feelings about themselves and develop confidence that others will like them. They will also develop the ability to realize what others expect of them and make choices about meeting those expectations in a flexible way without anxieties.

For some individuals, particularly teenagers, peer groups may be destructive to autonomy. This may be the case with teenagers whose experiences with peers have not enabled them to develop self-confidence. Under these circumstances, anxieties and a desire for approval or acceptance may lead to drugs, smoking cigarettes, or other destructive behaviors that seem to make the individual feel part of the group.

See also ANGER; CONTROL; FRUSTRATION; SELF-ESTEEM.

Johnson, D. S. and R. T. Johnson, "Peer Influences." In Corsini, Raymond, *Encyclopedia of Psychology.* (New York: Wiley, 1984), pp. 493–498.

May, Rollo, *Freedom and Destiny* (New York: W. W. Norton, 1981).

Vinack, W. E., "Independent Personalities." In Corsini, Raymond J. *Encyclopedia of Psychology*, Vol. 2. (New York: W. W. Norton, 1981), pp. 192–195.

autophobia   Fear of being alone, or fear of oneself.
See also BEING ALONE, FEAR OF; SOLITUDE, FEAR OF.

aversions   An aversion is a preparatory response to fear and could lead to anxiety responses. For example, many people have strong dislikes (rather than fears) of touching, hearing, tasting, or smelling certain things that most people are indifferent to or even enjoy. An aversion is not a phobia, because the feelings these people exercise are somewhat different from fear; aversions make one uncomfortable, perhaps feel cold and clammy, short of breath, and nauseated, not fearful. Fairly common aversions are the screechy sound of chalk against a blackboard, the scraping of a knife against a plate, the feel of fuzzy textures, wet wool, or rubber, the feel of raw seafood, or the taste or smell of other foods. Aversions, while not as disabling as fears and phobias, can influence a person's life. For example, a person who has an aversion to the sound of chalk on the blackboard may give up an ambition to be a schoolteacher. One who has an aversion to fuzzy textures may avoid touching the skin of fresh peaches and never eat fruits with fuzzy skins.

See also FUZZ AVERSION; SMELL, FEAR OF; TASTE, FEAR OF.

Marks, Isaac M., *Fears, Phobias and Rituals* (New York: Oxford University Press, 1987).
———, *Living with Fear* (New York: McGraw-Hill Book Co., 1978).

aversion therapy   A form of BEHAVIOR MODIFICATION to help the individual avoid undesirable behaviors or stimuli by associating them with unpleasant or painful experiences; also known as aversive therapy. This kind of therapy has been used to treat ALCOHOLISM, nail biting, BED-WETTING, smoking, fetishes, and many other "habit" problems as well as obsessive thoughts and compulsive behavior. The primary goal of the therapy is to enable the individual to make a connection between the behavior and the aversive reaction and thereby reduce the frequency of the undesirable behavior. Secondarily, alternative, acceptable behavior must be shaped and reinforced.

Electrical and chemical techniques have been used to create aversions. With electrical therapy, the therapist administers a mildly painful shock to the patient whenever the undesirable behavior, or its imagined equivalent, is elicited. With chemical therapy, the individual is given a drug to produce nausea and is then exposed to the deviant stimulus or is required to carry out the deviant act at the time the drug produces its maximal effect. Unfortunately, the drug effect cannot be paired with deviant behavior as precisely as electrical stimulation. The chemical method has been used most widely in treatment of alcoholism; the electrical method has been used predominantly in the treatment of sexual disorders.

There are limitations to aversion therapy, which is based on Ivan Petrovich Pavlov's classical conditioning theory, and therapists now place more importance on cognitive factors. A newer form of aversion therapy, based largely on modification of cognitive behavior, is known as covert sensitization. In this form of therapy, the patient is asked to imagine the deviant activity or stimulus and then to imagine some extremely undesirable consequence, such as nausea, shame, or pain.

See also BEHAVIOR THERAPY; CONDITIONED RESPONSE.

Blake, B., "The Application of Behavior Therapy to the Treatment of Alcoholism," *Behaviour Research and Therapy* 5 (1967): pp. 78–85.
Cautela, J., "Covert Sensitization," *Psychology Reports* 20 (1967): pp. 459–468.
Feidman, M. P., "Aversion Therapy for Sexual Disorders," *Psychology Bulletin* 65 (1966): pp. 65–69.
Lemere, G. and W. Voegtlin, "An Evaluation of the Aversion Treatment of Alcoholism," *Quarterly Journal of Studies of Alcohol* 11 (1950): pp. 199–204.
Rachman, S., and J. Teasdale, *Aversion Therapy and the Behavior Disorders* (Miami: University of Miami Press, 1969).

aviatophobia (aviophobia)   Fear of flying.
See also FLYING, FEAR OF.

avoidance learning   A procedure used to treat ANXIETIES and PHOBIAS by pairing a warning signal with an aversive event. After repetitions, the individual learns to respond to the signal alone and engages in avoidance behavior whether the aversive event occurs or not. The behavior is then maintained by negative reinforcement (avoidance of aversive stimulation). Fear reduction can result from avoidance responses, and avoidance responses can continue after the feared event no longer occurs. Although avoidance behavior is motivated by fear, it is reinforced by the presence of a new stimulus, indicating that relief has been achieved.

See also AVERSION THERAPY; NEUROTIC PARADOX.

avoidance response   An observable behavior resulting from an anxiety-provoking situation. For example, a person fearful of elevators might walk up 15 floors rather than enter the elevator. Avoidance occurs in anticipation of aversive stimulation, whereas escape is a response to aversive (anxiety-producing) stimulation. Where avoidance is not possible, a phobic individual might exhibit escape behavior, such as running away from the situation. Both kinds of responses help to reduce the individual's anxiety.

See also BEHAVIOR THERAPY.

avoidant personality disorder As classified by the American Psychiatric Association, the essential feature of this disorder is a pervasive pattern of anxiety, social discomfort, fear of negative evaluation, and timidity, beginning in early adulthood and present in a variety of contexts. Individuals with avoidant personality disorder have anxiety, depression, and anger at themselves for failing to develop social relations. Some individuals have social phobia as a complication, and others who have this personality disorder also have specific phobias. Some individuals who are agoraphobic show relatively pervasive avoidant behavior, but this is usually due to a fear of being in places or situations where help may not be available, rather than to a personality disorder.

Diagnostic criteria for Avoidant Personality Disorder, according to the American Psychiatric Association, are

- easily hurt by criticism or disapproval
- no close friends or confidants (or only one) other than first-degree relatives
- unwilling to become involved with people unless certain of being liked
- avoids social or occupational activities involving significant interpersonal contact; for example, refuses a promotion that will increase social demands
- reticence in social situations because of a fear of saying something inappropriate or foolish, or of being unable to answer a question
- fears being embarrassed by blushing, crying, or showing signs of anxiety in front of other people
- exaggerates potential difficulties, physical dangers, or risks involved in doing something ordinary but outside his or her usual routine; for example, may cancel social plans because he or she anticipates being exhausted by the effort of getting there.

See also AGORAPHOBIA; ANXIETY; PERSONALITY DISORDERS.

American Psychiatric Association, *Diagnostic and Statistical Manual of Mental Disorders,* 4th ed. (Washington, DC: American Psychiatric Press, 1994).

Ayurveda *Ayurveda* is derived from the Sanskrit words for "the science of health and knowledge." Over time, *Ayurveda* has come to mean "the science of life." While Western medicine works on illness, Ayurvedic medicine focuses on the person as a complex, multileveled individual. Anxiety and fears can be addressed by Ayurveda diagnosis and treatment.

Ayurvedic treatment is highly individualized for each person. For one who feels well, Ayurvedic activities make the most of one's mental, physical, and spiritual well-being, enabling better coping skills against the anxieties of daily life. When fighting illness or coping with specific anxieties, Ayurvedic therapy works by enhancing the healing potential within oneself.

Ayurvedic health care (in the United States) is meant to complement, not replace, standard medical treatment. Ayurvedic health care is considered a form of complementary therapy. Ayurvedic medicine was first recorded in the holy scriptures of the Vedas of India and is possibly the oldest recorded health science. Currently, Ayurvedic therapy addresses health in terms of body, mind, and spirit and may be helpful to some individuals experiencing stress.

Ayurveda is an art of insight that brings harmony to daily life and one's relationships. Believers say it can bring a quality of consciousness such that one can develop insight to deal with one's inner life and the anxieties of one's inner emotions—one's inner hurt, grief, and sadness.

Ayurvedic beliefs hold that life is a relationship between you and your body, mind, and consciousness. These relationships are life, and Ayurveda is a healing art that helps bring clarity to these relationships. Clarity in relationships brings compassion, and compassion is love; therefore, clarity is love. Without this clarity, there is no insight.

A characteristic element of Ayurveda is the determination of one's mind/body type. One's specific type is a combination of three fundamental principles, known as *doshas,* which govern thousands of mental and physical processes. These three principles *vata* (movement), *pitta* (metabolism), and *kapha* (structure), are the governing agents of nature. Permutations of the DOSHAS determine an individual's subtype; through careful observation over time and pulse diagnosis, a practitioner can determine imbalances of energy. Disease is diagnosed through questioning, observation, palpation, percussion, and listening to the heart, lungs, and intestines.

An ancient art of tongue diagnosis also describes characteristic patterns that can reveal the functional status of respective internal organs merely by observing the surface of the tongue. The tongue is the mirror of the viscera and reflects many pathological conditions.

Many factors affect the *doshas.* Disease can result from imbalanced emotions, such as unresolved anger, fear, anxiety, grief or sadness. Ayurveda classifies seven major causative factors in disease: hereditary, congenital, internal, external trauma, seasonal, natural tendencies or habits, and super-natural factors. Disease can also result from misuse, overuse, and underuse of the senses: hearing, touch, sight, taste, and smell.

Prana, the Ayurvedic term for "energy" has counterparts in Eastern medicine (*qi* or *chi*) and homeopathy (*vital force*). Pranic energy is mental and physical and can be changed by diet, exercise, herbs, or spiritual practices such as meditation. Pranic energy flows along specific paths, called *nadis,* which converge and cross in energy centers called *chakras* located along the length of the body. During an Ayurvedic examination, *chakras* are studied and *doshas* may be determined to be out of balance, leading to ill health.

In the United States, physician training in Ayurveda is under the direction of the Maharishi Training Program in Fairfield, Iowa, and directed by Dr. Deepak Chopra, who is also a contemporary writer about Ayurvedic medicine.

See also COMPLEMENTARY THERAPIES; IMMUNE SYSTEM; MIND/BODY CONNECTIONS; PSYCHONEURO-IMMUNOLOGY.

Kahn, Ada P., *The Encyclopedia of Stress and Stress-related Disorders,* 2nd ed. (New York: Facts On File, 2006).

babies, fear of Some people fear babies for many different reasons. For example, some parents fear holding a new baby because of its small size and apparent fragility. Parents have anxieties about first baths and hairwashings because the baby is slippery, squirms, and almost invariably cries. The fact that crying peaks at about the sixth week often causes anxieties for parents. The inability of a baby to communicate his or her feelings except by crying and the possibility of SUDDEN INFANT DEATH (SID) is frightening. A baby's fitful, noisy sleep pattern may make parents suspect that something is wrong or that the infant is not getting enough sleep. The appearance of a newborn baby may cause anxieties for parents who are not prepared for how newborns look. Newborns frequently have an oddly shaped skull, too much or too little hair, and discolored or wrinkled skin.

The psychological impact of a baby's arrival on both parents may cause anxieties. Parents may be frightened by their new responsibilities. New mothers often enter a period of DEPRESSION that is unpleasant for them as well as for the new fathers. A woman may feel that she has been replaced by the baby as the center of attention. A man's feelings of being on the fringe of events, which started with pregnancy, may continue. A couple naturally fears that the baby's birth may come between them and deprive them of the privacy and romance that had been present in their relationship.

The entrance of a new baby into a household also produces anxieties for parents because of the jealousy it produces. Older children and even pets may need special attention to keep them from resenting the presence of a new baby.

These fears usually subside with increased accommodation and experience with the newborn. If they do not, professional intervention may be required.

baby boomers The 76 million Americans born between 1946 and 1964. They represent the population explosion that began during World War II, peaked following the war, and lasted until the mid-1960s.

The baby boom has been attributed to several factors, including the wartime prosperity following the Great Depression, increased births as servicemen returned from the war, a lower marriage age than for previous generations, and a tendency to have children in quick succession early in marriage.

This generation has experienced many anxieties, both individual as well as societal. These anxieties have not been static but have been influenced by the changing times in which baby boomers have lived. As young adults, their protest against the Vietnam War labeled some hedonistic, rebellious, and undisciplined. When they reached college age, they were fighting for civil rights and were active in the women's movement. Improved birth control, more permissive sexual standards, and an emphasis on education for both sexes gave young women of the baby boom generation more choices. Resulting questions about pursuing careers, entering marriage, and having children are sources of anxiety that continue to haunt women in the 21st century.

A good job market and a rapidly expanding economy greeted many adult baby boomers and they were soon described as having materialistic tendencies that included acquiring possessions at an early age and "having it all." In reaction, baby boomers tended to become entrepreneurial and viewed a job as something that should be fulfilling and stimulating rather than simply a means to the end of supporting oneself and one's family. However, the sheer numbers of the baby boom generation created a population bulge that increased competition for jobs. A changing economy, downsizing, the looming failure of the Social Security System, rising health care costs, and the need to save for RETIREMENT have led to frustrations and additional anxieties for many.

See also BIOLOGICAL CLOCK; COMMUNICATION; INTERGENERATIONAL CONFLICTS; WORKING MOTHERS.

Silver, Don. *Baby Boomer Retirement: 65 Simple Ways to Protect Your Future* (Los Angeles: Adams-Hall Publishers, 1994).

bacilli, fear of   Fear of bacilli or of microorganisms in general is known as bacillophobia. Bacilli are a class of rod-shaped microorganisms, including many species of spore-forming bacteria.

See also CONTAMINATION, FEAR OF; GERMS, FEAR OF; PARASITES, FEAR OF.

bacillophobia   Fear of bacilli or of microorganisms in general.

See also BACILLI, FEAR OF; BACTERIA, FEAR OF.

back pain   Back pain has many causes. Anxiety, fear, and stress may be factors, as tension can contribute to a tightening of muscles and improper posture that leads to back pain and muscle spasms in the back. The stress that causes back pain may be physical or psychological. Many back pains begin during a particularly stressful time in life.

Back pain is feared because many workdays are lost because of it. People who do heavy lifting, carrying, sitting in one place, or are overweight often develop backaches that may be due to a ligament strain, a muscle tear, damage to a spinal facet joint or a disk prolapse. Understanding how one's work habits can lead to back pain and making appropriate changes is a step toward removing fear of chronic discomfort.

According to Richard Balderston, M.D., Section on Orthopedics at Pennsylvania Hospital, "Fifty to 80 percent of the population have back problems significant enough to cause them to be out of work at some point during their lifetime." Of those, only a handful of backache sufferers, perhaps 10 to 20 percent, ever discover a cause for their pain. Diag-

nosis often remains an unsolved mystery because the causes of back injury vary widely and the pain usually goes away on its own.

Anxieties caused by back pain affect the individual, family, and workplace. There are also many psychological implications, especially when one is diagnosed with "nonspecific back pain" and continues to suffer from it. Back pain is sometimes called a psychosomatic illness because is it hard to prove or disprove, is a lingering complaint, and often an "excuse" for avoiding work, social, or family obligations.

Treatment of Back Pain

Physicians often begin treatment by recommending conservative therapy for common backaches. For some pains, a few days of bed rest, anti-inflammatory or muscle relaxing medications, and the application of local heat to ease the pain and relax back muscles may be enough. Stretching exercises are important as soon as the back pain begins to improve. A light workout, stretching the lower back and hamstring muscles, may be helpful. In some cases, ACUPUNCTURE, massage, spinal manipulation, physical therapy, or wearing a back brace is recommended. An extra-firm mattress or a bed-sized sheet of heavy plywood under the mattress may also help. Consultation with a mental health worker or participation in a support group helps many people alleviate some of the anxieties of dealing with surgical treatments when they are necessary.

Tips for Preventing Stress on the Back

1. Stay in good physical condition and exercise regularly to keep muscles strong, particularly abdominal muscles, as they are important in back support.
2. Stand tall with your chin and abdomen tucked in and the curve of your lower back as straight as possible. When standing in one place for any length of time, put one foot up on the rung of a stool, box, or some other object to adjust your weight.
3. When sitting, sit well back in your seat with your back straight. Do not slouch. Change your position from time to time.
4. Sleep on your side with your knees bent, or on your back with only a small pillow under your

knees to release stress on your lower back. Avoid sleeping on your stomach.

5. When lifting objects, squat down with your knees and hips bent. Use your leg muscles to rise, keeping your back straight and elbows bent. Hold the object as close to your body as possible to avoid strain on other muscles.

Back Pain and Stress

When back pain persists over time, many individuals experience enough anxiety to lead to mild DEPRESSION and withdrawal. Persistent pain without relief makes one feel out of CONTROL of one's body. Taking a positive attitude and pursuing avenues of relief can increase one's feeling of control over the situation.

See also ALEXANDER TECHNIQUE; BODY THERAPIES; DEPRESSION; RELAXATION; STRESS.

bacteria, fear of   Fear of bacteria is known as bacteriophobia. Many individuals fear bacteria because some bacteria cause infections and can be seen only under a microscope or a magnifying glass. Bacteriophobics often fear many diseases and many have compulsions about hand-washing and cleanliness. Others may be obsessively concerned about coming into contact with germs. Howard Hughes, for example, took elaborate precautions against exposing himself to "germs." Bacteria are tiny, single-celled organisms that reproduce when each cell splits in half to form two completely new organisms. Although bacteriophobics fear many kinds of bacteria, only a few are dangerous to human beings. These, known as pathogens, are responsible for some serious infectious diseases, including tuberculosis, diphtheria, gonorrhea, typhoid fever, pneumonia, and tetanus (lockjaw). Some phobics with illness phobias fear these bacteria specifically. Bacteria also cause many skin infections, leprosy, boils, impetigo, folliculitis, and scarlet-fever blisters. Some who fear skin diseases also are bacteriophobic.

See also GERMS, FEAR OF; DISEASE, FEAR OF; ILLNESS, FEAR OF; OBSESSIVE-COMPULSIVE DISORDER.

bad men, fear of   Fear of bad men is known as scelerophobia or pavor sceleris. This term may refer to burglars, robbers, and others who attack or annoy unsuspecting victims. In urban areas where crime is prevalent, such fears are not totally unfounded, and individuals take precautions, such as locking their doors and cars and not walking alone in deserted areas. However, when these fears prevent an individual from going out and participating in normal activities, they can be considered phobias.

See also CRIME, FEAR OF; MUGGERS, FEAR OF; ROBBERS, FEAR OF.

bald, fear of becoming; baldness, fear of   Fear of becoming bald is known as phalacrophobia. This phobia may be related to a fear of loss of strength, fear of aging, fear of loss of attractiveness, or fear triggered by seeing one's own body. Baldness occurs when hair falls out and is not replaced by new hair growth. "Male pattern" baldness is the most common type of baldness and accounts for about 95 percent of all cases of baldness in men. Women also fear hair loss and hair thinning with age, and some seek assistance from beauticians or use artificial hairpieces.

Many people fear other types of temporary hair loss caused by infection, disease, some scalp disorders, and certain drugs (such as those used in chemotherapy). Hair loss may also occur after pregnancy; although this is somewhat frightening, normal regrowth will usually begin again after a few months. An individual who has had a hair loss from a disease will become less anxious about it when he or she realizes that the baldness is temporary.

Parents often become fearful if their babies develop temporary bald spots on the back of their heads caused by the friction of rubbing the head against bedding. Adults also sometimes develop bald spots if their work gear or rough clothing produces friction.

Another type of baldness that causes much anxiety is alopecia areata. In this condition, bald patches suddenly appear on the scalp and occasionally on other hairy areas such as the beard, eyelashes, and eyebrows. The cause of this disorder is unknown, but the hair generally regrows.

See also AGING, FEAR OF; BODY IMAGE; HAIR, FEAR OF.

bald people, fear of   Fear of bald people is known as peladophobia. Those who have this fear may be repelled by the sight of a shiny, bald head. They may also fear going bald themselves. Some who fear bald people may fear contracting the disease that caused the baldness. Other reasons for fearing bald people may be unique to the individual, such as having had a previously frightening experience with a bald person. In psychoanalytic terms, the bald head may be symbolic of eggs, fertility, or lack of fertility.

See also BALD, FEAR OF BECOMING.

ballistophobia   Fear of missiles.

See also MISSILES, FEAR OF.

barber's chair syndrome   Barber's chair syndrome includes the fear of obtaining a haircut or visiting a barber shop or beauty shop. The fear may be related to a fear of confinement and of restricted musculo-skeletal movement (being "trapped") because one must sit still for a period of time. Barber's chair syndrome includes some aspects of agoraphobia, because some individuals who fear going out also fear going to barbershops. The syndrome may be related to social phobia, because social phobics fear being seen in what they consider compromising situations, such as with their hair half cut or covered in the barber's wrap, which also may produce a feeling of confinement. Phobics may also have anxiety about trusting other people (in this case, the barber). Additional fears may relate to being cut with the barber's scissors or razor. Individuals who have barber's chair syndrome sometimes experience sweating, nausea, dizziness, weakness, increased muscle tension, headache, and palpitations. Many individuals have been treated for this syndrome, with varying degrees of success, by relaxation and desensitization therapy, in vivo desensitization, assertiveness training, and drug therapy.

See also AGORAPHOBIA; HAIRCUT, FEAR OF GETTING A; SOCIAL PHOBIA.

Erwin, William J., "Confinement in the Production of Human Neuroses: The Barber's Chair Syndrome," *Behavior Research Therapy* 1 (1963): pp. 175–183.

barbiturates   A group of psychotropic substances that are used as antianxiety drugs, SEDATIVES, anticonvulsants, and hypnotics. Derived from barbituric acid, these drugs depress the central nervous system. Some examples of barbiturates are pentobarbital (Nembutal), secobarbital (Seconal), butalbital (Fiornal), butabarbital (Butisol), talbutal (Lotusate), aprobarbital (Alurate), and phenobarbital (Luminal).

Shortly after the beginning of the 20th century, barbiturates replaced narcotics and other sleep-inducing drugs for many people. Until BENZODIAZEPINES became available in the 1950s, barbiturates were the largest and most widely used group of sedatives and hypnotics. They produce increasing sedation with increased dosage, causing poorer performance in vigilance tests, increased bodily unsteadiness, decreased intellectual performance, some loss of motor skills, and an underestimation of time.

The chronic use of barbiturates may lead to a tolerance, meaning that higher doses are needed to achieve the same result, as well as both psychological and physical dependence on the drug. Barbiturates used to be one of the leading causes of fatal drug poisoning. For this reason, physicians generally prescribe only small quantities of these drugs. Barbiturates are controlled drugs under the Controlled Substances Act.

Barbiturate addiction refers to the physical and psychological dependence on barbiturates. Some phobia sufferers who were prescribed barbiturates to diminish their anxiety symptoms have become addicted and some have experienced extreme withdrawal effects.

Some adults abuse barbiturates, whether prescribed to them or obtained through illicit means. According to data from the Monitoring the Future study of adults, in 2004, 7.2 percent of college students and 12.2 percent of their same-age peers reported having abused barbiturates.

See also ANXIETY; DRUGS.

Johnston, Lloyd D., et al., *Monitoring the Future: National Survey Results on Drug Use, 1975–2004. Volume II: College Students & Adults Ages 19–45.* (Bethesda, MD: National Institute on Drug Abuse, National Institutes of Health, 2005).

barophobia   Fear of gravity.
See also GRAVITY, FEAR OF.

barren spaces, fear of   Fear of barren spaces is known as cenophobia. Many who have this phobia also have AGORAPHOBIA. Some fear barren spaces while walking or driving a car; others can go through barren spaces in a vehicle but are afraid of walking through such an area. Fear of barren spaces may also be related to a fear of LANDSCAPE or certain types of landscape.
See also LANDSCAPE, FEAR OF.

basic anxiety   An anxiety characterized by vague feelings of loneliness, helplessness, and fear of a potentially hostile world. As conceptualized by German-American psychiatrist Karen Horney (1885–1952), basic anxiety is the source from which neurotic tendencies get their intensity and pervasiveness.
See also ANXIETY; FEAR.

basiphobia   Fear of walking. Also known as basophobia.
See also WALKING; STANDING UPRIGHT, FEAR OF.

basistasiphobia (or basostasophobia)   Fear of walking and standing upright.
See also WALKING, FEAR OF; STANDING UPRIGHT, FEAR OF.

bathing, fear of   Fear of bathing is known as ablutophobia. Some who have this fear also fear WATER. Some fear being seen in the nude. Some fear that their bodies will be criticized or compared with those of others. Some fear that harm will come to their skin from the water. Others fear warm water or cold water. This phobia extends to taking baths, taking showers, and swimming.
See also SKIN; WATER, FEAR OF.

bathophobia   Fear of depths. This fear may be noticeable in situations such as looking into a dark room or boating or swimming in deep water. A person who fears depths may be comfortable when he or she can see the bottom of the lake but not in deeper water. Similarly, such an individual may not fear a dark space when he or she is aware of the size of the room.
See also DEPTHS, FEAR OF.

bathroom phobia   Fear of the bathroom or toilet. Some children and some adults who have obsessive-compulsive disorders have this fear. They may be afraid of falling into the toilet, of being attacked by a monster coming from it, or of being infected. Bathroom phobia may also be related to a fear of dirt and germs, of using a toilet other than in one's own home, or of being seen or heard by others while urinating or defecating. Fears of urination or defecation in unfamiliar bathrooms are often not disclosed (or even assessed by surveys) but from clinical reports may be extensive. From the psychoanalytic viewpoint, bathroom phobia may involve ideas of castration.
See also CASTRATION FEAR; DEFECATING, FEAR OF; URINATING, FEAR OF.

Campbell, Robert J., Psychiatric Dictionary (New York: Oxford University Press, 1981).

batophobia   Fear of high objects, such as tall buildings.
See also HEIGHTS, FEAR OF; HIGH OBJECTS, FEAR OF.

batrachophobia   Fear of frogs. The term also sometimes applies to fear of reptiles.
See also FROGS, FEAR OF.

bats, fear of   Some people fear bats because in folklore, myth, and art bats have become symbolic of black magic, darkness, madness, peril, and torment. The bat has been thought to be a ghost and also a witches' familiar, capable of transporting evil spirits into and out of the human body. Some people believe in a superstition that bats are attracted to women's hair and that once entangled they can be cut out only by a man.

Most bats have gained their malevolent and fear-inducing reputation because of their ghastly appearance, avoidance of light, and ability to hunt in the dark. The vampire bats of Mexico and Central and South America deserve their bad name, as they actually do feed on the blood of humans and animals, sometimes choosing favorite individuals to attack. The bat can draw blood from a sleeping victim because its saliva apparently contains an anesthetic substance that deadens the pain of the bite.

See also FLYING THINGS, FEAR OF.

Breland, Osmond, *Animal Life and Lore* (New York: Harper & Row, 1972).

Jobes, Gertrude, *Dictionary of Mythology, Folklore and Symbols* (New York: Scarecrow Press, 1961).

Cavendish, Richard, *Man, Myth and Magic* (New York: Marshall Cavendish, 1983).

battle fatigue   Also known as shell shock. A more recent term for this is POST-TRAUMATIC STRESS DISORDER.

beards, fear of   Fear of beards, or of persons who have beards, is known as pogonophobia. In a classic study during the 1920s, John Watson was able to condition this fear in a young boy by classical conditioning methods. He found that the fear first conditioned to a rabbit generalized to other hairy objects such as beards, animals, and fur coats.

beating, fear of   Fear of beating or being beaten may have ritualistic or religious significance or, according to psychoanalytic theory, may be related to fantasies of sexual arousal. Freud discussed beating, or flagellation, as a fantasy related to masturbation. According to Freud, girls have three phases of beating fantasies; first the father beats a sibling, next the girl herself, and then boys who are not necessarily siblings. In boys, according to Freud, beating fantasies originate from an incestuous attachment to the father. The boy evades the threat of homosexuality by transforming the beating father into the beating mother, while the girl transforms herself in fantasy into a man and derives masochistic pleasure from what appears on the surface to be a sadistic fantasy. In our culture, fears of beating and personal violence are prevalent among young children and youths. Psychologists point out that we live in a violent society. Surveys of children find that fears of being attacked at home or on the street are very common.

See also FANTASIES; SEXUAL FEARS.

Deutsch, Albert, and H. Fishman, *The Encyclopedia of Mental Health* (New York: Franklin Watts, 1963), p. 75.

beauty shop, fear of   Some women fear going to a beauty shop because they fear going out (in the case of agoraphobics), because they fear that they will be judged unattractive by others in the shop (dysmorphophobia), or because they fear being confined in the beautician's chair. Some women fear being helpless during their visit to the beauty shop and fear that they may not be able to make a quick exit if they feel a need to leave the scene. Others fear being at the mercy of another person, in this case the beautician. Some fear that their appearance may be changed drastically by mistake; for example, too much hair cut off, their hair color changed unexpectedly, or the degree of curl not what they expected. Some women fear being seen by others in a vulnerable situation, such as while they are having their hair cut or colored. Fear of going to the beauty shop is related also to social phobia.

See also AGORAPHOBIA; BARBER'S CHAIR SYNDROME; SOCIAL PHOBIA.

bed, fear of   Fear of beds is known as clinophobia. Fear of beds and of going to bed may be related to sleep phobias or sleep disorders. Persons who fear going to bed may do so because of unpleasant past experiences such as chronic insomnia, night terrors, sleepwalking episodes, or fear of bed-wetting. Others may fear beds and going to bed because they are afraid that they will not wake up; for some, fear of going to bed is related to a fear of death.

See also BED-WETTING, FEAR OF; WAKING UP, FEAR OF NOT.

bed-wetting Bed-wetting, medically known as enuresis, means uninhibited or unconscious urination during sleep by a person over the age of three. The cause of the problem may be either emotional or physical. A child who fears having a urinary accident, who has perhaps been punished for or embarrassed by a past accident, may have nightmares about the accident or about going to the bathroom; during the dream he may urinate into the bed. A child who has had bed-wetting accidents at home may be fearful of visiting another child's home, of napping anyplace but at home, or of falling asleep in a car. The best way to relieve a child's fear of bed-wetting is through reassurance that if an accident happens, punishment and shaming will not ensue. Physical problems that may cause bed-wetting include infections or inflammation of the urinary tract, systematic diseases such as diabetes and hypothyroidism, and exhaustion; these should be treated medically. The child can be given less liquid in the two-hour period before bedtime; if bed-wetting occurs about two hours after the child has gone to sleep, he can be awakened a little before that time and accompanied to the bathroom. Gradually, he will develop the habit of waking himself when he feels an urge to urinate. If the cause is emotional (such as parental conflict), contributing factors can be identified and corrected. For example, the child can be retrained in his toilet habits. When an older child or adult urinates involuntarily during waking hours, the problem is known as incontinence. O. Hobart Mowrer developed a "bell and pad" device based on a two-stage classical conditioning model. This device effectively treats bed-wetting in almost 90 percent of all situations. The device is commercially available.

See also BED, FEAR OF; SLEEP.

bees, fear of Fear of bees is known as apiphobia or melissophobia. Fear of bees, which combines the anxiety of potential injury with a general fear of flying insects, often begins in the preschool or early school years. The fear may result from a child's own experience or from hearing frightening stories or seeing frightening movies. Bee phobics report that flying, stinging insects give the appearance of attacking them. The fact that fear of a tiny insect may seem ridiculous to others is often upsetting to the phobic but may be of assistance in treatment.

The consequences of a fear of bees may mean restricted travel (so as to avoid seeing bees), driving with the windows of the car up at all times, or even staying indoors during daylight hours.

See also FLYING THINGS, FEAR OF; STINGS, FEAR OF.

Melville, Joy, *Phobias and Obsessions* (New York: Coward, McCann & Geoghegan, 1977).
Sarafino, Edward P., *The Fears of Childhood* (New York: Human Sciences Press, 1986).

behavioral family therapy An approach to family therapy using techniques of behavioral therapy. Therapy includes modifying the ways in which the identified patient receives attention from the others in the family. Behavioral family therapy is often used in treating agoraphobia. The therapist helps identify the problem behavior, chooses reasonable goals and alternative adaptive behaviors, and directs and guides the family to change their patterns of reinforcement toward target behaviors.

See also BEHAVIOR THERAPY.

behavior analysis A study of the relationship of problem behaviors and their consequences. Behavior analysis is the first step in behavioral therapies, which are based on the principles of operant conditioning. During behavior analysis, the therapist will examine the interaction between stimulus, response, and consequence and plan a program according to the individual's needs. Behavior analysis is an ongoing process that ends only when the treatment goals have been reached.

See also BEHAVIOR MODIFICATION; DIAGNOSIS.

behavior constraint theory The theory that an individual may develop a helpless attitude or a phobic behavior when he or she cannot gain control over certain events.

See also LEARNED HELPLESSNESS.

behaviorism School of psychology associated with American psychologist John Broadus Watson (1878–

1958), who proposed that observable behavior, not consciousness, is the proper subject of psychology. OPERANT CONDITIONING evolved from this point of view, and the behavioristic approach led to many later techniques of behavior modification and methods for treating phobias. By this time, however, Watson had left psychology to pursue a career in advertising.

See also BEHAVIOR THERAPY.

behavior modification A type of psychotherapy used to treat phobias that stresses the effect of learning on behavior, uses active therapist and client involvement and *in vivo* practices, outlines explicit goals and desired new behaviors, and evaluates progress toward those goals. Behavior modification does not rely on diagnostic labels and deemphasizes the importance of the past in determining current behavior.

See also BEHAVIOR THERAPY.

behavior psychotherapy See BEHAVIOR THERAPY.

behavior rehearsal A behavior therapy technique in which the patient practices a new behavior in a controlled setting aided by the therapist. The therapist may use techniques of MODELING, coaching, feedback, positive reinforcement, and role playing. Behavior rehearsal is useful in treating SOCIAL PHOBIAS. A widely used form of behavior rehearsal is assertiveness training, in which inhibited, submissive individuals learn to behave more assertively, to express anger, to respond to another's anger, and to not feel guilty or anxious in doing so.

See also ASSERTIVENESS TRAINING; BEHAVIOR THERAPY; PHOBIAS.

behavior shaping See OPERANT CONDITIONING.

behavior therapy A form of psychological, emotional, and behavioral therapy that stresses learned responses; also known as behavior modification. Unlike a psychoanalyst, a behavior therapist does not regard phobias as symptoms of unconsciously

caused, "deeper" problems that require restructuring of the psyche. Behavior therapists regard panic, anxiety, and obsessive-compulsive behavior as something that has a learned component (as well as a biological component) and can be replaced with desirable behaviors. Behaviorists generally do not believe that other drastic symptoms will appear to replace the ones thus eliminated.

Behavior therapy is considered the most effective treatment for AGORAPHOBIA, social phobias, and other specific phobias, as well as for obsessions, compulsions, certain sexual problems, and alcoholism. Many therapists use behavior therapy to treat phobias, sometimes in conjunction with other forms of treatment.

Behavior therapy focuses on measurable aspects of observable behavior, such as frequency or intensity of particular behaviors like compulsive hand-washing, physiological response, and verbal reports. Verbal reports by the patients and self-rating scales are commonly used to describe details of behavior. Specific treatment techniques are tailored by the therapist to the needs of the individual.

Treatment goals are defined by the therapist in conjunction with the patient and the patient's family. In behavior therapy, the therapist is seen as an instructor or coach, and the patient chooses whether to try to learn a new behavior. The goal generally is to develop self-controlled behaviors and an increased repertoire of new, more adaptive behaviors.

Behavior therapy became fairly well established during the latter half of the 20th century. Important individuals in the development of behavioral techniques include Joseph Wolpe, Hans Jurgen Eysenck and Frederick B. Skinner, Ogden Lindsley, and Ted Ayllon, who based much of their work on the earlier works of Ivan Pavlov and John Watson. Lindsley coined the term "behavior therapy" in a research article in the late 1950s. Wolpe, in his book *Psychotherapy by Reciprocal Inhibition,* introduced many of the basic therapies used today, such as systematic desensitization, sexual therapies, and assertiveness training.

Behavior therapy includes many basic learning techniques, such as reduction of anxiety, desensitization, flooding, classical conditioning, modeling, operant conditioning, aversive therapy, and reciprocal inhibition. Therapists often use techniques that gradually expose the phobic individual to the feared objects or situations. Such exposure may take place in real life or in the individual's imagination. The gradualness of the exposure is considered important in making the treatment effective, combined with the simultaneous use of relaxation responses and cognitive changes.

A major development in the treatment of phobias was described in 1958 by South African psychiatrist Joseph Wolpe (1914–97), who had a background in learning theory. Wolpe reported excellent results in treating adults who had a variety of neuroses, including phobic anxiety, hysteria, reactive depression, and obsessive-compulsive disorder, with a procedure called "systematic desensitization," adapted from a technique developed in the 1920s for helping children overcome animal phobias. Based on the principle of "reciprocal inhibition," this technique trains the individual to relax the muscles, imagine increasing degrees of anxiety-producing stimuli, and then face increasing degrees of the fear-producing stimuli in vivo until the maximum stimulus no longer causes great anxiety.

Systematic desensitization requires the individual to learn deep-muscle relaxation and to rank situations that causes anxiety. For example, an individual who fears elevators might place at the top of the list of things that make him or her anxious riding to the top of a high building alone in an elevator; merely looking at the entrance to an elevator from the lobby of a building might rank at the bottom of the list of fear-producing stimuli.

After relaxing, the individual is then asked to imagine, in as much detail as possible, the least fear-producing item from the list. By relaxing while imagining the feared situation, the individual may weaken the association between the phobic situation and anxious feelings. Once he becomes comfortable imagining the least-threatening situation, he gradually moves up the hierarchy.

Some therapists believe that facing a feared situation in the imagination may be just as effective as facing it in reality. However, most therapists have found that there is a gap between imagination and reality. Once the individual has completed densensitization treatment and goes on to face the real fear, he or she is likely to regress slightly back down the list. For example, an individual who has learned to remain calm while riding an imaginary elevator to the top of a building may be able to enter an actual elevator but may not be comfortable riding in it right away. By taking a floor at a time, however, the individual will be able to master the fear and eventually ride to the top of the building alone.

During the late 1960s, another treatment for phobias was developed by Thomas Stampfl, called "implosion" or "implosive therapy." Implosion was a modification of a technique known as "imaginal flooding," or just "flooding."

Flooding

Flooding, like desensitization, involves the individual's experiencing fear-provoking situations in his or her imagination or *in vivo*. In flooding, the individual is exposed directly to a maximum level of the fear-producing stimulus without any graduated approach.

However, in flooding, the therapist, rather than the individual, controls the timing and content of the scenes to be imagined. The therapist describes such scenes with great vividness, in a deliberate effort to make them as disturbing as possible to the phobic person. The individual is not instructed to relax. Rather, the aim is for him to experience his fears and anxieties with maximum intensity, which gradually diminishes. The prolonged experience with these feared objects or situations is designed to help the individual to experience "extinction" of the anxiety response.

Implosive Therapy

This is a variation and extension of the flooding technique. The individual is repeatedly encouraged to imagine a fear-producing situation at maximum intensity in order to experience as intense anxiety as possible. Assuming there is no actual danger in the situation, the anxiety response is not reinforced and thus becomes gradually reduced through extinction. However, the therapist also begins to weave into the terrifying images fantasy-based images and thoughts drawn from psychoanalytic theory, presumably to also extinguish these unconscious factors. Implosive therapy was developed by Thomas Stampfl, an American psychologist, in the mid-1950s as a treatment for anxiety-related disorders and other negative emotional responses.

Like desensitization, both flooding and implosive techniques reduce phobic anxiety and behavior in persons with simple phobias, but desensitization appears to be more effective and more permanent. There is some evidence that small amounts of flooding are more effective with agoraphobics.

Exposure Therapy

This is a term used to describe a variety of behavioral therapies that have in common the use of gradual exposure to a feared situation (such as systematic desensitization), exposure at full intensity (flooding and implosive therapy), and exposure with cognitive modification (contextual therapy). Contextual therapy was developed by American psychiatrist Manual Zane (1913–   ). The focus of contextual therapy is to keep the person rooted to the present situation and to work with the anxiety-producing internal cues of the person.

Modeling and Covert Modeling

In this form of therapy, the phobic individual watches another person, often of the same sex and age as the phobic, successfully perform a particular feared action, such as crossing the street or taking an elevator. The phobic presumably experiences vicarious extinction of the feared response. Modeling is also called social learning or observational learning.

In "covert modeling" the phobic individual simply imagines that another individual is facing the same phobic situation and that anxiety reduction is experienced by the model. Such "vicarious" extinction processes have many potential applications in treatment.

COMPARISONS OF PSYCHOTHERAPY AND BEHAVIOR THERAPY

Psychotherapy	Behavior Therapy
1. Based on inconsistent theory never properly formulated in postulate form.	Based on consistent, properly formulated theory leading to testable deductions.
2. Derived from clinical observations made without necessary control observations or experiments.	Derived from experimental studies specifically designed to test basic theory and deductions made therefrom.
3. Considers symptoms the visible upshot of unconscious causes ("complexes").	Considers symptoms as unadaptive conditioned responses.
4. Regards symptoms as evidence of *repression*.	Regards symptoms as evidence of faulty learning.
5. Believes that symptomatology is determined by defense mechanisms.	Believes that symptomatology is determined by individual differences in conditionability and autonomic lability, as well as accidental environmental circumstances.
6. All treatment of neurotic disorders must be *historically* based.	All treatment of neurotic disorders is concerned with habits existing at *present;* their historical development is largely irrelevant.
7. Cures are achieved by handling the underlying (unconscious) dynamics, not by treating the symptom itself.	Cures are achieved by treating the symptom itself, i.e. by extinguishing unadaptive C.R.s and establishing desirable C.R.s.
8. Interpretation of symptoms, dreams, acts, etc. is an important element of treatment.	Interpretation, even if not completely subjective and erroneous, is irrelevant.
9. Symptomatic treatment leads to the elaboration of new symptoms.	Symptomatic treatment leads to permanent recovery provided autonomic as well as skeletal surplus C.R.s are extinguished.
10. Transference relations are essential for cures of neurotic disorders.	Personal relations are not essential for cures of neurotic disorder, although they may be useful in certain circumstances.

H. Eysenck, *Behaviour Therapy and the Neuroses* (London: Pergamon Press, 1960).

Operant Conditioning

This technique is based on the principle that individuals will either maintain or decrease the frequency of a particular behavior as a result of responses they receive from their environment. Thus behavior that produces reinforcing consequences is strengthened, while behavior that produces aversive consequences is weakened. Avoidance and approach behavior to feared stimuli are often considered under operant control and thus modifiable through operant shaping.

Hypnosis

Although hypnosis is not based on learning theory, it is classified as a behavioral technique because the role of the therapist is active, rather than passive, as it is in psychoanalysis. Hypnosis can be used to produce a hypnotic trance in which the individual becomes very receptive to suggestion. Through posthypnotic suggestion, an individual may learn to change behavior patterns, such as having phobic reactions to certain stimuli. Hypnosis by itself, however, is not an adequate form of treatment for phobias.

Biofeedback

Biofeedback, a technique to monitor psychophysiological events by electrical feedback, provides an anxious or phobic individual with a basis for self-regulation of certain processes, such as reaction to fearful situations. The technique is useful in many approaches to therapy for anxieties and phobias. It establishes a diagnostic baseline by noting physiological reactions to stressful events, enables therapists to relate this information to the individual's verbal reports, fills gaps in the individual's history, and encourages relaxation of the body part to which the biofeedback equipment is applied. Relaxation training is often suggested to assist the individual in controlling anxiety reactions.

See also AVERSION THERAPY; DESENSITIZATION; OPERANT CONDITIONING; PAVLOVIAN CONDITIONING; RECIPROCAL INHIBITION.

being alone, fear of　Fear of being alone is known as autophobia. The term taphephobia is also used for being alone, but usually refers to fear of being

BURIED ALIVE. Some agoraphobic individuals are also afraid of being alone, particularly when they leave the place where they feel secure. Infants and young children fear being alone, generally because they feel helpless and are afraid of being abandoned by their parents or other caretakers. Older people also fear being alone as they see others in their age group retiring and moving away or dying. A fear of being alone and a feeling of being far from anyone who cares about one may sometimes lead to DEPRESSION.

For people of all ages, fears are usually greater when individuals are alone. Even though people who have SOCIAL PHOBIA may avoid particular forms of social contact, they rarely like to be alone most of the time.

See also GROWING OLD, FEAR OF; SEPARATION ANXIETY.

Marks, Isaac M., *Fears, Phobias and Rituals* (New York: Oxford University Press, 1987), p. 52.

being enclosed, fear of　Fear of being enclosed in a very confined space is known as clithrophobia. Somewhat similar to claustrophobia, clithrophobia generally applies to a very small, well-defined space, whereas claustrophobia also can refer to fear of being in a large room without an easy or visible way out.

See also BEING LOCKED IN, FEAR OF; CLAUSTROPHOBIA.

being locked in, fear of　Fear of being locked in is known as claustrophobia. The term clithrophobia might also apply, if the space in which one is locked is very small as well as confining. Some individuals specifically fear being locked in an elevator, a closet, their car, or a room.

being looked at, fear of　Fear of being looked at, or stared at, is known as scopophobia. Fear of two staring eyes is common throughout the animal kingdom, including man. Particularly in individuals who have social fears, being looked at means being the object of another's attention and intention; the gaze of others thus may trigger acute discomfort in self-conscious persons. Many social phobics are afraid of being watched by others.

Realizing that eyes are looking at one may be instinctive. The eyes of another are one of the first figural entities perceived by the infant. Of all the features of the face, the eyes possess the greatest combination of those qualities that attract an infant's fixation—figure, color, movement, and light reflection. In human infants, two eyes are the minimal visual stimulus required to elicit the first human social response, the smile. The infant's smile and his fixation on the eyes of the person looking at him may be an instinctual response of the infant that itself elicits further approach and caring behavior by the mother.

The effect of being looked at has been studied in animals. For example, when rhesus monkeys see a human face observing them in the laboratory, they show a change in behavior and in electrical activity in the brain stem. Many species of mammals use their eyes and eye markings to intimidate intruders, and eyes and conspicuous eyelike markings are used by birds and insects as defense against attack.

See also EYES, FEAR OF.

being oneself, fear of   Some individuals live their lives to fulfill expectations of others and fear being themselves. Some individuals tend to mirror the lives of their same-sex parent. Some women are raised to be images of their mothers in terms of appearance, education, interests, and life goals. Such women grow up aspiring to be and have as much as, but no more than, their mothers. They may imitate their mothers even to the extent of having the same number of children. Similarly, some young men grow up following their father's sports, educational, and career examples. Such individuals become accustomed to subordinating their own desires to those of their parent. As adults, they look to their spouse for guidance in everyday decisions and fear following their own desires and making their own choices.

Often people who grew up under domineering parents raise their children to meet their own expectations and perpetuate the fear of being oneself in their children.

The existentialists say that people are afraid that they do not have a true self and live behind a facade. Most therapies, traditional and behavioral, emphasize reduction of the person's facade or conditioned aspects of their behavior.

being poisoned, fear of   Fear of being poisoned is known as toxocophobia. This fear may be related to a fear of contamination, dirt, or germs.

See also CONTAMINATION, FEAR OF; DIRT, FEAR OF; GERMS, FEAR OF; OBSESSIVE-COMPULSIVE DISORDER; POISON, FEAR OF.

being touched, fear of   Fear of being touched is known as aphenphobia, haphephobia, and haptephobia. This fear may be a social phobia. In some cases, fear of being touched may relate to sexual fears. Some people fear being touched because they fear contamination.

See also CONTAMINATION, FEAR OF; SEXUAL FEARS.

belching, fear of   Some individuals who have social phobias fear belching in front of others. Belching, or the common burp, occurs when one swallows air or when gas is produced in the stomach by the chemical reactions between food and digestive juices.

See also FLATULENCE, FEAR OF.

belonophobia   Fear of needles and pins is known as belonophobia or belonephobia.

See also ACUPUNCTURE, FEAR OF; NEEDLES AND PINS, FEAR OF.

bends, fear of   Divers and enthusiasts of scuba (self-contained underwater breathing apparatus) diving fear "the bends," which is also known as caisson disease or decompression sickness. Fear of the bends deters many sports enthusiasts from undertaking scuba diving. Fear of developing this condition motivates participants to learn their skills adequately before going underwater and to observe many safety precautions. The bends occur when a person has been under high atmospheric pressure for a prolonged period, usually a matter of hours, and is suddenly exposed to a lower pressure. When a person stays underwater at a considerable depth, body fluids and tissues conform to the pressure, and the individual may have difficulty if he does not decompress himself slowly while rising to the surface. This is a natural fear that is quite logical and adaptive. However, if one begins to excessively avoid scuba diving because of such a fear, then it might be called a phobia.

See also DIVING, FEAR OF; WATER, FEAR OF.

benzodiazepine drugs   A group of prescription medications that are widely prescribed to help relieve the symptoms of anxiety. These medications also act as muscle relaxants, sedatives, and anticonvulsants, and they are sometimes used to ease withdrawal symptoms from alcohol for individuals with ALCOHOLISM or to treat epileptic seizures. Different drugs in this class are approved for different conditions. For example, drugs such as ALPRAZOLAM (Xanax) and clonazepam (Klonopin) are approved by the Food and Drug Administration (FDA) for the treatment of panic disorder. Other benzodiazepines are prescribed for the general treatment of anxiety.

Some benzodiazepines are used to treat insomnia, such as estazolam (ProSom), temazepam (Restoril), and triazolam (Halcion).

Benzodiazepines are Schedule IV drugs, which means that they are controlled like narcotics, although the risk of addiction is significantly lower. Dependencies and fears during withdrawal make these drugs more appropriate for short-term use. These medications may be taken orally or by injection.

Benzodiazepine drugs have less toxicity and fewer drug interaction problems than both BARBITURATES and nonbarbiturate sedative-hypnotic drugs. Also, benzodiazepine drugs have a lower risk of cardiovascular and respiratory depression compared to barbiturates and, as a result, are often used before general anesthesia is administered. However, benzodiazepines are sedating, and individuals taking benzodiazepine drugs should avoid alcohol altogether because the combination of alcohol and drugs could result in a dangerous depression of the central nervous system.

Benzodiazepines can also cause slowed reaction time and decreased impulse control. In higher doses of benzodiazepines, blackouts and confusion may occur.

See also PANIC ATTACKS; PANIC DISORDER.

bereavement, phobia following   Phobias occurring after the loss of a loved one may be related to separation anxiety. In some individuals, such a loss brings back unresolved feelings from childhood caused by separation from one's parents.

See also DEATH, FEAR OF; GRIEF REACTION; SEPARATION ANXIETY.

beta adrenergic blocking agents   See BETA-BLOCKING AGENTS.

beta-blocking agents   More commonly referred to as beta-blockers, these drugs have been used to assist in the relief of anxiety symptoms. Primarily, beta-blockers tend to have a calming effect on the heart, reducing the heart rate and the force of the cardiac contraction. Some examples of beta-blocking drugs used to treat anxiety are atenolol (Tenormin) and propranolol (Inderal).

Beta-blockers are used to treat high blood pressure (hypertension), cardiac arrythmias, and, as mentioned, anxieties. These medications act on the physical symptoms of anxiety by preventing the racing heartbeat and quickened breathing which is caused by the adrenaline rush that accompanies anxiety.

Beta-blockers have been used effectively to prevent the anxiety that is associated with both public speaking and test-taking. In these particular situations, they are used on a situational basis only.

Some beta-blockers have been shown to cause DEPRESSION. Beta-blockers may also have other side effects, including fatigue, lightheadedness, drowsiness, and upset stomach. Some infrequent side effects are severe, such as shortness of breath, swelling of the feet, ankles, lower legs, or hands, fainting, or unusual weight gain.

In general, if a beta-blocker medication is to be either discontinued or replaced by another type of medication, the beta-blocker should not be stopped abruptly. Rather, it should be tapered off over a period of one to two weeks or more, depending on the advice of the prescribing physician. Use with anxiety reactions is situational and therefore discontinued immediately after the event.

See also ANXIETY DRUGS.

biased apperception   Seeing things as one wants to see them. The term was used by Viennese psychologist Alfred Adler (1870–1937). Adler believed that biased apperception is necessary for participation in society, because without it, individuals are anxious and indecisive. Individuals who fear making a move unless they are certain they are right are usually paralyzed by indecision. Well-adjusted, well-integrated personalities take chances and make choices without undue anxiety according to a subjective evaluation of each situation.

Bible   No conclusions can be drawn as yet regarding the impact of Bible and biblical teachings on anxiety. Generally, it is believed that the effects of religious works on anxiety depend on the individual. People who are able to cope well with anxiety usually respond more positively to the Bible, while individuals who have poorer coping skills tend to become more anxious in response to the same teachings. Interest in the effects of religion has increased since 1976, when the American Psychological Association officially recognized a group of religiously-oriented therapists.

Both the Old and New Testaments contain references to fear of God and fear of evil spirits, as well as commentary about music therapy, abnormal behavior, and possession by devils. Treatment for possession by devils included exorcism. For example, Jesus is said to have removed the evil spirit from two men and transferred it into pigs who subsequently fell over cliffs into a lake. David's playing the lyre for Saul was an early example of music therapy. Judas Iscariot is the only suicide mentioned in the Bible. Fears of the Bible may be related to fears of religious ceremonies and holy things.

See also HOLY THINGS, FEAR OF; PHOBIAS, HISTORY OF; RELIGIOUS CEREMONIES, FEAR OF.

bibliophobia   Fear of books.

See also BOOKS, FEAR OF.

bibliotherapy   See BOOKS AS ANXIETY RELIEF.

binge drinking   Episodic and excessive consumption of alcoholic beverages, a major factor in nearly all leading causes of death for youth. Binge drinking refers to the consumption of five or more drinks on one occasion in the past two weeks for men, and for women, the consumption of four or more drinks in the same time frame. In general, males are more likely to be binge drinkers than females. Binge drinking is common in college-age youths.

Binge drinking has been implicated in automobile crashes, homicides, suicides, and fatal injuries among young people, as well as in numerous injuries incurred by binge drinkers and others who are harmed by binge drinkers. Dangerous drinking is a source of STRESS and ANXIETY for parents, school and college administrators, and for young people themselves. It is also linked to an increase in anxiety disorders among adults.

According to Robert D. Brewer and Monica H. Swahn in their 2005 article on binge drinking in the *Journal of the American Medical Association,* about 75,000 deaths in the United States were caused by excessive drinking in 2001. Of these deaths, binge drinking accounted for more than half.

Studies have shown that one out of three American colleges has a majority of students who engage in high-risk drinking. More than two out of every five college students are binge drinkers, with excessive drinking accounting for an estimated 1,400 student deaths, 500,000 injuries, and 70,000 sexual assaults or date rapes every year, according to the National Institute on Alcohol Abuse and Alcoholism (NIAAA). Peer pressure plays a large part in binge drinking, but there are other forces at work as well.

"Today's college students face powerful social and commercial influences to drink. If we are to reduce the dangerous levels of campus drinking and its consequences, colleges and surrounding communities must cooperate to reduce the numerous environmental factors that contribute to alcohol abuse," said American Medical Association President-elect J. Edward Hill, M.D., in 2004.

Combating Binge Drinking

Traditional efforts to reduce underage drinking have focused primarily on youth education and prevention techniques, often simply trying to convince youths to avoid drinking altogether. Research has shown that this model has been only marginally successful.

To combat alcohol abuse among underage youth and college students and the significant health risks and societal harms associated with it, the American Medical Association (AMA) and the Robert Wood Johnson Foundation (RWJF) have joined forces to help communities throughout the country find solutions that go beyond simply admonishing youths to say "no" to alcohol. The AMA and RWJF are working to create solutions through two national programs: "A Matter of Degree: The National Effort to Reduce Underage Drinking Through Coalitions" and "Reducing Underage Drinking Through Coalitions."

"We are finally taking decisive action against a major public health crisis that has taken the lives and futures of young Americans," said Percy Wootton, M.D., past president of the AMA.

A Matter of Degree (AMOD). With funding from the RWJF and management by the AMA, the two entities have been working together since 1996 with 10 university-community coalitions in a national effort to reduce binge drinking among college students. A Matter of Degree (AMOD) is an $8.6 million, multi-year program designed to foster collaboration between participating universities and the communities in which they are located to address the issue of excessive drinking and improve the quality of life for all community residents.

Participants in the program identify those environmental factors that contribute to promoting the use of alcohol, such as alcohol advertising and marketing, institutional policies and practices, local ordinances, and social and cultural beliefs and behaviors that converge to encourage alcohol abuse, and then program participants work together to create positive changes. For example, coalitions may seek to curb the practice of alcohol discounting, such as two-for-one drink specials, inexpensive beer pitcher sales, and other promotions that encourage excessive drinking in their communities. They also work to limit alcohol-industry sponsorship of social events, including sports events and other celebrations.

According to an evaluation conducted by the Harvard School of Public Health, published in the

---

RATES PER 1,000 POPULATION OF SELECTED PSYCHIATRIC DISORDERS, BY SEX, ACCORDING TO FREQUENCY OF DRINKING FIVE OR MORE DRINKS FOR MEN OR FOUR OR MORE DRINKS FOR WOMEN IN A SINGLE DAY IN THE PAST YEAR, AMONG CURRENT DRINKERS, UNITED STATES, 2001–2002

Never Binged in the Past Year	Both sexes, age 18 and older	Males	Females
Panic disorder without agoraphobia	12.95	8.62	16.78
Panic disorder with agoraphobia	4.21	1.39	6.71
Social phobia	24.66	17.97	30.58
Specific phobia	67.67	38.06	93.84
Generalized anxiety	18.62	11.27	25.12
Binged 1 to 11 times in the past year	**Both sexes, age 18 and older**	**Males**	**Females**
Panic disorder without agoraphobia	21.25	10.41	34.26
Panic disorder with agoraphobia	7.38	3.22	12.38
Social phobia	36.51	27.37	47.47
Specific phobia	100.36	63.61	144.47
Generalized anxiety	28.47	12.89	47.16

Adapted from: National Institute on Alcohol Abuse and Alcoholism, *Alcohol Use and Alcohol Use Disorders in the United States: Main Findings from the 2001–2002 National Epidemiologic Survey on Alcohol and Related Conditions (NESARC)*, U.S. Alcohol Epidemiologic Data Reference Manual 8, no. 1 (January 2006), Bethesda, Md.: National Institutes of Health, January 2006, p. 213.

American Journal of Preventive Medicine in 2004, college students at universities that are participating in AMOD are less likely to miss their classes, to be assaulted by a drunken student, or to hurt themselves after drinking. The study also found a decline in the drinking rates at those colleges that incorporated the most AMOD policies or interventions.

Further, findings indicated that the five colleges that had achieved a high level of implementation by 2001 saw significant reductions, not only in the actual rates of drinking, but also in the rates of binge drinking and frequent drunkenness relative to the 32 comparison schools. In addition, the five participating colleges also had reductions in the direct and secondary harms of alcohol use, including reductions in students who were falling behind in their schoolwork, vandalizing school property, and experiencing unwanted sexual advances by someone who was drinking.

Binge Drinking and Psychiatric Problems

According to the National Institute of Alcohol Abuse and Alcoholism in a study released in 2006 and based on more than 43,000 subjects, binge drinkers have a higher rate of PANIC DISORDER, SOCIAL PHOBIA, SPECIFIC PHOBIA, GENERALIZED ANXIETY, and many other diagnoses, compared to those who have not binged in the past year. For example, among non-bingers, the rate of panic disorder without agoraphobia was 12.95 per 1,000 people, compared to a percent of 21.25 per 1,000 people among bingers. The rate of social phobia among nonbingers was 24.66 per 1,000, compared to 36.51 among bingers. (See the table on page 91.)

In addition, there were gender differences between bingers and nonbingers with psychiatric problems, with women (both nonbingers and bingers) at a higher risk for some disorders. For example, in considering the incidence of generalized anxiety, nonbinging women had a rate of 25.12 per 1,000, compared to the rate of 47.16 for binging women. The estimate of specific phobia among nonbinging women was 93.84 per 1,000, while the rate among binging women was 144.47 per 1,000. Clearly, binge drinking is very problematic for women and is associated with a significant risk for anxiety disorders, even more so than for men.

See also ALCOHOLISM.

Brewer, Robert D., M.D., and Monica H. Swahn, "Binge Drinking and Violence," *Journal of the American Medical Association* 294, no. 5 (August 3, 2005): pp. 616–618.

National Institute on Alcohol Abuse and Alcoholism, *Alcohol Use and Alcohol Use Disorders in the United States: Main Findings from the 2001–2002 National Epidemiologic Survey on Alcohol and Related Conditions (NESARC)*, U.S. Alcohol Epidemiologic Data Reference Manual 8, no. 1 (January 2006), Bethesda, Md.: National Institutes of Health, January 2006.

Weitzman, Elise R., et al., "Reducing Drinking and Related Harms in College: Evaluation of the 'A Matter of Degree' Program," *American Journal of Preventive Medicine* 27 (October 2004): pp. 196–197.

biodynamic psychology   A term that describes an approach to psychotherapy directed toward integrating the individual's physical and social and metapsychological needs. Biodynamic psychology was introduced by American psychoanalyst Jules Homan Masserman (1905). This approach is a holistic one, with a unified approach to the individual's mind, body, and spirit, using psychological, organic, and spiritual methods. A wide range of techniques are used to help an individual with anxieties and phobias. Masserman's "7 Pil-Rs" of therapeutic wisdom are: reputation (of the therapist), rapport, relief, review, reorientation, rehabilitation, and resocialization.

Masserman, J. H., *Principles and Practice of Biodynamic Psychotherapy: An Integration* (New York: Thieme/Stratton, 1980).

biofeedback   A technique to monitor psychophysiological events by electrical feedback. Biofeedback is useful in many approaches to therapy for anxieties and phobias. It provides an anxious or phobic individual with a basis for self-regulation of certain processes, such as autonomic system reaction to fearful situations. It establishes a diagnostic baseline by noting physiological reactions to stressful events, enables therapists to relate this information to the individual's reports, fills gaps in the individual's history, and encourages relaxation in the part of the individual's body to which the biofeedback equipment is applied. Relaxation training is often suggested to assist the individual in controlling anxiety reactions.

See also BEHAVIOR THERAPY.

Forgione, A. G., and R. Holmberg, "Biofeedback Therapy." In *Handbook of Innovative Psychotherapies*. Edited by R. J. Corsini (New York: Wiley, 1981).

biological basis for anxiety Researchers studying ANXIETY, including Freud, predicted that the brain and CENTRAL NERVOUS SYSTEM might function abnormally in persons who have serious ANXIETY DISORDERS. Much research focusing on the brain is under way on anxiety and related disorders focusing on the brain.

See also ADENOSINE; AGORAPHOBIA; ALPRAZOLAM; ANTIDEPRESSANTS; CAFFEINE; CARBON DIOXIDE SENSITIVITY; CHEMOCEPTORS; DIAZEPAM; DRUG EFFECTS; GAMMA AMINO BUTYRIC ACID (GABA); HYPERVENTILATION; LACTATE-INDUCTED ANXIETY; LOCUS CERULEUS; MITRAL VALVE PROLAPSE; MONOAMINE OXIDASE INHIBITORS; NEUROTRANSMITTERS; NOREPINEPHRINE; PANIC ATTACK; PREMENSTRUAL SYNDROME.

biological clock For the many women in their mid- to late thirties who hope to become mothers, the words *biological clock* refer to the limited period of time that they are biologically able to produce children. As their "biological clock" runs out, unmarried women as well as wives who are in their late thirties or early forties and who are having difficulty becoming pregnant experience a great deal of anxiety and concern. Statistics show that a woman's fertility is reduced and her ability to conceive becomes more difficult with age and birth defects occur more frequently in infants born to older mothers.

See also BABY BOOMERS; INFERTILITY; PARENTING.

McKaughan, Molly, *The Biological Clock* (New York: Penguin Books, 1989).

biological markers Biological markers include test results that can confirm a diagnosis, such as of depression. There are two basic tests relating to biological markers. One is the dexamethasone suppression test; the other is the thyroid-releasing hormone challenge test.

Dexamethasone Suppression Test (DST)

The dexamethasone suppression test was the first biologic marker for affective disorder. Dexamethasone is a synthetic glucocorticoid that has the effect of turning off the secretion of ACTH and, subsequently, cortisol. In normal persons, a dose of dexamethasone given at 11 P.M. reduces cortisol levels over the next 24 hours. In depressed individuals, however, the suppression effect of dexamethasone does not occur. The nonsuppression of cortisol is called a positive dexamethasone test.

While DST is considered a biological marker for mood disorders, it identifies only about 50 percent of clinically depressed individuals. A positive DST result confirms depression. However, a negative DST result does not rule out the diagnosis of major depression. Also, studies suggest a positive correlation between the severity of depression with the rate of DST nonsuppression. There is also a correlation between the DST nonsuppression index and risk of SUICIDE.

Individuals identified as nonsuppressors upon testing before antidepressant medication return to a normal suppression pattern when the treatment is successful. Individuals who show no reversal effect after treatment are at increased risk of relapse.

Thyrotropin-Releasing Hormone Challenge Test (TRH)

Indications for clinical use of the TRH challenge test are similar to those for DST. It is sometimes used as an aid in diagnosing depression and assessing thyroid status. A positive test result confirms diagnosis of major depression, but a negative test result does not eliminate the diagnosis.

When the two tests are used together, the increased sensitivity rate is 84 percent. The hypothalamic-pituitary-thyroid (HPT) axis is the thyroid gland link to the central nervous system. The hypothalamus releases thyroid-releasing hormone (TRH) from neurons which stimulate pituitary cells to release thyroid-stimulating-hormone (TSH) into the blood. TSH then stimulates release of other chemicals from the thyroid gland. Release of TRH is facilitated by dopamine and norepinephrine and is inhibited by serotonin. Levels of TSH have a CIR-CADIAN RHYTHM, with the highest levels of secretion from 4 A.M. to 8 A.M. Some individuals who are depressed have symptoms of hypothyroidism. A TRH test is used to determine if the HPT axis is functioning normally.

See also NOREPINEPHRINE; SEROTONIN.

biorhythms   Physiological functions, such as menstrual cycles, that follow a regular temporal pattern. These biological rhythms regulate psychological as well as physiological functions in the individual: energy level, hunger, sleep, and elimination can all be affected. These rhythms vary considerably from person to person and within a single individual at different times. Such external factors as travel and changing time zones or unpredictable and unfamiliar changes in routine can also disrupt biorhythms. Anxiety can result from bodily sensations produced by disruption of biorhythms and lead to anxieties.

To deal with the anxieties caused by disruptions in biorhythms, individuals develop their own techniques. For example, some travelers may prepare by waking earlier for several days before a trip, or getting more rest following travel. Some develop particular dietary patterns that they find helpful, such as eating small meals more often and drinking lots of water.

See also CIRCADIAN RHYTHMS; JET LAG; MENSTRUATION, FEAR OF; SHIFT WORK.

bipolar disorder   Bipolar disorder, also known as manic depression, is the most distinct and dramatic of the affective disorders (mood disorders). Unlike major DEPRESSION, which can occur at any age, bipolar disorder generally strikes in late adolescence or early adulthood even though signs are present from an earlier age. The psycholothymic disorders are a milder form of cyclic mood disorders.

Bipolar disorder can be very disabling and have a strongly negative effect on the individual's life. According to the National Institute of Mental Health (NIMH) individuals with bipolar disorder lose more than twice as many workdays as do those with major depressive disorder (depression), or 65.5 lost workdays per year for individuals with bipolar disorder compared to 27.2 lost workdays for individuals with depression. However, at the same time, bipolar disorder is among the most treatable of the mental illnesses. A combination of psychotherapy and medications returns the vast majority of individuals with bipolar disorder to productive lives.

About 2 million Americans ages 18 or older, or 1 percent of the population in this age group, have bipolar disorder, although many people are not diagnosed with the disorder for years. Many people who have bipolar disorder also suffer from PHOBIAS.

Depressive illnesses often run in families. In early 1987, researchers discovered a genetic marker among members of the Old Order of Amish that made them susceptible to bipolar disorder.

In a second study that year, scientists found an aberrant gene on another chromosome (the material that contains genes). The researchers emphasized that their findings do not account for every case of bipolar disorder because their results have not been repeated for other populations. However, these studies provide important early evidence toward identifying the precise genes linked to these genetic markers. Now scientists can work toward identifying the genetic defects in other forms of bipolar disorder among other populations. They also can work toward understanding the biochemical reactions that are controlled by these genes and that contribute to the disorder.

Some studies have suggested that environmental factors can trigger the illness. Comprehensive psychoanalytic studies in the past have indicated that individuals with bipolar disorder were reared to become achievers in order to bring honor to their families; however, at the same time, they were never allowed to become fully autonomous. Research suggests that these people grow up with a need to achieve and a contradictory need to depend on others. The failure to reach a goal or to maintain a needed relationship is believed to trigger the bipolar illness. However, environmental factors interact with genetic factors to produce a disorder and the family dynamics described here could also interact with genetics to cause bipolar reactions.

Some studies suggest that imbalances in the biochemistry that controls a person's mood could contribute to bipolar illness. For example, people suffering from either bipolar disorder or major depressive disorder often respond to certain hormones or steroids in a way that indicates that they have irregularities in their hormone production and release.

Other research suggests that bipolar patients' neurotransmitters—the chemicals by which the brain cells communicate—become imbalanced during various phases of the disease. Finally, some people who have depressive illnesses have sleep patterns in which the dream phase begins earlier in the night than normal. Such research helps scientists develop scientific theories about how medications work.

Symptoms and Diagnostic Path

What distinguishes bipolar illness from other depressive disorders is that the individual swings from depression to mania, generally with periods of normal moods in between the two extremes. A manic episode may typically last about a week. Phobias may come and go during these cycles. Some patients cycle from mania to depression and back within a few days and without a period of normal mood. People with this condition are called *rapid cyclers.*

In general, the signs and symptoms of a manic episode include

- extreme irritability
- increased activity, energy, or restlessness
- excessively good or euphoric mood state
- racing thoughts, causing the person to talk very rapidly and often unintelligibly
- little need for sleep
- excessive spending
- drug abuse, especially the abuse of cocaine, alcohol, or sleep remedies
- poor judgment
- unrealistic belief in one's own abilities
- aggressive or provocative behavior
- denial that there is a problem
- proneness to high-risk behaviors, such as sexual risks, financial risks, and so forth

When an individual experiences a manic phase, he or she will feel a sudden onset of elation or euphoria that increases in a matter of days to a serious impairment. The individual feels "on top of the world," and not even bad news will change his or her happiness. The mood is way out of bounds, given the individual's normal personality. Furthermore, clinical studies have shown that manic states still have depressive underpinnings.

A manic person lacks judgment and will express unwarranted optimism. Self-confidence may reach the point of grandiose delusions in which the person may think that he or she has a special connection with God, celebrities, or political leaders. He or she may think that nothing, not even the laws of gravity, can stop him or her from accomplishing any task. As a result, the person with bipolar disorder may feel capable of stepping off a building or out of a moving car without being hurt.

Other symptoms of bipolar disorder are hyperactivity and excessive plans or participation in numerous activities that have good chances for painful results. The manic person becomes so enthusiastic about activities or involvements that he or she often fails to recognize that there is not enough time in the day for all of them. For example, the individual may book several meetings, parties, deadlines, and other activities in a single day, feeling confident that he or she is able to make all of them on time. Added to the expansive mood, mania also can result in reckless driving, spending sprees, foolish business investments, or sexual behavior that is highly unusual for the person. Of course if such impulses are acted upon, the individual may become seriously injured or killed.

The manic person's thoughts race uncontrollably. When the person talks, his or her words come out in a nonstop rush of ideas that abruptly change from topic to topic. In its most severe form, the loud, rapid speech of the person with bipolar disorder is hard to interpret because the individual's thought processes have become so totally disorganized and incoherent.

The manic person will often experience a decreased need for sleep, allowing him or her to go with little or no sleep for days without feeling tired. The manic will also experience distractibility in which his or her attention is easily diverted to inconsequential or unimportant details. At times, the manic will become suddenly irritable, enraged, or PARANOID when his or her grandiose plans are thwarted or excessive social overtures are rebuffed.

As the manic episode abates, the individual may have a period of normal mood and behavior. But eventually the depressive phase of the illness will set in. This phase has the same symptoms as major or *unipolar* depression. Symptoms of a depressive episode may include as follows:

- sleep changes, in which the person sleeps much more or less than normal
- appetite changes, causing weight gain or loss
- loss of interest in previously enjoyed activities, including sex
- decreased energy and fatigue
- difficulty concentrating
- feelings of pessimism and hopelessness
- intense feelings of helplessness, guilt, and/or worthlessness
- chronic pain not caused by a physical illness or injury
- thoughts of death or attempts at suicide

In most cases, psychiatrists diagnose bipolar disorder, and the diagnosis is made based on the patient's current behavior and past history. There are no brain scans or laboratory tests for bipolar disorder. It is also best to check for thyroid disease, since many patients with bipolar disorder also have thyroid disease. In addition, hyperthyroidism may present as mania and thus the individual may be misdiagnosed and the thyroid disease will go untreated. In some cases, individuals with ATTENTION-DEFICIT/HYPERACTIVITY DISORDER who are hyperactive are misdiagnosed with bipolar disorder.

Some other physical and mental disorders mimic bipolar disorder. For example, an individual with symptoms of bipolar disorder might be reacting to substances such as amphetamines or steroids or could suffer from an illness such as multiple sclerosis. An individual who has symptoms of bipolar disorder should have a thorough medical evaluation to rule out any other mental or physical disorders and to ensure accurate diagnosis and appropriate treatment.

Treatment Options and Outlook

Individuals with bipolar disorder are treated with both psychotherapy and medications. Psychotherapy can enable individuals to understand the consequences of their actions and change their behavior; for example, cognitive-behavioral therapy may help the person with bipolar disorder to change any inappropriate or negative thoughts. Family therapy can help the family learn better ways of coping with the distress that the person with bipolar disorder often generates.

Mood-stabilizing medications can reduce the risk for rapid cycling and excessive acts. Medications such as lithium or valproate (Depakote) are approved by the Food and Drug Administration (FDA) for the treatment of bipolar disorder. Some physicians use anticonvulsants in an off-label treatment of the disorder.

In extreme cases, electroconvulsive therapy (ECT) may be used with the patient with bipolar disorder, particularly if the patient is psychotic or suicidal.

Risk Factors and Preventive Measures

Although the genetic picture of the disease is still far from complete, we do know that close relatives of people who have bipolar illness are 10 to 20 times more likely than the general population to develop either depression or bipolar disorder. Between 80 and 90 percent of individuals who have bipolar disorder have relatives who also have some form of depression. If one parent has bipolar illness, a child has a 30 percent risk of suffering from a depressive disorder; if both parents have bipolar disorder, the children have a 75 percent chance of developing a depressive disorder.

There is no known way to prevent bipolar disorder altogether. Once bipolar disorder is diagnosed, however, treatment can minimize the effect of the symptoms on both the individual and others who care about him or her.

See also ANTIDEPRESSANTS; BIOLOGICAL BASIS FOR ANXIETY; DEPRESSED PARENTS, CHILDREN OF; LITHIUM.

birds, fear of   Fear of birds is known as ornithophobia. Some bird phobics believe that the sudden, unpredictable movements of birds constitute an attack. Phobics commonly fear the swooping motions of birds and the sound and sight of flapping wings in an enclosed space. Other phobics mention the beady eyes and claws of birds as being particularly frightening. Pigeons are the phobic objects for many individuals, as pigeons gravitate toward buildings and people more than other birds do. Some individuals fear only the sight of a dead bird. Some bird phobics are less frightened by the sight of birds in the open and even may be fascinated by them in this situation. Alfred Hitchcock played on the duality of attraction to and revulsion of birds in his film *The Birds.*

This phobia, like many animal and common stimuli phobias, often severely limits the individual's functioning. Fear of birds, for example, in moderate to severe intensities, limits the person's range of movement outside, often restricting him to areas of few birds or to travel at night. Also, travel is accompanied by ANXIETY or dread at the possibility of seeing birds; windows must be tightly closed, and walking in open spaces is impossible. The individual may not even be able to look outside.

See also FLYING THINGS, FEAR OF.

Kent, Fraser, *Nothing to Fear: Coping with Phobias* (Garden City, NY: Doubleday, 1977).

Melville, Joy, *Phobias and Obsessions* (New York: Coward, McCann & Geoghegan, 1977).
Neumann, Frederic, *Fighting Fear* (New York: Macmillan, 1985).

birth control   The term *birth control* refers to controlling the number of children born by preventing or reducing the chance of conception by natural or artificial means. The issue produces anxieties for many people, including those making a choice of birth control methods or those whose religious convictions are counter to using birth control as a practical and economic plan for their families. Furthermore, side effects of birth control medication can lead to anxieties for some individuals.

Methods of Birth Control

Each method of birth control has advantages, disadvantages, and sources of anxieties. They should be discussed by couples before they engage in sexual intercourse. Women and men must weigh the factors relative to a birth control method, including effectiveness in preventing unwanted pregnancy, protection from a sexually transmitted disease, freedom from side effects, cost, or spontaneity of use.

METHODS OF BIRTH CONTROL*

The "pill" contains hormones that prevent conception.

Norplant—involves matchstick size synthetic rods that are inserted in the skin of a woman's upper arm. For five years at a slow, nearly steady rate, the rods release the hormone levonorgesterol, a form of progestin, which inhibits ovulation and thickens cervical mucus.

Depo-Provera, an injectable form of progestin administered every three months, has been used by 15 million women worldwide.

A diaphragm is a rubber disk with a flexible metal rim that is inserted to fit around the cervix. Spermicide placed inside the diaphragm kills most of the sperm in the area. The cervical cap is smaller and more rigid than the diaphragm but works the same.

Placed inside the uterus, an intrauterine device (IUD) is believed to set up a mild, harmless inflammation that impedes sperm and keeps any fertilized egg from implanting.

The condom, one of the oldest forms of birth control, is a simple sheath that covers the penis, blocking sperm from the uterus.

Available since 1993 in the United States, the female condom is a long polyurethane sheath that is anchored between the cervix and the vagina.

Medications known as the "morning after" pill, which can be used by women who engage in unprotected sex or who fear pregnancy. These medications are oral contraceptives taken in prescribed dosage no longer than 72 hours after intercourse, followed by another dose 12 hours later.

* No one method of birth control has proven to be 100 percent effective.

According to the 1995 National Survey of Family Growth by the National Center for Health Statistics, the most popular method of birth control is female sterilization (29.5 percent), followed by the birth control pill (28.5 percent), male prophylactics (17.7 percent), vasectomy (12.5 percent), the diaphragm (2.8 percent), the IUD (1.4 percent), and all other methods (4.9 percent). The numbers total more than 100 percent because some women use more than one method of birth control.

See also CONDOM; FAMILY PLANNING; PREGNANCY, FEAR OF; SEXUALLY TRANSMITTED DISEASES, FEAR OF; UNWED MOTHERS.

birthdays, fear of   Some individuals fear telling others their birthday and also fear celebrating their birthday in any way. This fear may be related to a fear of aging and fear of getting old. Some individuals fear telling anyone their correct age and consistently say they are younger than they really are. Some even fear celebrating the birthday of another; this may be related to a superstitious fear.

See also AGING, FEAR OF.

birthing a monster, fear of   Fear of birthing a monster is known as teratophobia. The term also relates to fear of giving birth to an infant with a severe birth defect. Some women fear pregnancy and childbirth because they have teratophobia, especially if they have been exposed to rubella or other agents known to cause birth defects.

See also CHILDBIRTH, FEAR OF; MENTAL DISORDER, FEAR OF; PREGNANCY, FEAR OF; RADIATION, FEAR OF; X RAY, FEAR OF.

birth order   A term introduced by Alfred Adler (1870–1937), a Viennese psychologist, to describe different effects in personality and behavior due to birth position. Studies of birth order have led to some generalizations about how a child's position in relation to his/her parents and siblings may affect his/her anxiety level, personality, and view of the world.

The first child born to a family has the advantage of undivided attention and resources. Whether that child becomes the only child of the family or its oldest child, he/she may tend to be more adult in behavior and more interested in goals and personal achievement. As a group, first children are strongly represented in the ranks of the successful and powerful. They also tend to score highest on intelligence tests.

Only children often have characteristics and resulting anxieties of their own. Having been the center of their parents' attention, they are in danger of becoming selfish and spoiled. Likewise, their parents' expectations for them to succeed at anything they do may be unreasonably high. With more exposure to adults, they may not relate well to other children and may have problems with sharing.

For older children, the arrival of a sibling, even though happily anticipated, has the ultimate effect of making them feel dethroned. They often assume a certain amount of responsibility for younger children in the family and may be responsible for setting a good example, showing younger children how to do things, and baby-sitting. Older children are frequently more aware of family difficulties and problems and their own parents' insecurities. As a result, they tend to be more anxious, conservative, and responsible than younger brothers and sisters.

The middle child position in the family has more variables since the ages and sex of siblings may have a profound effect on him or her. Middle children usually become good at sharing, but also guard their privacy. They may perceive that they are too young for the privileges of the oldest and too old for the coddling of the youngest. As a result, middle children may show off to get attention and may also seek rewarding relationships outside the family. The need to belong to a peer group is strong in middle children, and they are team players, frequently quite popular. To compete with an older sibling, a middle child will develop his abilities in an area quite different from the talents of his or her older brother or sister.

The youngest child of a family never has the experience of having his position usurped. Younger children tend to preserve and use childish characteristics such as crying, acting cute, or emphasizing their dependence and inadequacy to get what they want. Younger children frequently have very positive feelings about themselves because of their position in the family and tend to be charming and popular. They have the best sense of humor in the family. Their disadvantage is that they often obtain information and opinions from other children rather than adults and therefore lack the wisdom and realism they might gain from adult contact.

A very specific type of younger child is the "change of life" baby who arrives several years after the older siblings. This younger child is really more in the position of being the only child, but with several parents, since usually one or more of his or her siblings act as a parent. These children grow up with a great deal of attention and support, but may also have the additional stress of a confused sense of themselves from the variety of images and ideas from siblings they perceive as adult but who are, in fact, children.

Other positions in the family that can have long-lasting effects on personality are the "only daughter" or "only son" syndromes. Only daughters have traditionally had the "feminine" chores of the family and, in many cultures, are expected to take care of the parents as they grow old, even if it means personal sacrifice. "Only sons" were expected to enter the family business or succeed at some profession.

See also COMMUNICATION; FAMILIES; SIBLINGS RELATIONSHIPS.

Brownstone, David, and Irene Franck, *The Parent's Desk Reference* (New York: Prentice Hall, 1991).

Franklin, Deborah, "Why Are Siblings So Different?" In *Health,* March/April, 1991.

Richardson, Ron, and Lois A. Richardson, *Birth Order and You: How Your Sex and Your Position in the Family Affects Your Personality and Your Relationships* (Bellingham, WA: Self-Counsel, 1990).

birth trauma   A term coined by Otto Rank (1884–1939), an Austrian psychoanalyst, to describe his concept that ANXIETY has roots in the traumatic event of birth. According to Rank, factors in psychoanalysis represent birth SYMBOLS; for example, transference is the reenactment of the oneness with the mother, and the separation from the analyst at the end of the treatment corresponds to the expulsion from the mother's womb. A desire to return to the womb is seen as the universal neurotic wish,

and only when this is overcome is the analysis complete. More recently, natural childbirth advocates have expressed interest in the psychological effects of the birth process and have suggested that a calm separation of the baby from the uterus increases the infant's mental health and facilitates the bonding process with the mother.

See also ANXIETIES; ATTACHMENT THEORY; PRIMAL THERAPY.

black cats, fear of   Some individuals fear black cats because they are associated with witchcraft and superstition. Some people avoid letting a black cat cross their path out of superstitious fear of future misfortune. Some fear black cats but not cats of other colors, while other individuals fear only lighter-colored cats.

See also CATS, FEAR OF.

blennophobia   Fear of slime.

See also SLIME, FEAR OF.

blocking   Interruption of a train of speech before a thought or idea has been completed. After a period of silence, which may last from a few seconds to minutes, the individual indicates that he/she cannot recall what he/she has been saying or meant to say. Blocking should be judged as present only if the person spontaneously describes losing his thought or if, upon questioning, he or she gives that as the reason for the pause. Blocking is often due to low levels of ANXIETY that affect concentration.

Blocq's syndrome   Fear of standing or walking; also, a hysterical inability to stand or walk. The fear may be motivated by a desire for secondary gains of sympathy and support. Blocq's syndrome is also known as astasia-abasia. The syndrome was named for Paul Oscar Blocq (1869–96), a French physician.

See also SECONDARY GAIN.

blood (and blood-injury) phobia   Many individuals are afraid of the sight of blood. Fear of blood is known as hematophobia or hemophobia. While susceptible individuals may not say they have a fear of blood, when faced with the sight of their own or another's blood, they may recoil, close their eyes, or even faint. A reaction may occur on hearing a description of blood and gore, such as a war scene, or even imagining seeing someone bleeding. Blood phobia is different from some other phobias in that the individual does not perceive danger of injury or death.

Blood phobics may experience more nausea and faintness than fear or anxiety. They may avoid their phobic stimuli because they fear fainting, and their fear of fainting in turn can cause them anxiety.

With most phobias, the individual's pulse and breathing rate increase in response to the phobic stimulus. However, with blood phobia (and related blood-injury phobias, such as phobia of needles, injection, blood donation, etc.) there is often a sharp drop in heart rate and blood pressure, which is called a diphasic cardiovascular pattern. Why some blood phobics lose consciousness when faced with the stimulus is not clearly understood, but one hypothesis is that it is a "protective" biological mechanism that, in the event of actual injury, prevents the individual from doing anything that might cause further blood loss.

Like phobias of animals, those of blood and injury often begin during childhood. It appears to be relatively common in minor forms, and is excessive in very few instances. Epidemiological studies indicate that approximately 3.1 to 4.5 percent of the population report blood and blood-injury phobias. In one 1980 study, a high percentage of blood phobics (68 percent) reported that close relatives had the same fear.

Severe phobia of blood and injury can be seriously handicapping. For example, sufferers may avoid necessary medical procedures or avoid attractive careers as medical professionals. Blood-injury phobic women may even avoid becoming pregnant in order to avoid medical examinations and the sight of blood.

Benjamin Rush (1745–1813), American physician and author, said of blood phobia:

> There is a native dread of the sight of blood in every human creature, implanted probably for the

wise purpose of preventing our injuring or destroying ourselves, or others. Children cry oftener from seeing their blood, than from the pain occasioned by falls or blows. Valuable medicines are stamped with a disagreeable taste to prevent their becoming ineffectual from habit, by being used as condiments or articles of diet. In like manner, Blood-letting as a remedy, is defenced from being used improperly, by the terror which accompanies its use. This terror rises to such a degree as sometimes to produce paleness and faintness when it is prescribed as a remedy. However unpopular it may be, it is not contrary to nature, for she relieves herself when oppressed, by spontaneous discharges of blood from the nose, and other parts of the body. The objections to it therefore appear to be founded less in the judgments than in the *fears* of sick people.

See also DEATH, FEAR OF; FAINTING, FEAR OF; FAMILY INFLUENCE; INJURY, FEAR OF.

Beck, Aaron T., and Gary Emery, *Anxiety Disorders and Phobias: A Cognitive Perspective* (New York: Basic Books, 1985).

Ost, Lars-Goran, and Kenneth Hugdahl, "Acquisition of Blood and Dental Phobia and Anxiety Response Patterns in Clinical Patients," *Behaviour Research and Therapy* 23 (1985): pp. 27–34.

Runes, D. D., ed., *The Selected Writings of Benjamin Rush* (New York: The Philosophical Library, 1947).

blood donating, fear of Fear of donating blood, for many people, is a fear of the sight of their own blood, a fear of needles, or a combination of these fears. Some fear the pain of the needle or fear becoming weak or ill because of the loss of blood. Many blood-donating phobics do not realize that there is very little pain in the actual donation process. Those who have donated blood say that the needle feels something like a pinch on the arm. Some who fear donating blood use the excuse that their blood is not the right type. This usually is a cover-up for their fear, because every type is the right type. Some phobics say that they do not have any blood to spare, although an adult in generally good health has about 10 to 12 pints of blood in his or her body, and one can safely donate one pint of blood every eight weeks. Other phobics say they do not have time to donate blood.

During the 1980s, when the spread of acquired immunodeficiency syndrome (AIDS) increased, many individuals became fearful of donating blood because they feared the possibility of acquiring AIDS during the procedure. Authorities have assured donors that it is impossible to get AIDS by donating blood because all materials involved in the donation procedure are used only one time and are completely sterile and disposable.

See also BLOOD PRESSURE PHOBIA.

blood pressure, fear of high   Because high blood pressure (hypertension) is closely linked with heart disease, many people fear having high blood pressure. Many who have illness or disease phobia fear having high blood pressure. The term blood pressure, as used in medicine, refers to the force of the blood against the walls of the arteries, created by the heart as it pumps blood through the body. As the heart beats, the arterial pressure increases. As the heart relaxes between beats, the pressure decreases. High blood pressure is the condition in which blood pressure rises too high and stays there.

Normal blood pressure varies from moment to moment within each individual. Blood pressure may be higher at one time than another. It goes up when one exercises or experiences ANXIETY and goes down when one rests or sleeps. In otherwise healthy adults, however, the generally recognized normal range of systolic (pumping) blood pressure is from 90 to 120 mm HG; the diastolic (resting) blood pressure ranges from 55 to 90 mm HG. In determining whether an individual has high blood pressure, the physician will be concerned with the usual pressure in one's system. The physician may measure an individual's blood pressure more than once during a visit. For example, if one has hurried to the office, one may feel out of breath, which could contribute to a high reading. Later during the visit, as one relaxes, one's blood pressure may go down. Also, a physician may consider the average of several readings taken at different times before making a diagnosis of high blood pressure. If blood pressure is high on only one occasion, the physician will want to measure it again

under other circumstances to see if drug treatment is necessary.

Because so many people do not feel any symptoms with high blood pressure, the disease has been called "the silent killer." However, some people with advanced high blood pressure have persistent HEADACHES, DIZZINESS, fatigue, tension and shortness of breath.

Some individuals who have PANIC ATTACKS may have elevated blood pressure at times; they should be checked periodically to be sure that their average blood pressure is within a normal range.

See also HEART ATTACK, FEAR OF; ILLNESS PHOBIA; "WHITE COAT HYPERTENSION."

Kahn, Ada P., *High Blood Pressure* (Chicago: Contemporary Books, 1993).

blood pressure phobia   Fear of blood pressure, usually high blood pressure.

See also "WHITE COAT HYPERTENSION."

blood transfusions, fear of   During the 1980s, fear of blood transfusion became widespread when it was recognized that the human immunovirus (HIV), which is known to carry the dreaded acquired immunodeficiency syndrome (AIDS), can be spread through blood transfusions. Others fear blood transfusions because the procedure involves use of needles or tubes placed in the body. Still others who have blood phobia fear seeing blood or blood components being fed into their bodies.

While blood transfusions are feared by many, they are lifesaving for many others. Transfusions are given after great loss of blood in an accident or in a surgical operation, to treat the systemic shock and fluid loss caused by severe burns, in replacing the blood of an Rh-positive newborn infant, and to treat severe anemias.

Since the rapid spread of certain types of hepatitis and AIDS from blood transfusions, blood of donors is tested before it's drawn, and blood is tested again before it is transfused into a recipient. An understanding of how this is done will allay many fears.

See also BLOOD PRESSURE PHOBIA; DISEASE, FEAR OF; ILLNESS, FEAR OF.

blushing, fear of   Fear of blushing, or erythro-phobia, can be a painful and difficult symptom for therapists to treat. Fear of blushing is manifest only when other people are present. The phobic individual, most commonly a woman, is terrified that she will blush in the company of others and is convinced that in this state she will be very visible and consequently the center of unwanted, painful attention. If questioned, such an individual can-not say what is so dreadful about blushing, but it is often evident that shame (fear of disapproval of others) is an important component of her anxiety. A change of color may not be at all evident to the observer, despite the fact that the individual insists that she feels bright red; the force of her fear often leads the individual to a severe restriction of her social life.

Edmund Bergler, in 1944, writing in *Psychoana-lytic Quarterly,* suggested that blushing in psychiatric literature is usually considered a hysterical conver-sion symptom within the "embarrassment neuro-sis" and that blushing is a symptom of unconscious sexual fantasies as well as punishment for those fantasies. Blushing represents an increase in blood volume to the face and head. It is part of the sym-pathetic nervous system arousal pattern of anxiety/excitement. As with any emotional response, exter-nal stimuli, such as the presence of other people, can become conditioned quite easily.

See also NEUROSIS; SOCIAL PHOBIA.

Bergler, Edmund, "A New Approach to the Therapy of Erythrophobia," *Psychoanalytic Quarterly* 13 (1944): 43–59.

body image, fear of   Body image is the mental picture one has of one's body at any moment. Body image is derived from internal sensations, postural changes, emotional experiences, fantasies, and feedback from others. Fear of deformity of one's own body is known as dysmorphophobia. Some individuals have fears relating to their body image and fear that one or more parts of their body are unattractive and noticeable to others. A mispercep-tion of one's body image can lead to eating disor-ders, such as ANOREXIA NERVOSA or BULIMIA, in an effort to make oneself thinner.

See also DEFORMITY, FEAR OF; DYSMORPHOPHOBIA; EATING DISORDERS.

body language   A form of COMMUNICATION through facial expression, posture, gestures, or movements, accompanied with or without words. Both the com-municator and the listener may employ body lan-guage. It can be a device used to express emotion or a reaction to the meaning of communication.

EXAMPLES OF BODY LANGUAGE AS INDICATORS OF ANXIETIES

Action	Meaning
Toes pointed outward	Confidence
Toes pointed inward	Submission
A jutting chin	Belligerence
Lip and nail biting	Disappointment
Lip licking	Nervousness
Foot tapping	Impatience
Leaning backward	A relaxed attitude
Leaning forward	Interest
Open palms	Honesty
Rubbing hands together	Excitement

Body language may be an indicator of the anxiety that the communicator and the listener are experi-encing. According to Gay Turback in *The Rotarian* (April, 1995), "Without uttering a syllable, it's pos-sible to communicate love, hate, fear, rage, deceit, and virtually every other emotion in the human repertoire." The article goes on to describe how body signals have been around for more than a mil-lion years, with some researchers having catalogued 5,000 hand gestures and 1,000 postures, each with its own message. Says Turback, "Although some body language is nearly universal, much of it is an accouterment of one culture or another." Certain actions may have one meaning in Mexico, a differ-ent meaning in the United States, and no relevance in Canada. Other examples given in the article that are especially common among North Americans are shown above.

body odor, fear of   Fear of body odors is known as osphreisiophobia or bromidrosiphobia. Some individuals fear their own body odor and have an unfounded fear that others will notice it. Such individuals may avoid going into crowded places where they must be close to others, may use deodorants and antiperspirants excessively, may bathe, shower, or change clothes excessively, and may seek constant reassurance from family members that they cannot detect any odor. Fear of one's own body odor is considered a SOCIAL PHOBIA and usually responds to appropriate treatment.

See also DYSMORPHOPHOBIA; ODORS, FEAR OF CERTAIN; SOCIAL PHOBIAS.

body therapies A group of therapies that emphasize the role of physical factors in anxieties and phobias and the resolution of those anxieties and phobias by relaxation, breathing, body manipulation, massage, and changes in posture and position of body parts. Body therapies are used in holistic therapies, which recognize relationships between mind and body in helping individuals overcome anxieties and phobias.

Body therapies encompass ancient Eastern traditions of spirituality and cosmology along with contemporary Western neuromuscular and myofascial systems of skeletostructural and neuroskeletal reorganization. They postulate that the body holds memory of trauma and that therapy must address body sensations. In fact, all proven theories for trauma focus extensively on body sensations.

Ancient disciplines in the category of body therapies include YOGA, TAI CHI CHUAN, Zen, Taoism, and Tantra. In the 20th century, Wilhelm Reich observed that clinical patients with emotional disturbances all demonstrated severe postural distortions. This observation helped to uncover more connections between the body-psyche and led to the development of the Reichian school of body therapy.

Another modern pioneer in the field was Moshe Feldenkrais, who postulated that the human organism began its process of growth and learning with one built-in response, the "fear of falling." All other physical and emotional responses were learned as the human organism grew and explored. To attain the full potential of the body-mind-emotions-spirit, there must be, according to Feldenkrais, "reeducation of the kinesthetic sense and resetting of it to the normal course of self-adjusting improvement of all muscular activity." This would "directly improve breathing, digestion, and the sympathetic and parasympathetic balance, as well as the sexual function, all linked together with the emotional experience." Feldenkrais believed that reeducation of the body and its functions was the essence of creating unity of the being. His method has helped many people with problems of BACK PAIN, whiplash, and lack of coordination. The method is also used to help people who have TEMPOROMANDIBULAR JOINT SYNDROME (TMJ), which is a collection of symptoms, including pain, that affect the jaw, face, and head, often brought about by anxieties, stress, and tension.

Four Systems of Body Therapies

Although many systems overlap and encompass aspects of the others, body therapies can be divided into four general categories, based on their methods.

Physical manipulation systems include the connective tissue work of the Ida Rolf school (Rolfing) and the deep tissues release systems such as myofascial release used by John Barnes, an American physical therapist.

Energy balancing systems include Chinese ACUPUNCTURE and ACUPRESSURE, polarity, and Jin Shin Jystu.

Emotional release systems include bioenergetics, primal therapy, and rebirthing.

Movement awareness systems include those of Aston, Feldenkrais, Trager, and Aguado.

See also AYURVEDA; COMPLEMENTARY THERAPIES; MASSAGE THERAPY; MIND/BODY CONNECTIONS; YOGA.

Feldenkrais, Moshe, *Explorers of Humankind* (San Francisco: Harper & Row, 1979).
———, *Awareness Through Movement* (San Francisco: Harper & Row, 1972).
Feltman, John, ed., *Hands-On Healing* (Emmaus, Penn.: Rodale Press, 1989).

bogeyman, bogyman, bogey, and bogy An imaginary character possibly possessing supernatural powers. The word has been used to refer to an apparition, hobgoblin, ghost, or the devil. Children fear the bogeyman because they are told that this spirit will punish them for misbehaving. The word *bogy* may have derived from a southern American form of bug, object of terror, or bugbear; it appears often in 19th- and 20th-century literature, as early as 1825.

The words *boglie*, meaning haunted, and *boglesome*, meaning shy or skittish, have been developed from the original term.

In psychoanalytic terms, the bogeyman is interpreted as externalized presuperego; that is, a projection onto persons in the external world of the internalized parental prohibitions that are the forerunners of the superego.

See also ANXIETY DISORDERS OF CHILDREN; PSYCHO-ANALYSIS.

Campbell, Robert, *Psychiatric Dictionary* (New York: Oxford University Press, 1981).

Oxford English Dictionary (London: Clarendon Press, 1961).

Random House Dictionary of the English Language (New York: Random House, 1987).

Sarafino, Edward P., *The Fears of Childhood* (New York: Human Sciences Press, 1986).

Spears, Richard A., *Slang and Euphemism* (Middle Village, NY: David, 1981).

Wright, John, ed., *English Dialect Dictionary* (New York: Oxford University Press, 1970; reprint of 1905 edition).

bogyphobia   Fear of bogies, or the bogeyman. Bogyphobia can also refer to a generalized fear of demons, goblins, or spirits. It has no relation to boogyphobia, which is a fear of "getting down and rocking."

See also BOGEYMAN; DEMONS; GOBLINS; SPIRITS; WITCHES.

books, fear of   Fear of books is known as bibliophobia. Fear of the power of books is often expressed in terms less personal than those used for other fears. For example, government and religious officials rarely feel that reading a book is damaging to them personally but rather believe that society must be shielded from dangerous or obscene material.

Obsessive-compulsives will sometimes fear particular words or numbers or fear reading about particular behavior, thoughts, or emotions.

With the advent of printing and the spread of literacy, books fell into hands other than those of scholars and religious leaders. As a result, both government and church took various measures to control reading of what were considered heretical or treasonous ideas. The 18th century saw a relaxation of control and a guarantee of freedom of expression in the American Bill of Rights. In the 20th century, however, the burning of "unpatriotic" books was one of the most dramatic indications of the repressive influence of the Nazi regime in Germany. Concentration on obscenity and the efforts of various pressure groups to control publication and distribution of books have characterized recent history in the United States.

Too much or too little association with books also produces a certain type of stigma. Adult illiterates fear situations that will reveal that they cannot hold down a job or perform other daily tasks. On the other hand, to be considered bookish or a bookworm is not particularly complimentary.

See also BOOKS AS ANXIETY RELIEF.

Haight, Anne Lyon, *Banned Books, 387 B.C. to 1978 A.D* (New York: R. R. Bowker, 1978) pp. i–xxv.

Sills, D. E., ed., *International Encyclopedia of the Social Sciences* (New York: Macmillan, 1968) "censorship."

books as anxiety relief   Bibliotherapy is an interdisciplinary field that combines the skills of psychotherapists, librarians, and educators. In the course of a bibliotherapy program, books are selected to promote normal development and to change disturbed patterns of behavior. The books may be directly concerned with mental health or may be fiction or nonfiction works relating to and interpreting the readers' problems and concerns. It has been suggested that reading about a disturbing subject such as DEATH, divorce, or AGING gives the reader a sense of control over his problems, a way of working them out in his mind. Use of selected books with children may alleviate fears by clearing up misconceptions and giving information about the UNKNOWN. Reading may also give the child the comforting knowledge that others share his fears and may promote communication with his or her parents.

Rubin, Rhea Joyce, *Bibliotherapy Sourcebook* (Phoenix: Oryx Press, 1978).

Sarafino, Edward P., *The Fears of Childhood* (New York: Human Sciences Press, 1986).

borborygami, fear of Rumbling, gurgling, etc. in the stomach or intestines, produced by gas in the alimentary canal, and audible at a distance. Some individuals so fear that others will hear these sounds that they become social phobics and avoid situations where other people may hear these sounds.

See also PHOBIA; SOCIAL PHOBIA.

borderline personality disorder A personality disorder characterized by anxiety and unstable moods, behaviors, self-image, and interpersonal relationships. Moods may shift from normal to depressed, and the individual may show inappropriate intense anger or lack of control of anger. There may be impulsive moods, particularly with regard to activities that are potentially self-damaging, such as shopping sprees, psychoactive-substance abuse, reckless driving, casual sex, shoplifting, and binge eating. There may be an identity disturbance noticeable because of uncertainty about self-image, gender identity, or long-term goals or values. The individual may be chronically bored. During periods of extreme stress there may be symptoms of depersonalization. This disorder is more common in females than in males.

See also ANXIETY; DEPERSONALIZATION; PERSONALITY DISORDERS.

boredom, fear of Boredom is characterized by slow reactions, lack of productivity, wandering attention, and lessened emotional response. In extreme form, boredom may produce depression and hallucination. Boredom is a uniquely individual psychological condition in that what may be fascinating or soothing to one person may be boring or even anxiety-arousing to another. Boredom has been held responsible for ANXIETIES that lead to vandalism, violence, educational and vocational dropping out, marital unhappiness, and even SUICIDE.

Participants in an experiment using an artificial sensory-deprivation environment dropped out in spite of the fact that they were being paid well for doing nothing. Boredom is actually a type of punishment. Solitary confinement for prisoners is a dreaded condition.

Boredom, or lack of stimulation, can be a triggering stimulus for anxiety, particularly with agoraphobics. For example, many agoraphobics fear being alone, which is a state of too little social stimulation. Likewise, quietness, open spaces, and empty rooms are common anxiety triggers characterized by lack of stimulation.

An essential fact of boredom is that it is almost always the creation of the person who is bored. Things are only boring if someone judges them as boring. While some people seem bored with everything, others are bored with nothing. For some people, boredom is a self-imposed prison that keeps them from trying new things or having new, life-enriching experiences. Boredom often occurs with individuals who thrive on excessive stimulation and is not a function of environmental or social causes but of reduction in stimulation.

Some people view things as boring because they really are afraid of failure. In his book, *A New Guide to Rational Living*, Dr. Albert Ellis says: "Viewing failure with fear and horror, some people avoid activities that they would really like to engage in." The rationale of such people is: if life is boring, nothing is worth doing. Thus if nothing is worth doing, a person can hardly fail.

Overcoming Boredom

Overcoming boredom depends on whether people are bored because they cannot live without excitement or whether they are bored because they have chosen to remain in a shell of inaction. Life is not supposed to be thrilling all the time. If you crave continuous thrills, reduce your expectations for excitement. If you are encased by the stresses of boredom, try to face reality. Get out and do one new thing each day, such as talk to some new people, become a volunteer, or write letters. Carried to the extreme, boredom and lack of stimulation can lead to depression and anxiety.

See also DEPRESSION; GENERAL ADAPTATION SYNDROME; HOBBIES.

botonophobia   Fear of plants.

See also PLANTS, FEAR OF.

bound, afraid of being   Fear of being bound is known as merinthophobia. This fear is related to a fear of being out of control and a fear of being closed in without escape.

See also ENCLOSED SPACES, FEAR OF; TIED UP, FEAR OF BEING.

bradycardia   Extremely slow heart rate; the opposite of tachycardia (rapid heart rate). In many blood-injury phobics, bradycardia occurs as a secondary reaction, following an initial phase of rapid heartbeat. Bradycardia can lead to fainting.

brain disease, fear of   Fear of brain disease is known as meningitophobia.

brain imaging techniques   Brain imaging techniques, like biological imaging techniques in general (such as X rays), allow a physician or researcher to look inside the body without surgically opening it. Techniques include regional cerebral blood flow (RCBF) imaging, nuclear magnetic resonance (NMR) imaging, positron emission tomography (PET), computerized tomography (CT), single photon emission computed tomography (SPECT), and computerized topographic EEG (electroencephalograph) mapping.

Unlike the other imaging techniques, PET can measure body chemistry rather than simply anatomy. Because it measures tracer concentrations up to a million times better than other techniques, it allows the study of microscopic, virtually invisible processes—such as the passage of nutrients through a membrane—as they take place. Thus PET can measure the distribution of psychoactive drugs, such as ANTIDEPRESSANTS, in the brain as well as the sites of trauma from head injuries, brain cancers, strokes, and epileptic seizures.

See also BIOLOGICAL BASIS FOR ANXIETY; DIAGNOSTIC CRITERIA.

brainwashing   The process of inducing an individual to depart radically from his former behavior patterns, standards, and beliefs, and to adopt those imposed on him by others. It is not a technique used to treat phobias, although the intentions of the process are to change the individual's attitude and behaviors. The term has been used since the middle of the 20th century. Brainwashing is a technique feared by servicemen and spies. Although nothing is done directly to the brains of the individuals, much is done to their bodies, including starvation, beating, torture, isolation, prevention of sleep, endless interrogation, and often rewards for acting or speaking along lines indicated by the captors. Brainwashing is not a scientific application of any special psychological techniques and can be successfully done by virtually primitive people who have never heard of psychology. It is basically a physical-abuse technique in which a victim is deprived of health and vigor by the captors. The induction of fears and anxieties is a key element in the brainwashing process.

breakdown, nervous   See NERVOUS BREAKDOWN.

breast cancer   A malignant tumor in the breast tissue or area. Most sufferers are female, but some men contract breast cancer. A diagnosis of breast cancer brings extreme anxiety, including the fear of death and, for women, fear of the loss of a breast and the potential loss of perceived physical attractiveness and sexuality.

Breast cancer is the most common newly diagnosed cancer in women. According to the National Cancer Institute, an estimated 211,240 women develop new cases of breast cancer in each year, as do about 1,700 men. The most common type of breast cancer is ductal carcinoma, in which abnormal cells are located within the lining of the ducts. Lobular carcinoma is another type of breast cancer.

Most studies show that white women have the greatest risk for a breast cancer diagnosis. However, African-American women have a worse prognosis and higher mortality rate with breast cancer than women of other races, which may be related to the higher grade (more advanced) tumors that they are more likely to develop, as well as a diagnosis in a later stage of the disease.

When cancer is detected while the tumor is still localized in the breast, the disease can be treated, and many women will lead normal life spans after receiving treatment. However, if the tumor has metastasized (spread) to other parts of the body, such as the bones, lungs, liver, or brain, this type of cancer is more difficult to treat and is usually not curable.

The anxiety, fear, and apprehension that each woman faces when she or her physician discovers a lump in her breast are, if proven to be breast cancer, the beginning of a long, stressful period in her life. In addition, the diagnosis of breast cancer affects her family, as they fear her possible death as well as physical harm and illness. Marriages or relationships can be put under a terrific strain and often they do not last. For these women, the stress of maintaining a positive sense of BODY IMAGE and self-worth follows them throughout their lives.

Women diagnosed with breast cancer face difficult decisions, such as which treatment to have and whether to have a breast reconstruction or to have the entire breast removed. The physician will offer advice, but the decision is ultimately up to the woman.

Once a lump has been discovered, whether through self-examination, physician examination, or mammography, a woman enters a world of baffling terminology in which she must depend on medical professionals. She must deal with the anxieties of tests and procedures that are used to identify a breast symptom and also cope with the time lapse before a final diagnosis is made. If a malignancy is found, she must select from a variety of treatment options and find the right resources to assure that the best decision is made. The more information that she has, the easier it may be for a woman to determine the advantages and disadvantages of various therapies.

When treatment is completed, the woman who has had breast cancer is faced with the fear and continuing anxiety that she could experience a recurrence of the disease.

Symptoms and Diagnostic Path

Only a physician can accurately diagnose the presence of breast cancer. However, some common symptoms of breast cancer are

- a lump or thickening in or near the breast or in the underarm area
- a change in how the breast or nipple looks (a change in the size or shape of the breast; a nipple turned inward into the breast; or the skin of the breast, the areola, or nipple may be scaly, red, or swollen and have ridges or pitting that is similar to the skin of an orange)
- the presence of a nipple discharge of fluid in nonnursing women

Women should receive screening for breast cancer through monthly breast self-examinations, as well as an annual examination by a physician and mammograms. Women should keep in mind that it is normal to experience some breast changes, such as the swelling and tenderness that may occur prior to the menstrual period. With self-screening or screening by a physician, the breast should be checked as well as the underarm area. The physician will also check the lymph nodes near the breast for lumps.

Often lumps are as small as the size of a pea. Women age 40 and older should have mammograms every one to two years, depending on the frequency recommended by their physician. In addition, women who are younger than age 40 but who have risk factors for breast cancer (such as a family history) should ask their physician whether to have mammograms and how often to have them.

If a lump is identified, the physician will usually order X-rays and/or ultrasound. The doctor may also order a magnetic resonance imaging (MRI) scan of the breast. The physician will also order a biopsy to determine if the lump is malignant (cancerous) or benign. Sometimes lumps are masses of fatty tissue that are not cancerous; however, only a biopsy can determine whether cancer is present.

The biopsy is performed in one of three basic ways: a fine-needle aspiration, a core biopsy, or a surgical biopsy. With a fine-needle aspiration, a very thin needle is used to remove fluid from a breast lump. The pathologist will examine the fluid and check for cancer cells.

With a core biopsy, the doctor will use a thick needle to remove breast tissue, and this tissue will be checked by the pathologist for cancer cells.

With a surgical biopsy, the doctor will remove a sample of a lump or of the abnormal area, and the pathologist will evaluate the tissue for cancer.

Treatment Options and Outlook

Once breast cancer has been confirmed, a treatment plan is made and carried out. Before a plan can be made, however, the oncologist (cancer doctor) must *stage* the cancer, or determine the size of the tumor and whether the cancer is localized or has spread. X-rays and laboratory tests will help determine the stage of cancer.

Staging the cancer.   There are five basic stages of breast cancer. Stage 0 cancer is also known as *carcinoma in situ*. In this early stage, there are abnormal cancer cells that have not invaded breast tissue. If not treated, however, this cancer can become invasive.

With Stage I cancer, which is an early stage of invasive breast cancer, the tumor is two centimeters (3/4 of an inch) or less in size. Cancer cells have not spread beyond the breast at this stage.

With Stage II cancer, there are three possible circumstances. First, the tumor may be as small as in Stage I, but the cancer has spread to the underarm lymph nodes. Or, the tumor is two–five centimeters and cancer has spread to the underarm lymph nodes. Last, the tumor is greater than five centimeters but it has *not* spread to the underarm lymph nodes.

Stage III cancers include locally advanced cancers which may be large but they have not spread beyond the nearby lymph nodes or breast. This stage also includes other cancers that include a spread to the lymph nodes.

Stage IV, the most advanced stage of breast cancer, is distant metastatic cancer, which means that the cancer has spread to other parts of the body. When cancer has metastasized, it can be treated but it cannot be cured.

Surgery, radiation therapy, hormone therapy, or chemotherapy are the primary treatments for breast cancer. Often a combination of treatments is used, such as surgery and radiation. Biological therapy is another treatment option. The oncologist will advise which options are the best.

If surgery is the treatment, the woman may need a breast removal (mastectomy) or a breast-sparing surgery may be sufficient. (Breast-sparing surgery is also called *lumpectomy, partial mastectomy, or breast-conserving surgery*.) Some women who have had a mastectomy choose to have a breast reconstruction while others wear a breast prosthesis, while others take no action. If breast reconstruction is chosen, it can be done at the same time as the mastectomy or at a later date. Some women have saline or silicone implants inserted. Information on breast implants is available from the Food and Drug Administration at http://www.fda.gov/cdrh/breastimplants. In other cases, the surgeon may remove tissue from another part of the body to create a breast shape.

Often the underarm lymph nodes are also removed, whether mastectomy or breast-sparing surgery is performed.

Some questions which women facing surgery may wish to ask the doctor include

- What kinds of surgery can I consider? Is breast-sparing surgery an option for me?
- Which surgery do you recommend and why?
- How long will it take to recover from surgery?
- Will my lymph nodes be removed? If so, how many and why?
- Will I need to stay in the hospital after surgery? If so, for about how long?
- How will I feel after the surgery?
- Where will the scars be? What will they look like?
- If I decide to have plastic surgery later to rebuild my breast, how and when can that be done? Would you suggest a plastic surgeon I could contact?
- Will I need to do special exercises to help me regain motion and strength in my arm and shoulder? Will a physical therapist teach me these exercises?
- Will I need to learn how to care for myself or my incision when I get home?

If lymph nodes were removed from the under-arm area, this can slow the flow of lymph fluid, which can lead to swelling of the arm and hand. Experts recommend that women who have had lymph nodes removed from under the arm take the following actions for the rest of their lives:

- avoid wearing tight clothes or jewelry on the affected arm
- carry the purse or a suitcase with the other arm
- use an electric razor to avoid cuts when shaving under the arm
- have blood tests, shots, and other blood pressure readings taken on the other arm
- wear gloves to protect the hands when washing dishes or gardening
- avoid burns or sunburns to the affected arm and hand

Radiation therapy may be given and if women have breast-sparing surgery, radiation is often given. Radiation may be given by a large machine, often daily for several weeks. Implant radiation is another option, in which thin plastic implants with a radioactive substance are placed inside the breast for several days. This treatment is given in a hospital and the implants are removed before the patient goes home.

Loose-fitting clothes should be worn to treatment because the skin may be sore. The patient should not use any lotions or creams on the area unless they have been approved by the physician. Radiation therapy can cause fatigue. Some questions that patients may wish to ask about radiation therapy, to allay their anxiety, include

- How will I feel during treatment?
- Will I be able to drive myself to and from treatment?
- When will treatment start and end?
- How will we know if the treatment is working?
- Will treatment affect my skin?
- How will my chest look after treatment?
- Are there any long-term effects to radiation treatment?

- How often will I need checkups?
- What is the chance that cancer could come back in my breast?
- What can I do to take care of myself, before, during, and after treatment?

Hormone therapy is another treatment for breast cancer. It is given to deplete the hormones that help cancer cells grow. Tamoxifen is the most commonly used drug for hormone therapy, as of this writing. The drug may cause hot flashes and vaginal discharge, as well as irregular menstrual periods, headaches, fatigue, nausea, and vomiting among other side effects. Not everyone experiences these side effects. It is still possible (although inadvisable) to become pregnant while on tamoxifen, which can harm the fetus.

Chemotherapy involves the use of drugs to destroy the cancer. These drugs often cause nausea and vomiting and temporary baldness. (The hair will grow back when the course of chemotherapy is completed, but it may be a different color and texture than before treatment.) According to the National Cancer Institute, some questions to ask the physician if chemotherapy is the considered option include

- What drugs will I be taking? What will they do?
- When will treatment start? When will it end? How often will I have treatments?
- Where will I go for treatment? Will I be able to drive myself home afterward?
- What can I do to take care of myself during treatment?
- How will we know if the treatment is working?
- Which side effects should I tell you about?
- Will there be long-term effects?

Biological therapy is sometimes used to treat breast cancer. It is a therapy that helps the immune system fight back. Some women receive a drug called trastuzumab (Herceptin), which is a drug that binds to cancer cells. It is given to women with an excess of a specific protein called HER2. Many women experience chills and fever with the initial treatment. Some women have other side effects.

The side effects generally lessen after the first treatment. Herceptin can cause damage to the heart and lungs.

Risk Factors and Preventive Measures

Women with family members who have had breast cancer are at risk for developing breast cancer, especially if their mother, sister, or daughter has had breast cancer. These women should be even more vigilant than others about receiving regular examinations from their physicians. In addition, all adult women should perform regular self-tests and also see their gynecologist for annual checks.

According to the National Cancer Institute, regular screening mammography is a protective action that reduces the risk of dying from breast cancer by 17 percent among women in their 40s, and it further reduces the death risk by 30 percent among women between the ages of 50 to 69 years.

Age is another risk factor, and most cases of breast cancer occur in women who are older than age 60. Breast cancer is not common before the onset of menopause.

Women who have previously had breast cancer in one breast are at an increased risk for developing breast cancer in the other breast.

Other risk factors for female breast cancer include women

- who have never had children
- who take menopausal hormone therapy with estrogen plus progestin
- who had their first menstrual period before age 12
- who are overweight or obese after menopause
- who have had radiation therapy to the chest before age 30, such as women who have been treated with radiation for Hodgkin's lymphoma
- who went through menopause after age 55

In addition, some studies have shown that ALCO-HOLISM increases the risk for breast cancer in men and women.

See also BODY IMAGE; CANCER, FEAR OF, CHRONIC ILLNESS, FEAR OF.

National Cancer Institute, *What You Need to Know About Breast Cancer.* Washington, DC: National Institutes of Health, 2005. Available online. URL: http://www.cancer.gov/pdf/WYNTK/WYNTK_breast.pdf. Accessed April 25, 2006.

breathholding spells Childhood breathholding spells, a common and frightening phenomenon that occurs in healthy, otherwise normal children, are a source of stress and anxiety for adult and child alike. Treatment of children with breathholding spells has largely focused on providing reassurance to families after a diagnosis has been made.

Some children use breathholding as an act of rebellion or a demonstration of AUTONOMY. When children know that they can terrify their parents with this behavior, it becomes somewhat reinforced. According to Francis DiMario Jr., M.D., Department of Pediatrics, University of Connecticut Health Center, Farmington, "It is neither feasible nor helpful for parents to attempt to avoid circumstances that may provide emotional upset in their child. Even though pain and fear may serve as provocatives, simple frustration and the expression of autonomy are both normal and expected in young children."

If parental anxiety leads to continuous attempts at appeasement, the child may soon learn to manipulate the parent with the threat of crying. This does not imply a willful attempt at breathholding, since in some cases these spells are reflexive and unpredictable. There is, nonetheless, the potential for parents to reinforce behavioral outbursts if appropriate calm firmness is not displayed at times of customary disciplining.

Should a breathholding spell occur, have the child lie on his or her back, face upward, to protect the child's head from inadvertent injury and aspiration.

See also BREATHING; PARENTING.

Brownstone, David, and Irene Franck, *The Parent's Desk Reference* (New York: Prentice Hall, 1991).
Kahn, Ada P., and Jan Fawcett, *The Encyclopedia of Mental Health,* 2nd ed. (New York: Facts On File, 2001).

breathing The major features of breathing are respiration and ventilation. Respiration puts oxygen into body cells and ventilation removes the excess carbon dioxide. Poor breathing habits diminish the flow of gasses to and from the body, making it harder for individuals to cope with fearful situations or situations producing anxieties.

With increased awareness of how people breathe and by incorporating certain controlled breathing techniques into relaxation practice, they will be able to quiet thoughts, calm emotions, deepen relaxation, and control blood pressure and other physical functions. Although breathing seems very easy and very normal, relearning breathing techniques can help many individuals who suffer from PHOBIAS, anxieties, and PANIC ATTACKS. Some performers and athletes learn this technique in order to combat STAGE FRIGHT or PERFORMANCE ANXIETY.

Breathing is controlled by the automatic or involuntary nervous system. Breathing patterns change during different psychological states. For example, in a state of calm and relaxation, breathing becomes deeper and more rhythmic. Under stress, breathing is shallow and irregular. When frightened, an individual may even hold his/her breath. However, breathing patterns can be consciously controlled in order to influence the autonomic system toward relaxation, thereby interrupting the physiological arousal that can lead to stress-related disorders and high blood pressure.

Breathing Styles

Most people breathe in one of two patterns: one is chest or thoracic breathing, the other is abdominal or diaphragmatic breathing. Chest breathing, which is usually shallow and often rapid and irregular, is associated with anxiety or other emotional distress. When air is inhaled, the chest expands and the shoulders rise to take in air. Anxious people may experience breath holding, HYPERVENTILATION or constricted breathing, shortness of breath, or fear of passing out. When an insufficient amount of air reaches the lungs, the blood is not properly oxygenated, the heart rate and muscle tension increases, and the stress response is triggered.

Abdominal or diaphragmatic breathing is the natural breathing of sleeping adults. The diaphragm contracts and expands as inhaled air is drawn deep into the lungs and exhaled. When breathing is even and unconstricted, the respiratory system performs efficiently in producing energy from oxygen and removing waste products.

Symptoms of Inefficient Breathing

Many people who often feel very anxious also often have breathing-related complaints. Some can't seem to catch their breath or get enough air. Others may frequently sigh, yawn, or swallow. Some breathe too deeply and hyperventilate. Symptoms associated with hyperventilation resemble those of panic disorder. Researchers have noted the overlap between hyperventilation, anxiety, and stress symptoms. It has been found that patients will hyperventilate just by asking them to think back to unpleasant or anxiety producing events.

Physical conditions associated with breathing difficulties, particularly hyperventilation, include hypertension, ALLERGIES, anemia, angina, arthritis, arrhythmias, asthma, colitis, diabetes, gastritis, HEADACHES, heart disease, and IRRITABLE BOWEL SYNDROME.

Deep, diaphragmatic breathing is a cornerstone for many relaxation therapies. Many therapeutic techniques (many known as COMPLEMENTARY THERAPIES)

TIPS FOR DIAPHRAGMATIC OR ABDOMINAL BREATHING FOR STRESS REDUCTION

- Lie down comfortably on your back on a padded floor or a firm bed with eyes closed, arms at your sides and not touching your body, palms up, legs straight out and slightly apart, and toes pointed comfortably outward.
- Focus attention on your breathing. Breathe through your nose. Place your hand on the part of your chest that seems to rise and fall the most as you inhale and exhale.
- Place both of your hands lightly on your abdomen and slow your breathing. Become aware of how your abdomen rises with each inhalation and falls with each exhalation.
- If you have difficulty breathing into your abdomen, press your hand down on your abdomen as you exhale and let your abdomen push your hand back up as you inhale.
- Observe how your chest moves; it should be moving in synchronization with your abdomen.

and behavior therapies incorporate control of breathing as a basis because the cycle of stress can be altered with breath control. Individuals who have mastered these techniques find that as soon as they are aware of a stressor, they become aware of their breathing and try to control their stress by deep, slow breaths. By contrast, holding the breath, as well as shallow, irregular breathing, can initiate as well as augment many stressful feelings and physiological response. Posture can also affect breathing. Keeping the body in alignment allows greater lung capacity.

Breathing, Yoga, and Language

Yoga is a more than 2,000-year-old method for developing and unifying mind, body, and spirit. Yoga practitioners have long recognized the relationship between breathing and health and maintain that life force is carried in the breath. Exercises to control breathing are incorporated into yoga postures (*asanas*) and practices. Yoga practitioners believe that extending and deepening the breathing process draws breath all the way down to one's heels and that deep and slow breathing can increase longevity.

See also ASTHMA; BEHAVIOR THERAPY; BIOFEEDBACK; COMPLEMENTARY THERAPIES; GUIDED IMAGERY; HYPERVENTILATION; MEDITATION; PANIC ATTACKS AND PANIC DISORDER; YOGA.

Kerman, D. Ariel, *The H.A.R.T. Program: Lower Your Blood Pressure Without Drugs* (New York: HarperCollins, 1993).
"RX: Breathing for Health and Relaxation," *Mental Medicine Update* 4, no. 2 (1995).

bridges, fear of   Fear of bridges is related to fear of being trapped, similar to the fear of being stopped in traffic and unable to turn around. Fear of bridges is also related to fear of heights and narrow spaces. Bridge fear may be considered a fear of childbirth, according to some sources.

"The Angel of the Bridge," a short story by John Cheever, contains an excellent description of panic attack symptoms on a bridge:

"The seizure came with a rush. The strength went out of my legs. I gasped for breath, and felt the terrifying loss of sight. I was, at the same time, determined to conceal these symptoms. . . . I felt the sense of reality ebbing. . . . The loneliness of my predicament was harrowing."

See also FALLING, FEAR OF; HEIGHTS, FEAR OF; NARROW PLACES, FEAR OF.

brief focal family therapy   An approach to family therapy derived from focal psychotherapy and other brief psychoanalytic approaches to treatment developed at the Tavistock Clinic, London. The therapist develops a focal pattern to serve as a guide in contacts with the family, and the treatment plan is modified as treatment progresses. Treatment for ANXIETY and PHOBIAS would include the family as a unit, with the goal being alleviation of the anxiety by focusing on dynamics within the unit that cause or maintain the anxiety.

See also BRIEF PSYCHOTHERAPY; FAMILY THERAPY.

brief psychotherapy   A form of therapy in which sessions are limited to 10 or 15 in number and during which the therapist uses active and goal-directive techniques and procedures. Brief psychotherapy has been used in individual and group settings to treat phobias and anxieties but is not the treatment of choice for these disorders. Brief psychotherapy has been effective in "crisis management" situations.

See also BEHAVIOR MODIFICATION.

bromides   Bromides are drugs that produce sedation and reduce anxieties. They were first widely used during the mid-1800s. During the second half of the 20th century, however, as many new antianxiety drugs became available bromides have become less popular. Newer drugs avoid a side effect of bromides known as bromism (a subdelirious state).

See also ANTIANXIETY DRUGS; SEDATIVES.

bromidrophobia (bromidrosiphobia)   Fear of offensive odors of the body, either of one's own or of others.

See also PERSONAL ODORS, FEAR OF.

brontophobia   Fear of thunder; also known as astrophobia. Historically, man has dreaded allegedly demonical phenomena in nature, to which he assigned personalities. Fear of thunder, in psychodynamic terms, may be related to fear of real persons in positions of authority, and especially of the father or father figure.

Those who experience fear of thunder (and usually lightning as well) are restricted to interior sections of buildings (away from outside sight or sound) during storms. Sometimes they will retreat to movie theaters or even leave town as a way to avoid exposure to thunder and lightning.

See also STORMS, FEAR OF; THUNDER, FEAR OF.

bugging, fear of   Fear of bugging is a fear that one is being watched, listened to, or otherwise monitored by others. This is a 20th-century fear as highly technologic listening devices, popularly known as "bugs," have been developed and put into use by governments, industry, and others. While the fear is a realistic one in many cases, such as in governmental embassies, where extensive listening devices have been found, some individuals have delusions that they are being listened to by others. Some of these individuals believe that others are pursuing them or are trying to harm them. A fear of "bugging" may be related to OBSESSIVE-COMPULSIVE DISORDER if the individual becomes compulsive about repeatedly checking for listening devices. It could also be an integral part of a delusional system characteristic of paranoid individuals.

See also PARANOID.

bugs, fear of   Fear of insects and spiders is known as bug phobia. From the psychoanalytic point of view, such fears may represent a direct projection of one's own drives, as the tiny creatures may represent genitals, feces, or little children, such as brothers and sisters. More likely, however, fears of insects develop, as do most fears, by traumatic conditioning, repeated aversive exposure, modeling, etc. In its severe form, fear of insects (which is usually quite specific in nature) leads to excessive cleaning of living areas, regular spraying of insecticides (sometimes to an excessive degree), and, if the dreaded insect is seen, complete avoidance of that area, even moving to another living environment.

Many individuals fear bugs because they bite, cause itching, carry disease, and imply less-than-clean conditions. Fear of bugs may be related to a fear of dirt or fear of contamination by germs. Some individuals who have OBSESSIVE-COMPULSIVE DISORDER have obsessions about keeping their environment bug-free.

See also ANIMALS, FEAR OF; INSECTS, FEAR OF; SPIDERS, FEAR OF.

building, fear of passing a tall   Fear of passing a tall building is known as batophobia. This fear may be related to a fear of HEIGHTS, a fear of looking up at a high place, or a fear of FALLING. Some individuals who have one phobia relating to heights have another of this type.

bulimia   See EATING DISORDERS.

bulls, fear of   Fear of bulls is known as taurophobia. The bull as a frightening symbol has a long history. The bull's ancestor, the auroch, was a prime source of meat for Paleolithic and Stone Age man. Since hunting the auroch meant first killing the strongest and most powerful bull—the leader of the herd—the image of the bull as the ultimate adversary became prominent in the prehistoric mind. In many ancient cultures, bulls were a symbol of power and authority associated with kings or gods. The strength and temperament of the bull also created symbolic, mythological associations with other fears, such as fear of destruction and fear of natural forces such as THUNDER, LIGHTNING, and EARTHQUAKES.

See also APOCALYPSE, FEAR OF; SYMBOLS.

bupropion   An atypical antidepressant drug approved by the Food and Drug Administration (FDA) for the treatment of depression. Bupropion has properties that are similar to those of the tricyclic antidepressants but has more rapid therapeutic effects and apparently no cardiovascular or sedative side effects.

It is sometimes used as an off-label treatment for ATTENTION-DEFICIT/HYPERACTIVITY DISORDER as well as BIPOLAR DISORDER. Bupropion should be avoided in patients prone to seizures and should be used with caution in combination with tricyclic antidepressants, lithium, and some antipsychotics.

Rarely, bupropion can trigger mania. Common side effects include headache, dizziness, constipation, and loss of appetite, but these side effects may abate with time.

See also ANTIDEPRESSANTS; DEPRESSION.

bureaucracy, fear of   Many people fear bureaucracy and "red tape," which, to some, mean the same. Bureaucracy is feared because the individual is subordinated to the group or government and loses his own sense of autonomy. He feels a loss of control as he associates bureaucracy with complicated forms, high-handed officials, narrow thinking, failure to assign or accept responsibility, rigidity, lack of attention to the individual, paper shuffling, official blundering, conflicting orders and information, and empire building. Yossarian, the hero of Joseph Heller's antiwar novel, *Catch-22,* was a victim of military bureaucratic thinking. In his efforts to get out of combat duty, he encountered Catch-22, the requirement that a man must ask to be removed from combat duty on the grounds of insanity but that to do so defeated the purpose because a request indicating concern for safety in the face of danger is the product of a rational mind.

See also AUTHORITY, FEAR OF.

burglars, fear of   Fear of burglars is known as scelerophobia. In contemporary urban life, many individuals have a fear of burglars and hence take extra precautions to have adequate locks, elaborate burglar alarm systems, and guard dogs. Some obsessive-compulsives who fear burglars may repeatedly check to be sure they have locked their doors and windows. Recent studies indicate that young children's greatest fear is of someone coming into their home and hurting them.

See also BAD MEN, FEAR OF; OBSESSIVE-COMPULSIVE DISORDER.

buried alive, fear of being   A type of claustrophobia, or fear of being in ENCLOSED PLACES. Individuals fear being buried alive because they fear an inability to escape from such a situation. This fear is also related to a fear of SMOTHERING.

See also CLAUSTROPHOBIA.

burnout   *Burnout* is a contemporary term for the progressive loss of energy, purpose, and idealism that leads to frustration and boredom. It may result from ongoing, chronic anxiety, and it is also a cause of stress for the sufferer as well as his family and coworkers. It strikes anyone in any job—executives to mothers with small children. It has no relationship to intelligence or financial or social position.

Burnout begins slowly and progresses gradually over weeks, months, and years to become cumulative and pervasive. Physical symptoms of burnout include excessive sleeping, eating, or drinking, physical exhaustion, loss of libido, frequent colds, headaches, backaches, neckaches,

---

TIPS FOR COPING WITH ANXIETIES PRODUCED BY BURNOUT

- Recognize that no one job (or personal relationship) is a total solution for life. Strive for variety in work; avoid routine.

- Put priorities into perspective; stop trying to be "all things to all people."

- Differentiate between authentic personal goals and those foisted on you by others.

- Learn to accept reality and assume responsibility for yourself.

- Set aside personal time (no phone, no TV, no eating or reading) and answer the vital questions, "Where am I going?," "What do I want to achieve?," and "How am I going to do it?"

- Develop competence in simple tasks to enhance your self-confidence and self-esteem, increase optimism and lift depression.

- Create an "outside life" of family, friends, interests, and activities unrelated to your work.

- Develop a support system that emphasizes problem solving; for example, "How can I improve on this situation."

---

and bowel disorders. The burnout victim desires to be alone, is irritable, impatient and withdrawn, and complains of boredom, difficulty concentrating, and burdensome work. Fellow workers may notice indecisiveness, indifference, impaired performance, and high absenteeism. Intellectual curiosity declines, identity diffuses, and interpersonal relationships deteriorate. "Overloaded," "tired of thinking," and "I don't know what I'm doing anymore," express the inner agony and stress of burnout sufferers.

Burnout victims are often high achievers, workaholics, idealists, competent, self-sufficient, and overly conscientious individuals. Their common denominator is the assumption that the real world will be in harmony with their ideals. They often hold unrealistic expectations of themselves, their employers, and society, and often have a vague definition of personal accomplishment. In their attempt to gain some distance from their source of anguish, they contract their world down to the smallest possible dimension and/or take on more and more work.

Recovery from burnout is possible through rediscovery of true self and the formation of a revised outlook about one's life. Realistic goals and nurturing activities often help resolve burnout.

See also ANXIETY; BOREDOM, FEAR OF; CHRONIC FATIGUE SYNDROME; CONTROL; DEPRESSION; HOBBIES; RELAXATION; STRESS.

Kahn, Ada P., *The Encyclopedia of Stress and Stress-related Disorders,* 2nd ed. (New York: Facts On File, Inc., 2006).

Kahn, Ada P., and Jan Fawcett, *The Encyclopedia of Mental Health,* 2nd ed. (New York: Facts On File, 2001).

Riess, Dorothy Young, *Better Health Newsletter* 3, no. 1 (February 1987).

butterflies, fear of   Individuals who fear butterflies, moths, and other flying insects fear that the flying insect may attack them. Some phobics avoid enclosed areas out of fear that they may be trapped with the insect. Some phobics actually have accidents while trying to avoid butterflies and moths.

See also BEES, FEAR OF; FLYING THINGS, FEAR OF; INSECTS, FEAR OF.

Melville, Joy, *Phobias and Obsessions* (New York: Coward, McCann & Geoghegan, 1977).

"butterflies in the stomach"   The feeling of uneasiness in the stomach is often referred to as "butterflies." Caused by a contraction of the abdominal blood vessels, this is a common experience among those who must make a speech in public, perform before an audience, appear for a job interview, or participate in any other type of activity that causes feelings of nervousness or apprehension.

See also ADRENALINE; NERVOUS.

cacomorphobia   Fear of fat people.

cacophobia   Fear of ugliness.

caffeine   A naturally occurring substance in tea leaves, cocoa and coffee beans, and kola nuts, caffeine is sometimes added to food and drink. Excessive consumption of caffeinated products can lead to anxiety and PANIC ATTACKS. It can also cause a low level of physical and psychological dependency. Caffeine is probably the most popular drug in the world.

Caffeine is a stimulant of the CENTRAL NERVOUS SYSTEM, and it is primarily consumed in coffee and tea. It is also consumed in cola drinks, cocoa, some headache pills, diet pills, and patent stimulants, such as Caffedrine, NoDoz, Vivarin, and other products. Caffeine is naturally present in chocolate products, with significantly higher concentrations found in dark chocolate than in milk chocolate.

AMOUNT OF CAFFEINE IN COMMON FOODS AND BEVERAGES

Item	Estimated Milligrams
1 cup of brewed coffee	40–180 mgs
1 cup instant coffee	30–120mg
1 cup decaffeinated coffee	3–5 mg
1 cup brewed American tea	20–90 mg
1 cup instant tea	28 mg
Caffeinated soft drinks per 12 ounces	36–90 mg
1 cup cocoa	4mg
1 ounce of milk chocolate	3–6 mg
1 ounce of dark chocolate	25 mg

Source: National Institutes of Health. Available online. URL: http://www.nlm.nih.gov/medlineplus/druginfo/uspdi/202105.html. Downloaded May 26, 2006.

(See the table at left for the range of milligrams in many common caffeinated products.)

Most adults who consume caffeine receive about two-thirds of their daily consumption from coffee, while children receive about half of their daily caffeine consumption from soft drinks.

Caffeine belongs to the family of methylxanthines (1, 3, 7-trimethylxanthine). A naturally occurring alkaloid found in many plants throughout the world, caffeine was first isolated from coffee in 1820 and from tea leaves in 1827. Both *coffee* and *caffeine* are derived from the Arabic word *gahweh* (pronounced "kehveh" in Turkish).

When consumed in beverage form, caffeine reaches all body tissues within five minutes; peak blood levels occur in about 30 minutes. Normally caffeine is rapidly and completely absorbed from the gastrointestinal tract. Little can be recovered unchanged in urine, and there is no day-to-day accumulation of the drug in the body.

Pregnant women should carefully limit their consumption of caffeine, because excessive amounts may slow the growth of the fetus or in some cases lead to a miscarriage. At most, pregnant women should not exceed 300 mg of caffeine per day, according to the National Institutes of Health. In addition, breast-feeding mothers should limit their consumption of caffeinated products because the caffeine will be present in the breast milk and nursing babies may become jittery and have trouble sleeping.

Negative Side Effects of Caffeine

Caffeine increases the heart rate and rhythm, affects the circulatory system, and acts as a diuretic. It also stimulates gastric acid secretion. Excessive amounts, such as greater than 400–500 mg a day, can cause a dangerous elevation in blood pressure, especially during stress.

Caffeine inhibits glucose metabolism and may thereby raise blood-sugar levels, which is dangerous for people with diabetes. An excessive intake of caffeine can lead to urinary incontinence and bladder pain and spasms.

The regular use of high dosages of caffeine may cause chronic INSOMNIA, breathlessness, persistent ANXIETY, PANIC, DEPRESSION, mild delirium, stomach upset, and diarrhea.

Individuals who regularly consume caffeine will often suffer from HEADACHES and irritability when they do not consume caffeine. At the same time, the chronic heavy use of caffeine can induce frequent and even daily headaches. In one study of 36 children with chronic severe headaches who were heavy cola drinkers, reported in 2003 in *Cephalgia*, 33 of the children had a complete remission of their headaches once they were tapered off caffeinated soft drinks. It is best to taper off the use of caffeine, unless otherwise directed by a physician, because a sudden cessation of caffeine will often induce a severe headache among those who are dependent.

Caffeine is also a behavioral stimulant. Caffeine appears to interact with stress, improving intellectual performance in extroverts and impairing it in introverts. However, caffeine intake may interfere with sleep and may postpone fatigue. Many individuals can tolerate about 300 mg of caffeine per day although sleep can be affected by as low a dose as 200 mg. Individuals wishing to sleep should avoid caffeinated products within three to four hours before the time when they wish to sleep, although residual effects can last up to 10 hours.

When taken before bedtime, caffeine may delay the onset of sleep for some individuals, may shorten sleep time, and may reduce the average "depth of sleep." It also may increase the amount of dream sleep (REM) early in the night while reducing it overall.

Some individuals should carefully limit their consumption of caffeine, particularly those with the following medical problems

- agoraphobia
- anxiety
- heart disease
- hypertension
- panic attacks
- insomnia
- liver disease (which may increase the level of caffeine)

Positive aspects of caffeine

Many people enjoy caffeinated beverages in moderation. Some health benefits have also been demonstrated. For example, a study in a 2000 issue of the *Journal of the American Medical Association* analyzed the caffeine and coffee consumption of 8,000 Japanese-American men ages 45 to 68 enrolled in the Honolulu Heart Program. The researchers found a higher coffee and caffeine intake was associated with a lower risk for the development of Parkinson's disease, and the researchers believed that the caffeine was likely responsible for these results. It is unknown if this tendency is also present among females or in other racial or ethnic groups.

Citrated caffeine is used with premature babies to treat breathing problems.

In a study published in a 2004 issue of the *Journal of the American Medical Association* on Finnish middle-aged men and women, the researchers found a reduced incidence of Type 2 diabetes among the coffee drinkers.

Effect of Caffeine Among Individuals with Anxiety Disorders

Research teams at Yale University and the National Institute of Mental Health (NIMH) have reported that a dose of caffeine equal to about eight cups of coffee produces far greater increases in anxiety, nervousness, FEAR, NAUSEA, and restlessness among patients diagnosed for AGORAPHOBIA and PANIC DISORDER than among healthy volunteers.

Panic attacks are characterized by severe emotional and physical distress that usually lasts for a few minutes; 2 to 5 percent of the population have panic disorder—repeated panic attacks with no apparent external cause. As a result, persons who have panic attacks should avoid caffeine.

In addition to an increased risk for panic attacks with regular doses of caffeine, phobic effects are often heightened with the regular use of caffeine. Caffeine apparently blocks the action of ADENOSINE, a chemical that reduces the spontaneous firing of neurons in several brain regions. Both caffeine and yohimbine, a drug with similar anxiety-producing effects, may increase the flow of calcium into neurons, a process controlled by adenosine. More calcium may activate more brain cells, leading to greater anxiety.

Medication Interactions

Individuals should tell their doctors if they are heavy users of caffeine. According to the National Institutes of Health, this is particularly important with drugs such as pemoline (Cylert), which is sometimes given to treat ATTENTION-DEFICIT/HYPERACTIVITY DISORDER or the antidepressant sertraline (Zoloft). These medications, when combined with caffeine, can increase central nervous system stimulant effects and could cause seizures or changes in heart rhythms. In addition, it can be dangerous to combine large amounts of caffeine with monomaine oxidase (MAO) inhibitors, a category of antidepressants. Caffeine and an MAO inhibitor together can lead to very high blood pressure or dangerous changes in heart rhythms.

Overdosing on Caffeine

It is possible to consume too much caffeine, causing an intoxication or overdose. Some symptoms of caffeine overdose include

- abdominal pain
- agitation
- confusion or delirium
- convulsions
- dehydration
- fast or irregular heartbeat
- fever
- frequent urination
- headache
- increased sensitivity to pain
- muscle trembling
- ringing or other sounds in the ears

Gwinnell, Esther, M.D., and Christine Adamec, *The Encyclopedia of Addictions and Addictive Disorders* (New York: Facts On File, Inc., 2005).

Hering-Hanit, R., and N. Gadoth, "Caffeine-Induced Headache in Children and Adolescents," *Cephalgia* 23, no. 4 (2003): p. 332.

National Institutes of Health, "Caffeine." Available online. URL: http: www.nlm.nih.gov/medlineplus/druginfo/uspdi/202105.html. Downloaded May 26, 2006.

Ross, G. Webster, M.D., "Association of Coffee and Caffeine Intake with the Risk of Parkinson Disease," *Journal of the American Medical Association* 283, no. 20 (May 24/31, 2000): pp. 2674–2679.

Tuomilehto, Jaako, M.D., "Coffee Consumption and Risk of Type 2 Diabetes Mellitus Among Middle-aged Finnish Men and Women," *Journal of the American Medical Association* 291, no. 10 (March 10, 2004): pp. 1213–1219.

cainophobia: cainotophobia (neo-phobia)   Fear of newness or novelty.

See also NEWNESS, FEAR OF; NOVELTY, FEAR OF.

caligynephobia   Fear of beautiful women.

cancer, fear of   Cancer is one of the most feared of human diseases. Many individuals have anxieties regarding their health because they fear cancer. Many do not visit a doctor because they fear the worst, and many others make frequent visits to reassure themselves that they do not have cancer. Many people even fear saying the word. Some people do not want to go near a person known to have cancer; this is an unfounded fear, as cancer is not contagious. However, fear of cancer may motivate more people to obtain checkups and pay attention to the warning signals of cancer, to stop smoking, avoid excessive exposure to the sun, and avoid other activities known to cause the disease. In Freudian terms, fear of cancer may also represent a fear of castration or a fear of being devoured by an object inside oneself.

See also CASTRATION COMPLEX; DISEASE, FEAR OF.

carbon dioxide sensitivity   When some individuals inhale small amounts of carbon dioxide, they have symptoms of HYPERVENTILATION, trembling, facial flushing, blurring of vision, and dizziness. Carbon dioxide-provoked panic attacks may occur as a result of increased activity in the LOCUS CERULEUS (a small organ of the brain rich in neurotransmitters) in individuals who have an abnormal sensitivity to carbon dioxide. Such panic attacks occur in nearly all predisposed individuals but rarely in normal persons. (Doctors in the armed forces have observed that people who have chronic anxiety cannot tolerate wearing gas masks because the masks make them breathe in some of their own exhaled carbon dioxide.)

See also ANXIETY DISORDERS; CHEMOCEPTORS; LACTATE-INDUCED ANXIETY; NEUROTRANSMITTERS; PANIC ATTACKS.

cardiophobia   See HEART DISEASE, FEAR OF.

cardiovascular symptoms   Some of the most frightening and most prominent symptoms of panic disorder are cardiac symptoms. Those who seek consultation with physicians for their cardiovascular symptoms associated with panic disorder may constitute as many as one third of all cardiology patients.

See also MITRAL VALVE PROLAPSE.

caregivers   In today's society, caregivers include family members or friends of a child or of an elderly, ill, or disabled person who cannot completely care for him- or herself. The term also applies to individuals who are health care professionals or social workers.

The caregiver role can be fraught with anxieties because of its physical and emotional demands. For example, family members who are caregivers may feel powerless and depressed in the face of the suffering of a loved one. Professional caregivers may emotionally withdraw or perhaps allow the pain and suffering they see to overwhelm them.

Caregivers have considerable power, and work in a close, personal relationship with their charges, frequently with little or no supervision. Unfortunately, some situations of abuse have occurred involving elderly adults as well as children. Children are frequently victims of sexual abuse by their caregivers, while the elderly are often subjected to neglect or emotional and financial abuse. When an elderly person, disabled person, or child is entrusted to the care of another, credentials and references should be carefully checked and verified.

Special Anxieties: Caregiving to the Elderly
Increased longevity means that many spouses will be caring for one another. Social mobility and shrinking family size put some women in the sole caregiver role for both their own and their husbands' aging parents. The Older Women's League in Washington, D.C., reported that at least a third of all women over age 18 can expect to be continuously in the caregiver role from the birth of their first child to the death of their parents. At the same time, women are moving into highly responsible professional positions at the time in life that their parents need care.

Individuals who have elderly parents or are over the age of 65 may be able to relieve some anxieties by planning ahead. Planning and preparation can deter the emotional and financial stress that often accompanies caring for an elderly loved one.

Identify Needs of Disabled Children, Adults, or Elderly Persons
When an individual realizes that she or he will be in the caregiver role, anxieties can be relieved by identifying the kinds of assistance the disabled or elderly person wants and needs. Some needs that can be met by a family member or by outside sources include meals, shopping, cleaning, yard work, household repairs, financial, living arrangements, personal care, and home health care.

An elderly person or disabled child or adult may need services to help him or her maintain social interaction or participation in the community. For example, these may include transportation to the doctor, shopping, or church; psychological support; help with cutting through the red tape of health insurance policies and Medicare, Medicaid, Social Security, and other governmental bureaucracies and protective services such as safety devices. A disabled child may need home tutoring or special education.

If possible, the caregiver and disabled or elderly person can explore how needs, once identified, may best be met. Consider resources of other family members, and their willingness and ability to help. Look at possibilities for blending resources within the family with those from outside the family. When caregiving is a shared responsibility among family members and/or friends, it leads to the understanding and sharing of anxieties, development of positive relationships, and enhancement of communication. Community and social-service agencies, such as Meals on Wheels, respite programs, support groups, and elderly day care, can also supplement caregivers' efforts.

carnophobia   Fear of meat.
   See also MEAT, FEAR OF.

carpal tunnel syndrome   A chronic condition characterized by numbness, tingling, and pain in the thumb, index, and middle fingers and sometimes, by weakness in the thumb. It may affect one or both hands. This syndrome results from pressure on the median nerve where it passes into the hand via a gap (the "carpal tunnel" under a ligament at the front of the wrist). Symptoms lead to anxieties and fears of being able to continue to work in one's chosen field.

   Carpal tunnel syndrome is one of several possible repetitive stress injuries (RSIs) common to certain occupations in which the wrist is subjected to repetitive stresses and strains, particularly those involving gripping or pinching with the wrist held flexed. For example, computer operators, typists, carpenters, factory workers, meat cutters (meat cleaver's elbow), violinists, and even hobbyists such as golfers or canoers may develop carpal tunnel syndrome. This injury is stressful for some sufferers because they may experience confusion over whether to continue or quit a job or activity that contributes to their discomfort. Stress itself can intensify the effects of carpal tunnel syndrome. The number of workers with disorders caused by repeated trauma on the job is increasing. Some severely injured carpal tunnel victims qualify for help under the Americans with Disabilities Act. However, proof of the source of injury may be difficult, as two people may perform the identical job

with only one of them developing carpal tunnel syndrome.

   With appropriate treatment, the pain can be relieved and there may be no permanent damage to the wrist or hand. Resting the affected hand at night in a splint may alleviate symptoms. Some health professionals may recommend ACUPUNCTURE. If symptoms persist, a physician may inject a small quantity of a corticosteroid drug under the ligament in the wrist. If this does not help, surgical cutting of the ligament may be performed to relieve pressure on the nerve.

   In some cases, psychological or career counseling may also be helpful.
   See also WORK, FEAR OF.

case control   An experimental study design in which groups of phobic individuals are selected in terms of whether they do (cases) or do not (controls) have the particular disorder being studied.
   See also COHORT; LONGITUDINAL STUDY.

castration anxiety   Castration is removal of the male testes or female ovaries by surgery, or inactivation of those glands by radiation, infection, PARASITES, or drugs. Castration alters the hormonal function of the individual and generally reduces libido. Castration anxiety involves unconscious feelings and FANTASIES associated with being deprived of the sex organs. Freud believed that boys worry that their penis will be cut off by an angry and jealous father (Oedipal complex) due to sexual interest in the mother. In girls, according to Freud, the castration anxiety is a fantasy that the penis has been removed as a punishment, for which they blame the mother (Electra complex). When castration anxiety persists into adulthood, it may become the cause of a neurotic inability to engage in SEXUAL INTERCOURSE, fear of the opposite sex, impotence in a male and frigidity in a female, or sexual perversions. At the metaphoric level, castration fears relate to loss of contact with the life force and hence life itself.

   Castration anxiety was thought by Freud to be a central factor in many phobias. The classic case of LITTLE HANS demonstrated its importance in the etiology of PHOBIAS from the psychoanalytic perspective, although Joseph Wolpe was able to take this case and persuasively show that it actually fit a learning theory analysis.

See also ELECTRA COMPLEX; FRIGIDITY; IMPOTENCE; OEDIPUS COMPLEX; SEXUAL FEARS.

catagelophobia Fear of ridicule. This is related to a fear of criticism.

See also RIDICULE, FEAR OF.

catapedaphobia Fear of jumping from both high and low places.

See also HIGH PLACES, FEAR OF; JUMPING, FEAR OF.

cataract extraction, fear of As cataracts—the cloudiness that forms in the lens of the eye—develop, many individuals experience anxiety, depression, and an acute sense of loneliness. When the condition seriously affects vision, the lens is surgically removed, and vision is restored by an implanted plastic lens, contact lens, or special glasses.

catastrophic anxiety Another term for panic or anxiety produced by overwhelming, frightening events. Sometimes the term *catastrophic anxiety* is used to denote catastrophic thinking or preoccupation with potentially disastrous events, such as crashing in an airplane.

See also ANXIETY; ANXIETY DISORDERS; CATASTROPHIZE.

catastrophize The habit of imagining that the worst will occur. People who frequently catastrophize have little self-confidence, low SELF-ESTEEM, difficulties making positive and desirable life changes; many have SOCIAL PHOBIAS.

An example of catastrophizing, is saying to oneself, "If I go to the party no one will know me and I won't have a good time," or "If I take this new job I'll fail because I don't have the right computer skills."

Catastrophizing causes anxieties because it keeps people in situations they might really prefer to change, such as their social life, job, or environment. With positive SELF-TALK and learned techniques to improve self-esteem, the habit of catastrophizing can be overcome. In severe cases, various PSYCHOTHERAPIES may be helpful, particularly cognitive behavioral therapies.

See also BEHAVIOR THERAPY; COGNITIVE THERAPY; SELF-ESTEEM; SOCIAL PHOBIA.

catharsis Release of suppressed or inhibited emotions and tensions that provides temporary relief from ANXIETY. It was noted and named by Joseph Breuer, a colleague and friend of Sigmund Freud's who thought it to be a technique for symptoms removal. Breuer's work was the impetus for Freud's analysis of the psychic mechanism. Catharsis is often observed during individual and group therapy; it also occurs outside therapy. The word "catharsis" is derived from the Greek *katharsis*, meaning purification or cleansing. In psychodynamic therapies, catharsis is viewed as an alleviation of fears, problems, and complexes by making them conscious and giving them expression.

See also ABREACTION; CONVERSATIONAL CATHARSIS.

cathexis Psychoanalysts use this term to signify an individual's concentration or investment of mental energy in a certain direction—for example, toward some person or object—in an effort to reduce anxieties.

cathisophobia Fear of sitting.

See also SITTING, FEAR OF.

catoptrophobia Fear of mirrors.

See also MIRRORS, FEAR OF.

cats, fear of The term is derived from the Greek work *ailouros*, meaning cat. Fear of cats is known as aelurophobia, galeophobia, gatophobia, and cat phobia. In its most intense form, this phobia may cause one to become virtually homebound or confined due to fear of encountering a cat in the street or even seeing one from a vehicle. The term ailurophobia also refers to a dread of being scratched or bitten in the genital area. Shakespeare grasps the cat phobic reaction in *The Merchant of Venice* when he says: "Some men there are love not a gaping pig; some, that are mad if they behold a cat."

Fear of cats is known as aelurophobia, ailurophobia, elurophobia, felinophobia, galeophobia, or gatophobia. The characteristics of fear of cats are similar to those of fears of other animals. Generally, it is a fear of being injured or scratched by them. Some individuals react with shortness of breath, rapid heartbeat, or feelings of panic just at the sight of a cat. For other individuals, the fear is induced only if the cat comes very close or touches them. Some people fear cats' eyes staring at them. One psychiatric interpretation of fear of cats is that it is a repression of dread of injury to a particular part of the body. Henry III of France is said to have feared cats.

With regard to cat phobia, Benjamin Rush (1745–1813), an American physician and author, said: "It will be unnecessary to mention instances of the prevalence of this distemper. I know several gentlemen of unquestionable courage, who have retreated a thousand times from the sight of a cat; and who have even discovered signs of fear and terror upon being confined in a room with a cat that was out of sight."

See also ANIMALS, FEAR OF; BEING LOOKED AT, FEAR OF; BLACK CATS, FEAR OF.

Runes, D. D., ed., *The Selected Writings of Benjamin Rush* (New York: The Philosophical Library, 1947).

Marks, Isaac, M., *Living with Fear* (New York: McGraw Hill, 1978).

causality   A view that events, such as phobic reactions, are consequences of preceding events. As an explanation of anxieties and phobias, the causality approach suggests that there is always a distinct cause and effect. The causal approach differs from the purely descriptive approach and from the introspective methods. Within the behavioral approach, causality is not a critical issue. The focus is rather on variables that maintain or trigger responses.

See also ANXIETY; PHOBIAS.

cemeteries, fear of   Fear of cemeteries is known as coimetrophobia. The word is derived from the Greek work "koimeterion," meaning sleeping room or burial place. Individuals who fear cemeteries usually also fear going to funerals, looking at tombstones, looking at dead bodies, and even hearing about funerals. Some will drive distances out of their way to avoid passing cemeteries. Others will walk on the side of the street away from a cemetery to avoid being near one.

See also DEATH, FEAR OF; TOMBSTONES, FEAR OF.

cenophobia   Fear of empty rooms, open places, and barren spaces. This fear may be related to agoraphobia.

See also AGORAPHOBIA; BARREN SPACES, FEAR OF; EMPTY ROOMS, FEAR OF; OPEN PLACES, FEAR OF.

center of the row, fear of sitting in the   Some individuals fear sitting in the center of the row in theaters, movies, churches, and community meetings. Some who fear being closed in have this fear. Agoraphobics fear being in the center of the row because they fear being trapped and unable to get to a place of safety. Some who fear that they might have to use a toilet in a public place fear being in the center of the row because getting out might be difficult or embarrassing. Some who have social phobias fear being in the center of the row where they must pass many others before getting to their seat. Others fear that they will do something embarrassing, such as cough, sneeze, or vomit, and want to be sure of a safe getaway, which is more difficult from the center of the row.

See also AGORAPHOBIA; CLAUSTROPHOBIA.

centophobia   Fear of newness or novelty.

See also NOVELTY, FEAR OF.

central nervous system The part of the nervous system that is encased in bone and consists of the brain and spinal cord and to which all sensory impulses are transmitted and from which motor impulses originate; the central nervous system also supervises and coordinates the activities of the entire nervous system. Some drugs used to treat phobic reactions and agoraphobia, as well as antidepressants, affect the central nervous system.

See also ANTIDEPRESSANTS; DEPRESSION; DRUGS.

ceraunophobia (keraunophobia) Fear of thunder.

See also THUNDER, FEAR OF; THUNDERSTORMS, FEAR OF.

chaetophobia Fear of hair is known as chaetophobia. This includes fear of hairy objects, animals, or people.

See also HAIR, FEAR OF; HAIR DISEASE, FEAR OF.

change, fear of Fear of change or of anything new is known as neophobia. Fear of making changes is known as tropophobia. Many individuals feel secure in their daily lives by doing things in a certain routine. They fear introducing new ways of performing daily activities, a new job, new place of residence, or changes in family status. Some individuals who never move may fear moving, or changing residence. Some never travel, because they fear new places, or changing location. Some who remain single throughout life may also fear change. Those who have AGORAPHOBIA may fear change, such as the change in stimulation when going out of their house, where they feel secure.

See also MOVING, FEAR OF; TRAVEL, FEAR OF.

character analysis Therapy focused on defensive behavior that is an integral part of the personality. Character analysis is a term introduced by Wilhelm Reich (1897–1957), an Austrian-American psychoanalyst, to describe a process the therapist uses in helping an individual to liberate repressed psychic energy. Reich suggested that individuals have a built-in character armor that they use to repress sexual and social freedoms of expression. Some of these repressed freedoms may lead to ANXIETIES and PHOBIAS. Reich identified six character structures that frequently confront the therapist: the phallic-narcissistic male; the passive-feminine male; the masculine-aggressive female; the hysterical female; the compulsive character; and the masochistic character.

Character analysis also refers to psychoanalytic treatment of character disorders and to the study of character traits supposedly revealed by external characteristics, such as the shape of the jaw.

character armor This term refers to rigid character structures that prevent release of emotions and liberation of an individual's personality. The term was introduced by Wilhelm Reich, who believed that the analyst should identify the individual's character patterns that serve as defense mechanisms against anxiety that block the way to the unconscious levels of the personality. Examples of character armor are cynicism and overaggressiveness. Clues such as facial expressions or posture determine these mechanisms.

See also CHARACTER ANALYSIS.

checking (as a ritual) Some individuals who have OBSESSIVE-COMPULSIVE DISORDER spend hours checking ordinary situations out of fear of omission of an act—for example, checking that the doors and windows of their houses are locked. They may fear hairs they have dropped and check and recheck for loose hairs on themselves or in their household. Checking (as a ritual) is more common in men than women; overall, a little more than one third of all obsessive-compulsives exhibit excessive checking.

Marks, Isaac M., *Fears, Phobias and Rituals* (New York: Oxford University Press, 1987).

cheimaphobia (cheimatophobia) Fear of the cold, being cold, cold things, or cold air.

See also COLD, FEAR OF.

chemoceptors Substances in the brain that monitor acidity in the blood. In normal individuals, these chemoceptors signal serious changes, such as a buildup of carbon dioxide, which may indicate that oxygen is not reaching the organs of the body. The result is likely to be panic, which influences individuals to take action, for example, to avoid suffocation. However, in people with panic disorder, oversensitive chemoceptors create terror without any apparent reason.

See also CARBON DIOXIDE SENSITIVITY; LACTATE-INDUCED ANXIETY; PANIC.

chemotherapy, fear of Many people fear chemotheraphy—the treatment of mental and physical disorders through drugs or other chemicals—because the treatment is associated with CANCER. Cancer patients fear chemotherapy because of unpleasant side effects associated with it. Strong anticancer drugs often cause side effects of repeated episodes of NAUSEA and VOMITING, and this often conditions strong aversion to stimuli associated with chemotherapy, including FOOD eaten before treatments. Some patients begin to vomit even before the drugs are injected and retch as they get a call from the oncology nurse, get dressed, or travel to the hospital.

Although, in the case of mental disorders, chemotherapy addresses only the symptoms of a disorder, it has become a popular way of treating some individuals because it has the effect of at least making the individuals more manageable and amenable to other forms of therapy. The main categories of chemotherapy (drugs) used to treat anxiety disorders, manic–depressive illness, and obsessive-compulsive disorders are ANTIPSYCHOTICS, antianxiolytics, and ANTIDEPRESSANTS.

See also CANCER, FEAR OF; DRUGS, FEAR OF TAKING.

cherophobia Fear of being happy or of gaiety. Manifestations of this phobia are ANXIETIES that are triggered by experiences of being happy, or by fears that the happiness or gaiety are going to produce disaster or aversive events.

See also GAIETY, FEAR OF; HAPPINESS, FEAR OF.

chickens, fear of Fear of chickens is known as alektorophobia. These fears can include feathers, eggs, or live or dead chickens. Some people fear chickens because they peck, swoop, and roost above eye level or because they eat their food from the ground, which may contaminate it. Fears of chickens may be related to fears of other birds and feathered animals. It is interesting that such fears usually involve proximity to a live chicken. A cooked chicken or meal would be quite acceptable. Such specificity is common with phobics.

See also CONTAMINATION, FEAR OF; FEATHERS, FEAR OF.

child abuse Includes physical, sexual, and emotional abuse as well as neglect. Also known as *child maltreatment*. Child abuse can cause lifelong anxieties, POST-TRAUMATIC STRESS DISORDER and other psychological problems, such as DEPRESSION. Neglect can be more harmful to children than all other forms of abuse, particularly among infants and young children. In fact, children from birth to age three are the most likely to be victimized by some form of child maltreatment among all age groups of children in the United States, and neglect is the most common form of abuse that infants and young children experience.

Children and adults who have suffered from childhood abuse have an increased risk for the development of ANXIETY DISORDERS, DEPRESSION, learning disabilities, ATTENTION DEFICIT/HYPERACTIVITY DISORDER, and SUICIDE, compared to those individuals who were not abused. Studies have shown that childhood abuse nearly triples the risk of an individual suffering from an anxiety disorder or mood disorder in adulthood and more than doubles the risk of the development of PHOBIAS in adulthood. Experts report that adults who were abused as children have 10 times the risk of suffering from a PANIC DISORDER in their own adulthood. Physically abused children are about four times more likely to develop anxiety disorders than nonabused children.

Children who have experienced pain from abuse may fear disease, doctors, or surgical operations. Those who have been tied and/or placed in ENCLOSED PLACES may develop CLAUSTROPHOBIA and fears of DARKNESS.

Each year, the Administration on Children, Youth, and Families releases statistical data on child abuse in the United States, based on information provided by the National Child Abuse and Neglect Data System (NCANDS). According to these federal agencies, about 872,000 children were substantiated victims of child abuse or neglect in 2004. Most child victims (about 60 percent) were neglected, while about 18 percent were physically abused, 10 percent were sexually abused, and 7 percent were emotionally maltreated. About 15 percent of the children fell into the category of "other" types of maltreatment, depending on state law. Some children are victims of multiple forms of child abuse.

Both girls and boys were maltreated, but girls were slightly more likely to be abused than boys. With regard to sexual abuse, however, the majority of all reported victims were female.

Some children die from maltreatment, and, in 2004, it was estimated that 1,490 children died because of abuse or neglect. Of these deaths, nearly 36 percent of the children died from neglect, 30 percent died from multiple forms of maltreatment, and 28 percent died from physical abuse only. The other children died from psychological maltreatment, medical neglect, or sexual abuse.

More than 80 percent of the children who died in 2004 as a result of child maltreatment were younger than 4 years old. Infant boys younger than one year old had the highest fatality rate or 18 deaths per 100,000 population. The rate for infant girls was 17 deaths per 100,000 population.

Adults abused as children.   Adults who experienced childhood abuse have an increased risk for many problems in adulthood, such as a greater risk for psychiatric problems, substance use disorders, SUICIDE, the abuse of their own children, victimization by others, and marital problems.

Increased risk for substance abuse.   Adults who were abused as children have an increased risk for alcohol and drug use dependence. For example, women who were sexually abused during childhood have nearly three times the risk of drug addiction in adulthood as women who were *not* abused as children. Both men and women who were child abuse victims have an increased risk for alcohol abuse and ALCOHOLISM in adulthood.

Increased risk for suicide.   Sexual abuse that occurs in childhood increases the risk for suicide in adulthood. According to Shanta Dube et al., in a 2005 issue of the *American Journal of Preventive Medicine,* both men and women with a history of childhood sexual abuse had twice the risk of attempting suicide compared to individuals who were not abused as children.

Increased risk for committing child abuse.   Adults who were abused in childhood have an increased risk for abusing their own children when they become parents themselves. From one-third to as many as 40 percent of adults who were abused as children will repeat this negative behavior toward their own children. It should be noted, however, that the majority of adults abused as children do *not* abuse their own children.

Increased risk for continued victimization.   According to the National Violence Against Women study reported by the National Institute of Justice in 2000, women who were physically assaulted as a child were twice as likely to be physically assaulted in adulthood.

It is also true that the majority of those who are homeless as well as the majority of those who prostitute themselves in adulthood were abused as children. Both homelessness and prostitution increase the risk for further incidents of physical and sexual victimization against adults.

Increased risk for bad relationships and marital problems.   Research has shown that adults who suffered childhood sexual abuse experience a 40 percent greater risk of marrying an alcoholic than adults who were *not* sexually abused as children. They also have a 40–50 percent greater risk of having current marital problems than those adults who were not abused as children.

Administration on Children and Families, *Child Maltreatment* 2004. Washington, DC: U.S. Department of Health and Human Services, 2006.

Clark, Robin E., and Judith Freeman Clark, with Christine Adamec, *The Encyclopedia of Child Abuse,* 3rd ed. (New York, Facts On File, Inc., 2007).

Dube, Shanta R., et al., "Long-Term Consequences of Childhood Sexual Abuse by Gender of Victim," *American Journal of Preventive Medicine* 28, no. 5 (2005): pp. 430–438.

Office of Justice Programs, *Full Report of the Prevalence, Incidence and Consequences of Violence Against Women: Findings from the National Violence Against Women Study.* Washington, DC: United States Department of Justice, November 2000. Available online. URL: http://www.ncjrs.org/pdffiles1/nij/183781.pdf. Downloaded April 22, 2006.

childbirth, fear of   Many women approach childbirth with fear and apprehension. Horror stories from friends and relatives fuel many such fears. Some first-time mothers, in particular, are disturbed by what seems to be an encounter with the unknown. Women fear the LOSS OF CONTROL inherent in the childbirth experience and are often afraid that they will behave in an embarrassing manner during childbirth. The contemporary expectation that fathers will attend childbirth produces fears and anxieties in some expectant fathers.

Women also fear many of the practical details connected with the experience of childbirth. Some fear that they will not recognize the beginning of labor and that they will not get to the hospital on time. Some fear hospital procedures, such as the use of stirrups, shaving the pubic area, and the episiotomy. Others fear loss of elasticity due to stretching of the vagina, stretch marks on their abdomen, and sagging breasts as a result of pregnancy and childbirth.

The condition of the newborn and the use of a rating scale for infants produces anxiety for some new mothers. Temporary physical conditions of the newborn, such as a misshapen head, skin blemishes, excess hair, or no hair at all, often disturb many new parents.

Women who have cesarean section births have special fears. For example, some fear that the surgery may damage the baby or that a baby born this way will be exceptionally fragile. Some women also fear that the cesarean procedure will damage their body and that it denies them what they believe should be a natural experience for a woman.

Some women anticipate childbirth as a glorious, fulfilling experience and fear disappointment because of their high expectations. Some anticipate a sense of emptiness after a childbirth, a loss of their reason for existence while pregnant. While education for childbirth has generally had a positive influence for most women, in some women, preparation produces the feeling that childbirth is a type of performance with the accompanying implications of success and failure.

Fears of bearing a monster, of bearing a stillborn baby, of dying during childbirth, and of losing a baby to SUDDEN INFANT DEATH SYNDROME also cause anxieties for many women and men.

See also BIRTHING A MONSTER, FEAR OF; PREGNANCY, FEAR OF.)

de Beauvoir, Simone, *The Second Sex* (New York: Modern Library, 1968).

childhood, anxieties, fears, and phobias   Childhood fears are related to a child's age. Infants and toddlers have some fears that arise out of inborn fright reaction to PAIN, sudden loud noises, bright LIGHTS, and loss of physical support, as in FALLING. Infants are most likely to fear STRANGERS and will react with a startled response to an unfamiliar face. Infants over six months also develop "separation distress," which makes them fear being left by the persons they love and trust. When left alone they may cry and scream. When the mother or caregiver returns they will show ANXIETY by staying close to her, touching her, and watching her.

Young children have many more fears than adults that start with no apparent cause and subside and change for no clear reason as the child grows older. Childhood fears may be developmental. An example is when a child suddenly fears things it has experienced without fear or trauma, such as small animals or birds. Fear may also come from exposure to a new situation, such as school (viewed as unpredictable, unknown). Illness or stress may cause a child to regress and reexperience earlier, forgotten fears until he or she is well again.

Whereas infants and toddlers often fear tangible and immediate events, fears of preschoolers are more abstract. Preschoolers have an active fantasy life and may have difficulty in distinguishing between real and unreal events and people. Children develop the greatest number of new fears during the preschool and early school years. It is considered normal for children to have specific fears. They are universally sensitive to the familiar in an unfamiliar guise (for example, parents wearing a mask). At these times, they may have actual frightening encounters or learn about frightening experiences of others. Preschool children are warned about possible dangers and learn about monsters from books, movies, and television. Between two and six, many children fear being in the dark or being alone; fear imaginary creatures, such as ghosts and witches; and fear animals. Some of the most common sources of fear are:

animals (dogs are most common) and insects
dark (especially at bedtime)
death (separation, sometimes injury)
doctors and dentists
heights
monsters and imaginary creatures
nightmares
school
storms (and other natural events)
water (deep)

School-age children worry about their schoolwork as well as about acceptance by teachers and schoolmates. There are particular fears during middle childhood and adolescence, such as fears of physical injury, social relationships, individual competence, and nuclear war.

Two adult fears—blood and injury phobias and animal and snake phobias—usually begin in childhood.

School and Death Fears

Separation anxiety is the basis for two common childhood phobias, SCHOOL and DEATH. School phobia is an intense fear related to attending school. It can begin at any age, even preschool or kindergarten. School-phobic children may describe problems at school, such as being afraid of teachers or classmates. They may claim that special problems await them on the way to school, such as bullies. They may pretend to be ill, and in some cases may have physical symptoms of illness, such as vomiting. When school phobia occurs in older children, it may be related to home life, school performance, or relationships with classmates. In some cases, separation anxiety also may be related to death phobias.

Some children fear that one or both parents will die; these children fear being left alone without the care and love of their parents. Children's perceptions of death change between ages three and 10. Young children may consider death to be like living in another place; they anticipate the return of the deceased. At age five to six, some children believe that death is not inevitable, because, for example, they can outwit monsters. Between ages six and 10, children increasingly understand that death is final, and that it can involve pain, injury, and disease. Thus they begin to fear pain or injury from their imaginary "bogeyman." Around age 10, most children fully understand death as inevitable and final. There is a high incidence of school-phobic children who later develop AGORAPHOBIA.

Obsessive-Compulsive Disorder (OCD)

The chronic and debilitating course of OCD in children and adolescents has been well documented in the literature. However, this disorder had gone underreported and undertreated in children. Despite a great deal of epidemiological and pharmacological research on childhood OCD during the 1990s, effective psychosocial interventions are lacking.

Onset of OCD appears to occur earlier in boys than girls. The early onset of the disorder has also been confirmed by retrospective reports of adult OCD patients. Symptoms of OCD in children and adolescents are similar to those found in adults. Common are obsessions involving contamination, sexual themes, religiosity, or aggressive-violent images. Compulsions involve washing and checking. Ordering and rituals become difficult to hide from schoolmates as the rituals become elaborate and time-consuming. For example, homework may become overwhelming, as the child may spend hours with repeated erasing and rewriting. A multiple-choice test may bring on checking rituals, resulting in the child not completing the test in the allotted time. Rituals may keep an adolescent from engaging in usual activities, such as dating or driving.

Children and adolescents who have OCD may have other anxiety disorders and mood disorders. Also, a high rate of tics and Tourette's disorder are associated with the youthful OCD populations. Differential diagnosis of OCD in children is rarely straightforward, according to Albano, Knox, and Barlow. Children with OCD may frequently display phobic avoidance of objects or situations that trigger their obsessions. A child who fears contamination of germs may avoid using public restrooms or refuse to use classroom supplies shared by other students. Even touching a beloved family pet may evoke fear of germs and cause the child to avoid the animal. This behavior may resemble the avoidance of a specific phobia. In extreme cases, fears of contamination may result in school refusal behavior, giving the appearance of AGORAPHOBIA.

Post-traumatic Stress Disorder (PTSD) in Children and Adolescents

The effects of trauma on children have not been studied by many researchers, who focus instead on children who have been exposed to natural disasters, sexual assault, street violence, shootings, warfare, and accidents. PTSD may exist when a child has experienced a traumatic event that would be perceived as markedly distressing to anyone. In children, only one re-experiencing symptom is considered enough to meet the diagnostic criterion. Re-experiencing symptoms include recurrent and intrusive thoughts about the trauma, trauma-related dreams, flashbacks of the traumas, repetitive play with trauma-related themes, and intense distress when exposed to reminders of the trauma, according to Ribbe, Lipovsky, and Freedy.

The same researchers suggest that children who have PTSD symptoms may exhibit symptoms of avoidance, including avoiding thoughts or feelings associated with the trauma, avoiding reminders of the trauma, inability to recall some aspects of the event, decreased interest in previously significant activities, feeling detached from others, restricted affective expression, and sense of a foreshortened future.

Also, children who have PTSD may show increased arousal, manifest in sleep difficulties, irritability, difficulty concentrating, hypervigilance, and physiological reactivity when exposed to stimuli associated with the trauma.

Pharmacotherapy for Childhood and Adolescent Anxieties

Medications used in adults (anxiolytics) are largely underresearched in children and adolescents, although there are some guidelines suggesting possible uses, specific applications for their use and dosage. According to Reiter et al., medication should always be used to complement other therapeutic approaches, depending on associated disturbances in each case. When pharmacological treatment alleviates symptoms of anxiety, it allows the clinician to work with the child and family and improve familial dysfunctions and negative behaviors. Interventions that help the active mastery of anxiety symptoms are also important to prevent the return of symptoms after discontinuation of medication.

An expanding array of treatments and available medications increases treatment options, but also places more complex demands on the clinician. The overriding issue in child and adolescent psychopharmacology is when and how to use medications. When a comprehensive diagnostic assessment has been completed, and when the disorder seriously interferes with the individual child's development, family, school, and social adjustments, judicious use of pharmacotherapy may be appropriate.

Sex Distribution of Fears

Girls seem to have more fears than boys, but it is possible that the differences in number are due to our society's acceptance of different behaviors for boys and girls. Girls admit to more fears, are warned about more dangers, and are comforted when they are fearful. Boys tend to hide their anxieties behind a tough facade, but their anxieties often show up later in different ways. For example, boys outnumber girls in some childhood problems, such as stuttering, asthma, and bedwetting.

See also BOGEYMAN, FEAR OF; DEATH, FEAR OF; SCHOOL PHOBIA; SEPARATION ANXIETY.

Albano, Anne Marie, Lenna S. Knox, and David H. Barlow, "Obsessive-Compulsive Disorder." In *Clinical Handbook of Anxiety Disorders in Children and Adolescents* (Northvale, NJ: Jason Aronson, Inc., 1994).

Chambers, Janice Somerville, "Horror in the Halls." *The Rotarian,* March 1999, pp. 18–60.

Eisen, Andrew, Christopher A. Kearney, and Charles E. Schaefer, eds., *Clinical Handbook of Anxiety Disorders in Children and Adolescents* (Northvale, N.J.: Jason Aronson, Inc., 1994).

Marks, Isaac, *Fears, Phobias and Rituals* (New York: Oxford University Press, 1987).

Reiter, S., S. Kutcher, and D. Gardner, "Anxiety disorders in children and adolescents: clinical and related issues in pharmacological treatment." *Canadian Journal of Psychiatry* 37:432–438 (1992).

Ribbe, David P., Julie A. Lipovsky, and John R. Freedy, "Posttraumatic Stress Disorder." In *Clinical Handbook of Anxiety Disorders in Children and Adolescents.* Edited by Andrew Eisen; Christopher A. Kearney; and Charles E. Schaefer. (Northvale, NJ: Jason Aronson, Inc., 1994).

Riggs, D. S., and E. B. Foa, "Obsessive compulsive disorder." In *Clinical Handbook of Psychological Disorders.* Edited by D. H. Barlow (New York: Guilford, 1993).

Sarafino, Edward P., *The Fears of Childhood* (New York: Human Sciences Press, 1986).

children, anxiety disorders of See CHILDHOOD ANXIETIES, FEARS, AND PHOBIAS.

children, fear of Fear of children is known as pediophobia. Many adults fear that children will be destructive or messy, will leave finger marks, or will be noisy and create a nuisance. Some adults fear children because they do not understand them and their normal development. The fact that some children tend to be noisy, aggressive, emotional, uninhibited, blunt, constantly interrupting, and complaining, makes them unappealing to many landlords and proprietors of some businesses and recreational facilities, as well as to some parents, relatives, and those who come into unwanted contact with children, for example in restaurants or public transportation.

Throughout history, fears of children have taken various forms. Influenced by a strong belief in original sin, the Puritans thought that children were essentially evil and could fall into depravity if not disciplined and put to work. On the other hand, the Victorians saw childhood as an idyllic time. Children were not particularly welcome in adult society but were seen as innocents who could be irreparably damaged by any but the most tactful, gentle references to the body in general and sex in particular. Parents feared bad influences on their children.

A late 19th-century etiquette book laid down rules for privileged families that indicate that children were not thought to be fit company for adults. Children under the age of 13 ate dinner in the nursery with their governess, not with their parents. The only meal eaten with father at all was Sunday lunch. Young children were excluded from the drawing room except on special occasions.

Early 20th-century child development experts promoted the fear that children's behavior and bodily functions would deteriorate if not properly scheduled.

Social and technological changes of the mid-20th century seem to have created a fear that there is no good way to bring up children. The birth rate is falling, and children have become an economic disadvantage to some parents. When most of society was engaged in farming and small-business operation, children served a role as employees. As the possibilities for children to play this role have decreased the cost of raising and educating a child have increased. Because of mixed emotions, possibly including fear, on the part of parents, child abuse and neglect have increased since the 1960s.

The acceleration of change has made the younger generation frightening to the older. In 1970, Margaret Mead (1901–78) reflected the anguish many adults feel when they see a child eagerly and expertly playing with a computer. "Today nowhere in the world are there elders who know what the children know, no matter how remote and simple the societies in which the children live."

Albert, Linda, *Linda Albert's Advice for Coping with Kids* (New York: Dutton, 1982).

Cable, Mary, *The Little Darlings: A History of Child Rearing in America* (New York: Scribner, 1975).

China Fear of China, the Chinese language, and things relating to the Chinese culture is known as Sinophobia.

In ancient China, hypnosis and supernatural practices were included in therapy for mental disorders, such as possession by spirits and demons. Special institutions for the insane existed in Peking (now Beijing) as early as 300 B.C. Western methods of treating anxiety disorders began during the 19th century when medical missionaries arrived.

A 1970 study indicated that Chinese medicine classified mental disorders by cause, including "wind madness," "ghost evil," "possession by devil," "anxiety due to animus," "convulsive madness," "puerperal (postpartum) insanity," and "mental deficiency."

See also SINOPHOBIA.

Neki, J. S., "Psychiatry in South-East Asia." British Journal of Psychiatry 123 (1973): pp. 257–269.

chins, fear of   Fear of chins is known as geniophobia. Some individuals characterize personalities by the shape of chins. For example, some individuals believe that in men, a receding chin may be a sign of meekness, while a strong, protruding chin may be a sign of strength and aggressiveness, and perhaps something to be feared. Some people fear others who have double chins. Individuals who have obsessions about their own body and the shape of their body, particularly their face, may believe that changing the shape of their chin will help change their personality or their life. Some individuals seek cosmetic surgery to correct what they perceive as a misshapen chin.

See also BODY IMAGE, FEAR OF.

chionophobia   Fear of snow.

See also SNOW, FEAR OF.

chiropractic medicine   Chiropractic medicine deals with the relationship between the skeleton and the nervous system and the role of this relationship in restoring and maintaining health. Many people visit chiropractors to relieve anxieties and stress as well as physical discomforts.

According to chiropractic philosophy, the body is a self-healing organism and all bodily function is controlled by the nervous system. Abnormal bodily function may be caused by interference with nerve transmission and expression. This interference can be caused by pressure, strain, or tension on the spinal cord, spinal nerves, or peripheral nerves as a result of a displacement of the spinal segments or other skeletal structures.

The art of the chiropractic practitioner involves detecting and correcting problems of the vertebral subluxation complex. Subluxation refers to a slight dislocation or biomechanical malfunctioning of the vertebrae (bones of the spine). According to the International Chiropractors Association, subluxation can irritate nerve roots and blood vessels that branch off from the spinal cord between each vertebrae. The irritation causes pain and dysfunction in muscle, lymphatic, and organ tissue as well as imbalance in normal body processes.

Causes of subluxation include anxieties, stress, falls, injuries, trauma, inherited spinal weaknesses, improper sleeping habits, poor posture, poor lifting habits, obesity, lack of rest, and exercise.

Chiropractors restore misaligned vertebrae to their proper position in the spinal cord through procedures known as "spinal adjustments" or manipulation. The adjustment itself does not directly heal the body. Rather, it is the resulting alignment of misaligned spinal vertebrae that restores balance so that the body can function more optimally.

Choosing a Chiropractor

Before choosing a chiropractor, ask him or her to fully explain the benefits, risks, and costs of all diagnostic and treatment options. Interview more than one doctor of chiropractic medicine before making a decision about which practitioner to use.

See also COMPLEMENTARY THERAPIES.

Coulter, Ian, Alan Adams, Peter Coggan, et al., "A Comparative Study of Chiropractic and Medical Education." Alternative Therapies 4, no. 5 (September 1998).

McGill, Leonard, The Chiropractor's Health Book: Simple, Natural Exercises for Relieving Headaches, Tension and Back Pain (New York: Crown Trade Paperbacks, 1997).

Rondberg, Terry A., Chiropractic First: The Fastest Growing Healthcare First . . . Before Drugs or Surgery (Chandler, AZ: The Chiropractic Journal, 1996).

chlordiazepoxide   An antianxiety drug marketed under the trade name Librium. This antianxiety drug (or anxiolytic) falls into a group of drugs known as BENZODIAZEPINES. Chlordiazepoxide is generally one of several drugs of choice for relief of anxiety and tension. Like the other benzodiazepines, it is also useful in alcohol and drug withdrawal syndromes and as a muscle relaxant.

See also ANTIANXIETY DRUGS; ANXIETY.

chlorpromazine   Generic term for one of the most widely used MAJOR TRANQUILIZERS, sold under the name Thorazine. It was the first ANTIPSYCHOTIC agent marketed. It is frequently used to treat psychotics and sometimes incorrectly prescribed for ANXIETY, as it is one of the most SEDATIVE antipsychotic drugs. Tolerance to this effect develops rapidly. Individuals under 40 years of age experience the fewest side effects from the drug. In older patients, there is a high incidence of DIZZINESS, low blood pressure, and vision changes. Because of these major side effects individuals who are taking it should be monitored regularly and closely by their physician.

See also ADVERSE DRUG EFFECTS.

choking, fear of   Although both fear of choking and ANOREXIA NERVOSA are eating disorders, they are distinctly different. Individuals who fear choking may have no particular wish to be thin and often remain hungry despite their inability to eat. They gradually lose weight as they limit themselves to what they consider safe foods and safe places to eat. While tightness in the throat is a common symptom of panic disorder and grief, fear of choking may be the only persistent complaint when there are no other symptoms of PANIC DISORDER or DEPRESSION.

The individual may describe one specific time when he or she almost choked; this is probably the episode during which the phobia began because intense fear or panic was elicited. Later on, the individual may describe a history of episodes of rapid pulse, chest pain or tightness, dizziness, tremulousness, tingling and numbness in the arms and legs, and a sense of impending doom or LOSS OF CONTROL. Some have been diagnosed as previously having had HYPERVENTILATION syndrome. They may have other phobias such as the fear of CROWDS, CLOSED PLACES, HEIGHTS, or DRIVING A CAR. These fears may have led to other avoidance behaviors.

Most individuals with fear of choking while eating welcome treatment and respond well. Systematic desensitization and a variety of pharmacologic agents have been known to be helpful to individuals who have choking phobia.

See also DESENSITIZATION; DRUGS, FEAR OF TAKING; EATING PHOBIAS.

cholera, fear of   Cholera, a disease caused by contaminated water or food supplies that carry the microorganism *ivrio cholerae,* was widely feared during the 19th century. During the European epidemic from 1840 to 1849, cholera victims died in the streets, causing further fears and anxieties among the non-infected population. Cholera is still feared in southcentral and southeast Asia, where it is prevalent because of lack of sanitary conditions. Many individuals who travel to "third world" countries still fear cholera, and medical authorities often advise inoculations against cholera for some travelers to certain areas. Infection results in such symptoms as diarrhea, muscle cramps, vomiting, dehydration, and sometimes shock. The disease may resemble severe cases of food poisoning.

See also DISEASE, FEAR OF; ILLNESS PHOBIA.

cholesterol, fear of   Cholesterol is a fatty substance essential to the cells of the body. Many people fear eating foods high in saturated fats such as meats and egg yolks because a high cholesterol count has been linked with heart disease. Individuals who fear heart disease often fear having a high cholesterol level. High cholesterol levels sometimes lead to deposits of fatty material within the walls of blood vessels and a condition known as atherosclerosis. High blood pressure, heart disease, and other circulatory problems sometimes follow atherosclerosis. An individual who is anxious about cholesterol and the risk of heart disease can reduce his chance of developing heart disease by reducing intake of saturated fats, which are derived largely from meat, egg yolk, butter, high-fat dairy products, and coconut oil. An intake of largely polyunsaturated fats, on the other hand, will lower the cholesterol level. Likewise, high-fiber diets seem to lower cholesterol levels. Some cholesterol is essential to health. Drastic low-cholesterol diets should not be tried without reason or without a physician's recommendation.

HIGH CHOLESTEROL:
ONE OF SEVERAL RISK FACTORS FOR HEART DISEASE

High LDL cholesterol (Higher than 100 mg/dL)
Smoking
Age (A man 45 or older; a woman 55 or older)
High blood pressure (treated or untreated)
Hereditary (father, brother, or son had heart disease
    before 55; mother, sister, or daughter before 65)
Low HDL cholesterol (Lower than 35 mg/dL)

Understanding the importance of controlling one's cholesterol level is important for good health, as high cholesterol is one of several risk factors for heart disease.

What Should Your Cholesterol Level Be?

The National Cholesterol Education Program (NCEP) recommends that those who already have heart disease should have a total cholesterol level of 160 mg/dl or less, with the LDL level at 100 mg/dl or less. For those who don't have heart disease but have two or more risk factors in addition to high cholesterol, the level should be under 200 mg/dl, with LDL level under 130 mg/dl. For those who don't have heart disease but have fewer than two risk factors in addition to high LDL cholesterol, the overall level should be under 240 mg/dl with the LDL under 160 mg/dl.

Several types of cholesterol-lowering medications are available. Medications should always be used along with a low-fat, low-cholesterol diet. A physician will decide whether medication is necessary and which medication is best for each individual.

See also ATHEROSCLEROSIS; CORONARY ARTERY DISEASE; HEART DISEASE, FEAR OF; STROKE.

Giles, Wayne H., et al., "Cholesterol," *The Journal of the American Medical Association.* March 2, 1993.

Grover, Steven A., et al., "HDL Cholesterol Level Is Important Indicator of Potential Heart Disease." *The Journal of the American Medical Association,* September 12, 1995.

chrematophobia   Fear of money. Also known as chromophobia, and more commonly as chrema-

tomania. This phobia is often linked to obsessive concerns about cleanliness and avoidance of germs thought to be carried on much-handled money. Sufferers will eventually quit handling money or begin to wear gloves as a safeguard.

See also GERMS, FEAR OF; MONEY, FEAR OF; OBSESSIVE-COMPULSIVE DISORDER.

chronic fatigue syndrome (CFS)   Illness characterized by fatigue that occurs suddenly, improves, and relapses, bringing on debilitating tiredness or easy fatigability in an individual who has no apparent reason for feeling this way. It causes anxieties for the sufferer because the profound weakness caused by CFS does not go away with a few good nights of sleep, but instead steals a person's vigor over months and years. Anxiety often occurs because of loss of income and vitality in relationships. Because many individuals who have CFS experience frustration both before being diagnosed and on learning that there is no cure, DEPRESSION often accompanies the disease.

While the illness strikes children, teenagers, and people in their fifties, sixties, and seventies, it is most likely to strike adults from their mid-twenties to late forties. Women are afflicted about twice to three times as often as men; the vast majority of those who suffer this illness are white. Because young urban professionals were most afflicted during the 1980s, the term *yuppie flu* was attached to CFS. However, individuals regarded this term as trivializing their illness.

Symptoms and Diagnostic Path

CFS can affect virtually all of the body's major systems: neurological, immunological, hormonal, gastrointestinal, and musculoskeletal. According to the National Institutes of Health, CFS leaves many people bedridden, or with headaches, muscular and joint pain, sore throat, balance disorders, sensitivity to light, an inability to concentrate, and inexplicable body aches. Secondary depression, which follows from the disease rather than causing it, is just as disabling. However, knowing that there is a chemical basis for mood swings and that they are directly related to illness can be reassuring.

Symptoms wax and wane in severity and linger for months and sometimes years. Some individuals respond to treatment, while others must function at a reduced level for a long time. However, for all sufferers, the cumulative effect is the same, namely, transforming ordinary activities into tremendous stressful challenges. They cannot tolerate the least bit of exercise, their cognitive functions become impaired, and their memory, verbal fluency, response time, and ability to perform calculations and to reason show a marked decrease.

Disruption of sleep patterns cause the CFS sufferer additional stress. Despite constant exhaustion and desire for sleep, they rarely sleep uninterruptedly and awake feeling refreshed. Some have severe INSOMNIA, while others have difficulty maintaining sleep. There is often not enough rapid-eye movement (REM) sleep, which is considered necessary for a good night's rest.

Many CFS sufferers experience stressful disorders of balance or of the vestibular system, which is modulated by the inner ear. They sometimes feel dizziness, lightheadedness, or nausea. Even walking can be difficult, with sufferers tilting off balance or stumbling for no apparent reason. Some individuals who have balance disorders develop PHOBIAS, such as a fear of falling. Some who have this fear even become housebound.

CFS causes anxieties for sufferers, family, and friends. Those in their support circles can reduce their stress by being helpful, understanding, and available to listen. Sufferers are likely to feel estranged from some of their friends because they believe that no one really understands their feelings of emotional and physical exhaustion. This belief is exacerbated because many sufferers think that others do not take their illness seriously. In addition, some friends and family members may fear that CFS is contagious and try to maintain a distance from the sufferer. (Medical opinion seems to indicate that CFS is not contagious.) Spouses face the issue of reduced sexual activity, although both partners can satisfy their needs by engaging in sexual activity during peak periods of energy.

Diagnosing CFS produces anxieties for physicians as well as patients because many of the symptoms are like those of other disorders. Until the mid-1980s, many CFS patients were misdiagnosed as suffering from depression, accused of malingering, encouraged to undergo stressful, costly, and inappropriate laboratory tests, or simply pushed aside by the medical community because of lack of understanding of the disease. In recent years, however, studies on the immune system, viruses, and the physiological effects of stress have contributed to better understanding of CFS. Individuals with CFS no longer have to feel abandoned by their physicians or fear that they are "going crazy" because no one takes their illness seriously.

Treatment Options and Outlook

Many therapies have been tried on CFS sufferers. Usually a plan is devised for each patient, depending on symptoms. Pharmacological therapies include use of antidepressant drugs, pain relieving drugs, and muscle-relaxing drugs.

Other therapies that have been tried include deep relaxation, YOGA, BIOFEEDBACK, and visualization therapy to relieve anxieties and chronic pain. Nutritional therapies have included emphasizing certain vitamins, such as Vitamins A, B_6, B_{12}, C, and E, as well as zinc, folic acid, and selenium, all of which are said to have immune-boosting potential.

Oil extract from the seeds of the evening primrose plant is another medicine that some CFS patients have found helpful. The theoretical basis for its use (although not scientifically proven in known double-blind studies) is that evening primrose oil contains gamma-linolenic acid (GLA), which converts in the body to prostaglandin, a vital substance in the regulation of cellular function.

Role of Support Groups and Self-Help. Several nationwide organizations encourage research and political advocacy and also provide lists of local support groups. CFS sufferers may find relief from some stressors and help with practical and emotional needs through these organizations.

See also CHRONIC ILLNESS; DEPRESSION; SUPPORT GROUPS.

Jason, Leonard A., Wynee Wagner, Susan Rosenthal, et al., "Estimating the Prevalence of Chronic Fatigue Syndrome Among Nurses," *American Journal of Medicine*, September 28, 1998.

McSherry, James, "Chronic Fatigue Syndrome: A fresh look at an old problem," *Canadian Family Physician* 39 (February 1993).

chronic illness   Chronic illness describes a disorder or set of symptoms that has persisted for a long time with progressive deterioration. In addition to the anxieties and stresses of physical pain, chronic illness often brings with it emotional consequences that can be more far-reaching than the illness itself. These affect not only the patient but also cause anxieties for the immediate caregivers. Some, particularly close family members, let illness-related anxieties take over their lives and their depression arises from COPING with illness and the threat of possible long-term disability or death of a loved one.

Reactions to illness are similar to the stages of GRIEF after the death of a loved one. First there is the patient's shock and a feeling of many losses, of CONTROL, of AUTONOMY, and of the way things used to be. In addition, they experience physical losses ranging from having to give up their job or favorite sport to impaired speech or vision. Stress and symptoms of depression may follow, including hopelessness, self-blame, shattered self-esteem or withdrawal. Some ill persons may develop many fears. They may fear exercise and being active again, while others may deny the realities of their condition and overdo activities too soon.

The anxieties of pain and fears about disability and death lead some people who are ill to substance abuse as a form of escape. Anger, denial, or perceived helplessness lead others to abandon medical treatment or assume a "why me" attitude that gives them a pessimistic view of their world.

The crucial issue is "whether you can get past the stage of rage, sadness, and overwhelming anxiety," says Lloyd D. Rudley, M.D., an attending psychiatrist at The Institute of Pennsylvania Hospital, Philadelphia, "Will you resume the initiative for living or become psychologically paralyzed?" Many people become trapped by emotions that do not serve them well, according to Dr. Rudley.

Unfortunately, there are chronically ill people who do not comply with instructions from their physicians. This may take the form of not showing up for physical therapy, refusing medication, or driving a car against the physician's advice. Individuals with emphysema may continue to smoke. According to Dr. Rudley, "People want to think everything will be normal again if they follow the

doctor's orders. When things don't work this way and there is no magic formula, a patient may give up on treatment."

Some individuals neglect medical advice as a means of getting more attention. Others who harbor shame or guilt about their condition may punish themselves, in effect, by not complying with prescribed treatment. Forces of denial may be at work, too, in those who try to "bargain with illness" by following some recommendations, but not others.

How individuals coped with life stress before the illness will determine how well they respond when illness occurs. However, even when symptoms of illness go into remission or people have adjusted to their illness, a whole new set of external stressors may arise or family dynamics can change dramatically.

"Patients need to accept that chronic illness changes them permanently, that a change in lifestyle is necessary," advises Dr. Rudley. Healthy acceptance is achieved when people come to terms with the stresses of their illness as a part of who they are, a sort of coexistence with it," he says.

Some individuals feel certain "benefits" from being chronically ill. Such motivations are referred to as "secondary gains" and increase the likelihood of them continuing to be ill or to have symptoms. Common "benefits" of illness include receiving permission to get out of dealing with a troublesome problem, situation, or responsibility of life; getting attention, care or nurturing; and not having to meet their own or others' expectations.

Every area of a person's life is affected by ill health, including marriage, family, work, financial affairs, and future plans. Professional counseling can help individuals and their families adapt to stresses brought on by chronic illness. Counseling may also help individuals who feel a need to hide their illness, increase their use of drugs or alcohol, fail to follow treatment recommendations, or exhibit fear of resuming their activities. It can help those who have insomnia and disrupted sleep, experience prolonged depression, show negative personality changes, and have obsessive anxiety or preoccupation with death.

See also CAREGIVERS; GENERAL ADAPTATION SYNDROME; PAIN, FEAR OF.

Rudley, Lloyd D., "Conquering the Psychological Hurdles of Chronic Illness." *The Quill* (Fall 1991).

chronic obstructive lung disease and anxiety

Many individuals who have chronic obstructive pulmonary (lung) disease (COPD) such as chronic bronchitis and chronic emphysema frequently fear that they will suffocate, lose control, and die. They also fear having a breathless attack in public and the embarrassment of requiring emergency care. During an attack of obstructed breathing, they may have a panic attack in which they gasp for air, which only worsens their situation and anxiety. Some recall frequent periods of panic and may even have nightmares about being unable to inhale. Some who suffer from COPD have disabling anxiety because of their disease. They may avoid social situations because they fear an obstructed breathing attack and may become depressed and withdrawn.

An understanding of what happens to an individual who has COPD can help others around him or her cope with the anxieties the individual experiences. In many respiratory disorders, there is a narrowing of the bronchial tubes. In chronic bronchitis, the mucous membrane lining the main air passages (bronchi) of the lungs becomes inflamed, leading to breathlessness and heavy coughing. In chronic asthma, the muscles of the bronchial walls contract, leading to partial obstruction of the bronchi and the bronchioles (smaller air passages in the lungs). The individual has attacks of wheezing and difficult breathing. In asthmatics, such attacks may be brought on by stimuli to which they are allergic, or by exercise or stress. With chronic emphysema, the air sacs (alveoli) at the ends of the bronchioles are damaged. Because this is where oxygen and carbon dioxide exchange, the lungs become less and less efficient, and the primary symptom is difficult breathing, which gets worse and becomes more frightening as the individual ages.

chronic pain, fear of

Fear of chronic pain is associated with fear of certain diseases, such as arthritis and cancer, and with aging and growing old.

See also AGING, FEAR OF; CANCER, FEAR OF; PAIN, FEAR OF; PAIN AND ANXIETY.

chronophobia

Fear of time; also known as prison neurosis, because it may be the most common anxiety disorder in prison inmates. Chronophobia is characterized by panic, anxiety, and claustrophobia. Sooner or later, almost all prisoners suffer chronophobia to some degree and become terrified by the duration and immensity of time. This is often called going "stir crazy." Chronophobia appears suddenly, without warning. The introductory phase of imprisonment is ordinarily marked by hopes and plans for a new trial, by uncertainty, and by a studied indifference or carefree attitude. After the novelty of prison wears off, when the prisoner comes to grips with the real length of the sentence, chronophobia sets in. The prisoner goes into a panic, usually while in his cell, and fears his enclosure and restraint; this apparent claustrophobia arises from fear of time, as represented by the prison. After the first attack, the prisoner experiences more or less constant anxiety, restlessness, insomnia, dissatisfaction with life, numerous hypochondriacal complaints, and progressive inability to adjust himself to his surroundings. The intensity of the crisis usually passes within a few weeks or months, though mild relapses may occur. Later the prisoner becomes relatively indifferent to his surroundings and serves the rest of his sentence by the clock and lives wholly in the present, one day at a time.

See also ANXIETY; CLAUSTROPHOBIA; PANIC; TIME, FEAR OF.

Deutsch, A., and H. Fishman, *The Encyclopedia of Mental Health* (New York: Franklin Watts, 1963), pp. 110–111.

churches, fear of

Fear of churches is known as ecclesiaphobia. The term also refers to fear of clergypersons.

See also HOLY THINGS, FEAR OF.

cibophobia

Fear of food. This is commonly associated with a particular food or class of foods. Often there is a trauma-related onset and intense aversive conditioning. Sometimes even textures or smells are conditioned.

See also FOOD, FEAR OF.

circadian rhythms   Cycles of sleep and wakefulness coordinated by an inherent timing mechanism known as the body's biological clock. The circadian rhythm of a person's body temperature is a marker for those clocks. Body temperature rises and falls in cycles parallel to alertness and performance efficiency. When body temperature is high, which it usually is during the day, alertness and performance peak, but sleep is difficult. A lower temperature (generally during the night) promotes sleep, but hinders alertness and performance. Anxieties may result when tasks are attempted that are not in synchronization with circadian rhythms. Or, the individual may be more prone to develop anxiety when rhythms are dissynchronized.

Alertness and mental capability seems to be best when people follow their internal clocks, which are synchronized to the Sun's 24-hour cycle. For example, sunrise means waking and working, while sundown means dinner and sleep. However, individuals who work night shifts find that their "day" is reversed. Many shift workers go home to sleep during the day when their bodies want to be awake and they have to work at night when their bodies want to sleep, according to Charmaine I. Eastman, Ph.D., in her report *Insights Into Clinical and Scientific Progress in Medicine*.

Timothy Monk, director of the Human Chronobiology Program at the University of Pittsburgh School of Medicine, says that circadian rhythms affect many performances of mental feats. For example, different skills follow different cycles, so that at any time a person's mind is naturally sharp for certain tasks and dull for others. Memory varies though the day, and short-term memory is at its peak at nine in the morning while memorizing for the long term works best around three in the afternoon. Problem-solving peaks in the morning and falls during the afternoon and evening. However, reaction time improves throughout the day and finally peaks in the evening.

Readjusting to Jet Lag

Jet lag—the discrepancy between the individual's "internal clock" and the exaggerated passage of time brought on by air travel—is a well-known disruption of circadian rhythms. Physical stress occurs and anxieties may result from these body sensations or the weakened state. Symptoms of jet lag may include insomnia, headache, loss of appetite, or nausea. A conventional rule says that each time zone passed takes one day of recovery. Generally, recovering from jet lag is easier when one flies west, rather than east. That is because it seems easier to delay the body's schedule than force it to advance. Exposure to daylight can help the body resynchronize more quickly.

For similar reasons, most people have an easier time changing from daylight savings time back to standard time in the fall than the reverse in the spring. Setting clocks back in the fall allows an hour more of sleep. However, in the spring, when clocks are set ahead, and people have to get up an hour earlier than is customary, sleep deprivation may make them tired.

Adjusting to Night Work

People who work at night can adjust more easily and reduce anxieties if they have darkness during the day and bright light at night. Night workers can also adjust more quickly if they can maintain a schedule of work-sleep-leisure, rather than the work-leisure-sleep pattern of day workers.

See also BIOLOGICAL CLOCK.

circumspection-preemption-control (CPC) cycle   A cyclical process in which an anxious or phobic individual develops a system that enables him or her to interpret the environment and anticipate future events. When faced with a novel situation or new material to learn, the individual may approach it first by loosening his constructs (circumspection), then by tightening them (preemption), and finally, when the situation or material has been integrated, by developing new control. The term was introduced by George A. Kelly (1905–67), an American psychologist.

Kelly, G. A., *A Psychology of Personal Constructs* (New York: W. W. Norton, 1955).

circumstantiality   A term that describes an indirect speech pattern common among individuals who have obsessive-compulsive disorder. The individual delays reaching the point by introducing unnecessary, tedious details and parenthetical remarks. Circumstantial replies or statements may be prolonged for many minutes if the speaker is not interrupted and urged to get to the point. Therapists often respond to circumstantiality by interrupting the speaker in order to complete the process of history-taking. Such interruption may make it difficult to distinguish loosening of associations from circumstantiality. In loosening of associations, there is a lack of connection between clauses, and the original point is lost; but in circumstantiality, the clauses always retain a meaningful connection, and the speaker is always aware of the original point, goal, or topic.

classical conditioning   A form of learning by which some specific FEARS and PHOBIAS may develop. An understanding of the concept evolved from the work of Ivan P. Pavlov (1849–1936), a Russian physiologist, who conditioned dogs to salivate at a specific STIMULI, such as the sound of a bell. The procedure involves simultaneously exposing the individual to two different stimuli, one of which, known as the unconditioned (or unconditional) stimulus (UCS), automatically or reflexively brings about a specific response, known as the UNCONDITIONED (or unconditional) RESPONSE (UCR). The second stimulus, known as the CONDITIONED STIMULUS (CS), at first has no effect on the response in question. After repeated trials delivering the CS slightly preceding the UCS, the CS alone comes to elicit the response previously brought on by the UCS. If the response is brought about by the CS alone, it is known as a CONDITIONED RESPONSE (CR). This type of learning is by association or stimulus substitution.

John B. Watson (1878–1958), an American psychologist known as the founder of behaviorism, was one of the first and most influential proponents of the theory that classical conditioning could be used to account for acquisition of fears and anxieties.

There has been some controversy about general applicability of the classical conditioning theory to the development of all phobias. Many individuals with specific fears do not recall any conditioning experience associated with the beginning of their fears. Also, many people have phobias out of proportion to the stimulus. For example, fear of snakes is a generally prevalent fear, yet few phobic people have had direct contact with snakes. Fear of dentists is about half as prevalent as that of snakes, and although many people have received unpleasant stimuli on the DENTAL chair, most do not develop conditioned fear reactions. However, classical conditioning is still regarded as a source for some people's phobias and fears.

This particular learning model or method is applicable in situations in which traumatic events have occurred. For instance, people who have severe auto accidents often react to brakes squealing or traffic lights with intense anxiety. In this case, since brake lights or squealing (CSs) have been associated with the accident (and the pain and anxiety elicited by it), they become conditioned stimuli. Likewise, observation of a person in a painful/anxious/frightening situation (such as the shower scene in Alfred Hitchcock's movie, *Psycho*) can classically condition people to fear showers or showering while alone.

See also BEHAVIORISM; CONDITIONING THERAPY.

claustrophobia   Claustrophobia is an exaggerated fear of closed places, such as closets, subways, tunnels, telephone booths, elevators, small rooms, crowds, or other enclosed or confined spaces. The word is derived from the Latin word "claustrum," meaning bolt or lock. More people may suffer from claustrophobia than from any other exaggerated fear. *Claustrophoboid* is the term used to describe one who suffers from claustrophobia, or fear of being in an enclosed place.

Claustrophobia takes many forms. Some individuals fear being in a car or room in which they cannot open a window or in which the door is closed or the shades drawn. Others fear sitting in the center of a row in a church, theater, or airplane. Some cope with their fears, to some extent, by sitting at the end of the row or at the aisle. Some claustrophobics fear and avoid FLYING because they do not like to be in an enclosed place.

While most people dislike feeling hemmed in or trapped to any extent, claustrophobics react with severe PANIC and physiologic symptoms such as increased pulse when they feel closed in. Persons with this phobia often fear suffocation. There are many reasons why individuals have claustrophobic feelings. Some individuals who have claustrophobia may once have had a frightening experience while enclosed in a small space. While the experience itself is forgotten, the feelings associated with it remain and lead to the phobia. Such individuals tend to avoid, at all costs, being in situations that make them panic. Others may have had a frightening dream of being trapped in a closed place. While the dream is forgotten, the feelings of fear and panic remain.

Some whose phobias include being in tunnels may fear that the tunnel will cave in and they will be buried alive or be killed by the falling structure. While they travel through a tunnel, they imagine what might happen and may actually feel shortness of breath as though something was crushing their chests.

Claustrophobics who are afraid of elevators must make many life choices so that they can avoid taking elevators. This may affect where they work and where they live. Some who fear elevators fear that the elevator will get stuck between floors, that the doors will not open, that they will be trapped, and that they may starve or suffocate to death. Some claustrophobics have similar fears about airplanes.

Another form of claustrophobia is a morbid fear of being below ground level, such as in submarines or underground trains. Some servicemen have been rejected from submarine duty because of their panic at being underwater. Others avoid going in subways or underground trains by taking other means of transportation.

Many individuals who have agoraphobia were first claustrophobic. There is strong evidence that a claustrophobic tendency is an innate human potential that can become activated by (negative) experiences and become a conditioned response. Nevertheless, these reactions are avoidable, and improvement and recovery is possible with a proper treatment approach.

See also AGORAPHOBIA; COUNTERPHOBIA; ELEVATORS, FEAR OF; FLYING, FEAR OF.

cleaning (as a ritual) Fears of dirt and contamination lead many individuals to excessive cleaning rituals. Some sufferers feel contaminated, for example, each time they urinate, defecate, touch a pet, or pass a hospital. Afterward, they repeatedly wash their hands or disinfect objects they have touched while they feel dirty. Cleaning (as a ritual) appears in about half of all sufferers of OBSESSIVE-COMPULSIVE DISORDER.

See also OBSESSION; RITUAL.

cleptophobia A fear of stealing. Also known as kleptophobia.

See also STEALING, FEAR OF.

client-centered psychotherapy A therapeutic technique that stresses the uniqueness and personal growth of the individual. In this therapy, unconditional regard and communication of emphatic understanding are seen as conditions for self-actualization and greater personal acceptance. This therapy was developed by Carl Rogers.

See also BEHAVIOR THERAPY.

cliffs, fear of Fear of cliffs or precipices is known as cremnophobia. It is similar to bathophobia, which is a fear of DEPTH and of looking down from HIGH PLACES. It is also related to batophobia, a fear of being on or passing by HIGH OBJECTS such as skyscrapers.

See also ACROPHOBIA; BATHOPHOBIA; BATOPHOBIA; SIMPLE PHOBIAS.

climacophobia Fear of stairs or of climbing stairs.

See also STAIRS, FEAR OF.

climate, fear of Seasonal affective disorder (SAD) is a type of depression that seems to occur more in climates that have long periods of dark, gloomy weather. Individuals who suffer from the anxieties associated with SAD generally feel better during the brighter months of the year. Some people benefit from special treatments with lights used on a regular basis each day. In earlier times, scholars (including Robert Burton, author of *The Anatomy of Melancholy*) believed that cold, damp climates produced more insanity than warmer ones, but statistical studies have not been able to substantiate these concerns.

See also DEPRESSION; SEASONAL AFFECTIVE DISORDER.

clinical psychology The branch of psychology (study of behavior) that specializes in the study, diagnosis, and treatment of behavior disorders. Many individuals who have anxieties, fears, and phobias receive treatment from clinical psychologists. Clinical psychologists in most states must have a Ph.D. degree and a license in order to offer their services to the public. Graduate training for the Ph.D. emphasizes research knowledge and skills, academic coursework, and clinical practice and internship experiences. Clinical psychology came into prominence after World War II when its emphasis shifted from mental and personality testing to psychotherapy and research. Clinical psychologists are responsible for most of the major research on clinical methods/therapy, psychopathology, and the diagnostic system.

See also BEHAVIOR THERAPY; PSYCHOLOGY.

clinophobia Fear of beds or of going to bed.

See also BED, FEAR OF.

clocks, fear of Individuals who fear seeing clocks, hearing clocks, or thinking of clocks may fear the passage of time, or the infinity of time. Some have chronophobia, or fear of a long duration. Some prisoners develop this fear. Looking at clocks may be a COMPULSION for one who has OBSESSIVE-COMPULSIVE DISORDER. The person who watches clocks frequently may have a compulsion to be on time, or a fear of being late.

See also CHECKING; CHRONOPHOBIA; INFINITY, FEAR OF.

clomipramine A tricyclic ANTIDEPRESSANT that is the drug of choice in treating OBSESSIVE-COMPULSIVE DISORDER. It has been used for many years in Europe and Canada. Clomipramine is reportedly at least twenty percent effective in alleviating symptoms and in significantly helping those who can tolerate the drug.

See also MONOAMINE OXIDASE INHIBITORS (MAOI).

clonazepam An anticonvulsant drug of the benzodiazepine group marketed under the trade name Klonopin. It has been tried in the treatment of tardive dyskenesia (a drug-induced neurological disorder). It is also used to treat anxiety disorders in certain individuals. Adverse reactions to the central nervous system occur in many patients.

See also ANTICONVULSIVES; TARDIVE DYSKENESIA.

clonidine A drug used in the treatment of high blood pressure and relief of anxieties in some individuals. Clonidine (trade name: Catapres) is an adrenergic agonist that acts on the central nervous system and reduces the action of the sympathetic nervous system by altering the chemical balance within the brain. Effects in the brain slow the heart rate and decrease the action in some nerves that control blood vessel constriction. In studies during the early 1980s, clonidine was effective in alleviating anxiety in most patients who had GENERALIZED ANXIETY DISORDER (GAD) and PANIC ATTACKS. Clonidine was more effective in reducing ANXIETY ATTACKS than general physical symptoms. As a side effect, it may cause persistent drowsiness and dryness of the mouth, in which case physicians usually advise cutting down on the medication. Abruptly stopping this medication can trigger a sudden, dangerous rise in blood pressure. Methyldopa is a similar drug.

See also ADVERSE DRUG REACTIONS; HIGH BLOOD PRESSURE, FEAR OF.

closed spaces Fear of closed spaces, or being locked in an enclosed space, is known as clithrophobia, cleisiophobia, or cleithrophobia. This fear is a form of claustrophobia.

See also CENTER OF THE ROW, FEAR OF SITTING IN; CLAUSTROPHOBIA.

clothing, fear of Fear of wearing clothing, or the sight of clothing, is known as vestiphobia. This fear is usually associated with particular styles, textures, or colors of clothing.

See also COLORS, FEAR OF.

clouds, fear of   Fear of clouds is known as nephophobia. People who experience this phobia will not look up in the sky at clouds. Occasionally, pilots will feel anxious when flying over clouds or through clouds, whereas they are comfortable in clear skies. This fear may be related to other fears concerning weather, such as impending rain, thunderstorms, or lightning. Some people who feel depressed on gray days also fear clouds, because they anticipate an episode of depression. Some depressions are seasonally related, and for those whose depression occurs during the cloudier months, clouds can be particularly threatening.

See also FLYING, FEAR OF; LIGHTNING, FEAR OF; RAIN, FEAR OF; THUNDERSTORMS, FEAR OF.

clovaxamine   An antidepressant drug.

See also ANTIDEPRESSANTS; DEPRESSION.

clozapine   A medication to treat SCHIZOPHRENIA. After preliminary trials, clozapine appears to be an effective treatment for a substantial number of schizophrenics who do not respond to other drugs. Clozapine rarely causes movement disorders—for example, muscle jerks or cramps, tremors, muscle rigidity, restlessness, or the severe movement disorders known as TARDIVE DYSKENESIA—associated with other ANTIPSYCHOTIC drugs. However, weekly blood tests are necessary to check for a potentially fatal weakening of the immune system in response to the drug. Clozapine does not cure schizophrenia, but it improves symptoms enough so that individuals can function in the community and benefit from rehabilitation services. Clozapine has been tried unsuccessfully as a treatment for anxiety.

See also DRUGS.

cnidophobia   Fear of stings. The term applies to stings of bees, wasps, mosquitoes, and other insects.

The fear may relate to a fear of flying things and insects that may look threatening to an individual.

See also BEES, FEAR OF; STINGS, FEAR OF.)

coaching   The way in which a behavior therapist teaches an anxious or phobic individual or family to develop new behaviors. The procedure helps the individual move toward the defined treatment goal by shaping behavior. While this is a term that comes from family therapy, coaching is also very evident in fieldwork and in *in vivo* desensitization or exposure treatments.

See also BEHAVIOR THERAPY; FAMILY THERAPY.

cocaine, fear reactions from   Cocaine is a stimulant drug that affects the CENTRAL NERVOUS SYSTEM, inducing feelings of euphoria and many other psychological and physical effects. It is a Schedule II drug under the Controlled Substances Act and is only legally used by physicians in treating some diseases of the eye and nose. Cocaine can be taken orally or injected. A more concentrated form of cocaine, crack cocaine, is smoked. Cocaine is an addictive drug.

In 2004, according to the National Survey on Drug Use and Health, about 1 million people used cocaine for the first time. Most new users (66 percent) were ages 18 and older, and the average age for new users was 20 years. The number of people receiving treatment for a cocaine abuse problem at a specialty facility increased significantly from 276,000 people in 2003 to 466,000 individuals in 2004.

According to the National Survey on Drug Use and Health, in 2004 there were 2 million current users of cocaine in the United States. Of these, 467,000 used crack cocaine. Another annual study, the 2004 *Monitoring the Future* study of students in the 8th, 10th, and 12th grades, found that 16 percent of all Americans have tried cocaine by age 30. Of these cocaine users, 8 percent had tried cocaine by their senior year in high school.

Many people who abuse cocaine also abuse other drugs, particularly alcohol. The simultaneous use of both alcohol and cocaine is risky to an individual's health because the two drugs combine to form a substance known as cocaethylene. This substance can boost the euphoria caused by cocaine, but it also increases the risk for sudden death.

Effects of Cocaine

The effects of cocaine are similar to the effects of the natural substance ADRENALINE and the manufactured stimulants AMPHETAMINES. Small doses may cause the following effects

- extreme euphoria
- delusions of increased mental and physical strength and sensory awareness
- a decrease in hunger, pain, and the need for sleep
- panic attacks

Large doses significantly magnify these effects, sometimes causing irrational behavior and aggression. In heavy users, the heightened euphoria of cocaine abuse is often accompanied by an intensified heartbeat, sweating, dilation of the pupils, and hyperthermia (an extreme rise in body temperature). A period of euphoria can be followed by irritability, DEPRESSION, INSOMNIA, PANIC, and an extreme condition of PARANOIA. Formication, or the belief and feeling that insects are running up and down, either on or underneath the skin, is common. In some cases, a condition similar to amphetamine poisoning may occur, and the user will not only appear extremely restless and nervous but will experience delirium, HALLUCINATIONS, muscle spasms, and chest pain.

Male users of cocaine may become impotent or incapable of ejaculation. If the drug is injected, abscesses may appear on the skin. Many of the symptoms can be reversed simply by stopping the drug.

Because of its high cost in the 20th century, cocaine abuse was confined primarily to the upper strata of the economic ladder, particularly to people in the sports and entertainment fields. However, in the latter part of the 20th century, cocaine became more accessible to many individuals and steadily gained acceptance among young adults, including many college students, and in many blue- and white-collar circles as well. As a result, many individuals and their families have been affected by cocaine abuse and addiction.

See also ADDICTION, FEAR OF; DRUG ABUSE.

Gwinnell, Esther, M.D., and Christine Adamec, *The Encyclopedia of Drug Abuse.* (New York: Facts On File, Inc., 2007).

cockroaches, fear of Cockroaches are feared worldwide. They are agents in spreading cholera, dysentery, and many species of parasitic worms. Although cockroaches, unlike lice and mites, do not present any physical harm to humans through direct contact, they do feed on food and human feces. Because of this, they often become infected with disease-producing organisms, which they later excrete onto food, thereby spreading disease. Cockroaches are associated with dirt and garbage and are difficult to kill. Cockroaches develop immunities to pesticides easily and can live for days without food and water. They are sensitive to air currents and can run quickly to flatten their bodies and hide in tiny dark cracks, causing frustration and anxiety to the humans trying to rid their living space of the pest. As scavengers, cockroaches can live on such seemingly inedible materials as glue, leather, hair, paper, and starch in bookbindings.

See also DIRT, FEAR OF; CONTAMINATION, FEAR OF.

Encyclopedia Americana, "Cockroaches" (Danbury, CT: Grolier, 1986).
Goldman, Jane, "What's Bugging You?" *New York*, May 27, 1985.
Osmond, Breland, *Animal Life and Lore* (New York: Harper & Row, 1972), p. 313.

codependency A condition in a relationship between a person with the identified problem (such as ALCOHOLISM or drug dependence) and the codependent who seeks to make up for the shortcomings of the person with the problem. Another word for a codependent person is an *enabler*. Codependency is often seen in individuals with panic disorders with AGORAPHOBIA. Spouses and parents are the most likely attachment object.

The codependent is specifically characterized by a strong need to be needed. Codependent relationships bring about anxieties for one or both of the partners. In many cases, the individual would like to eliminate the anxieties caused by the codependent relationship, but he or she is too committed to the existing situation to change.

An example of a codependent relationship is one in which the husband covers up for his wife's alcoholism or supports her agoraphobia because it continues to keep her dependent on him. This may be an unconscious motivation, as the husband both believes and tells himself that he is helping his wife. In this case, the husband performs household chores, drives the children to their activities, and explains the wife's problem to others as an *illness*. There are also many female enablers who make up for the serious shortcomings of their husbands or partners who are alcoholics, drug addicts, child abusers, and so forth.

Often the enabler regards him- or herself as critically important to the life and happiness of the other person and does not realize that the other person would be far better off if his or her problem were acknowledged, treated, and overcome.

When parents frequently compensate for or cover up a child's difficulties in school or with the law, thinking that they are protecting the child, this is also an example of codependent behavior. Therapists may interpret the parental behavior as persisting because the parents wish to keep the child dependent on them and preserving the child's flaws and immaturity will achieve that goal. However, the parents may sincerely believe that they are helping the child by their actions.

Since codependency is viewed as a type of addiction, advocates of the codependent theory feel that these tendencies can be overcome with a process similar to the recovery process used by Alcoholics Anonymous.

Motivations of enablers. In his book *Introduction to Addictive Behaviors,* Second Edition, author Dennis L. Thombs said that there were six key characteristics of psychological distress experienced by most people who are codependents. First is low self-esteem. Codependents may come from alcoholic families or they may have been physically or emotionally abused in the past.

Next, codependents rate their own personal value in terms of how well they care for others. Third is an urge to change others, and the codependent person believes that (irrationally) he or she can help the other person overcome the problem, whatever it is.

The willingness to suffer is the fourth trait. Often the enabler believes that this willingness validates that he or she really cares about the other person, unlike others who are not willing to suffer.

The fifth characteristic of codependents is a resistance to change, and, for example, the belief that leaving the addict is not a viable consideration. Last, the enabler fears change, and believes that any change in the current circumstances would be worse than the current difficult situation.

See also ADDICTION, FEAR OF; ALCOHOLISM; RELATIONSHIPS.

Thombs, Dennis L., *Introduction to Addictive Behaviors,* 2nd ed. (New York: The Guilford Press, 1999).

coffee   See ANXIETY; CAFFEINE; GUIDED IMAGERY; HEADACHES; INSOMNIA, FEAR OF; MEDITATION; RELAXATION.

cognitive appraisal   A process by which the individual attempts to evaluate and consider potential consequences of an upcoming event. The initial components of fear might begin at this point, especially if the individual is unsure of the outcome or expects it to be unpleasant. This appraisal process is also referred to as anticipatory anxiety. An example is starting to feel fearful just after learning that the date for an important examination has been set. The term is also used in the literature about stress to point out that what is stressful is in the "eye of the beholder." That means that cognitive appraisal of a situation is usually what identifies it as stressful.

See also ANXIETY; FEAR.

cognitive-behavioral approach   See COGNITIVE BEHAVIOR THERAPY.

cognitive behavior therapy A type of therapy based on learning theory. Cognitive behavior therapy is used to help some individuals who have anxieties and phobias by examining the irrational exaggerated thoughts that lead to anxiety reactions. For example, if a person feels that "everyone" criticizes them they will experience resultant anxiety. The individual's own statements are stimuli.

Cognitive behavior therapy includes self-instructional training, STRESS INOCULATION, and COPING SKILLS interventions. Three prominent innovators in this field are Albert Ellis, Donald Meichenbaum, and Aaron Beck.

See also BEHAVIOR MODIFICATION; BEHAVIOR THERAPY.

cognitive dissonance A state of conflict and discomfort that occurs when one's existing beliefs or assumptions are challenged or contradicted by new evidence. The individual usually seeks to relieve the discomfort by various means such as denying the existence or importance of the conflict, reconciling the difference, altering one of the dissident elements, or demanding more and more information. An example is smokers, who, when faced with evidence that cigarettes are hazardous to health, say the evidence is not enough. The term was coined by Leon Festinger, an American psychologist. Cognitive dissonance comes into play as phobic individuals begin to improve substantially. Attitudinally, they often hold to views of self as avoidant and fearful of a situation when in fact the emotional and physiological component may have diminished greatly.

See also BEHAVIOR THERAPY.

Festinger, L., A Theory of Cognitive Dissonance (Stanford, CA: Stanford University Press, 1957).

cognitive restructuring A behavior therapy technique in which one learns to change the way one thinks about life so that one may change one's behavior; often used in treating agoraphobia and many social phobias. Cognitive restructuring is also an important treatment for depression.

See also AGORAPHOBIA; BEHAVIOR THERAPY; PHOBIA; SOCIAL PHOBIA.

cognitive structure The unified structure of beliefs and attitudes about the world or society an individual holds. Phobias and anxieties may be part of an individual's cognitive structure. The term cognitive structure was introduced during the mid-1970s, and the concept predates cognitive behavior therapy. Cognitive structure is also an individual's mental pattern that maintains and organizes information in a learning situation.

See also BEHAVIOR MODIFICATION; BEHAVIOR THERAPY; COGNITIVE BEHAVIOR THERAPY; COGNITIVE RESTRUCTURING.

cognitive therapy A therapeutic approach based on the concept that anxiety problems result from patterns of thinking and distorted attitudes toward oneself and others and that one can alter one's behavior by changing one's thinking. Cognitive therapy is used to treat depressed individuals and others who have anxieties and phobias. One innovator during the late 1970s was Aaron Beck, an American psychiatrist. Earlier forms of cognitive therapy were introduced by Albert Ellis in the late 1960s under the name RATIONAL EMOTIVE THERAPY, or RET.

Cognitive therapy, like behavior therapy, has the goal of helping the individual change his unwanted behavior. It differs from radical behavior therapy in that it rejects focus only on overt behavior for therapy. Instead, cognitive therapy emphasizes the importance of the individual's thoughts, feelings, imagery, attitudes, and hopes and their causative relationship to behaviors.

See also BEHAVIOR THERAPY; COGNITIVE BEHAVIOR THERAPY; DEPRESSION.

cohabitation Situation of unmarried individuals living together. This arrangement can lead to anxieties when one of the partners desires marriage and the other does not, or when after living together for a number of years, the couple decides to separate. As in a DIVORCE, there may be additional anxieties and stress when division of property, including real estate, and consequent legal arrangements occur.

There have been dramatic increases in cohabitation during the last decades of the 20th century. Greater approval and societal acceptance of living together without benefit of marriage has resulted from general attitudinal changes, including fears of permanent commitment, effectiveness of contraception during a long-term sexual relationship, and the havoc raised by divorce.

Many couples sign a cohabitation contract, which is intended to remove some of the stresses in the practicalities of the living together arrangement. The cohabitation contract is a legal document in which unmarried partners agree to specified arrangements, such as how much each partner pays toward specified expenses. It may also specify division of belongings, should the couple separate.

See also DIVORCE; LIVE-IN; MARRIAGE, FEAR OF.

cohort   A group of individuals gathered together for an epidemiologic study. For example, cohorts (groups) of phobics and individuals who have anxiety disorders are brought together for research purposes to test hypotheses regarding the cause of their disorder. In a cohort, the group or groups of persons to be studied are defined in terms of characteristics evident before the appearance of the disorder being investigated; for example, they may be individuals of the same sex, same age, or identical educational background who became agoraphobic during their mid-twenties. Individuals in a cohort may be observed over a period of time to determine various factors related to their disorder.

See also CASE-CONTROL; CROSS-SECTION; LONGITUDINAL STUDY.

cohort effect   A term used in cross-sectional and longitudinal studies in which group differences may be due to cohort grouping rather than effects of an independent variable. For example, differences in sexual behavior between twenty-year-olds and sixty-year olds would be due to differences in developmental and cultural experiences rather than age per se.

See also COHORT; LONGITUDINAL STUDY.

coitophobia   Fear of sexual intercourse, or coitus. Coitus means sexual intercourse through the vagina between male and female. In medicine, the words coitus, copulation, cohabitation, and sexual intercourse are used synonymously, although the words have somewhat different meanings in their original context. A wide variety of fears regarding sexual intercourse have been reported, including impotence, inability to achieve and maintain an erection, inability to ejaculate, intercourse without orgasm, coitus interruptus, rectal penetration, vaginal penetration, oral penetration, pain during intercourse, vaginismus or tightening of the vaginal muscles to impair penetration, and intercourse with animals. The best treatment for this is behavioral sex therapy, which involves a gradual desensitization of the fear response to sexual arousal and enhanced stimulation, relaxation, and sexual excitement.

See also COITUS MORE FERARUM; COITUS ORALIS; FEMALE GENITAL FEARS; PAIN; PREGNANCY; PSYCHOSEXUAL ANXIETIES; SEXUAL FEARS; SEXUAL INTERCOURSE.

coitus more ferarum, fear of   A term derived from the Latin words meaning sexual intercourse in the manner of wild beasts. Although the term is obsolete, the fear of the situation, and the anxieties produced by it, are not. The term applies to the act of heterosexual intercourse in the position usual in lower animals, with the male inserting the penis into the vagina from the rear, and usually with the female on hands and knees. When the penis is inserted into the rectum, the act is called anal intercourse. This latter practice is called pederasty when the partner is a boy. Although coitus more ferarum is not sodomy, it is often thought of as primitive. The axis of the vagina, in this position, is in direct correspondence with the axis of the penis in erection, which might indicate its primitive biological congruity.

See also SEXUAL FEARS; SEXUAL INTERCOURSE.

coitus oralis, fear of   Fear of sexual relations using the mouth. The term is now obsolete, but relates to fellatio, which involves inserting the penis into the partner's mouth. The act of the male using his mouth, lips, and tongue to stimulate the female's vaginal area is known as cunnilingus. Some individuals, whether heterosexual or homosexual, fear sexual relations involving the mouth.

See also SEXUAL FEARS; SEXUAL INTERCOURSE.

cold, fear of   Fear of cold or cold objects is known as cheimaphobia, cheimatophobia, cryophobia, frigophobia, and psychrophobia. Individuals who fear cold may fear being in a cold climate, being outdoors in winter, or not having enough heat indoors, and they may tend to dress too warmly for the circumstances. Such individuals may even avoid cold drinks and particularly ice in their beverages.

colic   The causes for colic are unknown, although there are reasons to believe that it is due to a spasm in the newborn baby's intestines. It appears around the third or fourth week of life and usually goes away on its own by the age of 12 weeks. Signs that the baby is experiencing colic are irritability, excessive screaming, and tightening of the body. Colic may be related to traumas at birth.

There are few solutions to the problem, and parents face the anxieties of trying to make the baby comfortable. Feeding, cuddling, or changing diapers doesn't seem to help. Because episodes of colic seem to be worse in the evenings, both parents and baby suffer from sleep deprivation.

Handling the Colicky Baby

Parental anxiety may make the infant even more irritable. Feeding the baby when he or she cries could worsen the situation by causing the stomach to bloat. Rhythmic, soothing activities, such as rocking the baby, carrying the baby in a front sling or pouch, or taking the baby for a ride in the car usually work best.

To avoid compounding the stress caused by the situation, new parents should try to avoid fatigue and exhaustion. They may find it helpful to sleep in shifts, one parent dealing with the baby while the other gets rest.

See also PARENTING.

collective unconscious   Ideas that are common to mankind in general. Carl Jung (1875–1961), Swiss psychiatrist and philosopher, introduced the term, believing that the collective unconscious is inherited and derived from the collective experience of the species. The collective unconscious transcends cultural differences and explains behavior observed in some individuals who have never been exposed to certain ideas. Certain fears, such as snakes and heights, may be part of the collective unconscious in western civilization.

colors, fear of   Fear of colors is known as chromophobia, chrematophobia, and chromatophobia. Some individuals fear specific colors; others have fears of any items that are not specifically black or white.

Studies have determined that colors have certain psychological and physical effects on the human body. Under certain circumstances, color can produce stress or induce relaxation. For example, red is the strongest and most stimulating of colors. It has been shown to increase hormonal activity and to raise blood pressure. Red stimulates creative thought and is a good mood elevator, but is not conducive to work. Orange shares many of the qualities of red, but it is considered more mellow and easy to live with.

Blue has the opposite effect of red. It lowers bodily functions and creates a restful atmosphere, although, if used too extensively, may have a depressing effect. Participants in psychological tests, when surrounded by blue, tend to underestimate time periods and the weight of objects. Purple, a combination of red and blue, has a neutral effect. When used in large amounts, for instance as a typeface, the eye does not focus on purple easily.

Having the characteristic of visibility, yellow is useful for road safety signs. Green and blue-green promote an atmosphere of relaxation, concentration, and meditation. Monotonous use of the same color has been found to be more disturbing than a variety of colors.

With age, attraction to colors and their stressful and soothing effects seem to change somewhat. Babies tend to be attracted to yellow, white, pink, and red. Older children are less attracted to yellow and tend to like colors in the order of red, blue, green, violet, orange, and yellow. With adults, blue tends to become a favorite color, possibly because of changes in the eye itself and the way it sees color.

Colors carry with them anxiety-producing psychological associations that are expressed in language. For example, we are "green with envy," "see red," and "have the blues." Certain clear shades of red, orange, and yellow are associated with food and are very appetizing, while tinting foods with blue, violet, or mixtures of colors has the adverse effect, making them unappetizing. Color aversion is usually the result of aversive conditioning.

Throughout history, mystical and healing properties have been ascribed to color. For example, the ancients associated colors with the houses of the zodiac and with the elements. They were highly important in the practice of magic. Some superstitious people believe that blue and green divert the power of the evil eye. Part of a religious symbolism and ritual, red, blue, purple, and white have been considered divine colors in Judaism, while green, the color of life and rebirth, is important in Christianity and Islam. In many cultures, surrounding a patient with red clothing, red furniture and coverings, and giving him red food and red medicine was thought to aid the healing process.

Color Blindness

Inability to recognize any colors or certain colors; usually a genetic defect located in the cones, small color-sensitive cells in the retina of the eye. Some individuals who are color blind may not be aware of their condition and experience anxieties when mistaking signs and symbols. They confuse color changes with dark and light shades, not understanding the nature of colors they have never seen. People who are color blind reduce the anxieties of the disability by training themselves to use other visual clues. For example, they learn shapes and sizes of safety signs and memorize vital information such as that the red traffic light is usually located above the green light.

Other disorders of the eye may result in temporary or permanent color blindness, including degeneration of the optic nerve due to neuritis or anemia, and infectious diseases such as syphilis or malaria. Malnutrition and ingestion of poisonous chemicals or drugs can also cause color blindness or a limited perception of colors. While cataracts and other eye diseases that result in opacities (nontransparent areas) of the lens and cornea will reduce color vision, when underlying diseases are relieved, color vision may improve.

See also RED, FEAR OF THE COLOR; WHITE, FEAR OF THE COLOR.

combat fatigue, battle fatigue, combat neurosis Anxieties occurring after the extreme stresses of war or battle. The term has been replaced in contemporary usage with POST-TRAUMATIC STRESS DISORDER (PTSD). Veterans of World War I were said to have "combat fatigue," while Vietnam veterans with the same symptoms are said to have PTSD.

See also ANXIETY DISORDERS; POST-TRAUMATIC STRESS DISORDER.

combined therapy A form of psychotherapy in which the individual is involved in both individual and group therapy with the same or different therapists. Combined therapy is often used to help agoraphobic individuals; the individual, their spouses and families in therapy.

See also FAMILY THERAPY.

comets, fear of Fear of comets is known as cometophobia. A comet is a celestial body, observed only in the part of its orbit that is relatively close to the sun. A comet is thought to consist chiefly of ammonia, methane, carbon dioxide, and water.

See also FLYING THINGS, FEAR OF; METEORS, FEAR OF.

commitment phobia A term introduced by Steve Carter and Julia Sokol in their book, *Men Who Can't Love: When a Man's Fear Makes Him Run from Commitment and What a Smart Woman Can Do About It* (New York: M. Evans and Company, 1987). The authors see the avoidance of commitment as a true phobia similar to claustrophobia, the fear of being trapped in a small enclosed place. Sustained closeness intensifies this fear since it creates conflict over priorities, work and leisure preferences, and relationships.

communication   Process through which meanings are exchanged between individuals. When individuals feel understood, they are communicating effectively: they are in control of events; other people trust and respect them; in work settings, they feel valued. Communicating effectively enhances health and self-esteem, nurtures relationships, and helps people cope with anxieties.

Failure to Communicate

When individuals do not communicate well, they feel misunderstood, frustrated, distressed, defensive, and often hostile, which increases their level of anxiety. Faults and flaws in communication habits, or communication gaps, cause stress to many people, those they love, and those with whom they interact on all levels, from the most intimate to the most distant of acquaintances. People who don't communicate effectively are more vulnerable to disease; they can be hostile and confrontational and are at increased risk for heart disease. People who feel misunderstood report more depression and more mood disorders of the kind shown to weaken their immune function. When communication breaks down, heart rate speeds up, cholesterol and blood sugar levels rise, susceptibility to headaches and digestive problems increases, and sensitivity to pain becomes more acute. In work settings, communication gaps can reduce produc-

tivity, make workers irritable, and even increase the risk of accidents.

Differences in Male-Female Communication Styles

According to Bee Reinthaler, a personnel communications specialist, in business, differences between communications styles of male and female managers can cause problems in efficiency and in accomplishing goals. Males in the corporate world often use a complex combination of business, sports, and military jargon. Their behavior is action-oriented and competitive. On the other hand, women generally are more demonstrative and express their feelings. Many women frame their speech with qualifiers, questions, and questioning intonations. They express doubts and uncertainties more frequently than men.

According to Reinthaler, when women wait for men to speak first, they create an image of incompetence. "Men may then fall into the stereotypical role of treating women as incompetent and the stereotypical interaction continues in a destructive way. It would be more effective if both genders of managers would 'speak the same' language."

"Many women attempt to crack the male communication code in the workplace until something happens that shows they have underestimated its complexities," says Candiss Rinker, an expert in the science and practice of change management. She

---

OVERCOMING ANXIETIES BY AVOIDING COMMUNICATION GAPS

- *Learn to cope with criticism.* Receiving criticism causes anxieties. The impact on our mood and body depends more on how we describe the negative feedback to ourselves. Ask yourself: Does this seem reasonable? Is it fact or opinion? Are there others who might confirm or dispute this view? How would others have behaved?

- *Learn to listen.* Listening is an active process requiring openness and receptivity. Keep your mind free of distracting reactions, responses, judgments, and questions and answers.

- *Observed your own body language.* Research shows that more than half of what we communicate is conveyed by BODY LANGUAGE. Smiling, frowning, sighing, touching, or drumming fingers give out strong messages. Women tend to smile more than men, nod their heads, and maintain more continuous eye contact while listening and speaking than men. Under stress or in new situations, this tendency becomes even more pronounced.

- *Recognize and respect differences in conversational styles.* Styles of conversing play a major role in triggering misunderstanding. For example, women tend to ask more personal questions than men. Men more often give opinions and make declarations of fact.

- *Become more assertive.* Speak and act from choice and stand up for your rights without being aggressive.

- *Learn to say no when you want to.* Avoid feeling resenful, frustrated, or guilty. Take time before you respond to a request. You need not give lengthy explanations for saying no.

explains that women have been socialized from childhood to avoid direct communication about difficult issues, so they often use a sugar-coated approach that other women understand but men do not.

Deborah Tannen, linguistics professor, says gender differences put women in a double bind at work that is not as evident in personal relationships. "Workplace communication norms were developed by men, for men, at a time when there were very few women present. The situation is aggravated when women hold positions of authority. If they talk in ways expected of women, they may not be respected; if they talk in ways expected of men, they may not be liked," says Tannen, author of *Talking from 9 to 5: How Women's and Men's Conversational Styles Affect Who Gets Heard, Who Gets Credit and What Gets Done at Work.*

Removing the Anxiety and Stress from Your Communication Style

Individuals should apply the old "golden rule" in communicating with others. They should speak the way in which they would like to be spoken to and listen to others the way they hope others will listen to them. It is important that they learn to express their likes and dislikes in a tactful and diplomatic way. They will find that when they are more direct, other people will be more responsive. With slight adaptations, these suggestions may be useful in communicating with children, siblings, parents, coworkers, bosses, or acquaintances and should be helpful in most situations.

See also ASSERTIVENESS TRAINING; BODY LANGUAGE; IMMUNE SYSTEM; RELATIONSHIPS; SELF-ESTEEM.

Kahn, Ada P., and Sheila Kimmel, *Empower Yourself: Every Woman's Guide to Self-Esteem* (New York: Avon Books, 1997).

Reardon, Kathleen Kelley, *They Don't Get It, Do They?: Communication in the Workplace—Closing the Gap Between Women and Men* (New York: Little, Brown, 1995).

Reinthaler, Bee, "Verbal Communications," *The Professional Communicator* (Fall 1991).

Tannen, Deb, *Talking from 9 to 5: How Women's and Men's Conversational Styles Affect Who Gets Heard, Who Gets Credit and What Gets Done at Work* (New York: William Morrow, 1994).

Tingley, Judith C., *Genderflex, Men and Women Speaking Each Other's Language at Work* (New York: Amacom, 1995).

commuter marriage   See MARRIAGE, FEAR OF.

compensation   A defense mechanism by which the individual, either consciously or unconsciously, tries to make up for an imagined or real deficiency, physical or psychological, or both. For example, a person with social phobias or feelings of incompetence may excel in music, art, or drama.

competition   One of the many dichotomies present in American life today that induces stress. It encourages individual achievement and the need to win. As such, it is the extreme opposite of another American concept—teamwork—which teaches us to respect others, appreciate their strengths and weaknesses, share our skills and knowledge, and help others meet their goals.

Early in life, children on the playing field experience the contradiction of competition and teamwork. Thus begins a source of stress we carry through much of our adulthood. Competition encourages comparisons between ourselves and others, both on a social and economic level; this in turn affects our feeling of self-esteem.

See also AUTONOMY; CONTROL; SELF-ESTEEM; TYPE A PATTERN.

complementary therapies   A set of practices that, depending on the viewpoint, either complement or compete with conventional medicine in the prevention and treatment of stress-related disorders as well as other diseases. Complementary therapies are often referred to as "alternative" therapies.

According to David Edelberg, M.D., writing in *The Internist* (September 1994), the terms *complementary* or *alternative therapies* commonly refer to anything that is not conventionally practiced or taught in medical school. In 1994, there were more than 200 fields of alternative medicine. Alternative fields can be divided into four broad categories: traditional medicine, such as Chinese or Native American; hands-on bodywork; psychological or psychospiritual medicine; and many holdovers from the 19th century, such as chiropractic and homeopathy.

Complementary therapies for dealing with anxieties and healing mind as well as body, include emotional release therapies with or without body manipulation, emotional control or self-regulating therapies, religious or inspirational therapies, cognitive-emotional therapies, and emotional expression through creative therapies. Some of these have been known by such names as encounter groups, gestalt therapy, primal therapy, EST, bioenergetic psychotherapy, ROLFING, TRANSCENDENTAL MEDITATION, and BIOFEEDBACK.

It is important to note that complementary therapies are not subject to scientific scrutiny through controlled efficacy studies with placebo or comparisons of treatments. They are accepted and promoted as helping on the basis of "anecdotal evidence" stemming from individual reports of success. Some may be truly helpful while others may be useless or ineffectual.

Many individuals find relief for anxiety-induced conditions from one or combinations of complementary therapies either along with or after seeking traditional care. For example, mental imagery is rated one of the six most commonly used alternative treatments among cancer patients and is believed by physicians as well as patients to reduce both the pain and distress of symptoms. However, as with other medical conditions, individuals should not overlook traditional psychiatric or medical treatments in favor of alternative therapies because they may be robbing themselves of valuable time as their condition progresses.

Complementary v. Conventional Care

Conventional medical practitioners adhere to scientific models and methodologies that many complementary medical practitioners believe focus too exclusively on reductionist and physiochemical explanations of biological phenomena. Proponents of alternative medicine suggest that this approach shows limited understanding of health and disease and, in particular, of interactions between mind-body connections, psychological, social and biological factors that influence coping with stress and disease processes.

Advocates of complementary approaches, in recent decades known also as "holistic" (or "wholistic") medicine, regard the influence of psychological factors and cognitive processes as equal to, if not more powerful than, the insights and methods of conventional medicine in coping with stress and disease and improving clinical outcomes.

For most of the 20th century, the generally accepted model for understanding biological phenomena and intervening therapeutically was the allopathic method. It achieved scientific, economic, and political primacy over the competing models, such as osteopathic medicine, homeopathy, and chiropractic, as well as other alternative approaches. However, the public's interest in complementary therapies has grown tremendously during the last two decades of the 20th century and the first decade of the 21st century.

In a survey conducted by Harvard Medical School, researchers reported that more than a quarter of the people they interviewed saw a physician regularly but were also employing another treatment, usually with their doctor's knowledge. One in ten respondents were relying on nontraditional treatments exclusively. The study emphasized the widespread acceptance of "alternative medicine," a variety of unrelated practices from acupuncture to yoga that are promoted as having healing benefits. The common factor between them is that they have not yet been subjected to scientific review, the process most of the Western world uses to determine whether a treatment is safe and effective.

A landmark study published in 1993 in the *New England Journal of Medicine* showed that far more people visited providers of complementary therapies—an estimated 425 million in 1990—than visited primary care physicians (388 million) during the same time period. The study, conducted by David Eisenberg and colleagues, found that one-third of Americans used alternative medical treatments. In addition, most of the expense for these visits, $10.3 billion, was out-of-pocket.

Herbal and "Folk" Therapies

In many cultures, herbs and other natural and botanical products are used to relieve anxiety-induced health conditions instead of modern diagnostic techniques and pharmacological treatments. Herbs are used both to cure specific illnesses, improve health, lengthen life, and increase sexual vigor and fertility.

Herbal medicine may have begun with the Greeks and spread across Europe with the Roman conquests. However, the development of an organized approach to using herbs took place in central Europe and the British Isles. Practices and beliefs in folk medicine are preserved in isolated, traditional cultures such as Appalachia and Native American tribes. Folk medical treatments have developed by trial and error, and serendipity without benefit of the scientific method. Since folk cultures generally mix religious or spiritual beliefs with concepts of health and illness, they attribute disease to causes other than to the natural causes recognized by conventional medicine. In folk beliefs, mental or physical illness may be caused by divine retribution for transgression or by the will of spirits or other magical beings. Folk healers pass down techniques from one generation to the next and may jealously guard their secrets.

Because of immigration to the Western world at the end of the 20th century, many practitioners of Western medicine are learning about folk medicine, so that they may better communicate with patients from other cultures.

Increasing Interest by Government and Insurers

In 1991 the Office of Alternative Medicine (OAM) was created within the National Institutes of Health. It was later renamed the National Center for Complementary and Alternative Medicine (NCCAM). The goal of the NCCAM is to research and evaluate many alternative or unconventional medical treatments.

Increasingly, some health insurers are paying for complementary therapies, removing some of the financial stress involved in seeking these treatments. A study reported in the *Journal of Health Care Marketing* (vol. 15, no. 1 [Spring 1995]) included insurers from government, third-party insurance companies, and HMOs; results indicated the mechanisms through which each of three complementary therapies (chiropractic, acupuncture, and biofeedback) gained some credibility and acceptance by insurers. Results indicated that these therapies have each achieved at least moderate success in obtaining third-party reimbursement.

Choosing Alternative Therapies

Individuals who decide to take an unproven therapy should let their physician know what they are doing. He or she will need to take the effects of that treatment into account when evaluating their care. Be wary when encountering claims that a treatment works miracles, such as rejuvenating skin or curing cancer with no pain or side effects. Watch out for contentions from proponents of a treatment that the medical community is trying to keep their "cure" a secret from the public. Also, be wary of any demands by the practitioner that a complementary treatment be substituted for a currently accepted practice. According to *Harvard Women's Health Watch* (June 1994), while there may be little harm in adding an alternative practice such as MEDITATION or massage therapy to a therapeutic regimen, replacing a valid treatment with one that has no proven efficacy may have serious consequences.

Watch out for claims that the treatment is better than approved remedies just because it is "natural." Natural products are not necessarily more benign than agents synthesized in a laboratory. A drug is any substance that alters the structure or function of the body, regardless of its source. It is important to remember that many plants contain toxic substances that can be harmful when taken in uncontrolled doses.

See also ACUPUNCTURE; AYURVEDA; BIOFEEDBACK; CHIROPRACTIC MEDICINE; CROSS-CULTURAL INFLUENCES; GUIDED IMAGERY; HOLISTIC MEDICINE; MEDITATION; MIND/BODY CONNECTIONS; MASSAGE THERAPY; RELAXATION.

Goldberg, Burton Group, eds., *Alternative Medicine: The Definitive Guide* (compiled by the Burton Group) (Puyallup, WA: Future Medicine Publishing, 1993).

Goleman, Daniel, and Joel Gurin, eds., *Mind Body Medicine: How to Use Your Mind For Better Health* (Yonkers, N.Y.: Consumer Reports Books, 1993).

Eisenberg, D., et al., "Unconventional medicine in the United States: prevalence, costs, and patterns of use. *New England Journal of Medicine* 1993, 328:246–252.

Facklam, Howard, *Alternative Medicine: Cures or Myths?* (New York: Twenty-First Century Books, 1996).

Morton, Mary, and Michael, *5 Steps to Selecting the Best Alternative Medicine* (Novato, Calif.: New World Library, 1996).

Weil, Andrew, *Eight Weeks to Optimum Health: Proven Program for Taking Full Advantage of Your Body's Healing Power* (New York: Knopf, 1997).

complex A group of connected conscious and unconscious ideas and feelings that affect an individual's behavior. The most well-known complex may be the Oedipus complex (or Electra complex in girls) as identified in Freudian psychoanalysis, and the superiority and inferiority complexes, as identified by Adler. The oedipus complex begins during the phallic stage of psychosexual development (approximately age three to five), in which the child experiences the conflict of sexual desire for the opposite-sex parent and sees the same-sex parent as a rival. This psychic conflict causes the child anxiety as he or she fears punishment (castration) from the same-sex parent and realizes the inability to fulfill his or her desires. To resolve this conflict, the child represses feelings for the opposite-sex parent and identifies increasingly with the parent of the same sex. This identification with the presumed "aggressor" is an anxiety-reducing mechanism and helps sexual roles and the superego develop.

Resolution of the Oedipus conflict (or the Electra conflict in girls) involves adoption and internalization of social mores and values, and the beginning of the SUPEREGO.

Other well-known complexes are the superiority complex and inferiority complex, which were named by Alfred Adler.

Bootzin, R., et al., *Psychology Today* (New York: Random House, 1983).
Davison, Gerald C., and John M. Neale, *Abnormal Psychology* (New York: Wiley, 1986).

compulsion Seemingly purposeful, repetitive behavior that an individual performs according to certain internal, idiosyncratic rules or in a stereotyped fashion. The behavior is not an end in itself but is designed to produce or prevent some future state of adverse affairs to which it may not be connected in a realistic way or for which it may be clearly excessive. The person performs the act with a sense of subjective compulsion coupled with a desire to resist it (at least initially). Performing the particular act is not pleasurable, although it may afford some relief of tension and this is definitely an impetus for performance of compulsive behavior. Often people dissociate when engaged in compulsive behaviors. An example is when a person feels compelled to wash his/her hands every time he/she shakes hands because of an excessive fear of contamination. Compulsions are characteristic of OBSESSIVE-COMPULSIVE DISORDER.

compulsive personality A personality type characterized by inability to relax, extreme inhibition, overconscientiousness, and rigidity. Many phobics have compulsive personalities; individuals who have obsessive-compulsive disorder also have compulsive personalities.

See also NEUROSIS; OBSESSIVE-COMPULSIVE DISORDER; PERSONALITY TYPE.

computers and anxiety Fear, distrust, or hatred of computers is known as *cyberphobia*. However, some experts, such as Mark Kenwright and Isaac Marks, M.D., have used computers to help individuals become desensitized from the things they fear, as discussed in the *British Journal of Psychiatry* in 2004.

In this study, experts used computer-aided help over the Internet with 10 patients with phobia and panic. (The study is small and larger studies should be performed in the future.) The patients improved significantly at a one-month follow-up, and their gains were clinically significant. Kenwright and his colleagues said the Internet users were generally satisfied, although three of them said they would have preferred face-to-face help. Said Kenwright et al., "Computer-aided self-exposure guidance using the internet [sic] at home, with brief advice from a clinician on a live helpline, may help some people with phobia or panic disorders to overcome barriers to treatment such as the scarcity of qualified therapists and having to travel to see the therapist in person."

Obviously those who are computer-phobic could not use the Internet to deal with their phobias.

Some individuals who are faced with the need to learn to use computers or to learn new programs on their computers will show symptoms of classic phobia, such as nausea, dizziness, cold sweat, and high blood pressure. Many computer phobics hide their fears because of heavy work and peer pressure to make efficient use of computers. Individuals who fear computers can overcome their phobia by gradually exposing themselves to electronic calculators, games, and eventually to simple computer programs. Coaching and feedback (from an expert) are good ways to improve the learning curve for mastering electronic devices.

See also CARPAL TUNNEL SYNDROME; TECHNOLOGY, FEAR OF.

Kenwright, Mark, Isaac M. Marks, Lina Gega, and David Mataix-Cols, "Computer-Aided Self-Help for Phobia/Panic via Internet at Home: A Pilot Study," *British Journal of Psychiatry* 184 (2004): pp. 448–449.

condensation   A psychological process often present in dreams in which two or more concepts are fused so that a single symbol represents many components. For example, one symbol may represent several phobic objects or situations. Or, a phobia itself may be symbolic of many situations.

conditioned response   A learned or acquired response to a stimulus that originally did not elicit the response. A conditioned response, also known as a conditioned reflex, is elicited by a conditioned stimulus. In classical conditioning theory, the conditioned response is brought about as a result of the pairing of a neutral and an unconditioned stimulus. For example, the salivation response that occurred in Pavlov's dogs following the ringing of a bell (conditioned stimulus) is a conditioned response.

See also BEHAVIOR MODIFICATION; CONDITIONED STIMULUS; CONDITIONING.

conditioned stimulus   A stimulus, or cue, that elicits a response as a result of learning or conditioning. In classical conditioning, the pairing of a neutral stimulus with an unconditioned stimulus produces a conditioned stimulus. The conditioned stimulus is capable of producing approximately the same response as

that of the unconditioned stimulus. For example, a child who fears loud noises could be conditioned to transfer that fear to a white rat. The white rat is the conditioned stimulus; after several exposures of the pairing of the noise and the rat, the fear associated with the loud noise is transferred to the rat.

See also BEHAVIOR THERAPY; CONDITIONED RESPONSE; CONDITIONING.

conditioning   Procedures to change behavior patterns. Conditioning techniques are used in therapy for phobias and anxieties. There are three main types of conditioning: classical, operant, and modelling. In classical or Pavlovian conditioning, two stimuli are combined: one adequate, such as offering food to a dog to produce salivation (an unconditioned response), and the other inadequate, such as ringing a bell, which by itself does not have an effect on salivation. After the two stimuli have been paired several times, the inadequate or conditioned stimulus comes to elicit salivation (now a conditioned response) by itself. In operant conditioning, consequences are introduced that strengthen or increase the rate or intensity of the desired activity (reinforcement) or weaken or decrease the rate or intensity of the undesired activity (punishment). Partially reinforcing or punishing the activity will increase its resistance to extinction. Unlike classical and operant conditioning that require repeated trials for new learning or behavior, modelling results in behavior acquisition by observation. Subsequent performance of the new behavior may rely on operant reinforcement and the past history of the observer.

See also BEHAVIOR MODIFICATION; CONDITIONING.

conditioning therapy   A term sometimes used for BEHAVIOR THERAPY.

See also CONDITIONED RESPONSE; CONDITIONED STIMULUS; CONDITIONING.

condom   A cylindrical sheath of rubber or synthetic material that is placed on the penis prior to sexual intercourse so that it will capture the seminal fluid and thus prevent a pregnancy. If there is a tiny tear in the condom or semen is deposited near the vaginal tract, fertilization can occur. Most individuals use condoms out of fear of causing a pregnancy and/or acquiring a sexually transmitted disease. However, some couples say that a condom interferes with their enjoyment of sexual intercourse, although many new types of condoms have been developed in recent years to enhance sexual pleasure.

Some women carry condoms in their purse in case their partner forgets to purchase them. In some cases, a man refuses to use a condom and insists on having sex without protection. This is not a good idea unless there is evidence of no sexually transmitted diseases (STDs) in either partner.

In the 1980s and 1990s, with the escalating prevalence of ACQUIRED IMMUNODEFICIENCY SYNDROME (AIDS) and the fear that surrounded it, condoms were promoted by the government and many physicians as a SAFE SEX measure and a means of reducing the risk of the spread of AIDS and SEXUALLY TRANSMITTED DISEASES (STDs). Because treatment has been developed for individuals who are infected with the human immunodeficiency virus (HIV) that leads to AIDS, as well as for individuals with AIDS, some experts believe that the fear of contagion has subsided significantly, and perhaps too much. There is still no cure for AIDS, but the "cocktail," or mixture of various viral-inhibiting drugs, has proven successful in retarding its intensity and spread.

The condom should be placed on the penis before any sexual contact occurs and should be properly removed and discarded after ejaculation. If correctly used, condoms are more effective than other forms of birth control, with the exception of the birth control pill. However, if the male scrotum is infected, condoms are not always effective in preventing the spread of some sexually transmitted diseases.

Advantages of a condom as a contraceptive include the relatively low cost, the availability without a physical examination or prescription, and some protection against STDs. Disadvantages are the inconvenience, the perceived lack of feeling that occurs with direct contact, and the care with which condoms must be used.

The condom may have been invented by Dr. Condom, a physician in the court of Charles II of England (1650–85). However, the first published report of the use of a condom to prevent sexually transmitted disease was included in the work of the Italian anatomist Fallopius in 1564.

confinement, fear of Fear of confinement, or of being in a closed space, is known as CLAUSTROPHOBIA.

See also AGORAPHOBIA; BARBER'S CHAIR SYNDROME; ELEVATORS, FEAR OF; FLYING, FEAR OF.

conflict resolution A means by which disagreements between parties to a conflict are resolved. The anxiety caused by anger and confrontation are minimized, and those participating are able to be heard and to express their position and their needs.

TECHNIQUES TO AVOID ANXIETIES IN CONFLICT RESOLUTION

- Think before speaking.
- Say what you mean and mean what you say.
- Listen carefully to the other person.
- Do not put words in the other person's mouth.
- Stick to the problem at hand.
- Refrain from fault-finding.
- Apply the same rules to handling personal and business conflicts.

See also COMMUNICATION.

Kahn, Ada P., *The Encyclopedia of Stress and Stress-related Disorders*, 2nd ed. (New York: Facts On File, 2006).

confrontation A therapeutic technique that requires the individual to face his own attitudes and perceived shortcomings, such as anxieties and phobias. It encourages the individual to face the way he or she is perceived by others and the possible consequences of his or her behavior. The therapist may offer feedback, make interpretations, or attack the individual's defense mechanisms. Confrontation as a technique is used in psychoanalytic therapy, Adlerian therapy, group therapy, existential psychotherapy, encounter groups, and other therapies.

See also ENCOUNTER GROUPS; EXISTENTIAL THERAPY.

congestive heart failure   The end result of many different types of heart disease where the heart cannot pump blood out normally. This results in congestion (water and salt retention) in the lungs, swelling in the extremities, and reduced blood flow to body tissues. Living with congestive heart failure is a very anxiety-producing situation for the sufferer as well as those around him or her. Medical treatment can improve the quality of life for many of these patients.

See also CHOLESTEROL, FEAR OF; CHRONIC ILLNESS; CORONARY ARTERY DISEASE; HEART ATTACK, FEAR OF; HIGH BLOOD PRESSURE, FEAR OF.

conjoint therapy   A type of marriage therapy. Also called triadic or triangular, as two individuals and one therapist work together. The therapist sees the partners together in joint sessions; conjoint therapy may be helpful when one spouse has AGORAPHOBIA.

conscience   Synonymous with SUPEREGO. The part of the individual that judges one's own values and performance. Conscience plays a role in self-esteem, self-image, and development of some SOCIAL PHOBIAS. Conscience may involve negative evaluations (such as guilt and shame) or positive evaluations (pride, self-pleasure) of behavior.

See also SELF-ESTEEM.

conscious   The part of the mind that is immediately aware of the environment at any time. The conscious is differentiated from the preconscious and the UNCONSCIOUS. Their divisions can best be viewed as degrees of availability of cognitive and emotional material. An individual's functions of reality testing, perception, observation, and evaluation are all conscious activities. Expansion of con-sciousness is a term and training that is associated with 20th-century psychology and spirituality.

See also EGO.

consensual validation   Ongoing comparison of the thoughts and feelings of members of a group toward one another; the process tends to modify and correct distortions of interpersonal relationships and to alleviate social fears and ANXIETIES. The term was introduced by Harry Stack Sullivan, an American psychiatrist (1892–1949), to refer to the therapeutic process between therapist and patient. Previously, Trigant Burrow, an American psycho-analyst (1875–1951), used the term "consensual observations" to describe this process, which results in effective reality testing.

constipation, fear of   Fear of constipation is known as coprastasophobia. Constipation is difficult, incomplete, or infrequent evacuation of the bowels. Some individuals fear constipation if they do not have one or more bowel movement every day. Some who become obsessed with the notion that this is necessary resort to taking laxatives regularly, which leads to a dependence on laxatives for complete evacuation. Fear of constipation may be related to a fear of painful bowel movements (defecalgesiophobia).

See also GASTROINTESTINAL SYMPTOMS; IRRITABLE BOWEL SYNDROME.

contamination, fear of   Fear of contamination is known as misophobia, mysophobia, and molysomophobia. Contamination is a state of being impure or being in contact with unclean or disease-producing substances. Those who fear germs or contracting a disease by touching something also usually fear contamination. Individuals who have OBSESSIVE-COMPULSIVE DISORDER, with frequent hand-washing as a symptom, often fear contamination and thus wash their hands frequently. Contamination obsessions include disease, dirt, germs, mud, excrement, and sputum. It may extend to animals and objects regarded by some as unclean, such as chickens, rats, mice, and insects.

In psychiatry, the term "contamination" also applies to the combining of a part of one word with a part of another, usually resulting in a word that is unintelligible.

content, latent   See LATENT CONTENT.

contextual family therapy   See TRANSGENERATIONAL FAMILY THERAPY.

contextual therapy   A form of BEHAVIOR THERAPY. Contextual therapy is also known as *in vivo* therapy, because it takes place in real life, as opposed to in the imagination. After a phobic individual has been through a series of sessions in the therapist's office during which he vividly imagines himself facing a feared situation, he actually ventures out to face the situation itself. Sometimes the therapist or a trained assistant accompanies the phobic individual. In some cases of AGORAPHOBIA, the agoraphobic's spouse is trained to accompany and assist the individual in facing the feared situation. The individual is trained to focus on his "phenomenology" or direct experience in the moment. The task of the therapist is to help direct attention to the ongoing internal and external context in which anxiety occurs. Contextual therapy was developed by American psychiatrist Manuel Zane (1913–   ).

contingency management   The therapist's process of changing an individual's possible responses by control (introducing or removing consequences to a behavior) in order to change the rate of intensity of the behavior. For example, by their very nature, anxiety responses are usually aversive to the individual (that is, the individual will work to reduce or eliminate them). Avoidance of anxiety-arousing stimuli becomes a behavior that is reinforced by the ensuing diminishment of anxiety, thus making it very difficult to modify. Behavior therapists using exposure therapies will introduce the phobic individual to anxiety-arousing stimuli in small doses that do not stimulate a lot of anxiety. In this way,

approaching (rather than avoiding) the stimulus becomes reinforced.

See also BEHAVIOR THERAPY; OPERANT CONDITIONING; REINFORCEMENT.

contraception   See BIRTH CONTROL.

contreltophobia   Fear of sexual abuse, or of being touched or fondled by another person, usually involving genital stimulation. The term is derived from the Latin word "contrectare," which means "to handle" or "to take hold of."

See also CHILD ABUSE; SEXUAL ABUSE.

control   A means of directing the course of everyday events. While life is going well, most people do not consciously think about their level of control. However, when that sense of control is threatened, they become anxious, leading to ANGER and FRUSTRATION. Lack of control and lack of predictability almost always induce anxieties.

Loss of control causes people who could help themselves no to do so. They may lose motivation as a result of previous failures or may be experiencing what psychologist Martin Seligman called LEARNED HELPLESSNESS. They feel that whatever they do will not make any difference. Their learned response is to not try to gain control over their lives. But they continue to feel the stress of the anger, frustration, and hostility, which may lead to physical problems.

The anxieties some people face on the job is caused by lack of control over the pace of work, the work environment, or decision making. People living in institutions or in other such controlled environments are frustrated because they cannot change their situation and feel that things are being done to them or for them. An example is patients in hospitals who feel that their sense of control and autonomy has been taken away from them by the hospital routine. Other people do not recognize their own options for making decisions and feel trapped by invisible forces. People who always try to please others in an effort to gain validation and self-esteem are an example of this. Some who fear flying do so because they feel totally out of control in the hands of the pilot.

Although individuals cannot always control events occurring around them, they can learn healthier responses to stressful situations. RELAXATION, BREATHING, or BIOFEEDBACK techniques can help a person gain a feeling of control.

control group   The group in which a condition or factor being tested is deliberately omitted during an experiment. For example, in a study of the effects of a new drug on ANXIETY, the control group may be given a PLACEBO instead of the new drug.

conversational catharsis   See CATHARSIS.

conversion   The term conversion applies to an unconscious mental conflict that the individual converts into a physical symptom; the physical symptom may represent a disguised drive gratification or wish fullfillment, or both. Freud said that conversion neuroses are "conversion hysteria" and "pregenital conversion neuroses," and that fixations on the later or early anal stages may lie at the root of these illnesses.

A conversion symptom is a loss or alteration of physical functioning that suggests a physical disorder but that is actually a direct expression of an unconscious psychological need or conflict. Such a disturbance is not under voluntary control and, after examination, cannot be explained by any physical disorder. Conversion symptoms, seen in conversion disorder, are relatively rare in their true form. However, as common knowledge about medical conditions improves, conversion symptoms have become more sophisticated. The tendency to develop conversion symptoms is related to stress, past medical history, and observation or personal experience with the particular symptom and a reinforcement in the current environment either through stress reduction, social status, or attention.

See HYSTERIA; NEUROSES; SCHIZOPHRENIA.

coping   The psychological as well as practical solutions that people must find for anxiety-producing, as well as everyday, situations. Examples of these situations are dealing with cancer, caring for an aging relative, readjusting after the death of a loved one, facing unemployment, and dealing with RANDOM NUISANCES. Different individuals develop different ways of coping and learn to adapt their responses and reduce their stress and anxieties.

Stone and Porter, writing in *Mind/Body Medicine* (March 1995), defined coping as "constantly changing cognitive and behavioral efforts to manage specific external and/or internal demands that are appraised as taxing or exceeding the resources of the person."

To some, "coping" means getting on with life and letting things happen as they may. To others, it is consciously using the skills they have learned in the past when facing problem situations. Coping can mean anticipating situations, or it can mean meeting problem situations head on. For example, some managers who are able to handle employees in everyday situations become nervous and jittery anticipating giving a public speech. In a serious medical crisis, some people cannot cope with their own illness but manage to muster strength when they need to care for a loved one.

Individuals can learn new coping skills from psychotherapists as well as those who practice alternative or COMPLEMENTARY THERAPIES such as meditation and RELAXATION training. Relaxation and deep BREATHING techniques can help overcome the stress involved in a difficult situation.

Better Coping for Better Health

When Hans Selye (1907–82), an Austrian-born Canadian endocrinologist and psychologist, wrote his landmark book *The Stress of Life*, he described the GENERAL ADAPTATION SYNDROME. The secret of health, he said, was in successful adjustment to ever-changing conditions.

Research studies have shown that people who cope well with life's stresses are healthier than those who have maladaptive coping mechanisms. In his book *Adaptation to Life*, George Valliant, a Harvard psychologist, summarized some insights about relationships between good coping skills and health. He found that individuals who typically handle the trials and pressures of life in an immature way also tend to become ill four times as often as those who cope well.

Stone and Porter reported that coping efforts may have direct effects upon symptom perception and may have indirect effects on physiological changes and disease processes as well as mood changes, compliance with physician's instructions, and physician-patient communication.

Selye, Hans, *The Stress of Life* (New York: McGraw Hill Book Co., 1956).

———, *Stress Without Distress* (Philadelphia, J.B. Lippincott Company, 1974).

coping behavior Any ADAPTATION that reduces ANXIETY in a stressful situation. Individuals who have anxieties and PHOBIAS can learn new coping behaviors to keep their fears under control. Coping behaviors are also known as COPING MECHANISMS. Coping behaviors include taking a detour to avoid crossing a BRIDGE or ordering groceries by telephone to avoid going out. Some coping behaviors are unproductive, such as REGRESSION, in which the individual resorts to behaviors learned at an earlier developmental stage, or the adoption of the SICK ROLE, which has as its aim the unconscious wish to avoid a situation, or denial, the mental process through which the individual tries to make the anxiety-producing situation disappear. Coping behavior also includes problem solving, choice of alternative methods of coping, selection of one of them, and taking appropriate steps to put it into effect.

See also BEHAVIOR THERAPY; COPING SKILLS INTERVENTION.

coping mechanism See COPING BEHAVIOR; COPING SKILLS INTERVENTION.

coping skills intervention Techniques that a therapist uses to help an individual develop coping behaviors that can be useful in a variety of anxiety-producing situations. Coping skills intervention focuses on ways to teach the individual to face stress rather than reduce or avoid it. The procedures include covert modeling, a modified form of systematic desensitization in which the individual is taught to cope with, rather than avoid, anxiety-producing imagery, relaxation training, anxiety management training, and stress inoculation.

See also ANXIETY MANAGEMENT TRAINING; BEHAVIOR THERAPY; COPING BEHAVIOR; COPING MECHANISMS; COVERT MODELING; STRESS INOCULATION; SYSTEMATIC DESENSITIZATION.

coprophobia Fear or revulsion of feces or dirt. Also known as scatophobia and koprophobia. This phobia is interpreted psychoanalytically as a defense against anal erotism, or coprophilia.

See also CONSTIPATION, FEAR OF; DEFECATION, DIRT, FEAR OF; FECES, FEAR OF.

corners, fear of Some individuals fear sitting in the corner of a room or fear bumping into corners. Those who fear sitting in corners may be fearful of CONFINEMENT or of being in an enclosed space with no easy exit. Some who have AGORAPHOBIA or CLAUSTROPHOBIA may feel this way. Some who fear injury or ILLNESS may fear bruising themselves with furniture or counters that have corners. Some parents are very fearful when their infants and young children get too close to sharp corners.

See also CLOSED PLACES; ILLNESS/INJURY, FEAR OF.

coronary artery bypass anxiety, postoperative Many people are likely to experience anxiety or DEPRESSION following a coronary artery bypass operation. This type of anxiety is now fairly common, as about 427,000 such operations were performed in the United States in 2004 according to the National Center for Health Statistics. An anxiety reaction can bring about serious variations in heartbeat (arrhythmia). Antianxiety drugs that do not adversely affect a postoperative heart patient are often helpful. ALPRAZOLAM (Xanax) is one such antianxiety drug.

Desensitization procedures are often helpful in alleviating this form of conditioned anxiety.

See also HEART ATTACK, ANXIETY FOLLOWING.

coronary artery disease Caused by atherosclerosis, hardening of the arteries that supply blood and oxygen to the heart. The disease is an anxiety to the sufferer as well as those who are caregivers. It is preventable to a great extent by lifestyle modifications and dietary changes.

See also ATHEROSCLEROSIS; CHOLESTEROL, FEAR OF; CONGESTIVE HEART FAILURE; HEART ATTACK, FEAR OF; HIGH BLOOD PRESSURE, FEAR OF; TYPE OF BEHAVIOR PATTERN.

coronary-prone Type A behavior   Coronary-prone type A behavior is characterized by generally aggressive, driven, and competitive behavior. Type A individuals are usually racing against the clock and have little time for relaxation. Type B behavior, on the other hand, is characterized by more easygoing, generally less aggressive behavior. Most individuals are not simply Type A or Type B, but are a combination of both. People exhibiting predominantly Type A behavior are statistically more prone to develop coronary heart disease and suffer heart attacks. The critical element appears to be anger and poor management of anger. Behavior modification can be successful in shifting an individual closer to the Type B end of the continuum. There is some suggestion that there are at least two types of Type A behavior patterns, one with and one without the aggressive component.

See also HEART ATTACK.

corpses, fear of   Fear of corpses, or dead human bodies, or bodies of animals, is known as necrophobia. This fear extends to looking at cadavers and carcasses of animals. Fear of corpses may be related to a fear of death, and many individuals who fear viewing a corpse also fear going into a cemetery, looking at tombstones, or even attending a funeral.

See also CEMETERIES, FEAR OF; DEATH, FEAR OF.

corrective emotional experience   Reexposure to a previously difficult emotional situation under favorable circumstances. Considered a technique of short-term psychotherapy, it may be useful in helping phobic individuals. Corrective emotional experience was advocated by Hungarian-American psychoanalyst Franz Alexander (1891–1964), who suggested that the therapist temporarily assume a particular role to generate the experience for the individual and facilitate insight and change.

See also BRIEF PSYCHOTHERAPY.

correlation   Correlation is the extent to which two measures vary, or a measure of the strength of the relationship between two variables, such as the treatment of phobias with certain techniques of behavior therapy and the age of the individual. Correlation is expressed by a coefficient that varies between ×1.0, indicating perfect agreement, and -1.0, indicating a perfect inverse relationship. A correlation coefficient of 0.0 would mean a perfectly random relationship. The correlation coefficient signifies the degree to which knowledge of one score of a variable can predict the score on the other variable. Such results are useful to researchers and therapists in planning treatment for phobic individuals. However, a high correlation between two variables does not necessarily indicate a causal relationship between them; the correlation may occur because each of the variables is highly related to a third unmeasured factor. For example, there is a correlation between sex and age of a person and onset of anxiety. However, is it unknown from a correlation if these are causative factors.

cortisol   A hormonelike secretion (a corticoid) from the adrenal cortex, which responds to STRESS. Cortisol is sometimes referred to as a biochemical marker of distress.

See also AUTONOMIC NERVOUS SYSTEM.

cosmetic surgery   Procedures performed by plastic and reconstructive surgeons to improve a patient's appearance. Many people undergo cosmetic surgery to overcome negative feelings about parts of their face or bodies that lead to anxiety, particularly social and performance anxieties. Some individuals who have DYSMORPHOPHOBIA, or a fear of a specific defect that is not noticeable to others, may seek cosmetic surgery. Others with feelings of low SELF-ESTEEM may view cosmetic surgery as a way to like themselves better. Some individuals expect, unrealistically, that all their problems will be resolved once a cosmetic defect is corrected, and they are disturbed after recovery from surgery to discover that they still have problems, although not related to the cosmetic issue.

In a society that worships youth and beauty, older and middle-aged adults are waging their battle against wrinkles and other signs of aging. In addition, some younger women with small breasts have procedures to enlarge their breasts. Both men and women have rhinoplasty, a surgery to improve the appearance of the nose. These are part of a broad array of procedures performed by cosmetic surgeons.

According to Dr. Gwinnell and Christine Adamec in their book, *The Encyclopedia of Addictions and Addictive Disorders,* some individuals have repeated and unnecessary cosmetic procedures and are addicted to cosmetic surgery. "The patient feels compelled to have surgery to correct real or imagined imperfections. However, once the procedure occurs and if the supposed defect is corrected, the patient finds yet another problem to obsess about and subsequently desires correction of this newfound defect through cosmetic surgery. Both women and men may have this problem, although it is more commonly noted in women."

Choosing a Cosmetic Surgeon

The consumer considering cosmetic surgery can alleviate some of the anxiety of the situation by following a few guidelines. First, it is important to identify a physician who has a great deal of experience in performing the procedure, and this surgeon should be certified by the American Board of Plastic Surgery. This certification means that the surgeon has had at least five years of surgical training after medical school, including a minimum two-year plastic surgery residency.

Next, a personal meeting with the physician is essential. Also, whenever possible, talk with other patients on whom the doctor has operated. Because of patient privacy issues, the doctor cannot release the names of others without their permission, but some individuals may offer such permission and be willing to talk to prospective patients.

See also BODY IMAGE, FEAR OF.

Gwinnell, Esther, M.D., and Christine Adamec, *The Encyclopedia of Addictions and Addictive Disorders.* (New York: Facts On File, Inc., 2005).

co-therapy A form of PSYCHOTHERAPY in which more than one therapist works with a phobic or anxious individual or a group. Co-therapy is also known as combined therapy, cooperative therapy, dual leadership, multiple therapy, and three-cornered therapy.

coulrophobia Fear of clowns.

counseling Professional services available to individuals seeking help in some area of their life, such as with concerns about anxiety. These services may range from those of a trained social worker to a psychiatrist. Individuals, couples, and families can find counseling services appropriate to them. They may be provided through a school, the workplace, a hospital or clinic, or a community center.

To seek counseling, call a local hospital or look in the yellow pages of the telephone directory under "psychologists" or "psychiatrists." Some listings have the heading "counselors." There are also many community self-help and support groups in which members share their experiences. For participants in these groups, sharing means they are not alone with their problems, and they learn from one another to problem-solve.

Before beginning therapy with any counselor, ask what his or her credentials are and whether he or she is certified by any state agency or professional board. As with any professional, one may meet an individual's needs better than another. Individuals should not be afraid to change counselors if they feel their needs are not being met. Generally, "counselors" have less training than social workers, psychologists, or psychiatrists. The term *counseling* refers to methods for dealing with adjustment problems rather than serious mental health concerns.

See also BEHAVIOR THERAPY; MARITAL THERAPY; PSYCHOTHERAPY; SUPPORT GROUPS.

counterconditioning   Relearning by reacting with a new RESPONSE to a particular STIMULUS. Counterconditioning is achieved by strengthening a response that is antagonistic to or incompatible with an undesirable response, such as a phobic reaction. It is commonly believed that relaxation acts as counterconditioning to ANXIETY, assertiveness to SHYNESS and inhibition, sexual arousal to impotence, etc. The counterconditioning view has been an alternative explanation for Wolpe's "reciprocal inhibition" theory.

See also BEHAVIOR THERAPY; DESENSITIZATION; RECIPROCAL INHIBITION.

counterphobia   A preference by the phobic individual for the fearful situation.

See also FEARS; PHOBIAS.

countertransference   An emotional response by the therapist to an individual under treatment. Such a relationship may reinforce the phobic or anxious individual's earlier traumatic history.

See also PSYCHOANALYSIS; TRANSFERENCE.

covert rehearsal   A visualization technique in which an individual in therapy is asked to imagine him- or herself effectively doing a task that produces or alleviates anxiety. Often this rehearsal is done in hierarchical fashion so as not to desensitize the client. The individual may repeat the visualization many times and consider different alternatives. This procedure often follows covert modeling, in which the individual imagines or observes another person successfully performing a particular behavior or action. The goal of covert rehearsal is to motivate the individual to believe that he or she can face the situation or do the task with a reduced level of anxiety.

See also BEHAVIOR THERAPY; MODELING; PSYCHOTHERAPY.

covert sensitization   A form of AVERSION THERAPY in which the individual is asked to imagine a situation or object (to which they are attracted) at the same time as he or she calls up unpleasant feelings by imagination. This fear induction procedure or fear aversive conditioning is used for treatment of addictions. This is an internal mental process, and thus referred to as "covert."

See also BEHAVIOR THERAPY; COVERT MODELING.

creativity   Unusual association of ideas or words and ingenious methods of problem solving. It may involve using everyday objects or processes in original ways or it may involve using an imaginative skill to bring about new thoughts and ideas. Some creative ideas are ahead of their time and may never be appreciated or not appreciated until after their creator's death. Those creative people may experience feelings of inadequacy and lack of SELF-ESTEEM. On the other hand, there are those who overestimate their creativity and experience anxieties from feeling undervalued and underappreciated.

Creativity and Careers

While creativity is strongly associated with the arts, it is equally important in such fields as science, business, or manufacturing. People who try to be creative and cannot, feel anxious. This is particularly true of those whose job depends on their creativity.

The Creative Process

Biographers and researchers of creative individuals have identified certain stages in the creative process. Often the scientist or artist identifies an area of work or a project but, after approaching it, feels dissatisfied and returns to less creative endeavors. Suddenly during this incubation period, a solution or artistic concept emerges. It then must be fleshed out, elaborated, or tested.

Creativity has been found to correlate with certain personality and intellectual characteristics. Although intelligence and creativity are thought to be separate mental gifts and not all intelligent people are creative, intelligence does seem to be necessary for creativity. Creative people have been found to be leaders and independent thinkers. They are self-assured, unconventional, and have a wide range of interests. Since they are frequently involved in their own thoughts and inner life, they tend to be introverted and uninterested in social life or group activities. Passion for their field of work and a sense that what they do will eventually be recognized and make a difference are also qualities that support creativity.

The Creativity Theory

Many behaviorists have adopted the position that there is no such thing as a creative act, that what appears to be new is, in fact "old wine in new bottles," or arrived at by luck and random experimentation. For example, Shakespeare created dramatic masterpieces without using original plots. Others have come up with the theory that a necessary element of creativity is its relation to reality. A work of art may be original but not truly creative unless it relates somehow to the experiences, feelings, or thoughts, even though previously undefined, of the observer.

Mental health professionals have been interested in creativity for years. For example, J. P. Guilford (1897–1987), who explored this area in the 1960s, described two areas of thinking: convergent or narrow, focused thinking and divergent thinking, which allows the individual to let his mind roam and explore a broad spectrum of ideas. Guilford felt that the latter type of thinking was most creatively productive. Stimulating and increasing creativity has also interested researchers. It has been found that people's creativity may increase or decrease according to their environment and work habits. For example, certain people can be more or less productive at work according to the atmosphere, the time of day, and even the clothing they wear.

Benson, P. G., "Creativity Measures," in Corsini, Raymond J., ed., *Encyclopedia of Psychology.* Vol. 1 (New York: John Wiley, 1984, p. 307).

Kahn, Ada P., and Jan Fawcett, *The Encyclopedia of Mental Health.* (New York: Facts On File, 1993).

Weisberg, Robert, *Creativity, Genius and Other Myths.* (New York: W. H. Freeman and Company, 1986).

cremnophobia   Fear of precipices or cliffs.
See also CLIFFS, FEAR OF; PRECIPICES, FEAR OF.

crime, fear of   Fear of crime has become a fact of life, particularly in urban areas. Crime is feared much more now than it was a generation ago, and fear of crime is one of the most frequent fears of children.

Kadish, Sanford H., et al., *Encyclopedia of Crime and Justice* (New York: The Free Press, 1983).

Pasternak, Stefan, *Violence and Victims* (New York: Spectrum, 1978).

crisis   A turning point for better or worse in an acute disease or mental illness, or an emotionally significant event or radical change in status in a person's life. The anxiety involved in a crisis situation may result from a combination of the individual's perception of an event as well as his or her ability or inability to cope with it. Some people will cope with a crisis situation better than others.

Crisis Intervention

Crisis intervention is often necessary to provide immediate help, advice, or therapy to individuals with acute stress or psychological or medical problems. Many crisis intervention centers utilize telephone counseling. For example, in cities throughout the United States, there is a suicide hot line for those contemplating ending their lives. In some cases, a rape victim's first step toward seeking professional assistance is to call a rape crisis hot line. When a bombing or shooting occurs in a public place, crisis intervention services are provided for survivors who witnessed the event in an effort to prevent the onset of or ameliorate POST-TRAUMATIC STRESS DISORDER.

The goal of crisis intervention is to restore the individual's equilibrium to the same level of functioning as before the crisis, or to improve it. Many different types of therapists and self-help groups provide crisis intervention. Therapy may include talking to the anxious individual and appropriate family members or short-term use of appropriate prescription medications. However, crisis intervention is not a substitute for longer term therapy. The individual may learn to immediately modify certain environmental factors as well as interpersonal aspects of the situation causing the crisis. Emphasis should be on reducing anxiety and fears, promoting self-reliance, and learning to focus on the present.

Longer term therapy is helpful after the individual has regained some degree of composure and coping skills.

See also COPING; CRIME, FEAR OF; GENERAL ADAPTATION SYNDROME; RAPE, FEAR OF; SELF-HELP, SUICIDE; SUPPORT GROUPS.

criticism, fear of   Many social phobics fear criticism and scrutiny by others. Some fear being criticized for the way they look, talk, act, or eat. They feel that they may be criticized because their hands tremble as they hold their fork or cup. Some may experience this fear most intensely in a crowded restaurant, and some fear even their spouse's criticism of their eating habits and thus cannot eat in front of their spouse. Some fear shaking, BLUSHING, SWEATING, or looking ridiculous on a bus or train. Some fear leaving home during the daylight because they might be seen by others and criticized. Some avoid talking to superiors. Others avoid performing or speaking in public. Some fear criticism of their body shape and avoid swimming so that others will not see their bodies. Those who fear criticism of handwriting may do all their banking by mail. Individuals who fear criticism usually have a low sense of self-esteem.

Fear of being criticized makes many individuals reluctant to do or try certain activities. For example, when children receive negative criticism regarding singing ability from a teacher, they may carry this message for the rest of their lives. Self-criticism can be just as harsh. After judging themselves as failures at public speaking, some adults will not try it again. Often, criticism can produce anxiety for the critic as well. In employment settings, for example, there are supervisors who find it difficult to criticize employees.

An ability to accept criticism that is appropriate and then alter behavior associated with that criticism is considered self-improvement. Children thrive on encouragement, even when it is tinged with criticism, particularly when they receive it from a parent or teacher. On the other hand, some people take criticism very badly and the experience results in anxiety, defensiveness, or feelings of helplessness and low self-worth. Constant criticism can lead to an INFERIORITY COMPLEX, charac-

terized by feelings of inadequacy in most social situations.

Constructive criticism should genuinely explain and define what is desirable as well as what is not. Focusing criticism on the task or skill rather than on the person is useful.

See also ANXIETY DISORDERS; INFERIORITY COMPLEX; PHOBIAS, HISTORY OF; SELF-ESTEEM; SOCIAL PHOBIA.

Kahn, Ada P., and Sheila Kimmel, *Empower Yourself: Every Woman's Guide to Self-Esteem* (New York: Avon Books, 1997).

cross-cultural influences   Beliefs and behaviors that may not be concordant with those of currently practiced Western-style biomedicine. This is an area of concern to therapists who treat phobias, fears, and anxieties as the influx of immigrants into American society adds new dimensions to skills needed to treat these individuals. Therapists and patients often hold different models of health and illness that may affect COMMUNICATION during a clinical visit as well as outcome of treatment. For example, there may be significant differences in the ways anxiety is described and experienced. Friedman suggests that the range of symptoms included in DSM-IV should be expanded to make the manual applicable across cultures, and that perhaps diagnostic criteria may also need modification.

Pachter (*JAMA,* March 2, 1994) defines a "cultural group" as a group of people who share common beliefs, ideas, experiences, knowledge, attitudes, and behaviors. Most clinical encounters can be regarded as an interaction between two cultures—the culture of medicine and the culture of the patients. Therapists and patients may have different explanatory models for sickness. An explanatory model is the way an individual conceptualizes a sickness episode, including beliefs and behaviors concerning etiology, course and timing of symptoms, reasons for becoming sick, diagnosis, treatment, and roles and expectations of the sick individual.

Personal experiences, family attitudes, and group beliefs affect one's decision making during illness or treatment for anxiety disorders. Communication is maximized when the patient and health care provider share beliefs about the illness. Discrepancies in beliefs and behaviors are often greatest when the practitioner and patient have different cultural orientations. Also, gender differences between therapist and client often must be considered in therapy with culturally diverse populations.

Depression and Fears Across Cultures

People of various cultural backgrounds experience symptoms of depression and anxiety. However, depression, fears, anxieties, and phobias are viewed in different ways in different cultures. For example, studies have indicated agitation as a more common symptom among Japanese, South Indian, and North Indian depressives than among Western depressives. Feelings or delusions of guilt are somewhat less common among Indians than Westerners, while fugitive impulse is more common.

Indian studies during the 1970s indicated a fairly high degree of hypochondriasis, which is noticeable as bowel consciousness and concern about sexual potency and the genital organs. Chinese studies during the 1940s described the "Shook Yang," in which an individual fears retraction of the genitals and death because of this process.

In comparison studies of Indian and British depressed persons (1970s), certain differences were noted that may reflect cultural influences. For example, the Indians complained more about physical symptoms than the British. Physical symptoms have also been observed in studies of African depressives.

In determining choice of symptoms, expectancy by the individual concerning what local medical people consider an illness plays a role. Purely psychological symptoms are often dismissed as not of much consequence in less sophisticated groups. Thus rural Indians may use the body to express inner tensions and anxieties. Differences in such symptoms were noted among British and Indian soldiers under extreme stress during World War II.

Interpretation of guilt among depressives varies between cultures. For example, some Indians attribute their present suffering to possible bad deeds in a previous life. In the Indian social system, conformity is highly valued and the assumption of self-responsibility for one's acts is less well developed. Thus the individual fears failure because he is con-

cerned what others will say rather than fear of loss of self-esteem.

Contrarily, most Westerners assume a higher degree of individual responsibility, and their guilt may come from a sense of self-failure, causing feelings of shame.

Symptoms of obsession and paranoia appear more frequently in Western studies than among Indian depressives. This may be because rituals are well accepted daily practices in some Indian socio-religious systems, and thus such systems are not considered irregular by the individual or his relatives. Also, Westerners tend to be more competitive than Indians, and this tendency may explain a higher degree of suspicious paranoid attitude.

Following are some specific differences across cultures:

Mourning practices differ between cultures, and the process of grief influences the occurrence of depression. For example, in some societies, religion promises continued interaction with the deceased and the possibility of reparation for whatever wrong may have been done. However, acceptance of loss may be inhibited, if customary rites and beliefs lose significance in rapidly acculturating groups. Whether mourning leads to depression depends on the degree of ambivalence of the individual's relationship to the lost person or object. Such relationships are affected by the interaction between parent and child, and particularly the relationship of father to child in patriarchal, traditional societies, which differs from that in most Western cultures.

Shame and guilt influence depression and anxieties. Depression may be rare among illiterate Africans because of the lack of self-reproach and self-responsibility, fatalistic attitude, and a lack of individual competition. Researchers during the 1950s and 1960s agreed that in Africa, depression is relatively light and short, without feelings of sin and guilt. There is a relative infrequency of manic symptoms and a very low suicide rate.

Early missionary reports indicated that Japanese guilt feelings were not related to sexual and sensual bodily expressions but instead connected with family obligations. The Japanese (according to a 1960 study reported by Yap) have a term that literally means repaying one's parents; infractions of this obligation cause feelings that Westerners call guilt. Different individuals feel guilty about different things, depending on their culture.

In Japanese literature, more first-born than last-born males are among those who become depressed. This may occur because in the Confucian system, the eldest son has a heavy responsibility, especially when the father dies.

Projection (a defense mechanism by which unacceptable impulses are attributed to others or personal failures are blamed on others) is used in many cultures. In some societies in which religion teaches that the individual is evil because of a supernatural cause, there is also a mechanism for absolution, atonement, and relief of guilt in the individual. In the Orient, rites of worship or reverence serve a similar function. Some individuals will project guilt and depression to some evil "personality" that possesses one. These are alternative reactions to depression and are influenced by differences in education and social class.

Sick role of depressed individuals varies between cultures. For example, the "lost soul" belief in South America may also give cultural support to the depressed person in the condition called Susto, which does not call for medical attention. Illiterate groups, including the lower classes in advanced cultures, tend to define the sick role in physical terms and visit doctors with physical problems instead of psychological ones.

Child training influences how depression, anxieties, and fears are expressed in later life. Guilt feelings may be influenced by parental severity in child training. Withholding of love and affection may increase self-aggression, and aggression seems to turn inward more readily when the mother rather than the father gives punishment. Variables in societies include type of parental dominance, use of verbal, love-oriented techniques or of physical punishment, the size of the family, number of siblings, presence of mother surrogates, and finally, social class or culture pattern.

Folk Practices

Individuals from some cultures may go to biomedical practitioners for relief of symptoms while simultaneously using a folk therapist to eliminate the cause of the illness. Therapists should be aware of folk illness belief because some folk practices and treatments may be potentially hazardous. According to Pachter, one example is marijuana tea, which is occasionally used to treat asthma by some West Indian patients. Geophagia—the ingestion of earth or clay—is a folk practice that has been noted in Africa and in the American South.

Another group of practices has a different type of potential risk, in which the folk therapy produces skin lesions that may be mistaken for signs of abuse. According to Pachter, most widely recognized are the Southeast Asian practices of "coining," the Chinese practice of moxabustion, and the Mexican-American and Southeast Asian practice of "cupping." Coining involves placing warm oil on a child's trunk and briskly rubbing the area with the edge of a coin or spoon; this practice is thought to relieve fevers. Moxabustion involves touching the skin with burning herbs or incense. Cupping consists of placing a heated glass or cup on the skin; as it cools, it creates negative pressure that produces an area of redness.

There is a high prevalence of POST-TRAUMATIC STRESS DISORDER among refugee groups from Southeast Asia and Central America who fled violence and terror. Researchers studying these groups have found a high co-occurrence of depressive disorder and dissociative experiences. The term *cultural bereavement* has been proposed as a diagnosis that more fully captures the nature of the syndrome of traumatic losses experienced by refugees.

In Japan, a type of social phobia *(taijin kyofusho)* has been identified in which the primary symptom is the fear of embarrassing others rather than oneself.

In New Guinea and Melanesia, "cargo anxiety" occurs out of a belief that ancestral spirits will arrive, bringing valuable cargo. Locals destroy existing food supplies in expectation of better items to come. Insecurity and dissatisfaction with the existing way of life are thought to lead to such delusions.

Phobias in India

One recent study comparing phobic individuals in India and those in the United Kingdom indicated several differences. The British sample contained more individuals with agoraphobia and social phobias. The Indian sample contained more individuals who had phobias of illness and sudden death. The lower incidence of agoraphobia among the Indians may be explained by the fact that while agoraphobia generally occurs more among females than males, Indian women are traditionally housebound, and an inability to venture out by themselves may not be considered unusual behavior.

More important, this difference may be explained by the differences in social structure between India and the United Kingdom. In India, for example, social life is defined by one's roles, such as son, husband, father, grandson, or neighbor, whereas in Western cultures the focus is on individuality and independence. Thus the Indian may feel less social pressure than Westerners, and this lack of social pressure may play a role in the incidence of agoraphobia and social phobias. It may also be that fear of social situations is not recognized as a condition requiring medical help. Also, poor health education and less-than-adequate health services

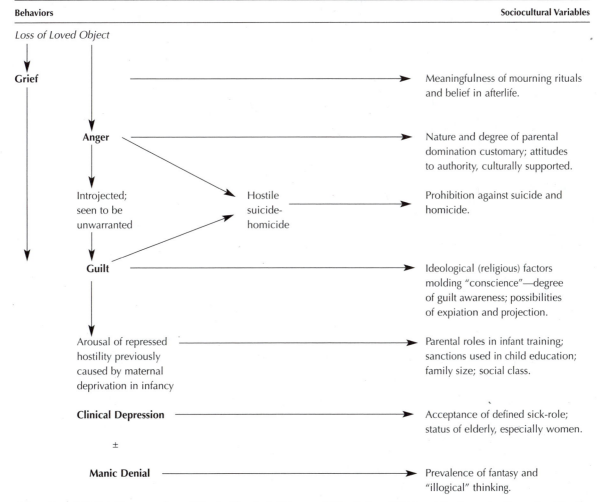

POSSIBLE RELATIONSHIPS OF SOCIOCULTURAL VARIABLES TO DEPRESSION

Behaviors   **Sociocultural Variables**

Loss of Loved Object

Grief ————————————————————————→ Meaningfulness of mourning rituals and belief in afterlife.

Anger ————————————————————————→ Nature and degree of parental domination customary; attitudes to authority, culturally supported.

Introjected; seen to be unwarranted   Hostile suicide-homicide ——————→ Prohibition against suicide and homicide.

Guilt ————————————————————————→ Ideological (religious) factors molding "conscience"—degree of guilt awareness; possibilities of expiation and projection.

Arousal of repressed hostility previously caused by maternal deprivation in infancy ——————→ Parental roles in infant training; sanctions used in child education; family size; social class.

Clinical Depression ——————————————————→ Acceptance of defined sick-role; status of elderly, especially women.

±

Manic Denial ——————————————————————→ Prevalence of fantasy and "illogical" thinking.

Adapted from P. M. Yap, "Phenomenology of Affective Disorder in Chinese and Other Cultures," CIA Foundation Symposium/Transcultural Psychiatry (London, 1965), p. 98.

in general may heighten anxieties about illness and death.

Culturally Sensitive Care Is Necessary

Pachter encourages "culturally sensitive" health care. This means a system that respects the beliefs, attitudes, and cultural lifestyles of its patients. It is a system that acknowledges that culturally constructed meanings of illness are valid concerns of clinical care.

According to Friedman, many areas of cross-cultural influences in treating phobias, fears, and anxieties need further study. These include qualitative studies of indigenous belief systems, efficacy of traditional psychotherapeutic treatments, such as those used in Caribbean populations, use of antianxiety medications, and how help from spiritists helps or hinders treatment and recovery. Additionally, there is a need for more clinical research on anxious African Americans. Information concerning African-American families perceptions of mental illness, help-seeking, and behavior, can contribute to the therapist's knowledge and effective treatment of anxious African-American clients. Also, there is a need for more research on dosages of psychotropic medications such as benzodiazepines, antidepressants, and antipsychotics in patients of other populations, particularly Asians.

See also ACCULTURATION, FEAR OF; CURSES, FEAR OF; DEMONS, FEAR OF; EVIL EYE, FEAR OF; EXORCISM; FOLK HEALERS; MIGRATION; SATAN, FEAR OF; VOODOO, FEARS IN; ZOMBIE, FEAR OF.

Chambers, J., et al., "Phobias in India and the United Kingdom." *Acta Psychiatrica Scandinavica* 74 (1986): pp. 388–391.

Friedman, Steven, *Cultural Issues in the Treatment of Anxiety* (New York: The Guilford Press, 1997).

Howells, J. G., and M. L. Osborn, *A Reference Company to the History of Abnormal Psychology* (Westport, CT: Greenwood Press, 1984).

Neki, J. S., "Psychiatry in South-East Asia." *British Journal of Psychiatry,* 123 (1973): pp. 257–269.

Pachter, Lee M., "Culture and Clinical Care." *Journal of the American Medical Association* 271, no. 9 (March 2, 1994).

Teja, J. S., et al., "Depression across cultures," *British Journal of Psychiatry* 119 (1970): pp. 253–260.

Yap, P. M., "Phenomenology of Affective Disorders in Chinese and Other Cultures." CIA Foundation Symposium/Transcultural Psychiatry, London, 1965.

crossing a bridge   See BRIDGES, FEAR OF.

crossing the street, fear of   Fear of crossing the street is known as dromophobia.

See also AGORAPHOBIA; STREETS, FEAR OF CROSSING.

crowds, fear of   Fear of crowds, or of a large number of people gathered together, is known as demophobia, enochlophobia, and ochlophobia. Many who have AGORAPHOBIA also fear crowds. Fear of crowds may also be related to a fear of being con-

PATTERNS OF DEPRESSION IN THREE CULTURES			
	West	**Nigeria**	**India**
Incidence	Common	Rare (artifact?)	Common
Sick role	Acknowledged	Not acknowledged (no word for depression)	Acknowledged
Hypochondriasis	Less common	Common	Common
Paranoid symptoms	Uncommon	Most frequent	Rare
Guilt feelings	Frequent	Almost absent	Rare
Retarded/agitated	R > A	A > R	A > R (artifact?)
Fugitive impulse	Not described	Common (wander into jungle)	Frequent (renunciation)
Suicide	Common	Rare	Less common

Adapted from J. S. Neki, "Psychiatry in South-East Asia," *British Journal of Psychiatry,* 123 (1973): 257–269.

fined, because in a crowd there may be no quick way for the anxious individual to get to a place he or she regards as safe.

See also CLOSED PLACES, FEAR OF; CONFINEMENT, FEAR OF.

crucifixes, fear of   Fear of crucifixes, or the image of Christ on a cross, or of items in the shape of a cross, is known as staurophobia. This fear may be related to religious fears, superstitious fears, or fear of the supernatural.

See also SUPERNATURAL, FEAR OF.

crying, fear of   Some individuals who are quick to cry in uncomfortable situations may avoid those situations because they fear others will see them cry. They may fear criticism for their tearful reactions. This is a type of social phobia and can be treated with behavior therapy.

See also BEHAVIOR THERAPY; SOCIAL PHOBIA.

cryophobia   Fear of extremely cold temperatures, cold objects, or ice. Also known as psychrophobia and frigophobia.

See also COLD, FEAR OF; ICE, FEAR OF.

crystallophobia   Fear of glass.

See also GLASS, FEAR OF.

cult   A group devoted to a leader, usually a religious leader, who claims ultimate wisdom. Cults usually have a rigid power structure and regulations.

Recent cults share certain similarities. They seem to have arisen the 1960s, a period of social unrest when values were questioned and criticized. Depending on the cult, new recruits are people who may not be emotionally stable, may lack family and close friends, and are searching for relief from the confusion and anxieties of modern life. Cult leaders welcome new members with an attitude of caring and acceptance, creating a strong emotional experience for them. The moral behavior and attitudes of the cult are dictated by strong peer pressure. Mem-

bers are made to feel that there are continually higher levels of commitment or sanctity that they can attain. Leaving or questioning the values of the group is looked upon as evil or sinful. Members are reminded that to return to the outside would be to return to the confusion and anxiety they had formerly faced. Some cults also may have social and political reform or terrorism as their goals. Family and friends of cult recruits find affiliations by their loved ones a source of anxiety. Some new cult members sever all close ties and disappear without warning.

Deprogrammers who specialize in trying to extricate cults members are often hired by their families. These deprogrammers may use force or coercion to remove members from the cult environment and, then, implement BRAINWASHING techniques similar to those used by the cults in their indoctrination.

culture shock   See CROSS-CULTURAL INFLUENCES; MIGRATION.

cupping   See CROSS-CULTURAL INFLUENCES.

curses, fear of   In many cultures, individuals fear that harm will come to them because of verbalizations of such wishes from others. Ancient Greeks and Romans publicly put curses on offenders against the government, traitors, and enemies of the country. William Shakespeare is said to have put a curse on anyone who might disturb his grave. Fears of curses are associated with fears of witchcraft and Voodoo.

See also EVIL EYE, FEAR OF; VOODOO, FEAR OF; WITCHES AND WITCHCRAFT, FEAR OF; ZOMBIE, FEAR OF.

cyberphobia   Fear of computers, computerization, or things related to computers.

See also COMPUTER PHOBIA.

cyclones, fear of   Fear of cyclones is known as anemophobia. Individuals who fear cyclones may also fear strong winds or air movements.

See also AIR, FEAR OF; CLIMATE, FEAR OF; WIND, FEAR OF.

cyclophobia   Fear of bicycles.

cyclothymia   A chronic mood disturbance in which the individual regularly experiences alternating moods of elation and DEPRESSION, usually unrelated to external circumstances. It is sometimes considered a milder type of BIPOLAR (MANIC-DEPRESSIVE) DISORDER. A cyclothymic individual has had at least two years of this disorder (one year for children and adolescents) and many periods of depressed mood or loss of interest or pleasure not as severe as the criteria for a major depressive or a manic episode. Cyclothymia differs from DEPRESSION and manic episodes in that the individual is not markedly impaired in social or occupational activities during the hypomanic episodes. However, many cyclothymic individuals experience difficulties in their social relationships, in school, and at work because of recurrent cycles of mood swings and the anxiety that comes about because of the rapid changes in mood. The disorder, which usually begins in adolescence or early adult life and sometimes develops into bipolar disorder, is apparently equally common in males and females. Major depression and bipolar disorder may be more common among first-degree biologic relatives of people who have cyclothymia than among the general population.

See also PERSONALITY TYPES.

American Psychiatric Association, *Diagnostic and Statistical Manual of Mental Disorder* (Washington, DC: American Psychiatric Press, 1987).

cymophobia   Fear of waves or wavelike motions. Derived from the Greek word *kymo* meaning wave. Also known as kymophobia.

See also MOTION, FEAR OF; WAVES, FEAR OF.

cynophobia   Fear of dogs or fear of rabies; also known as kynophobia. The term is derived from the Greek word *cyno*, meaning dog.

See also DOGS, FEAR OF.

cyprianophobia   Fear of prostitutes; also known as cyprinophobia.

See also PROSTITUTES, FEAR OF; SEXUAL FEARS.

cypridophobia   Fear of sexually transmitted diseases. The term is derived from the Greek word *kypris*, meaning Venus, the goddess of love. Cypridophobia also means fear of sexual intercourse.

See also SEXUAL INTERCOURSE, FEAR OF.

daemonophobia   See DEMONOPHOBIA.

dampness, fear of   Fear of dampness, wetness, moistness or excessive humidity is known as hygrophobia.

dance therapy   Dance therapy permits release of anxieties and expression of emotion through body movement. It can be used effectively with a wide variety of individuals, from those who have mild anxiety symptoms to those who have severe mental health disorders. Many individuals who will not speak about their anxieties will indicate something about them with movement. Movement also helps the client be "in touch" with their body and release tensions stored in the body.

Therapists who use this technique are usually trained in dance and body movement as well as psychology. Dance therapy alone does not relieve symptoms associated with anxiety disorders, but may be used in conjunction with other therapies or medication.

See also CREATIVITY.

dancing, fear of   Fear of dancing is known as chorophobia. Fear of dancing may be a SOCIAL PHOBIA that can be overcome by taking dancing lessons, or it may have more deep-seated causes, such as fear of coming into close contact with another person, being touched, or touching another person, particularly one of the opposite sex. This fear may be related to fears of the opposite sex or sexual fears.

See also SEXUAL FEARS.

darkness, fear of   Fear of darkness is also known as achluophobia, lygophobia, myctophobia, nyc-

tophobia, and scotophobia. Fear of darkness is associated with feelings of uncertainty, helplessness, the inability to see what one is doing, and a sense of unfamiliarity because things look different in the dark. Children often develop a fear of darkness at about two years of age. Their first fears of darkness are associated with separation from their parents. Fear of the dark may be partly produced by the sense of being alone. At older ages, children commonly say they hear noises or see images and may imagine ghosts or monsters. As children get older, most lose their fears of the dark, but if they do not outgrow their normal fear, the fear may develop into a phobia in which darkness has unconscious symbolic significance or is associated with danger and threat. Many individuals feel more secure with a night-light on during the night; they can assure themselves that they will not bump into anything if they arise in the dark. Some individuals fear darkness when driving; others will only ride in cars and not walk in the dark.

Fear of darkness in children and adults has been successfully treated with behavior modification approaches.

Fear of darkness is the opposite of fear of daylight, which is known as phengophobia. Many agoraphobics feel more comfortable in the dark than in the light.

Individuals who are hearing-impaired have particular fear of darkness, as they depend so much on visual stimuli. They may fear being alone in dark places, fear being robbed, or fear being attacked in dark situations.

See also NIGHT TERRORS.

dasein   A term used in the existential approach to PSYCHOTHERAPY. Dasein is derived from the German word meaning "being there." The term was used originally by Martin Heidegger (1889–1976), a German philosopher, to describe aspects of an individual's experience of awareness of self, others, environment, choices in deciding how to act upon the environment, and limitations by history and culture. The individual struggles between freedom and limitation, which may lead to anxieties and fears. Heidegger's approach held that, faced with the inevitability of death, man must find meaning in life, not through outer conformity and adaptation to others, but through self-understanding and self-analysis. By drawing on the uniqueness of experience and the pattern of our potentialities, each individual will develop his or her own kind of life and relief from ANXIETIES.

dasein analysis   Dasein analysis is a form of existential PSYCHOTHERAPY that utilizes classical psychoanalytic technique for relief of ANXIETIES and other psychological concerns. Dasein analysis is particularly associated with the work of Medard Boss, Swiss psychiatrist and author of *Psychoanalysis and Dasein-analysis.* Boss acknowledged the role of the past and the future in influencing the individual's current behavior. Boss, like HUMANISTIC therapists and other EXISTENTIAL therapists, viewed the therapeutic relationship as requiring full participation of both parties. As in client-centered therapy, Boss stressed the curative power of the enduring, unshakable, benevolent, and tactful devotion that an individual receives from the analyst and believed that his relationship, rather than interpretations, leads the individual to relief from anxieties and phobias.

See also, EXISTENTIAL THERAPY; PSYCHOANALYSIS.

Boss, M., *Psychoanalysis and Dasein-Analysis* (New York: Basic Books, 1963).
———, *Existential Foundations of Medicine and Psychology* (New York: Jason Aronson, 1971).
Walrond-Skinner, Sue, *A Dictionary of Psychotherapy* (London: Routledge & Kegan Paul, 1986).

dating   A social process by which individuals become acquainted with one another and perhaps develop a relationship that may lead to friendship,

---

TIPS TO REDUCE ANXIETIES IN DATING

- Know something about the person's background before the date.
- Accept "blind" dates only arranged by people you know and trust.
- Seek out people who treat others with respect.
- Date people who agree with your values.
- Avoid people who are overly critical or abusive.

---

romance, sex, and/or marriage. Dating is stressful for participants of all ages. Individuals who have SOCIAL PHOBIAS find dating very difficult because they may fear meeting new people, criticism, embarrassment, or other results of social encounters.

For young people, dating is a rite of passage from childhood to adulthood. Some young people begin dating during their teen years, while others wait until their college years. There are often issues of SELF-ESTEEM, and many are often held back from dating because of negative feelings about themselves. Others may have the additional anxieties of CRITICISM of their dates by their parents. Additionally, peer pressure can make young people drink, smoke, or enter sexual relationships before they are ready and they may suffer the anxieties of pain and guilt because of their actions.

Individuals who are divorced or widowed find themselves back in the dating scene. Many concerns of young people hold true for older people as well, such as self-esteem and concern about appearance. For single parents, dating presents particular anxieties, as young children often "screen" their parents' dates. Some children ask embarrassing questions, such as "are you going to marry my Daddy?"

Despite the anxieties inherent in dating, the process allows people a socially acceptable way of getting acquainted with others.

See also CRITICISM; DIVORCE; INTIMACY; PUBERTY; RELATIONSHIPS; REMARRIAGE; SELF-ESTEEM; SOCIAL PHOBIA.

dawn, fear of   Fear of dawn is known as eosophobia. Fear of dawn may be related to fear of daylight or light. Some agoraphobics fear being out during daylight, or after dawn, but are comfortable going out in the dark. Others who fear dawn and daylight may fear being seen by others or fear criticism about their appearance or their actions.

See also DAYLIGHT, FEAR OF; LIGHT, FEAR OF.

daydreaming When people daydream, they are awake and experiencing a pleasant reverie, usually of wish fulfillment. Daydreaming occurs during idle moments or when people are unconcerned about the activity around them. In these ways, daydreaming, which may be a form of relief from anxieties, differs from serious, logical, and controlled thinking, which is done in a more deliberate manner.

Some people may daydream about developing great ideas or inventions or taking new directions in life; in daydreaming, their mind is free to roam without inhibition and self-censorship. Different outcomes of looking at work and family situations are often developed during moments of daydreaming, because daydreams are usually concerned with ends, not means.

People of all ages daydream. Young and old may be caught staring out the window, putting down a book and gazing at nothing in a trancelike state. Unless they share their dream, it is difficult to tell if they are lost in revery or just bored.

See BOREDOM; CREATIVITY.

daylight, fear of Fear of daylight is known as phenogophobia or phengophobia. Manifestations of this fear involve secluding oneself in curtained rooms where sunlight cannot enter and permitting only illumination by artificial light. Usually the individual can exit at night and move around at night.

Fear of daylight may be related to a fear of being seen in public, being watched, or of criticism by others for behavior or appearance. Some agoraphobics go out only at night because they are fearful of being seen having a panic attack during the daylight.

Feydeau, the French playwright, is said to have feared daylight; he practically never went out during the day. Fear of darkness is more common than fear of daylight.

See also DAWN, FEAR OF; LIGHT, FEAR OF.

daymare A term roughly related to ANXIETY ATTACK or PANIC ATTACK and which is produced by an ongoing thought or image.

dead bodies, fear of Fear of dead bodies, corpses and cadavers is known as necrophobia. Individuals who fear looking at dead bodies may indirectly fear that they will also die or that there may be some "contagion." Some necrophobes may also be fearful of disease or injury.

See also CORPSES, FEAR OF; DEATH, FEAR OF.

deadlines The time within which something must be completed. Most people have experienced anxieties in meeting or failing to meet a deadline. Once they have fallen behind, it is difficult to catch up. They find that rushing tends to add to the anxiety level and decrease effectiveness. Ineffectiveness leads to frustration. Some people become moody, emotional, and blame themselves or others for the deadline failure.

The key to avoiding anxieties produced by deadlines is setting realistic time schedules, enlisting the help needed when deadlines go awry, and negotiating new deadlines when it appears that for one reason or another, deadlines are going to be missed. For individuals to keep a positive outlook, they should break deadlines down to a series of small steps. As each step is completed, they will feel some success, and that success, in turn, will keep them motivated toward their final goal.

See also AUTONOMY; CONTROL; WORKPLACE.

deafness Loss of hearing, either complete or partial. Hearing loss becomes a source of anxiety for many individuals who begin to lose their hearing. While hearing aids help many individuals, some are embarrassed to wear them or find them uncomfortable. Some try to draw attention away from their loss or otherwise conceal it. Some people associate loss of hearing with aging, and hence postpone getting a hearing aid to preserve their image of youthfulness.

Deafness and hearing loss is a major societal problem. Estimates are that about a quarter-million persons in the United States are completely deaf and about 3 million have major hearing problems.

Causes of Hearing Difficulties

Hearing difficulties are related to many things, including problems within the ears themselves, overall body health, emotions, and external environment. People tend to shut off certain sounds at certain times and will hear only what is interesting or significant. For example, a man may hear all of a sports newscast but not hear a request to fix something around the house. In some nursing homes, it has been observed that individuals say they cannot hear, but when asked whether they want ice cream they are able to answer. The term *psychogenic deafness* pertains to such mental "shutting off" of hearing carried to an extreme. Some patients may have such a strong subconscious desire not to hear, they become completely deaf yet have physically normal ears.

The term *psychosomatic deafness* relates to situations in which actual physical deterioration occurs in the ear as a reaction to a mental or emotional problem. There also may be combinations of both physical and psychologically induced hearing difficulties.

See also DISABILITIES.

death, fear of   Fear of death, or thanatophobia, is one of the most universal fears, and may be the basis for many phobias. For example, individuals who fear darkness, choking, suffocation, enclosed places, flying in an airplane, epidemics, having a heart attack, developing cancer or acquired immune deficiency syndrome (AIDS), indirectly fear death under the other feared circumstances. Those who fear having panic attacks also fear death, because at the times when their hearts beat fast and they have difficulty breathing, they are afraid that they will die. Many agoraphobics fear death. The commonly used term "scared to death" probably came about because some individuals are so frightened by circumstances—or their own reactions—that they fear they will die.

Historically, philosophers and psychoanalytic thinkers have considered man's preoccupation with and fear of death, and most religions have incorporated teachings about death into their belief systems. Some people fear death because of its unknown aspects. Some fear their own death and worry that it will be painful and unpleasant. Others fear death because of what might happen to them after the end of life. For those who believe in a hereafter, they worry about where they will go after death. Fear of death and retribution for possible sins during life may influence some individuals toward good behavior.

Others fear the death of a loved one, which would result in the survivor's being left alone. For example, when a spouse does not return when expected, some individuals start fearing an accident or a mugging. Many children fear the death of a parent, because the children fear being left alone. It is not uncommon for a young child to anticipate the return of a dead parent, because young children do not comprehend the finality of death.

Fear of death is common among children, particularly adolescents. Adolescents aged 15 to 18 are more anxious about death than younger children or older adults, while among 12- to 18-year-olds, the most common fear is of nuclear war (a fear of death by nuclear war).

In the United States, many people fear talking about death. As an example, many do not use the words "death," "dying," or "died." Some prefer to refer to another's death as "passing on," or "passing away" or "going to one's reward." People fear death because it is the ultimate unknown. Part of the reason our cultural attitudes about death continue from generation to generation may be that we hide the topic from children. Many adults view death as unspeakable.

In the last decade, however, death has become more commonly talked about out of necessity because of technology that has developed to keep terminally ill patients alive, the development of legal as well as medical definitions of death, questions about euthanasia (mercy killing), organ donation, and the movement toward hospice care for the dying.

The fear of blood and injury is related to a fear of death, as some phobic individuals associate blood, illness and injury with death. Those who fear needles, injections, or having dental work done may also indirectly fear that they will die as a result of the procedure. However, through exposure therapy, by gradually facing the feared circumstance, the individual can learn to reduce these fears. Exposure therapy helps many individuals overcome fear of dentistry and medical examinations to the point where they are able to relax adequately for necessary procedures.

Some of the factors that influence an individual's fear of death are the age of the person, the individual's psychological maturity, and the level of threat of death. Fear of death often becomes more common after age 40. Individuals dread not only the physically destructive aspects of death, but also the expected loss of consciousness, self-control, and aloneness that death implies.

Soldiers in combat are afraid of dying but learn to control or repress their fears. Some use defensive coping techniques including the adoption of a fatalistic attitude or the thought that they are invulnerable or immortal. During wartime, fear of death contributes to soldiers' alertness and readiness to use weapons. Because of continually facing this acute fear over a period of time, some servicepeople develop POST-TRAUMATIC STRESS DISORDER, during which they relive their fears of death, even years after active duty.

See also CHILDHOOD ANXIETIES, FEARS AND PHOBIAS; CLAUSTROPHOBIA; DEATH ANXIETY; DEATH-RELATED FEARS; DENTAL ANXIETY; INJECTION, FEAR OF; PANIC ATTACK.

Becker, Ernest, *The Denial of Death* (New York: Macmillan, 1975).

Choron, Jacques, *Death and Western Thought* (New York: Macmillan, 1963).

Henden, David, *Death As a Fact of Life* (New York: W. W. Norton, 1973).

death anxiety　Fear of death and anxiety over dying; also known as thanatophobia.

See also CEMETERIES, FEAR OF; DEATH, FEAR OF; ILLNESS, FEAR OF.

death-related fears　A fear hierarchy, or arrangement of fears relating to death, from maximum to minimum, is sometimes used during therapy for an individual who has a death phobia. The individual may be asked to name the situation that arouses maximum anxiety; that fear will be given a rating of 100. The situation that causes the least anxiety

is given a 5. A fear hierarchy or death-related fears for an individual might be:

Seeing a dead man in a coffin
Being at a burial
Seeing a burial assemblage from a distance
Reading the obituary notice of a young person who died of a heart attack
Driving past a cemetery (the nearer, the worse)
Reading the obituary notice of an old person
Being inside a hospital
Seeing a hospital
Seeing an ambulance

See also CEMETERIES, FEAR OF; DEAD BODIES, FEAR OF; SYSTEMATIC DESENSITIZATION; TOMBSTONES, FEAR OF.

Wolpe, Joseph, *Our Useless Fears* (Boston: Houghton Mifflin, 1981).

decapitation fear　Fear of having one's head cut off. Some psychiatric points of view consider decapitation fear a form of castration anxiety, or fear of having one's genital organs cut off. This bizarre and unlikely concern is usually part of a delusional pattern of obsessive fantasy.

See also CASTRATION ANXIETY; SEXUAL FEARS.

decaying matter, fear of　Fear of decaying matter is known as septophobia. Individuals who have this phobia may be afraid of disease.

See also CONTAMINATION, FEAR OF; DIRT, FEAR OF; FILTH, FEAR OF; GERMS, FEAR OF; INFECTION, FEAR OF.

decisions, fear of　Fear of making decisions is known as decidophobia. Some anxious individuals find it difficult to make choices in life, ranging from simple choices, such as what to wear, to major decisions, such as whether to get married or not, or where to live. Some individuals who fear NEWNESS or NOVELTY have difficulty making decisions regarding changes. ANXIETIES about decision-making are related to FEARS about one's own capabilities and feelings of self-confidence.

See also MOVING, FEAR OF.

deconditioning A behavior therapy technique in which learned responses such as phobias are "unlearned," or deconditioned. For example, a person who has a phobic reaction to water following a near-drowning experience could be deconditioned by going wading with a trusted friend, taking a small step at a time in very shallow water, and gradually going into deeper water. Desensitization is another term for the deconditioning process.

See also BEHAVIOR THERAPY; DESENSITIZATION.

deep places, fear of See DEPTH, FEAR OF.

defecalgesiophobia See DEFECATION, FEAR OF; DEFECATION, FEAR OF PAINFUL.

defecation, fear of Fear of defecation, or having bowel movements, is known as coprophobia. For some, the fear extends only to the times when the individual perceives that someone is watching or is aware of what is happening, such as in a public bathroom facility. For others, there is a fear of losing part of the body through defecation. Another interpretation is that the individual may have regressed, or perhaps never advanced, from an earlier stage of development in which his or her own feces were considered prized possessions.

See also ANAL STAGE; DEVELOPMENTAL STAGES.

defecation, fear of painful Fear of having pain during a bowel movement is known as defecalgesiophobia. This fear may be long-standing or may occur at times such as following surgery or during illness, where the pain may be real and not imaginary.

See also DEFECATION, FEAR OF.

defense mechanisms Patterns of feelings, thoughts, or behaviors that are relatively involuntary and arise in response to perceptions, psychic danger such as ANXIETY, internal conflicts, unacceptable impulses, GUILT, or other threats to the EGO. The term defense mechanisms was first used by SIGMUND FREUD in 1894. Examples of defense mechanisms are AVOID-ANCE, COMPENSATION, DENIAL, DISPLACEMENT, RATIONALIZATION, REPRESSION, and substitution. Defense mechanisms may be useful or harmful, depending on their severity, their inflexibility, and the context in which they occur.

See also DISSOCIATION; PROJECTION; SUPPRESSION.

American Psychiatry Association, *Diagnostic and Statistical Manual* (Washington, DC: American Psychiatric Association, 1987).

deformed people, fear of Fear of deformed people is known as teratophobia. Some individuals have a phobic reaction to deformed people when they see them on the street. Others have anxious reactions just by imagining or thinking of deformed individuals. Some fear giving birth to a deformed child. Fear of becoming deformed oneself is known as DYSMORPHOPHOBIA.

deformity, fear of Fear of a cosmetic defect in one's appearance is known as dysmorphophobia. The individuals who have this condition are in fact well within normal limits in their appearance but complain about some external physical defect they think is noticeable and upsetting to other people. Some individuals are continually concerned with a specific part of the body, e.g., genitals, mouth and smile, breasts, nose, ears, eyes, chin, bald head, buttocks, arms, legs, eyebrows, stomach, etc. Thoughts may be connected with feelings of inferiority. Dysmorphophobia, likeliest to occur in individuals who have sensitive or insecure personalities, may be an early symptom of obsessive-compulsive disorder or schizophrenia.

The term dysmorphophobia was coined in 1886 by Morselli, who described cases of patients concerned over small hands, a dimple on the chin, etc. Pierre Janet in 1908 described patients who had unwarranted feelings of dissatisfaction with their physical appearance. He thought these individuals were neurotic and stressed the obsessional side of their symptoms.

See also NEUROSIS; OBSESSIVE-COMPULSIVE DISORDER; SCHIZOPHRENIA.

Hay, G. G., "Dysmorphophobia," *British Journal of Psychiatry* 116 (1970): pp. 344–406.

deipnophobia   See DINING, FEAR OF.

déjà vu   An illusion in which the individual experiences a new event for a moment as something already experienced; such an event may be ANXIETY-producing or cause a PHOBIC REACTION. The word is French and means "already seen." The familiar feeling may be due to resemblance between the present and the past scenes, or to a similar scene pictured in a daydream or night DREAM. Some believe that déjà vu experiences are due to events in a previous lifetime.

delusion   An unshakable belief or system of belief based on a faulty premise and maintained in spite of rational evidence to the contrary. The delusion is not a belief ordinarily accepted by other members of the person's culture or subculture; it is not an article of religious faith. Delusions may cause the individual great anxiety and even panic reactions.

Individuals with mental illnesses often suffer from delusions; for example, individuals with schizophrenia may suffer from the delusion that others are plotting against them (paranoia). Some illegal drugs may induce delusions in the user, such as the excessive use of cocaine, amphetamines, methamphetamine, or hallucinogenic drugs. Some drug abuse causes long-lasting mental illness from which the individual may not recover, including delusional behavior. Alcoholics who are undergoing withdrawal may suffer from delusions.

Delusions may be transient and fragmentary or they may be highly systematized and superficially convincing, as in paranoid states, although most delusions fall between these two extremes. Though logically absurd and symptoms of psychosis, delusions sometimes have a purpose, such as to relieve an individual's anxiety or to counteract feelings of inferiority or insecurity and fill the need to blame others for their failures. In other cases, delusions have no discernible purpose.

Delusions should be distinguished from HALLUCINATIONS, which are false sensory perceptions. A delusion should also be differentiated from an overvalued idea, an unreasonable belief, or an idea that is not as firmly held as a delusion.

There are many common types of delusions. For example, delusions of being controlled by others involve feelings, impulses, thoughts, or actions that are experienced by the deluded individual as having actually originated elsewhere and as being imposed upon them by some external force. A typical case of this type of delusion is the man who claims that his own words were those of his father. Some deluded individuals believe that they are receiving coded messages through the television set and that characters in a television program are talking directly to them.

Grandiose delusions involve an exaggerated sense of one's importance, power, knowledge, or identity. Delusional jealousy may occur, for example, when a person has the delusion that his or her sexual partner is unfaithful. Nihilistic delusion involves the theme of nonexistence of the self or part of the self, others, or the world. An example is the person saying, "There is no need to eat, because I have no insides." The central theme of a persecutory delusion is that the person or group of which he or she is a member is being attacked, harassed, cheated, persecuted, or conspired against. A somatic delusion pertains to the function of the body. An example is the belief a woman has that she is pregnant, despite being postmenopausal.

Delusional thinking is not necessarily present in anxiety states; however, people who develop delusions have a severe sense of personal vulnerability and unrecognized fears that they may project outward.

See also ANXIETIES; COCAINE, FEAR REACTIONS FROM; PARANOIA; PSYCHOSIS.

demons, fear of   Fear of demons is known as demonphobia, demonophobia, daemonophobia, and phasmophobia. Demons, once considered companions or lesser devils of Satan at the time of his fall from heaven, were feared even before the Middle Ages (1220–1400), when church people and later judges and civil authorities sought to detect and rout the devil and other demons that were believed to take over some human bodies and cause diseases and other catastrophes. Those who feared demons feared that powerful forces got inside the human body and that these forces directly caused the possessed person to commit bizarre acts. The victims of demonic possession were not considered responsible for their disturbing mental and physical symptoms, which resemble what are now considered to be attacks of HYSTERIA and SCHIZOPHRENIA. To help the individual, someone or something had to get through to the inner forces, weaken them, and drive them out.

During the Middle Ages, demons were thought to have great knowledge and power. In addition to their potential control over human behavior, they could influence the stars, control weather, and produce earthquakes. Certain areas of learning, such as alchemy, were considered to be the province of demons. Demons were described as being able to assume any form they chose, sometimes having actual physical form, usually that of an animal or a powerful, striking human being.

In some periods, people thought to have made a pact with the devil were considered witches. The procedure for hunting down, detecting, and trying witches included various torturous exorcisms to induce the witches or wizards (male) to recant and break their bonds with the devil. In most cases the presumed witches and wizards possessed by demons were killed. Many individuals were unjustly accused of witchcraft, creating considerable anxiety in the innocent population, many of whom were identified as accomplices or witches themselves, in confessions by torture victims.

In modern therapy, figurative "demons" are driven out when the therapist understands and attempts to change the internal forces that cause observed undesirable behaviors, such as phobic reactions.

See also EXORCISM; WITCHES AND WITCHCRAFT, FEAR OF.

demophobia Fear of crowds.
See also CROWDS, FEAR OF.

dendrophobia Fear of trees. This fear may be related to fear of forests, or fear of landscape.
See also LANDSCAPE, FEAR OF; TREES, FEAR OF.

denial A DEFENSE MECHANISM in which the person fails to acknowledge some aspect of external reality that is apparent to others—for example, the existence of a phobia-provoking situation or anxiety-producing event. Denial can be a positive or negative force, depending upon how it is used. For example, in denying that a threat exists, the individual deludes himself or herself into relative calmness and possibly a better ability to cope. Soldiers in battle may use the denial mechanism in this way. An example of a negative adaptation of denial is an agoraphobic who denies that his or her fear of going out of the home may interfere with his or her own economic capacity and may be burdening other family members with chores.

Freud suggested that women's lack of a penis and the anxiety this realization causes in men and women was the basis for the denial mechanism.

See also EGO DEFENSE MECHANISMS.

dental anxiety Dental anxiety, or fear of dentists and dentistry, is sometimes referred to as dentophobia. Dental fear is an important clinical problem that seriously interferes with the provision of oral health care. A morbid fear of dental treatment is often traceable to at least one traumatic dental experience in childhood but also may be associated in many cases with a lower-than-normal pain threshold, and in some cases with strong personality factors that affect the situation. Dental anxiety ranges from a mild fear of dental treatment to extreme ANXIETY that leads an individual to avoid contact with a dentist entirely. Mild to high dental anxiety may surface as a mild queasy feeling in the stomach, a dryness in the mouth, an increased pulse, sweaty palms, or trembling hands. Persons with extreme dental anxiety may experience difficulty in breathing, dizziness or lightheadedness, choking, chest pain, diarrhea, and PANIC ATTACKS. Some even bolt from the chair during a dental procedure. Most frequently cited fears are the sight of the anesthetic NEEDLE and the sight and sound of the dentist's drill. Dental anxiety often occurs on its own, but it may also be associated with more general fears of BLOOD, INJURY, PAIN, DOCTORS, and HOSPITALS. While many advances in dentistry during the latter part of the 20th century have greatly reduced the anxieties most people have about dentistry, there are still many fearful individuals.

Studies show that persons with high dental anxiety, compared to those with little or no dental anxiety, may have lower pain thresholds or an increased sensitivity to pain.

As with many anxieties, in addition to the stress from the anxiety itself, the potential harm resulting from minor or otherwise preventable problems may become quite serious. Avoiding routine dental care can lead to more severe problems and complications, such as severe tooth decay or periodontal disease. Poor oral health may result in unsightly teeth and thus a reduction in self-esteem. If a dental abscess goes unchecked, the results may even be fatal; as many as 800 people die each year when unchecked bacterial infections travel to and attack other parts of their bodies.

Prevalence of Dental Anxiety

Getka and Glass report that up to 80 percent of the adult population in the United States admits to some anxiety concerning dental treatment, with 5 to 6 percent experiencing anxiety of such intensity that they are unable to obtain the dental treatment they feel they need. Often, in an emergency these individuals must have dental work done in a hospital under full anesthesia.

Steward Agras, in his large-scale study of anxiety prevalence, found that 19.8 percent of sampled individuals reported moderate anxiety, and an additional 2.4 percent reported intense reaction. Similar results were obtained by Ronald Kleinknecht and associates in a questionnaire survey of 920 persons (see summary table). Furthermore, Kleinknecht found that 44.5 percent of his sample had put off making a dental appointment due to anxiety and

PERCENTAGE OF RESPONSES TO THE QUESTION "ALL THINGS CONSIDERED, HOW FEARFUL ARE YOU OF HAVING DENTAL WORK DONE?"

Response %	Male %	Female %	Total* %
Not at all	29.1	21.8	25.4
A little	40.3	32.7	36.6
Somewhat	19.6	21.6	20.5
Much	6.11	13.7	10.2
Very much	4.0	10.1	7.3

*N = 920

that 4.7 percent had done so "nearly every time" an appointment was due or needed.

In this survey, the most feared events were seeing and feeling the needle and hearing, feeling, and seeing the drill. The lack of personal contact, anticipation of pain, feelings of vulnerability and embarrassment, and lack of confidence in the dentist or auxiliary personnel were also contributing factors to the reaction.

Sources of Dental Anxiety

Some dental anxiety is undoubtedly acquired through direct experience with painful or frightening dental situations. These traumas can produce conditioned emotional reactions so that dental tools or procedures become conditioned stimuli, generalizing further to the dentist, the dental office, and so on. How the patient perceives the dentist's demeanor and reacts personally to him or her also seems to contribute to fear acquisition. For example, if the patient feels embarassed or belittled, or feels little control of the situation, fear can be heightened. There also seem to be strong cognitive elements of catastrophic or anxiety-engendering thinking that contribute to the reaction.

While various psychoanalytical speculations as to underlying reasons for dental anxiety (some built upon themes of oral fixation or Oedipal authority conflicts) may be valid, the more common line of reasoning is to view dental anxiety as a learned or behavioral response to real, imagined, or anticipated dental stimuli. Firsthand painful or negative experiences during dental treatment are one of the better-documented origins of dental anxiety. Such experiences are certainly subjective and may be perceived as real even if they are not. When origins are not traceable to an unpleasant firsthand experience, they probably lie in vicarious experiences. For many people, dental anxiety is essentially a culturally learned fear. Dental "horror stories" told by friends or relatives or in the media are quite common, as are cartoons or fictional accounts depicting frightening circumstances. Stories told by childhood friends are a significant origin of dental anxiety. Dental "torture" scenes such as those portrayed in *Little Shop of Horrors* or *Marathon Man* are likely to have lasting effects or to reinforce a current dental anxiety. A family member with dental anxiety (most often the mother) might be another cause of an individual's own dental anxiety. In addition, anyone who has had a negative or painful medical experience is likely to generalize that experience to dental treatment. Whether acquired firsthand or vicariously, dental anxiety most often begins in childhood or adolescence.

Women and Dental Anxiety

A study of female patients reported by Walker, Milgrom, Weinstein, et al., found associations between dental fears and prior sexual, physical, and emotional trauma. The women in the study described concerns for their safety, such as the risk of dental anesthesia. They reported having fears of being trapped in the dental chair, feeling claustrophobic, being unable to breathe or experiencing choking or severe gagging that interfered with treatment. For these patients, a sense of helplessness and lack of control appeared to be underlying problems.

Women with high dental fear scores had significantly higher odds of having experienced several forms of childhood and adult trauma, and women reporting histories of trauma had significantly higher

---

SAMPLE ANXIETY HIERARCHY FOR TYPICAL DENTAL PHOBIA

Anxiety-Provoking Situation	SUD (0–100)
1. Being reminded you need a dental appointment	20
2. Calling for an appointment	25
3. Seeing the calendar that shows only 1 day left before appointment	32
4. Driving to the dentist's office	39
5. Entering the waiting room	45
6. Hearing the drill sounds while in the waiting room	54
7. Being taken into the dental chair	60
8. Seeing the dentist walk in	68
9. Dentist uses explorer (probe) to examine your teeth	73
10. Feeling vibrations from the drill on your mouth	80
11. Seeing the local anesthetic syringe	90
12. Dentist begins injection	95

Ronald A. Kleinknecht, *The Anxious Self* (New York: Human Sciences Press, 1986), p. 157.

---

dental fear scores. The researchers concluded that development and maintenance of dental fear is a complex process involving interaction of several factors, such as previous dental care, early family environment, and current social support and coping skills. They suggested that collaborations between dentists and mental health care providers may be useful in dealing with patients who have these fears. In some patients, resolution of dental fear may involve investigation by a trained mental health care provider into the patient's history of adverse experiences, followed by the development of a treatment plan combining supportive psychotherapy, behavior desensitization, and restoration of a sense of CONTROL to the patient.

Components of Anxiety: Dental Fear Surveys

From the dentist's point of view, it may be difficult to tell who suffers from anxiety and who does not. Many people do not outwardly display their fears; they may even go to great lengths to hide them, to avoid the fear of embarrassment. An understanding of the components that make up an individual's dental anxiety can be helpful in deciding which methods might best be employed to break down and treat the anxiety. A number of dental fear surveys have been developed, some for use by dentists or psychologists, others more for use by patients and their dentist together. Such questionnaires, filled out prior to an individual's first appointment, could indicate to the dentist or psychologist how that person would be likely to respond to a dental procedure and what steps might help the person overcome his or her anxiety.

A typical questionnaire assigns point values to specific elements of dental fear. A five- or ten-point scale gauges the range from no reaction or fear to intense reaction or fear. Questions concern the anticipation and avoidance of dentistry, physiological responses to dentistry, fear of individual experiences during specific phases of dental treatment (such as the sight of the anesthetic needle or sitting in the waiting room), general fear of dentistry, and reactions of family or peers to dentistry.

Using such a scale, Ronald Kleinknecht and D. A. Bernstein found that persons who score high anxiety prior to a dental appointment also report more anxiety when in the office and sweat more during treatment.

SAMPLE ITEMS FROM THE DENTAL FEAR SURVEY

Has fear of dentistry ever caused you to cancel or not appear for a dental appointment?

1	2	3	4	5
Never	Once or twice	A few times	Often	Nearly every time

When having dental work done:
My muscles become tense:

1	2	3	4	5
Not at all	A little	Somewhat	Much	Very much

My heart beats faster:

1	2	3	4	5
Not at all	A little	Somewhat	Much	Very much

How much fear do you experience when: Being seated in the dental chair?

1	2	3	4	5
Not at all	A little	Somewhat	Much	Very much

When seeing the anesthetic needle:

1	2	3	4	5
Not at all	A little	Somewhat	Much	Very much

Ronald A. Kleinknecht, *The Anxious Self* (New York: Human Sciences Press, 1986), p. 101.

Treatment Options and Outlook

Management of dental anxiety may include simple communication and explanation of dental treatments, chemical intervention (such as local or general anesthetics, analgesics, or sedatives), behavioral or psychological intervention (ranging from simple relaxation techniques to options such as biofeedback, hypnosis, or psychological consultation), or even acupuncture. Because the mouth is a very sensitive and private part of the body, dental work is likely to be viewed as an aggressive act with the dentist as the aggressor. Dental patients may feel distrust or even hostility toward their dentist. They may hide their anxiety out of embarrassment or fear of criticism. For these reasons, the dentist must be open and communicative; he must encourage patients to view and trust him as a person, not just a clinician. A dentist who is perceived as being critical, judgmental, or insulting will only increase a dental patient's anxiety. People are less likely to anticipate pain from a dentist whom they trust. Because a patient often feels loss of control while undergoing dental treatment, use of hand signals or a pushbutton to get the dentist to stop whatever he is doing can return this element of control and allay that component of anxiety. It is also important for the dentist to appear to be in control. Surprisingly, some people will accept their dentist's authority to the point where their anxiety can actually be reduced simply by the dentist's command. A straightforward explanation of the proposed treatment by the dentist will also lead to a greater feeling of knowledge and control on the part of the dental patient. These basic elements of explanation, understanding, and control are often all that is necessary to relieve dental anxiety for some individuals.

Relaxation and distraction techniques work on opposite principles. Relaxation reduces or inhibits anxiety, while distraction masks anxiety by keeping a person preoccupied. With both techniques, people still report feeling the pain, although not to the same extent. Using relaxation techniques, a person can focus his or her attention on relaxation through a series of muscle-relaxation and deep-breathing exercises. BIOFEEDBACK may also be used. In biofeedback, a machine is used to monitor the individual's state of relaxation or excitation. By a visible or audible signal, the machine relays this information to the person, who in turn concentrates on and responds to the machine's signals and learns to relax. An extension of the relaxation technique is SYSTEMATIC DESENSITIZATION, in which the person first relaxes and then imagines the anxiety-producing situation. The visualized dental treatment thus becomes associated with relaxation.

Distraction techniques focus a person's attention away from the dental work—through, for example, popular music played through headphones; a movie, such as a comedy; or cartoons for children. A video game mounted above the dental chair ensures active participation on the part of the dental patient and thus achieves a greater degree of distraction. In the MODELING technique a person observes someone else receiving dental treatment through a visual presentation, such as a film, slides, pictures, or in person. While the anxiety-producing situation is portrayed, the "model" shows no fear. Modeling leads a person to imitate the same response as the model. This is an excellent preventive technique when it is used with children on their first dental appointments.

HYPNOSIS, or hypnodontics, is capable of providing very deep relaxation in many patients. Despite the popular image created by fiction and magic shows, there is nothing mystical about hypnosis, nor does it cause a person to lose control. There are two major limitations: 1) Only about one-fifth of all dentists have been trained to use hypnosis, and 2) not everyone is equally able to achieve a trance state.

ACUPUNCTURE may be the most controversial technique for relieving dental pain. Only recently has it even been considered seriously to have real analgesic and anesthetic results. If the patient's anxiety is not increased by the use of needles, the apparent pain-relieving effects of acupuncture may help to reduce dental anxiety. Due to the underlying mystery of acupuncture (it is far from clearly understood—the traditional explanation involves yin and yang and energy balance), it is hardly a widespread technique in the U.S. One study suggests that acupuncture's results might be entirely due to a placebo effect.

Not surprisingly, evidence appears to indicate that treating the anxiety and not just the pain is more likely to help an individual free him- or herself from dental anxiety. A study has shown a higher incidence of kept appointments in persons who received behavioral modification than persons who received general anesthesia.

Dentists and fearful patients are not alone when it comes to combating dental anxiety. Recently, many dental fear clinics have opened. These clinics teach behavioral modification techniques to help people get over their dental anxiety. Self-help audiocassette programs and books are also available. In instances of extreme dental anxiety that a dentist is unable to manage or treat, consultation with a behavioral therapist may be helpful. Such persons may refuse sedation, act irrationally or with hostility, or exhibit symptoms of compulsive neurosis.

It is not very surprising that the dental patient's anxiety also affects the dentist. Not only is it likely to make his work more difficult, but it contributes to the dentist's unfortunate high incidence of stress-related diseases and suicide.

Getka and Glass reported that anxious patients may require up to 20 percent more chair time than patients who are relaxed. In fact, dentists regard patient anxiety as one of their most troublesome sources of professional stress.

Self-Help Approaches to Dental Anxiety

Direct experiences that help reduce fear and anticipatory reactions:

1. Expose yourself to a dental office, procedures, instruments, etc., in a nontraumatic way. Visit a dentist to talk, sit in the chair, look at instruments, become acquainted with procedures and personnel; these activities can be helpful in desensitizing yourself to these situations. Begin exposure while relaxed. Several exposure trials may be necessary.
2. Control in the dental situation is advised so that you can learn to stop or delay procedures until you are ready or can cue personnel when you need rest or recovery time.

Indirect experiences:

3. Observe others undergoing cleaning or nontraumatic dental procedures (live or on video) to reduce dental anxiety.
4. Obtain information on modern dental treatment. Develop coping skills to apply in the dental situation.

5. Learn to relax during dental treatment.
6. Learn to pace yourself and breathe to attain relaxation.
7. Develop positive, coping self-statements.
8. Minimize or avoid negative "catastrophizing" self-statements.
9. Learn to distract yourself.
10. Speak up to exercise control if needed.

See also BEHAVIORAL THERAPY; BLOOD-INJURY FEARS; GAGGING, HYPERSENSITIVE: RELAXATION TRAINING; TOOTHACHE, FEAR OF.

Getka, Eric J., and Carol R. Glass, "Behavioral and Cognitive-Behavioral Approaches to the Reduction of Dental Anxiety." *Behavior Therapy* 23 (1992): pp. 433–448.

Jongh, Ad De; Peter Muris; Guusje Ter Horst, et al., "One session cognitive treatment of dental phobia: preparing dental phobics for treatment by restructuring negative cognitions." *Behav. Res. Ther* 33, no. 8 (1995): pp. 947–954.

Sokol, Sokol, and Sokol, "A Review of Nonintrusive Therapies Used to Deal with Anxiety and Pain in the Dental Office," *JADA,* February 1985.

Walker, Edward A., Peter Milgrom, Philip Weinstein, et al., "Assessing Abuse and Neglect and Dental Fear of Women," *JADA,* April 1998.

dentophobia   See DENTAL ANXIETY.

dependent personality disorder   A personality disorder classified by the American Psychiatric Association. The essential feature of this disorder is a pervasive pattern of dependent and submissive behavior. Anxiety and depression are common. Individuals with this disorder usually lack self-confidence and tend to belittle their abilities and assets. They may at times seek, or stimulate, overprotection and dominance by others. Frequently, individuals with this disorder also have another personality disorder, such as avoidant personality disorder, or histrionic, schizotypal, or narcissistic personality disorders. Dependent personality disorder usually begins in early adulthood and shows up in a variety of contexts, as indicated by *at least five* of the following:

- Unable to make everyday decisions without an excessive amount of advice or reassurance from others
- Allows others to make most of his or her important decisions—for example, where to live, what job to take
- Agrees with people even when he or she believes they are wrong, due to a fear of being rejected
- Has difficulty initiating projects or doing things on his or her own
- Volunteers to do things that are unpleasant or demeaning in order to get other people to like him or her
- Feels uncomfortable or helpless when alone, or goes to great lengths to avoid being alone
- Feels devastated or helpless when close relationships end
- Frequently is preoccupied with fears of being abandoned
- Is easily hurt by criticism or disapproval

See also ANXIETY; AVOIDANT PERSONALITY DISORDER; DEPRESSION; PERSONALITY DISORDERS.

American Psychiatric Association, *Diagnostic and Statistical Manual* (Washington, DC: American Psychiatric Association, 1987).

depersonalization   A feeling of unreality or being removed from oneself and the environment. Depersonalization sometimes occurs in agoraphobia. The individual may feel that he or she is someone else or is watching himself, usually from above. Depersonalization may be a "cutoff" mechanism when anxiety, stress, or fatigue reaches an unacceptable level for an individual. It is a temporary condition, lasting a few seconds or minutes or, rarely, several hours.

Depersonalization is also a characteristic of depersonalization disorder, and may also occur in schizotypal personality disorder and schizophrenia.

See also DEPERSONALIZATION DISORDER; SCHIZOPHRENIA.

depersonalization disorder   A disorder characterized by one or more episodes of DEPERSONALIZATION that are severe enough to impair an individual's social and occupational functioning. Onset of depersonalization is rapid and usually shows up in a sensation of self-estrangement, a feeling that one's extremities have changed in size, a sense of being mechanical, perceiving oneself at a distance, and, in some cases, a feeling that the external world is unreal.

See also NEUROSIS.

depersonalization neurosis   See DEPERSONALIZATION DISORDER.

depressants   Agents that diminish or slow down any function or activity of a body system or organ. Types of depressants include ALCOHOL, BARBITURATES, and TRANQUILIZERS.

depression   An emotional state that is marked by great sadness and apprehension, feelings of worthlessness and GUILT, withdrawal from others, changes in patterns of sleep, appetite, and sexual desire, and either lethargy or agitation. Depression affects an individual both at work and at home. It is also known as *major depressive disorder* or *major depression*. A less intense but chronic form of depression is called *dysthymia*.

Depression usually occurs without psychosis (loss of reality), but it can occur in conjunction with psychosis. The depressed person may have many personal, work, or family problems or may have no apparent problems. Many individuals with anxiety disorders also suffer from depression. For example, many individuals who have AGORAPHOBIA also have some depression.

Depression is one of the most common and treatable of all mental illnesses, according to the National Institute for Mental Health (NIMH). In their 2006 report on the numbers of people with mental disorders in the United States, NIMH reported that major depressive disorder was the leading cause of disability among individuals ages 15–44 years in the United States. It is estimated that 14.8 million adults ages 18 and older in the United States, or 6.7% of the adult population, suf-

fer from depression in any given year. Individuals of any age, including children and adolescents, can develop depression, but the median age of onset is 32 years according to the NIMH.

About 80 percent of those who suffer from depression fail to recognize the illness and consequently receive no treatment for it. Many attribute the physical and emotional symptoms of depression to "the flu" or "stress." It is interesting to note that most cases of depression subside within one year without treatment of any kind. However, treatments tend to hasten this natural recovery.

Many depressed individuals who have not been treated have mental and physical feelings that never go away, appear to have no end in sight, and cannot be alleviated by happy events or good news. Some people are so disabled by their depression that they cannot build up sufficient energy to call a doctor. If someone else calls for them, these depressed individuals may refuse to see a mental health professional or physician because they are so hopeless that they think there is no point in seeking help.

The family, friends, and coworkers of depressed people may become frustrated with victims of depression because their efforts to help and comfort are to no avail. Often the depressed person will not follow advice, refuses help, and denies comfort. However, persistence is essential, because many doctors believe that depression is the illness underlying the vast majority of suicides in the United States. The best prevention for suicide is to recognize and treat the depression. However, it should be noted that even when individuals have begun taking antidepressants, there is still a risk for suicide, particularly in the early part of therapy. Any mention of suicidal thoughts or plans should be reported immediately to the treating physician, whether the person is taking antidepressants or not. Depressed individuals are at much greater risk of suicide than nondepressed individuals.

Scientists say that no single cause gives rise to depression in all individuals. However, many studies have found family links to depression. For example, if one identical twin suffers from depression or manic-depression (BIPOLAR DISORDER,) the other twin has a 70 percent chance of also having the illness. Other studies that have looked at the rate of depression among adopted children supported this finding. Depressive illnesses among children's adoptive family had little effect on their risk for the disorder; however, among adopted children whose biological relatives suffered from depression, the disorder was three times more common than the norm.

Some medications are known to cause some kinds of depression. During the 1950s, doctors realized that some people taking reserpine, a medication for high blood pressure, suffered from depression. Likewise, depression has been noted as a side effect of DIAZEPAM (Valium), ALPRAZOLAM (Xanax), and many other kinds of tranquilizers.

Recent research indicates that people suffering from depression have imbalances of neurotransmitters, which are natural biochemicals that allow brain cells to communicate with one another. Two particular biochemicals that tend to be out of balance in depressed people are *serotonin* and *norepinephrine*. Some scientists think that an imbalance of serotonin may cause the sleep problems, irritability, and anxiety from which many depressed people suffer. Likewise, an improper amount of norepinephrine, which regulates alertness and arousal, may contribute to the fatigue and depressed mood of the illness.

Other body chemicals also may be out of balance in depressed people. Among them is CORTISOL, a hormone that the body produces in response to stress, extreme cold, anger, or fear. In normal people, the level of cortisol in the bloodstream reaches a peak in the morning, and then the blood levels decrease as the day progresses. In depressed people, however, cortisol peaks earlier in the morning and does not level off or decrease in the afternoon or evening.

Scientists say that the environment also plays an important role in depression. Historically, depression has been viewed as either internally caused (endogenous) or externally related to environmental events (exogenous). Current thinking, however, views depression from the point of view of the interaction of both biological and environmental factors.

Symptoms and Diagnostic Path

Individuals who suffer from depression usually have pervasive feelings of sadness, helplessness, hopelessness, and irritability. Often they do not admit to experiencing these symptoms to themselves or others but they frequently withdraw from normal human contact and exhibit signs and symptoms of depression. Other symptoms may include the following

- a noticeable change of appetite with either significant weight loss from eating significantly less (without attempts at dieting) or weight gain caused by excessive eating
- a noticeable change in sleeping patterns, such as fitful sleep, inability to sleep, or sleeping too much
- the loss of interest in activities formerly enjoyed
- the loss of energy and fatigue
- feelings of worthlessness
- feelings of inappropriate guilt
- an inability to concentrate or think
- indecisiveness
- recurring thoughts of death or suicide, wishing to die, and, in some cases, attempts suicide
- melancholia (defined as overwhelming feelings of sadness and grief) accompanied by waking at least two hours earlier than normal in the morning, feeling more depressed in the morning, and being significantly slower in motor skills.
- disturbed thinking develops in some individuals

Treatment Options and Outlook

Between 80 to 90 percent of all depressed people can be effectively treated, according to the American Psychiatric Association.

Note that many people with depression require the assistance of a mental health professional to cope with their depression. Failing to handle depression by oneself is not a sign of weakness. There are a variety of therapies and medications that help many depressed people, such as psychotherapy, medications, and electroshock therapy. Some individuals benefit from self-help, such as learning how to deal with the depression themselves or attending support groups for people with a particular problem or situation.

Many people effectively deal with their depression with a combination of psychotherapy and medications. Electroshock therapy is limited to patients who are severely depressed and to those who are psychotic and depressed.

Psychotherapies.   There are a number of talk therapy treatments for depression, including psychoanalysis and cognitive-behavioral therapy (CBT). Research has indicated that cognitive/behavioral therapy and interpersonal therapy are effective.

Interpersonal psychotherapy is based on the philosophy that disturbed social and personal relationships can cause or contribute to depression. The illness, in turn, may make these relationships more problematic. The therapist helps the individual understand his or her illness and how depression and interpersonal conflicts are related.

Cognitive/behavioral therapy seems to be the most effective psychotherapeutic treatment for depression, based on the understanding that people's emotions are controlled by their views and opinions of the world. Depression results when individuals constantly berate themselves, expect to fail, or make inaccurate assessments of what others think of them. They may overvalue a situation, catastrophize, and have a negative attitude toward the world and the future. The therapist uses various techniques of talk therapy to alleviate negative thought patterns and beliefs.

Psychoanalysis, initially developed by Sigmund Freud in the early 20th century, is based on the concept that depression is the result of a significant loss of others or loss of sense of self and past conflicts that patients have pushed into their unconscious. Therapists work to identify and resolve the patients' past conflicts that have given rise to depression in later years. Psychoanalysis can require years of therapy.

Electroshock therapy (ECT).   Some years ago, electroconvulsive therapy (ECT) was used to treat depression. As more effective medications have been developed, the use of ECT has declined. However, ECT is still used for some patients who cannot tolerate medications. ECT is generally considered as a treatment when all other therapies have failed or when a person is suicidal. ECT has also proven effective as a treatment for psychotic and involutional depression (a major depression that occurs after age 50, usually in a sudden onset), but medications are usually as good or better at alleviating symptoms.

Medications.   During the 1950s, several pharmaceutical medications were developed to treat depression. The effectiveness of the medication depends on an individual's weight, overall health, metabolism, and other unique characteristics. Several trials of a medication or a combination of medications may be needed to learn which drugs work best for each individual. Generally, antidepressant medications become fully effective 10 to 28 days after an individual begins taking them.

Usually one of several major types of medication is used to treat depression. These include tricyclic antidepressants, selective serotonin reuptake inhibitors (SSRIs), serotonin norepinephrine reuptake inhibitors (SNRIs), monoamine oxidase (MAO) inhibitors, and lithium. There are also other drugs used to treat depression, such as BUPROPION (Welibutrin, Wellbutrin SR, and Welibutrin XL), an atypical antidepressant approved by the Food and Drug Administration (FDA) for the treatment of depression. Alpha 2 antagonists are sometimes used, such as mirtazapine (Remeron).

Tricyclic antidepressants may be prescribed for individuals whose depressions are characterized by fatigue; feelings of hopelessness, helplessness, and excessive guilt; an inability to feel pleasure; and a loss of appetite with resulting weight loss. Some examples of tricyclics are imipramine (Tofranil), nortripytline (Pamelor), amitriptyline (Elavil), desipramine (Norpramin), Serzone (nefazodone), Desyrel (trazodone), and maprotiline (Ludiomil).

Another type of antidepressant is the selective serotonin reuptake inhibitor (SSRI). Drugs in this category allow for the increased retention of serotonin and thus improved mood. Individuals with many types of depression are prescribed SSRIs. Some examples of SSRIs are fluoxetine (Prozac), escitalopram (Lexapro), citalopram (Celexa), paroxetine (Paxil), sertraline (Zoloft), and fluvoxetine (Luvox). Fluvoxetine is also approved by the FDA for the treatment of OBSESSIVE-COMPULSIVE DISORDER (OCD). Another antidepressant, fluoxetine, is FDA-approved for the treatment of OCD, PANIC DISORDER, SOCIAL PHOBIA, and POST-TRAUMATIC STRESS DISORDER. Escitalopram is FDA-approved for the treatment of GENERALIZED ANXIETY DISORDER (GAD).

Serotonin norepinephrine reuptake inhibitors are newer medications which allow for the retention of both serotonin and norepinephrine. These drugs may also be helpful to those with chronic pain that is associated with depression, particularly duloxetine (Cymbalta).

MAOs are prescribed for individuals whose depressions are characterized by excessive sleepiness and anxiety, phobic and obsessive-compulsive symptoms in addition to the depression. However, MAOs have many side effects and a strict diet must be followed by those who take them. As a result, they have fallen out of favor among mental health professionals. Examples of MAOs are phenelzine (Nardil) and isocarboxazid (Marplan).

Lithium is a naturally occurring salt that is generally limited to treating people who have BIPOLAR DISORDER. Occasionally, it is prescribed for people who suffer from depression without mania. Those most likely to respond are depressed individuals whose family members have manic-depression or whose depression is recurrent rather than constant.

Antidepressant medications may have a variety of different side effects, depending on the particular medication that is taken, and these side effects often discourage the individual from either using a full clinical dose or from taking their medications at all. In some cases, side effects wear off with time, while in other cases, they are sufficiently severe to cause the individual to cease taking the medication. Individuals should consult with their physicians about possible side effects of a medication before they begin a course of therapy.

Self-help Several techniques have been found effective in prevention of and self-care for depression. These include

1. A regular program of exercise, starting with brief periods and gradually expanding to at least one half hour per day.
2. Interpersonal contact with others, rather than separation and alienation. Support groups may be useful.
3. Efforts to cope with exaggerated thoughts that occur, such as self-deprecation, catastrophizing, and overvaluation, by introducing more realistic thoughts and supporting them.
4. Increased activity, gradually adding activities to the day's schedule.

Risk Factors and Preventive Measures

Women are about twice as likely to suffer from depression as men; however, the rate of depression also increases dramatically among older men. One supposition is that some men lose their sense of identity and self-worth when they retire. Among people of all ages, major changes in the environment, such as a move or job change, or any major loss, such as a divorce or death of a loved one, can bring on depression. Feeling depressed in response to these changes is normal; however, depression can become a long-term problem that may require treatment.

See also ANTIDEPRESSANTS; BIPOLAR DISORDER; DEPRESSION, ADOLESCENT; SEASONAL AFFECTIVE DISORDER.

National Institute of Mental Health, "The Numbers Count: Mental Disorders in America," 2006. Available online. URL: http://www.nimh.nih.gov/publicat/numbers.cfm#readNow, Rockville, Maryland, National Institutes of Health. Downloaded November 15, 2006.

Stahl, Stephen M., *Essential Psychopharmacology: The Prescriber's Guide.* (Cambridge: Cambridge University Press, 2005).

depression, adolescent For many people, adolescence is a period of complicated and demanding conflicts that lead to ANXIETIES, FEARS about SELF-ESTEEM, and fears regarding the future. Many become overwhelmed by the many changes and pressures and develop depression. Adolescents, neither children nor adults, may experience more loneliness than other age groups; some feel powerless and isolated. Failure in school can lead to a feeling of rejection, a lack of challenge can create BOREDOM, social expectations may be unrealistic, and conflicting messages from family may magnify the struggle for independence.

Depression during adolescence is more than a feeling of being "down in the dumps" or "blue." Depression is an illness and should be treated as such with available help. Recognizing depression in oneself or in one's children or students is important.

Symptoms

Factors relevant to adolescent depression include:

Feelings of helplessness or hopelessness
Death wishes, suicidal thoughts, suicide plans or attempts

Sadness

Extreme fluctuations between boredom and
  talkativeness

Anger, rage, verbal sarcasm, and attack

Overreaction to criticism

Guilt; feelings of being unable to satisfy ideals

Poor self-esteem and loss of confidence

Intense ambivalence between dependence and
  independence

Feelings of emptiness in life

Restlessness and agitation

Pessimism about the future

Rebellious refusal to work in school or cooperate
  in general

Sleep disturbances

Increased or decreased appetite; severe weight
  gain or loss

Adolescent depression may be difficult to diagnose.
Depression in a young person may be somewhat different from that in an adult in several ways. Adolescents do not always understand or express feelings
well. Some of their symptoms are often dismissed as
"just growing up." The young person, unaware of
the concept of depression, may not report anything
wrong. Also, there is a strong tie between "getting
into trouble" and feeling depressed. It is difficult to
sort out if the teenager is depressed because of being
in trouble, or in trouble because of being depressed.
Depression in the adolescent has been linked to poor
academic performance, truancy, delinquency, ALCO-
HOL and DRUG ABUSE, disobedience, self-destructive
behavior, sexual promiscuity, rebelliousness, grief,
and running away. The young person may have suffered an increase in the severity of life events, high
stress, a number of mental or physical illnesses, a lack
of support from family and other significant people,
and a decrease in the ability to cope. Adolescents
may attempt to escape from depression by denying a
need for relationships, or denying that loneliness or
depression exist.

Treatment

The most common ways of treating depression in
adolescence are medication, psychotherapy, or a
combination. For some individuals, the medication
(ANTIDEPRESSANTS) is useful in treating symptoms,
and a mental-health professional can help them
understand why they are depressed and how to

handle future stressful situations. PSYCHOTHERAPY
is effective in treating stress-related depression. In
this treatment, an individual has the opportunity
to explore painful events or feelings that might
have contributed to the depression. The therapist
helps the individual look beyond the problem and
explore these feelings. Contemporary therapies
also focus on the thought processes that contribute
to adolescent depression—for example, exaggerated concerns, misperceptions, and continual self-
criticism. Cognitive behavior therapies focus on
these processes. To increase acceptance and a sense
of belonging, adolescents who have depression
are advised to try to make new and more friends,
explore and make better use of existing social connections, and increase their activity in school, community, sports, or job. However, for many young
people, these changes are not possible without professional help. Help is available from many community resources, school counselors, and religious
advisors. The National Mental Health Association
can help interested individuals locate appropriate
services locally (in the United States).

See also DEPRESSION; GUILT; SCHOOL PHOBIA; STRESS
MANAGEMENT; SUICIDE; SUICIDE, ADOLESCENT; TEST
ANXIETY.

(Adapted with permission from "Adolescent
Depression," National Mental Health Association
Information Center, Alexandria, Virginia.)

depth, fear of   Fear of depths is known as bathophobia. The term commonly refers to fear of losing
control of oneself while in a high place. It is a fear
of falling from the height and of thus being killed.
The fear, common among many people, is considered excessive when the anxiety is intense and
lasting and leads to measures to avoid high places.

See also FALLING, FEAR OF; HIGH PLACES, FEAR OF.

depth psychology   A psychological approach that
emphasizes unconscious mental processes as the
source of emotional symptoms and disturbances
such as ANXIETIES, PHOBIAS, personality, and attitudes. Freudian psychoanalysis is an example of
depth psychology. Other therapies historically have
used a depth approach, notably Adler, Horney, Jung,
and Sullivan. Depth psychology includes other tech-

niques that explore the unconscious, such as hypnoanalysis, psychodrama, and narcosynthesis.

See also PSYCHODRAMA.

dermatitis Inflammation of the skin, sometimes due to allergy but sometimes occurring without any known reason. Dermatitis is one of many skin conditions feared by people who have dermatophobia, or dermatopathophobia, both involving fears of skin diseases and skin lesions. Dermatitis can result in painful itching and the distress of extreme discomfort. For some individuals, if the itching persists without relief, dermatitis leads to a feeling of helplessness and anxiety. Dermatitis can also result from anxiety. It also can intensify anxieties, particularly social anxiety.

Many types of dermatitis are better known as eczemas, such as atopic, common in babies; nummular, cause unknown, dermatitis which occurs in adults; and hand dermatitis, the result of household detergents and cleansers.

Other types of dermatitis include seborrheic dermatitis, which appears on the face, scalp, and back and develops during stress, and contact dermatitis, a reaction to something that comes in contact with the skin.

See also ALLERGIES; CHRONIC ILLNESS; DEPRESSION; HIVES; ITCH, FEAR OF.

dermatopathophobia Also known as dermatosiophobia.

See also SKIN DISEASE, FEAR OF.

dermatophobia See SKIN LESION, FEAR OF.

desensitization See SYSTEMATIC DESENSITIZATION.

developmental stages There is some question and debate in scientific circles about whether humans proceed through regular, predictable stages of development. At the physical level, it appears that development occurs in phases or stages, but questions persist about the psychological level.

The two most dominant state theories are those of Sigmund Freud and Erik Erikson. Freud elaborated stages of "intrapsychic" development to sexual (libidinal) energies and to some extent for aggressive (Thanatos) energies. Freud's psychosexual stages, however, became the best-known developmental phases. Erikson, a student of Freud, concentrated on the interpersonal and emotional effects of what he called psychosocial stages of development. Neither Freud nor Erikson emphasized anxiety, but they did conclude that it could develop as a result of frustration at any of the stages.

DEVELOPMENTAL STAGES		
Phase	**Freud**	**Erikson**
Birth to first year	*Oral stage.* Oral activity is source of psychic energy. Infant needs nurturing physically or deprivation develops with fixations that affect ability to give and receive love, as well as greediness and dependency.	*Infancy: Trust versus mistrust.* The mode of interaction is incorporative (to get and to take). Insufficiency of meeting physical and emotional needs results in sense of mistrust of others, insecurity, and anxiety.
Age 1–3 years	*Anal stage.* Anal activity is source of psychic energy. Retention and elimination become prototypes for power, independence, and self-control. Fixation can lead to stinginess obstinacy or disorderliness, impulsivity, and cruelty. Obsessive-compulsive characteristics result from frustration in this stage.	*Early childhood: Autonomy versus shame and doubt.* Child needs to explore, inquire, and test self. Holding on and letting go are modes of activity. Under- or over-gratification results in a sense of self-doubt, inhibition, shame, and feelings of inadequacy to control events. Adequate resolution results in internal locus of control.

(table continues)

DEVELOPMENTAL STAGES

Phase	Freud	Erikson
Age 3–6 years	*Phallic stage.* Basic conflict develops around incestuous feelings toward opposite-sex parent (Oedipal complex for males and Electra for females). Resolution produces superego and sense of sexuality. Many anxiety reactions stem from inadequate resolution of this stage.	*Preschool age: Initiative versus guilt.* This is an intrusive mode in which self-initiated exploration and discovery are important. Over- and under-gratification stifle initiative and lead to guilt, poor self-concept, and lack of self-worth. Confidence in oneself results from adequate experience. Exploration and discovery are important. Over- and under-gratification stifle initiative and lead to guilt, poor self-concept, and lack of self-worth. Confidence in oneself results from adequate experience.
Age 6–12 years	*Latency stage.* Sexual energies diminish, resolution of previous stages is possible, efforts are focused outward, and socialization begins.	*School age: Industry versus inferiority.* Understanding of outer world expands, sex role identity develops, achievement and attainment of goals and sense of adequacy develop.
Age 12–18 years	*Genital stage.* Extends from puberty to old age. Ideally, sexual energy should stem from genital sources but may be restricted by previous fixations. Sublimation into socially acceptable activities occurs, as well as sexual role identification.	*Adolescence: Identity versus role confusion.* Self-identity, life goals, and direction develop, as well as breaking of dependency (leaving home) and accepting personal responsibility. Previous frustration or difficulties at this age can lead to an *identity crisis* (an unclear sense of self).
Age 18–35 years	Genital stage continues	*Young adulthood: Intimacy versus isolation.* The task here is to develop intimacy, connection, and commitment to others in the capacity for both love and work. Inadequate resolution results in aloneness, separateness, and denial of need for closeness.
Age 35–60	Genital stage continues	*Middle age: Generativity versus stagnation.* This is a time to focus on the next generation, to adjust to differences between one's dreams and actual achievements, and to achieve a sense of productivity. Inadequate resolution leads to self-indulgence and futurelessness.
Age 60+	Genital stage continues	*Later Life: Integrity versus despair.* Ego integrity is the ability to look back without regret and to feel personally worthwhile and whole. Disappointment and feelings of futility result from inadequate resolution.

The chart on pages 187–88 compares Freud's psychosexual and Erikson's psychosocial stages through the life cycle.

See also PHALLIC STAGE; REGRESSION.

devil, fear of the Fear of the devil, also known as the supreme evil spirit, has had both a disciplinary and an explanatory role in the Judeo-Christian tradition. In early Judaism, Satan was viewed as God's righthand man. He was an obstructor, a tempter, and a negative force, but not an antagonist to God's power. Satan began to acquire a more intensely evil character as Judaism came into contact with the Persian beliefs in Zoroastrianism, a set of religious belief that separated the other worldly powers into forces of good and evil.

Christian belief made Satan into the angel who led a heavenly revolt and, because of his pride and jealousy, was ejected from heaven and fell into the underworld. The medieval church developed the threatening, grotesque image of the devil with horns and a tail, along with terrifying stories of his ability to tempt the weak and sinful. The Reformation strengthened the image of Satan's evil with its emphasis on the sinfulness of the physical world. Satan's existence became a way of rationalizing the belief in a loving God with the presence of illness, misfortune, and lust in the world. Witches were thought to have gained their power from a pact with the devil. It is believed that many mentally and emotionally disturbed people were identified as witches and burned at the stake. The idea that a man could obtain worldly success by selling his soul to the devil became somewhat widespread. However, at the same time, the devil was thought to be a punisher of evildoers. So great was the fear of the devil that the name Lucifer or "light bearer" was applied to him in the belief that using his real name would offend or summon him.

See also DEMONS, FEAR OF; WITCHES AND WITCHCRAFT, FEAR OF.

Brasch, R., *Strange Customs* (New York: David McKay Co., 1976).

Thomas, Keith, *Religion and the Decline of Magic* (New York: Charles Scribner's Sons, 1971).

dexamethasone suppression test (DST) This test is currently used as a diagnostic tool for identifying depression. The DST measures the degree to which the neurochemicals ACTH and cortisol are suppressed in the brain by the introduction of the synthetic drug dexamethasone. In normal people, dexamethasone suppresses these neurochemicals. Some studies show that depressed people fail to show such suppression. However, the validity of these studies is controversial. Also, dexamethasone suppression in panic-disorder patients has not been shown to be significantly different from that in normal people.

See also ANTIDEPRESSANTS; DEPRESSION; DIAGNOSIS; DRUGS.

dextrophobia Fear of objects at the right side of the body or fear of the right side.

diabetes, fear of Fear of diabetes is known as diabetophobia. Diabetes is a metabolic disease that develops due to the body's lack of ability to manufacture insulin or to make appropriate use of the foods one eats. Diabetes is not contagious, and there is no need to fear contact with anyone who has diabetes. Normally the food one eats is converted into glucose, which cells use as a source of energy. Glucose causes an increase in blood glucose level, which in turn signals release of the hormone insulin from islet cells of the pancreas, a gland in the abdomen. Insulin regulates the level of glucose in the blood and assists in utilizing and storing glucose in the body. Without enough insulin, glucose is not used by cells and thus builds up in the blood. Diabetes can be controlled but can also be life-threatening. Among the possible consequences of uncontrolled diabetes are poor circulation, high blood pressure, hardening of the arteries, and nerve damage. Having diabetes puts one at greater risk of having heart or kidney disease. Anxiety is also common with diabetics due to bodily reactions and glucose changes.

Kahn, Ada P., *Diabetes* (Chicago: Contemporary Books, 1983).

diabetophobia See DIABETES, FEAR OF.

diagnosis The art of distinguishing one disorder from another, and determining the nature or cause of the disorder. There are many types of diagnoses, such as biological diagnosis, determined by tests performed; clinical diagnosis, based on symptoms shown; and differential diagnosis, determining which one of two or more diseases or conditions an individual suffers from, by systematically comparing and contrasting their symptoms. The word diagnosis come from the Greek words "dia," meaning "through," and "gnosis," meaning knowledge. In cases of anxieties and phobias, diagnosis includes a period of study and evaluation of the individual, including problems, history, and environment, and the individual's own attempts at dealing with problems.

Various professionals have attempted to differentiate FEAR, PHOBIA, and ANXIETY and describe their unique characteristics for diagnostic purposes, although they often differ in their diagnoses because of the intertwining and close appearance of many symptoms. Phobias were first given a separate diagnostic label in the International Classification of Diseases in 1947 and by the American Psychiatric Association in 1952. A standardization of diagnostic criteria is found in the American Psychiatric Association's book, *Diagnostic and Statistical Manual III-R* (Washington, DC: American Psychiatric Press, 1987). Criteria for diagnosis continue to evolve.

Diagnostic procedures for anxieties and phobias depend largely on the type of therapy that will be used and the style of the therapist. For example, behavior therapists might use one or more of a series of tests to measure level of fear before embarking on a course of treatment. A diagnostic label would not be a part of the behavior therapy. Diagnosis would be a process of discovering the exact eliciting stimuli and response to such stimuli.

In differentiating simple phobias from other disorders, therapists will consider the presence or absence of other symptoms. For example, if the individual has DEPRESSION or OBSESSIVE-COMPULSIVE symptoms, fear may be a symptom of the major disorder. Sometimes fears will precede depressive illness. The diagnosis of SIMPLE PHOBIAS is based on two general findings, PHOBIC ANXIETY and/or AVOIDANCE and exclusion of other definable diagnostic entities. Diagnosing AGORAPHOBIA is more complex. The agoraphobic syndrome is characterized by clinical and psychophysiological similarities to the anxiety neuroses. A clinical difference

is that there is a great deal of avoidance behavior in agoraphobia and may be fairly little in anxiety neurosis. There are also personality factors used to diagnose agoraphobia, such as emotional suppression. There is a fine line in diagnosing depression in agoraphobia. This is because agoraphobia restricts an individual's activities, making the person fairly helpless and discouraged. These factors may appear to be depression, but most agoraphobic individuals lack characteristics of an endogenous (self-induced) depression. The individual has not lost his or her interest (which is characteristic of endogenous depression) but is frustrated by not being able to do all the things he or she would like to do. Also, the agoraphobic may be active and productive at home or in his or her restricted environment or when accompanied.

Various researchers during the second half of the 20th century have differed on diagnosing anxieties, fears, phobias, and obsessive-compulsive disorders because of the intertwining and close appearance of many symptoms. A standardization of diagnostic criteria is found in the American Psychiatric Association's book, *Diagnostic and Statistical Manual of Mental Disorders*.

Diagnosis, as we commonly use it for psychiatric purpose, is based on the concept of "topology"—that is, behaviors that are similar in form are categorized together. For example, "depression" is a topological term involving numerous behaviors that are similar in their form (lack of sleep, eating difficulty, etc.) and are symptoms of depression. Likewise, "anxiety" has many topological or symptom categories. The "topological model" or "medical model" is based on the view that these various symptoms derive from a common underlying source (such as childhood trauma, intrapsychic conflict, incongruities, repression, etc.). The underlying cause produces symptoms, which, in turn, can be grouped together or clustered into syndromes, disease entities, or diagnostic categories. Where there is great speculation regarding possible underlying causes, no such causes have been found after almost a century of massive research efforts.

The use of this model has been questioned by many scientists—behavioral therapists as well as psychologists and psychiatrists who have used it for diagnosis. Questions of reliability of diagnosis (which is quite low on some subgroups) and validity have been raised for decades. Others argue that the basic assumptions of this model are flawed, and that a better model—such as the learning-theory approaches of the behavioral scientists—should be developed. Since models are only approximations to reality, they are and should be replaced by more powerful models that afford better prediction and control.

One clear and present danger in the use of these diagnostic categories is that individual differences in etiology and manifestation of psychopathology are ignored or minimized. Yet it is the variations that require a response if treatment is to be effective and the individual is to gain from the experience with the disorder.

These are important issues and should be noted in talking about the diagnostic system.

See also CLASSIFICATION OF ANXIETIES; CLASSIFICATION OF PHOBIAS; *DIAGNOSTIC AND STATISTICAL MANUAL OF MENTAL DISORDERS*.

Marks, Isaac, *Fears and Phobias* (New York: Academic Press, 1969).
Mavissaklian, M., and D. Barlow, *Phobia: Psychological and Pharmacological Treatment* (New York: Guilford Press, 1981).
Morris, R. J., and T. R. Kratochiwill, *Treating Children's Fear and Phobias* (New York: Pergamon Press, 1983).

Diagnostic and Statistical Manual of Mental Disorders, Fourth Edition A categorical guide for classification of mental disorders published by the American Psychiatric Association in 1994. Mental disorders are grouped into 16 major diagnostic classes, e.g., anxiety disorders and mood disorders. The book is used for clinical, research, and educational purposes. It is used by psychiatrists, other physicians, psychologists, social workers, nurses, occupational and rehabilitation therapists, counselors, and other health and mental health professionals who wish to base a diagnosis of mental disorders, including anxieties and phobias, on standardized criteria. It was planned to be usable across settings including inpatient, outpatient, partial hospital, consultation-liaison, clinic, private practice, and primary care, and with community populations.

Efforts were made in the preparation of *DSM-IV* to incorporate material that may be useful in culturally diverse populations in the United States and internationally. Thus *DSM-IV* includes three types of data specifically related to cultural considerations. First, there is a discussion of cultural variations in the clinical presentations of certain disorders not included in the *DSM-IV* classification. Next, there is a description of culture bound syndromes that have not been included in the *DSM-IV* classification, and finally, there is an outline to assist the clinician in systematically evaluating and reporting influences of culture on a patient.

The first edition of the book appeared in 1952. The early categories were voted on by members of the American Psychiatric Association. The recent edition was revised over a period of nearly seven years and prepared by teams of physicians and researchers, including those from the National Institute of Mental Health (NIMH), National Institute on Drug Abuse (NIDA), and the National Institute on Alcohol Abuse and Alcoholism (NIAAA). Categories were formed by empirical studies. Field trials helped bridge the boundary between clinical research and clinical practice by determining how well suggestions for change that are derived from clinical research findings apply in clinical practice.

The editors of *DSM-IV* acknowledge that the title *Diagnostic and Statistical Manual of Mental Disorders,* unfortunately implies a distinction between "mental" disorders and "physical" disorders. Literature documents that there are physical aspects to mental disorders and vice versa.

American Psychiatric Association, *Diagnostic and Statistical Manual of Mental Disorders.* 4th ed. (Washington, DC, 1994).

diagnostic criteria Because anxieties, fears, and phobias are highly individual matters, unique to each individual, precise diagnosis of a person's condition is likely to be less than specific. However, the American Psychiatric Association, in its third *Diagnostic and Statistical Manual of Mental Disorders* (DSM-III-R), first provided specific diagnostic criteria as guides for making diagnoses, in the belief that such criteria enhance diagnostic reliability. The APA emphasized, however, that for most of the categories, diagnostic criteria are based on clinical judgment and have not yet been fully validated by data about such important correlates as clinical course, outcome, family history, and treatment response.

diaphragmatic breathing   See BREATHING.

diarrhea (as a symptom of anxiety)   Diarrhea—frequent, loose, watery stools—is one of many gastrointestinal symptoms anxious individuals experience due to arousal of the AUTONOMIC NERVOUS SYSTEM. When facing or thinking about a feared situation, some may experience stomachaches, diarrhea, weakness, and feeling faint. Those who have test anxiety may experience episodes of diarrhea before taking a test in school or at work. Some who have performance anxiety may experience diarrhea before a performance. Social phobics may have episodes of diarrhea when anticipating a type of social occasion or situation that they fear. Diarrhea induced by anxiety, sometimes referred to as functional diarrhea, can be treated with therapy known as fantasy desensitization, as well as antianxiolytics and medications that act on the gastrointestinal system.

See also ANXIETY; ANXIOLYTICS, BEHAVIOR THERAPY; DEFECATION, FEAR OF; DESENSITIZATION, GASTROINTESTINAL COMPLAINTS; IRRITABLE BOWEL SYNDROME; NAUSEA; VOMITING.

diazepam   An antianxiety drug that has sometimes been a drug of abuse. It is a sedating drug. Diazepam was first marketed under the trade name Valium in 1963, and it has been used and abused more extensively than other BENZODIAZEPINES, the class of drugs to which it belongs. Diazepam is a controlled drug under the Controlled Substances Act. According to the 2004 National Survey on Drug Use and Health, about 6 percent of individuals of all ages in the United States have abused diazepam.

Continued use of almost any dose of diazepam may result in psychological and physical dependence. Withdrawal effects from diazepam can be pronounced and, at times, dramatic (such as with

seizures or HALLUCINATIONS). Diazepam is not toxic, but dependence and addiction quickly develop. Part of the addictive process is because withdrawal from diazepam involves heightened anxiety responses and these are scary to people with anxiety disorders and usually leads to return to use of the drug.

Pregnant women should not use diazepam because diazepam crosses the placenta during labor. An increased risk of suicide is associated with this drug.

See also ANTIDEPRESSANTS.

Substance Abuse and Mental Health Services Administration, *Results from the 2004 National Survey on Drug Use and Health: National Findings.* (Rockville, MD, Department of Health and Human Services, September 2005).

dibenzepin   An antidepressant drug.
See also ANTIDEPRESSANTS; DEPRESSION.

didaskaleinophobia   SCHOOL PHOBIA, or fear of going to school.

dieting   Generally refers to following a special or modified diet for the purpose of losing weight. For some people, dieting is related to phobias or anxieties, such as fear of being fat, or fear of having a certain body shape (DYSMORPHOPHOBIA). It also causes anxieties because many people perceive themselves as overweight, whether this is the case or not.

Thin models unrealistically motivate many people, particularly women, to begin dieting. Dieting brings about anxieties because losing weight is not easy; it means setting realistic goals. It requires time—often a year for some people—for positive results. It means hard work, both to lose weight and to keep it off.

Some dieting approaches involve extensive behavior modification. These programs offer SUPPORT GROUPS and education about good NUTRITION and exercise. Most important, they offer help in altering the individual's behavior in order to limit food intake, increase physical activity, and reduce the anxieties of the current social pressures to be thin.

There are dangers involved in dieting. Donna Ciliska, in *Canadian Family Physician* (January 1993), noted: "The drive for thinness in women as they strive to be what our culture demands has contributed to poor nutrition, an increase in EATING DISORDERS, a decrease in SELF-ESTEEM, discrimination against overweight people, and a diminished bank account. Paradoxically, overweight is more common in men and poses more of a health risk; the social pressure for them to be thin is less severe than for women. Fewer men seek weight loss programs."

Individuals who believe they are overweight should have a physical examination from their physician to determine whether they are actually overweight or are weight-, shape-, or food-obsessed. If overweight, further assessment is necessary; if not overweight, they need supportive strategies to help them feel better about themselves and referral to community resources to help them with their anxieties.

See also BODY IMAGE; DYSMORPHOPHOBIA; EATING DISORDERS; OBESITY; SELF-ESTEEM.

Ciliska, Donna, "Women and Obesity," *Canadian Family Physician*, January 1993.

Hamilton, Michael, et al., *The Duke University Medical Center Book of Diet and Fitness* (New York: Fawcett Columbine, 1991).

Thomas, Patricia, ed., "Dieting May Be a Losing Proposition." *Harvard Health Letter* 19, no. 10 (August 1994).

dikephobia   Fear of JUSTICE is known as dikephobia.

dining (or dinner) conversation, fear of   Fear of conversation while dining is known as deipnophobia. Individuals who have this fear usually eat their meal in silence and request silence from their companions at the table. Such individuals may suffer from any of a number of related fears, such as choking, talking with their mouths full, looking ridiculous while they are opening their mouths to talk, saying something ridiculous, or being criticized.

See also CHOKING, FEAR OF; CRITICISM, FEAR OF; LOOKING RIDICULOUS, FEAR OF; SOCIAL PHOBIA.

dinophobia   Fear of DIZZINESS or WHIRLPOOLS.

diplopiaphobia   Fear of DOUBLE VISION.

dipsophobia   Fear of DRINKING: this usually relates to alcoholic beverages.

See also ALCOHOLISM, FEAR OF.

dirt, fear of   Fear of dirt is known as mysophobia or rhypophobia. Many individuals who fear dirt fear CONTAMINATION or INFECTION. Some obsessive-compulsives who wash their hands frequently fear dirt.

See also GERMS, FEAR OF; ILLNESS, FEAR OF.

dirty, fear of being   Fear of being dirty is known as automysophobia. Frequent hand-washing is a symptom of this phobia.

See also CONTAMINATION, FEAR OF; DIRT, FEAR OF; GERMS, FEAR OF.

disabilities   A disability refers to a temporary or permanent loss of faculty. It may refer to physical disabilities such as loss of a leg or of hearing or mental capabilities, such as retardation or autism. COPING with a disability causes fears and anxieties for the one who has the disability and also for parents, siblings, and children who face caring for the disabled person.

Persons who become disabled often struggle with the anxiety of trying to be like everyone else. Because of their disability they may feel a loss of SELF-ESTEEM compounded, in many cases, by the limitations of the living situations that they encounter. According to Reverend John A. Carr of the Yale-New Haven Medical Center, who was born with the congenital absence of both hands and one foot, "Coping with a handicap will depend on how human interactions occur, to allow more or less progress toward meaningful life. In the book, *Coping with Crisis and Handicap*, Reverend Carr recommends that open dialogue between those who are disabled and those who are not is essential because, "In denying our efforts to fight for a world more open to the handicapped, whether we refer to architectural or attitudinal barriers, we may be denying ourselves accessible avenues we will need later."

Coping with a Disability in the Family

Mary S. Challela, director of nursing and training at the Eunice Kennedy Shriver Center for the Mentally Retarded, defines *parental coping* as "managing the day-to-day activities of meeting the disabled child's needs, the parents' needs, and those of other children in the family, in a realistic manner. Before parents can be expected to assume any of these tasks effectively, they must be allowed and encouraged to respond emotionally to the crisis of disability." How parents react, she explains, is influenced by how and when they are told of the abnormality, their degree of social isolation, the type and severity of the disability, social class and education, attitudes of families and friends, and information received from and attitudes of professionals. Parents need emotional support and counseling in dealing with the initial and subsequent crises, education in learning how to care for the child's special needs, guidance in dealing with other family members, and continued interest and encouragement.

According to Allen C. Crocker, Children's Hospital Medical Center, Boston, there are many emotions generated in the sister or brother of a disabled child, including "anxiety, concern, curiosity, protectiveness, frustration, sorrow, grief, longing, unhappiness, jealousy, and resentment. The elements of stress assuredly exist and are troubling to consider."

Many professionals urge special support for siblings, and value the role of self-help groups for parents, siblings, and other family members. Such groups can help resolve problems and feelings, serve as a socializing agency for all concerned, and provide a way to reach out to others in similar situations. Also, these SUPPORT GROUPS provide an important exchange of resources and often become an important force for obtaining services through legislation and social pressure.

In some cases, it may be an elderly parent who becomes disabled. Coping mechanisms for relieving the anxieties of the situation include obtaining professional guidance and social support.

See also COPING; GENERAL ADAPTATION SYNDROME; PARENTING; SELF-ESTEEM.

Milunsky, Aubrey, ed., *Coping with Crisis and Handicap* (New York: Plenum Press, 1981).

disease, fear of Fear of disease (or illness) is known as nosemaphobia or nosophobia.

See also CANCER, FEAR OF; HYPOCHONDRIASIS; ILLNESS PHOBIA.

disease, fear of definite Fear of a definite disease is known as monopathophobia.

See also HYPOCHONDRIASIS; ILLNESS PHOBIA.

dishabillophobia Fear of undressing in front of someone.

See also UNDRESSING IN FRONT OF SOMEONE, FEAR OF.

disorder, fear of Fear of disorder or disarray is known as ataxiophobia. Some obsessive-compulsives have this phobia.

See also OBSESSIVE-COMPULSIVE DISORDER.

disorientation A state of mental confusion with respect to time, place, objects, or identity of self or other persons. Disorientation sometimes occurs in ANXIETY and AGORAPHOBIA.

displacement An unconscious DEFENSE MECHANISM by which one transfers an unacceptable idea or impulse to an acceptable one. For example, a man who fears his own hostile impulses might transfer that fear to knives, guns, or other objects that might be used as weapons. Displacement in psychoanalytic terms is the mechanism by which unconscious fears are transferred to neutral or nonthreatening (but often symbolic) objects, people, or situations.

dissociation A mental process in which thoughts and attitudes unconsciously lose their normal relationships to each other or to the rest of the personality and split off to function somewhat independently. Psychoanalytically, this is a defense mechanism that prevents conflict between logically incompatible thoughts, feelings, and attitudes. It is common for phobic individuals to have the experience of dissociation during periods of intense anxiety and panic. A chronic state of dissociation is usually regarded as pathological. Dissociative disorders are a group of disorders characterized by a sudden, temporary alteration in normal functions of consciousness. These include multiple or "split" personality, depersonalization disorder, certain delusional symptoms, somnambulism (sleepwalking), and hysterical amnesia.

See also DEPERSONALIZATION; NEUROSIS; SCHIZOPHRENIA.

dissociative identity disorders   See MULTIPLE PERSONALITY DISORDER.

dis-stress   Hans Selye (1907–82), an Austrian-born Canadian endocrinologist, differentiated between the unpleasant or harmful variety of stress called *dis-stress* (from the Latin *dis,* "bad," as in *dissonance, disagreement*), and *eustress* (from the Greek *eu,* "good," as in *euphonia, euphoria*). During both dis-stress and eustress the body undergoes virtually the same nonspecific responses to various stimuli acting upon it. However, certain emotional factors, such as frustration and hostility are particularly likely to turn stress into dis-stress. Anxieties and fear reactions are also likely to be associated with feelings of dis-stress. Ironically, Selye preferred the term *strain* to describe what we have come to call the "stress" reaction, but his translation skills were not sufficient to recognize this subtle difference in meaning.

See also EUSTRESS; COPING; GENERAL ADAPTATION SYNDROME; STRESS.

Selye, Hans, *Stress Without Distress* (New York: Lippincott, 1974).
———, *The Stress of Life,* Rev. ed. (New York: McGraw Hill, 1978).

diversity   Relates to any group of people that is mixed in terms of race, religion, ethnicity, and gender. Because diversity may be perceived as an approach to quotas in schools or in the workplace, the concept can be a source of anxiety for those involved. Anxieties can also arise between individuals from diverse backgrounds because of cultural differences. Respect for, and understanding of, these differences can make diversity a successful concept in business, religious, or community activities.

It is effective for businesses to have diversity in their workforces because no business can afford to ignore any population segment. Companies dependent on direct sales to customers must pay attention to the differing cultures in their marketplace. Additionally, the business management process can benefit from the imagination and creativity generated from diverse viewpoints.

Conducting diversity awareness workshops is one way companies have introduced the idea of valuing personal differences. However, these workshops are only a first step in creating an environment in which previous prejudices are erased and a true sensitivity to diverse employee needs prevails.

See also ACCULTURATION; COMMUNICATION; CULTURAL INFLUENCES; WORKPLACE.

diving, fear of   Fear of diving may be related to a fear of WATER, fear of DEPTHS, fear of swimming, or fear of DROWNING. It may also be related to a fear of the UNKNOWN because often the diver does not know the depth of the water he may enter. Fear of diving for deep-sea divers is related to a fear of getting the "bends," a physical condition that occurs when a diver surfaces too quickly.

The "deep dive" in literature (e.g., the dive taken by the whale in *Moby Dick*) is a universal symbol of moving into the unconscious, dark side, or mysterious aspects of one's life that are frightening because unknown.

See also BENDS, FEAR OF.

divorce   The legal ending of a MARRIAGE, a situation from which numerous anxieties and fears usually arise. Husband, wife, children, and even grandparents are affected by the dissolution of a marriage in the family. Divorce is a serious social problem in the United States; during the 1990s, about half of all U.S. marriages ended in divorce.

Women and men who seek divorce do so because they have one or more of many sources of anxiety in their marriage, such as infidelity, poor sexual relations, difficulties in communicating with each other, differences in goals, or financial problems. Feelings of failure are common when a marriage breaks up; lack of success in the marriage should not reflect on a partner's sense SELF-ESTEEM, but it does. While many divorced individuals learn from their experiences and bring new insights to new relationships, some will experience second or third divorces.

Divorced people are commonly angry with each other, feel that perhaps they have been exploited, treated badly, and suspect infidelities. Depending on what triggered the ANGER, it may not be easy to forget. However, if appropriately contained, one's anger will not interfere with adjusting to a new life.

According to Ada P. Kahn, in "Divorce: For Better Not for Worse," published by the Mental Health Association of Greater Chicago, studies show that when parents are incompatible, children do not feel that keeping the marriage together on their behalf is a gift. There is no advantage for children when parents stay in a marriage in which they are constantly stressed and cannot resolve basic issues.

Kahn advises telling children why you are getting a divorce, that it was a rational decision by both parties, deliberately and carefully undertaken with reluctance and with full recognition of how stressful it would be. Children have the right to know why, with an explanation suited to their age and level of understanding. Parents should try to communicate what divorce will mean for the children, specifically, how it will affect their visiting and living arrangements. They should be assured that they have parental support, permission to love both parents, and that both parents will continue to love them. Assurances that the children are not responsible for the rupture and that they are not responsible to heal the rupture should come from both parents. More complex explanations are in order in cases of desertion or abuse.

As a consequence of divorce, many children feel a diminished sense of being parented, because their parents are less available, emotionally, physically, or both. Children may feel that they are losing both parents. This is a predictable aspect of the divorce experience. In most instances, it is temporary, but in a significant number of families, it is a feeling that lasts a long time.

The most serious long-range effect is that children feel less protected in their growing up years and may become fearful that they will repeat their parents' inability to sustain a relationship. To address this issue, parents should talk about it or be ready to talk when children ask questions. They should not continue to fight with their ex-spouse, and should never criticize former mates in front of the children. Parents should realize that they remain role models after divorce.

Divorced individuals do marry again. However, according to the Center for the Family, Corte Madera, California, in the mid-1990s, 60 percent of second marriages failed, particularly if one or more of the mates brought children into the marriage.

DATING and meeting new people after divorce brings anxieties about acquiring a sexually transmitted disease, because of the prevalence of AIDS (ACQUIRED IMMUNE DEFICIENCY SYNDROME) and STDs (SEXUALLY TRANSMITTED DISEASES).

Rebuilding life after divorce may be stressful, complicated, and difficult. The best advice is to take one step at a time and start by choosing one step you really need or would like to take. Newly divorced people can seek out resources for their particular anxieties in their community, where there are churches, synagogues, and community mental health agencies that may be able to help.

Divorce differs from annulment, in which a court declares that a marriage has been invalid from its beginning; reasons for annulment vary between states and countries.

See also COMMUNICATION; COPING.

Kahn, Ada P., and Holt, Linda Hughey, *The A–Z of Women's Sexuality* (Alameda, Calif.: Hunter House Publications, 1992).

Wallerstein, Judith S., *Second Chances: Men, Women, and Children a Decade After Divorce* (New York: Ticknor & Fields, 1989).

dizziness, fear of   Fear of dizziness is known as dinophobia. Many who experience dizziness as a result of phobias fear the dizziness as much as the frightening event that brings it on. Dizziness may also be part of a combination of anxiety-induced gastrointestinal effects, which include nausea and possibly diarrhea and vomiting. It is also a prime symptom of HYPERVENTILATION.

Dizziness as a symptom of anxiety has been treated with behavior therapy and, at times, appropriate medication. Dizziness may be related to a disturbance of the inner ear; therapy may include diagnosis and treatment by an otolaryngologist (eye, ear, nose, and throat specialist).

Dizziness involves a feeling of being unsteady, lightheaded, or faint and a sensation of spinning, turning, falling in space, or of standing still while objects around are moving. During a phobic reaction or a PANIC ATTACK, an individual may HYPERVENTILATE (breathe more than they need to). This results in a drop in the carbon dioxide in the blood, causing constriction of blood vessels in the brain, leading to dizziness or fainting. Hyperventilation is sometimes caused by a physical condition, but is often the result of stress, anxiety, worry, or panic attacks. Chronic jaw tension can also cause dizziness.

Dizziness also may accompany seasickness. Some sailors advise keeping one's eyes on the horizon to give one a steady spot to watch. In most cases, dizziness disappears when the individual sets foot on land. Dizziness as a result of intoxication with alcohol usually subsides after a period of sleep.

There are prescription drugs as well some over-the-counter remedies available to help control dizziness. When dizziness occurs often, a physician should be consulted, as it may be a symptom of a condition requiring medical treatment.

See also MOTION, FEAR OF; NAUSEA, FEAR OF.

doctors, fear of   Fear of doctors is known as iatrophobia. Some people who have blood-injury phobias fear doctors because they fear that the doctor may give them a shot or take a sample of their blood. Some who fear undressing in front of others may fear doctors because they are often required to disrobe and cover themselves only with a sheet during a physical examination. Some become so anxious just by being in the doctor's office that their blood pressure increases, a phenomenon known

as "white coat" hypertension. Some fear doctors because they associate doctors with illness or injury and with authority figures. Some fear getting germs or a disease from others in the waiting room. Many individuals who fear doctors and doctors' offices also fear hospitals.

Benjamin Rush (1745–1813), American physician and author, commented on doctor phobia: "This distemper is often complicated with other diseases. It arises, in some instances, from the dread of taking physic, or of submitting to the remedies of bleeding and blistering. In some instances I have known it occasioned by a desire of sick people to deceive themselves, by being kept in ignorance of the danger of their disorders. It might be supposed that, 'the dread of a long bill' was one cause of the Doctor Phobia; but this excites terror in the minds of but few people; for who ever thinks of paying a doctor, while he can use his money to advantage in another way! It is remarkable this Doctor Phobia always goes off as soon as a patient is sensible of his danger. The doctor, then, becomes an object of respect and attachment, instead of horror."

See also HOSPITALS, FEAR OF; WHITE COAT HYPERTENSION.

Runes, D. D., ed., *The Selected Writings of Benjamin Rush* (New York: The Philosophical Library, 1947).

dogs, fear of   Fear of dogs is known as cynophobia. Many people are afraid of dogs because of their jackal and wolf ancestry, their tendencies to be noisy, destructive, and dirty, or because of childhood experiences of being bitten or fearing being bitten. The bark of a dog is frightening to many people, although reassuring to the master who uses the dog, with his protective loyalty, as a burglar alarm. Because of the dog's potential ferocity, combined with the ability to form rapport with humans, dogs are used extensively in police work, instilling fear in all targets of the hunt.

Society has long had a somewhat ambivalent attitude toward dogs, seeing them as both fearsome, unpleasant animals and friend and protectors. Some biblical references reinforce these ideas. Passages in the Old Testament reflect a feeling that the dog is unclean, sinful, and stupid, and Christian tradition sometimes associates dogs with heresy and paganism. On the other hand, medieval Christian art depicts dogs as symbols of watchfulness and fidelity. Dogs are associated with several of the saints.

See also ANIMALS, FEAR OF.

dogs as anxiety therapy   Recent research has reinforced what many people have known for thousands of years: that dogs and other pets can help reduce anxieties in humans and contribute to the human's improvement in physical and mental health. Studies in nursing homes with dogs as pets have indicated reductions in blood pressure and faster recoveries from illnesses when individuals care for or regularly observe the actions of a pet. Dogs provide comfort and stability, and the love they offer is unquestioning and unconditional, unlike close human relationships. Caring for a dog provides the owner with an opportunity for exercise and an object of affection that is totally dependent on and devoted to him. In many cases, the dog gives the owner a sense of self-worth and identity that might otherwise be missing from life. Also, the gluttonous, lustful, comic behavior of dogs is not only entertaining but also allows the inhibited human master to experience release and humor.

dolls, fear of   Fear of dolls is known as pediophobia. The fixed, staring eyes of a doll frighten some people. This feeling may be related to a common fear of being stared at or a sense that the lifeless eyes of a doll resemble those of a corpse. Doll phobia frequently extends to fear of other lifeless models of the human figure, such as mannequins, wax figures, statues, and ventriloquists' dummies. Fear of dolls may also stem from certain magical practices and beliefs. A very ancient practice of Voodoo and witchcraft involves trying to cause harm to an enemy by piercing or burning a doll made to resemble him or her.

See also VOODOO, FEAR OF.

domatophobia   Fear of being in a house.

See also HOUSE, FEAR OF.

domestic violence   Abuse of spouses, children, or parents. This may take the form of wife-battering, child abuse, INCEST, or elder abuse. Abuse may also be verbal or emotional. All of these situations produce anxieties for the victims as well as others in the family. The abuser may behave violently as a response to particular anxieties in his or her life.

Domestic violence happens in all strata of society, and there are many more cases than official records indicate because it is a subject often covered up out of fear and shame. Characteristics of persons who are victims of family violence include ANXIETY, powerlessness, GUILT, and lack of SELF-ESTEEM.

Professionals who treat victims of family violence are concerned with getting the victims, usually women or children, away from the abuser and into therapy before the abuse becomes too severe and additional stressors arise. Some perpetrators as well as victims of family violence compound their difficulties with use of alcohol or drugs.

Battered Women

Battered women are victims of physical assault by husbands, boyfriends, or lovers. Battering may include physical abuse sometimes for purposes of sexual gratification, such as breaking bones, burning, whipping, mutilation, and other sadistic acts. Generally, however, battering is considered part of a syndrome of abusive behavior that has very little to do with sexual issues. Drug and alcohol-related problems are more common among families with battering behaviors. Women who selected and choose to remain in abusive relationships were also often abused as children. Many women stay in such relationships without reporting the abuse and without seeking counseling. Batterers often were abused themselves as children.

Women who are abused by their husbands or boyfriends not only sustain injuries from physical beatings but also suffer from many mental and emotional scars, including POST-TRAUMATIC STRESS SYNDROME, DEPRESSION, and anxiety.

Help for battered wives is available. First, physical protection, often provided by women's shelters within the community, must be assured for the woman and her children. Second, social support services must provide economic protection, since women often stay in abusive relationships due to lack of practical economic alternatives. Finally, psychotherapeutic intervention should be aimed at both batterer and victim to trace antecedents of the violent behavior, correct substance abuse problems, and substitute positive coping mechanisms for violent behavior patterns.

Most abused women do not seek help until beatings become severe and have occurred over a period of time, often two to three years. Some women are too embarrassed or believe that if they report the beating to police they will not be taken seriously. The majority of women who seek help because of family violence are between age 20 and 60. In 75 percent of households in which abuse takes place, the husband or boyfriend is an alcoholic or on drugs.

A study at the University of California—San Francisco during 1992 indicated many details about living conditions and circumstances surrounding battered women. According to the study, the battered women who were interviewed did not depend on their violent partner for most of their financial support; almost 30 percent had jobs and many had income from families, welfare, Social Security, and other sources.

Among other findings, 40 percent of the women had to be hospitalized for injuries. One in three of the women had been attacked with a weapon, most often a knife or a club; four had been shot. One in 10 was pregnant when beaten; 30 percent of the group said they had been abused before they were pregnant. In about half the cases, the husbands or boyfriends drank heavily or abused drugs; 86 percent of the women had been beaten at least once before.

According to Kevin J. Fullin, M.D., St. Catherine's Hospital, Kenosha, Wisconsin, as many as one in two women has suffered from an episode of domestic violence sometime in her life. Due to such a high rate, physicians and health care workers are developing new approaches to domestic violence in order to increase its detection. The goal is to properly identify anyone who comes to a hospital with a domestic abuse situation. The woman, child, or adult who is suspected of being abused is questioned in a nonthreatening, nonjudgmental manner without any other family members present. The goal of this confidential questioning is to find the real cause of the problem and do something to stop the abuse.

WHAT BATTERED WOMEN CAN DO

Leave the scene of the abuse; stay with a friend or family member who will be supportive emotionally and provide a safe haven.

Leave the home when the abuser is absent to eliminate confrontation.

Take bank records, children's birth certificates, cash, and other information documents along with clothing and personal items.

If possible, photograph or videotape any consequences of abuse, such as injuries to yourself or damage to the home. These could be important for possible later court proceedings.

Call the police and file a police report. Obtain an order of protection as soon as possible.

Seek counseling for yourself and your children; join a SUPPORT GROUP along with others who have been victims of family violence.

Battered Child Syndrome

Battered child syndrome includes rough physical handling by caregivers resulting in injuries to a baby or child. This can result in failure to grow, a disability, and sometimes death of the baby or child. Studies have shown that parents who repeatedly injure or beat their babies and children have poor CONTROL of their own feelings of AGGRESSION, or may have been abused or psychologically rejected as children.

The syndrome is found among people with stable social and financial backgrounds as well as in parents who are mentally unstable, or alcoholic, or drug-dependent. In most states, laws require physicians to report instances of suspected willfully inflicted injury among young patients. When it appears that the children will continue to be battered, steps are taken to remove them from the home.

See also ADDICTION; ALCOHOLISM; CODEPENDENCY; COPING.

Domical   See AMITRIPTYLINE.

doorknob phobia   Fear of touching a doorknob. A doorknob may produce an avoidance reaction because the individual may believe that it is dirty, or that it has germs on it. Doorknob fear may be a fear of contamination. Also, an individual may fear something that may be on the other side of the door, such as a crowd, darkness, a feared object, etc. From the psychoanalytic point of view, the individual who avoids touching doorknobs is protecting himself against an anal-erotic wish to be dirty or to soil. In magic, the characteristics of an object are communicated by touching it.

See also ANAL STAGE; CONTAMINATION, FEAR OF; DEVELOPMENTAL STAGES; DIRT, FEAR OF; FREUD, SIGMUND.

Campbell, Robert J., *Psychiatric Dictionary* (New York: Oxford University Press, 1981).

dopamine   A precursor of the neurotransmitter NOREPINEPHRINE. The role of dopamine in producing anxiety has been studied less than other NEUROTRANSMITTERS. However, some research indicates some role for dopamine in the cause of anxiety.

doraphobia   Fear of the SKIN OF ANIMALS.

dothiepin   An antidepressant drug.
See also ANTIDEPRESSANTS; DEPRESSION.

double-bind theory   A theory proposed by Gregory Bateson (1904–80), a British-American anthropologist and philosopher, to explain causes of anxieties, phobias, and schizophrenia. A double bind is a breakdown in communications—for example, a situation in which a child receives contradictory messages from one or both parents and is therefore torn between conflicting feelings and demands. According to Bateson, there are at least two levels of communication present in every message. One of these is the content level, and the other is the intuitive feeling component that is nonverbal. In healthy dialogue, these levels are compatible, whereas in unhealthy dialogue involving a double bind they are inconsistent and contradictory.

See also NEUROSIS.

double-blind   A research term used in some studies of ANXIETIES and PHOBIAS. A double-blind study is one in which a number of treatments, usually one or more drugs and/or a placebo, are compared in such a way that neither the individual treated nor the persons directly involved in planning the treatment know which preparation is being administered. An example of a double-blind study is one in which depressed, phobic individuals with many common characteristics are divided into two groups; one group is treated with an antidepressant drug that has known effects and the other group is treated with a newer, experimental drug. Many pharmaceutical products for anxieties and DEPRESSION, as well as many other medical conditions, are evaluated in double-blind studies. While the double-blind is a minimum condition for drug studies, it is often insufficient in that treatment groups may show an obvious drug reaction whereas control (placebo) groups show no behavior.

double vision, fear of   Fear of double vision is known as diplopiaphobia. The fear may be founded on a feeling of losing control of one's environment. Double vision may be due to a muscle imbalance or to paralysis of certain eye muscles as a result of inflammation, hemorrhage, or infection. Double vision can be demonstrated by holding two objects straight in front of the eyes, one behind the other. Focusing on the more distant object makes the near object appear double; focusing on the near object makes the more distant object appear double. Double vision can usually be overcome with eye exercises, appropriate eyeglasses, or, in severe cases, muscle surgery.

Unusual fears such as this are sometimes also delusional manifestations of underlying psychosis.

See also EYES, FEAR OF; PSYCHOSIS.

downsizing   Refers to employee cutbacks (layoffs) and the practice of not filling the positions vacated. Downsizing causes anxieties for the managers who must decide who will go and who will stay and for the employees who are asked to leave.

In many cases, the anxieties involved in downsizing leave workers vulnerable to ANGER and

DEPRESSION. To help workers avoid and/or handle anger, such issues as job category, seniority, and performance, must be addressed. Equally important issues include treatment of dismissed employees, positive employee recommendations, and dealing with surviving employees.

Most companies now consider downsizing or employee cutbacks as a routine part of business. As they become more and more an everyday occurrence, the very idea of downsizing brings about anxieties for many workers. In 1994, an American Management Association (AMA) survey of 713 companies showed that 30 percent of companies reporting a downsizing planned to repeat the exercise. Respondees gave business downturn, improved staff utilization, transfer of production or work, automation or other new technology, merger or acquisition, and plant or office obsolescence as reasons for downsizing.

With downsizing, workers at all levels are affected, no matter how long they may have worked for the organization, no matter how well they perform their job, or how effectively they have managed their budget and staff. Of the 430,000 identified jobs eliminated by AMA respondents since July 1988, half belonged to hourly workers and half belonged to salaried workers.

Signs of impending downsizing include a hiring freeze, pessimistic budget projections, closed-door meetings, decreasing sales, and consolidation of operations. Middle managers should be particularly alert to requests for department justification and work plans based on budget reductions.

See also WORKPLACE.

Meyer, G. J., *Executive Blues: Down and Out in Corporate America* (New York: Franklin Square Press, 1995).

drafts or draughts, fear of   Fear of drafts is known as aerophobia or anemophobia. Individuals who fear drafts may fear movement, or movement of air, or wind. They may also fear illness, because many people believe that they can get a cold or influenza from sitting in a draft.

See also AIR, FEAR OF; ILLNESS PHOBIA; WIND, FEAR OF.

dreams, fear of   Fear of dreams is known as oneirophobia. Dreaming is a type of thinking that goes on when one is asleep. Dreams are characterized by vivid sensory images, mostly visual, but also involving hearing, motion, touch, and even taste or smell. Since a dreamer accepts a dream as real while he is experiencing it, dreams are a form of hallucination. People are afraid of particular dreams or of nightmares or a sense of losing willful control at night. Fear of dreams can also be connected with nightmare experiences or fright upon awakening.

Psychiatrists believe that dreams serve as a safety valve, permitting partial discharge of repressed, instinctual drive energies, especially the unconscious wishes from the infantile past. Further, Freud believed that dreams preserve sleep through many mechanisms, including displacement and condensation, inhibiting and suppressing disturbing emotions.

Pavor nocturnus are anxiety dreams in the form of nightmares; they are common in young children. For adults and children, phobias may emerge during dreams.

Freud designated a number of dreams that almost everyone has dreamed, and they seem to have the same meaning for everyone. Included in this category are embarrassing dreams of being naked, dreams of the death of loved ones, dreams of flying and falling, examination dreams, dreams of missing a train, tooth extraction, and water and fire dreams.

Dreams are an important part of one's psychic and physical life. Psychically or psychologically, they represent conscious and unconscious preoccupations, conflicts, unresolved fears, and events that either have happened or are to happen. They are symbolic monitors of one's psychological life and therefore can provide important information and direction to those who ponder their symbolic relevance.

Physically, the dream occurs during times of rapid eye movement (REM). Each person goes through three or four periods of REM or dream sleep each night. Depression, stress, drug use, and sleep deprivation or disruption often interfere with REM time or occurrence, and REM time has to be recovered at another sleep period. Important biochemical changes occur at REM and non-REM times that are necessary to normal daytime functioning.

See also CONDENSATION; DISPLACEMENT; DREAM SYMBOLS; INCUBUS; PAVOR NOCTURNUS; POST-TRAUMATIC STRESS DISORDER; SUCCUBUS; WET DREAMS.

dream symbols   In psychoanalytic terms, images in dreams are symbols of unconscious things, objects, or functions. For example, a snake appearing in a dream is conscious, but its meaning is unconscious. Dream symbols may refer to the male and female sexual organs, to birth, death, family members, and primary body functions. Water often symbolizes birth, the mind, and the unconscious. Through interpretations of symbols, a therapist may assist an individual in understanding the causes of his or her phobias and anxieties. Carl Jung pointed out that many dream symbols have universal or archetypal meaning. He pointed out that all the mental energy and interest devoted today by western man to science and technology were, by ancient man, once dedicated to the study of mythology.

See also DREAMS; PSYCHOANALYSIS; SYMBOLISM.

drink, fear of   Fear of taking a drink, or drinking, is known as potophobia. The individual fears swallowing liquid and possibly choking and losing the ability to breathe.

See also CHOKING, FEAR OF; SWALLOWING, FEAR OF.

drinking alcohol, fear of   Fear of drinking alcohol is known as dipsophobia, dipsomanophobia, alcoholophobia, and potophobia. The fear is of ill effects and the body changes that are uncontrollable.

driving a car, fear of   Many adults have anxieties while driving. Some individuals actually become phobic about driving and cannot get into the driver's seat without experiencing rapid heart rate, higher blood pressure, faster breathing, and sweating. Some individuals fear driving alone; some fear driving in the dark, on deserted roads, on open highways, or on crowded expressways. Some fear merging into fast-moving freeway or expressway lanes. Fears related to driving a car can be overcome with appropriate behavior therapy. Fears of driving a car may be related to agoraphobia, particularly if they relate to traveling a distance from a safe place such as home. Fears of vehicles are known as amaxophobia or ochophobia.

The fear of driving can occur after an accident or with traumatic conditioning or as part of an agoraphobic symptom. Fear of driving is prevalent in the United States but less common in countries that rely on other forms of transportation. For example, the fear of trains is more prevalent in England.

Fear of driving may be specific to freeways, busy surface streets, or any street (even quiet residential). In its most severe forms, the individual cannot even sit in an automobile without experiencing anxiety.

See also AUTOMOBILES, FEAR OF DRIVING.

dromophobia   Fear of crossing streets or wandering about is known as dromophobia.

See also STREETS, FEAR OF CROSSING.

drowning, fear of   Fear of drowning is a common fear of individuals who fear WATER. Some fear drowning so much that they will not enter a swimming pool or body of water. Some will not go out in boats. Even if life jackets are available to them, drowning phobics avoid situations in which they might become immersed in water. Some have a PANIC ATTACK when their head goes underwater or even if they get water in their nose or mouth. Fear of drowning is related to a fear of being out of control; most drowning phobics are not good swimmers and fear not being able to save themselves. However, some excellent swimmers have severe fears of drowning and will only swim when others are nearby or will swim only in shallow water. Some swimmers fear DIVING because they fear they will drown. Fear of drowning is a fear of DEATH.

See also LOSS OF CONTROL, FEAR OF.

drug effects   Because we now have a better understanding of how the brain works, drugs have been developed that can alter specific aspects of brain chemistry. Three classes of drugs are known to relieve panic attacks. Two are ANTIDEPRESSANTS—

MONOAMINE OXIDASE INHIBITORS (MAOIs) and TRI-CYCLIC ANTIDEPRESSANTS—and the third is a newer category, BENZODIAZEPINES (for example, alprazolam and diazepam). In research situations, individuals who suffer panic attacks experience less fear if they receive these drugs before they receive lactate infusions because the drugs may change the individual's metabolism, eliminating their abnormal sensitivity to lactate. MAOIs and tricyclics increase levels of the neurotransmitter norepinephrine. Most tricyclic antidepressants decrease activity of the LOCUS CERULEUS (an organ in the brain containing many neurotransmitters), perhaps due to increased availability of noradrenaline at autoreceptor sites. However, because antidepressants affect a wide range of NEUROTRANSMITTERS, many of which have been implicated as causes of anxiety, this mechanism cannot be proved. Antipanic drugs relieve anxiety symptoms, but they may have some undesirable side effects, such as high blood pressure or drowsiness.

The benzodiazepines are used for treating generalized anxiety disorder and have effects resembling those of classical sedatives, such as barbiturates or meprobamatelike drugs. These effects include muscle relaxation, anticonvulsive action, and sedation proceeding to hypnosis.

Drug Abuse

Some individuals turn to drugs in the belief that they can better cope with their anxieties or depression by using drugs to change their moods and attitudes. Generally, drug abuse occurs when individuals self-prescribe; however, some individuals also misuse substances prescribed by physicians by taking too many doses, or taking them in combination with other medications. Because drugs used to relieve symptoms of anxiety and depression have strong effects on neurotransmitters in the brain, close monitoring by a physician is necessary.

Drug Dependence

Individuals who depend on drugs to help them cope with their anxieties, phobias, or depression may develop a dependence on drugs. Dependence refers to a craving or compulsion to continue using a drug because it gives a feeling of well-being and satisfaction. The term habituation is frequently used interchangeably with the term psychological

dependence. An individual can be psychologically dependent on a drug and not physically dependent; the reverse is also true. Dependence can occur after a period of prolonged use of a drug, and the characteristics of dependence vary according to the drug involved.

See also ALPRAZOLAM; ANTIDEPRESSANTS, NEW; CARBON DIOXIDE SENSITIVITY; LACTATE-INFUSED ANXIETY; NORADRENERGIC SYSTEM.

drugs, fear of new   Fear of new drugs is known as neopharmaphobia. Individuals who have this fear do not want to take any medication that is categorized as experimental. They feel safer taking drugs that have been tried and proven effective for their particular disorder. They may fear toxic effects, or adverse interactions with other drugs. Such individuals may question their physicians closely about the track record of drugs being prescribed. Many drugs used for anxiety and depression are relatively new. Fearful people can be assured that such new drugs would not be commercially available if they had not first passed fairly rigorous scrutiny during clinical testing with large numbers of patients.

drugs, fear of taking   Fear of taking drugs is known as pharmacophobia. Some individuals have this fear because they are afraid of becoming dependent on drugs, or they fear that the drugs may cause them some harmful side effects, or they fear swallowing pills. A fear of taking drugs may be related to a general fear of doctors, hospitals, and health professionals.

See also DOCTORS, FEAR OF; ILLNESS PHOBIA.

drugs as treatment   See ANTICHOLINERGICS; ANTICONVULSIVES; ANTIDEPRESSANTS; ANTIHISTAMINES; ANXIETY DRUGS; DRUG EFFECTS; LITHIUM; MONOAMINE OXIDASE INHIBITORS (MAOIS); TRICYCLIC ANTIDEPRESSANTS; WITHDRAWAL EFFECTS OF ADDICTIVE SUBSTANCES.

dry mouth   Dry mouth is a common symptom of fear, along with a "lump in the throat." In many cultures, there was a test for witchcraft that consisted of asking the suspect to put a pebble in the mouth; if the pebble was dry when it was taken out, it indicated fear and thus the guilt of the suspect.

Dry mouth is a common side effect of some medications, particularly certain ANTIDEPRESSANTS. The sensation may make the patient uncomfortable and lead to NAUSEA or lack of interest in eating. Dry mouth can be helped, to some degree, by sucking on mints or drinking fluids frequently.

See also ADVERSE DRUG EFFECTS.

dryness, fear of   Fear of dryness and dry places is known as xerophobia. This fear may be related to a fear of lack of water or of landscape.

See also AIR, FEAR OF; LANDSCAPE, FEAR OF.

DSM IV-R   See *DIAGNOSTIC AND STATISTICAL MANUAL OF MENTAL DISORDERS.*

dual-sex therapy   A form of PSYCHOTHERAPY developed by William Masters and Virginia Johnson to treat a particular sexual disorder or fear. In a "round-table session", the male and female therapy team suggest specific exercises for the couple to diminish fears felt by both sexes. Therapy also includes suggestions for improvement in communication in sexual and nonsexual areas. The use of "dual" therapists helps clients feel more at ease since for each partner there is a same-sex therapist.

See also FRIGIDITY; IMPOTENCE; PSYCHOSEXUAL ANXIETIES; SEX THERAPY; SEXUAL FEARS.

duration, fear of   Fear of the duration of an event, or a long block of time, is known as CHRONOPHOBIA. This is a common fear of persons who are imprisoned, or those on long trips. Some have this fear during a school semester or a long academic program.

See also TIME, FEAR OF.

dust, fear of   Fear of dust is known as amathophobia or koniophobia. Some phobics who fear contamination and germs also fear dust. Some who fear dust may keep the windows in their houses closed at all times and install elaborate air-filtering equipment. Some wipe surfaces in their homes frequently and clean their homes thoroughly. Fear of dust may become an obsession with some individuals and may be a symptom of OBSESSIVE-COMPULSIVE DISORDER.

dying, fear of   See DEATH, FEAR OF.

dysfunctional family   This term indicates that the developmental and emotional needs of one or more members of a family are not being met, which may lead to anxieties for all concerned.

Research has shown that people raised in dysfunctional families—where alcohol or drug abuse, emotional or physical abuse, neglect, incest, marital conflict, or severe workaholism were present—carry varying vestiges of these problems well into adulthood. These issues generally surface in intimate relationships and on the job. Since these are places where other kinds of anxieties and stress can be found, unresolved family issues can compound the mental health issues.

People from dysfunctional families usually are excellent employees. They are hard workers, dependable, resourceful, loyal, kind—attributes that have helped them survive their earlier experiences. However, because people from dysfunctional families have often not learned to feel good about themselves, they may have poor SELF-ESTEEM, compensate by working longer hours than others, try for PERFECTION, and take on more than they can handle. This leads to even more stress that impacts their job performance and physical health.

Causes of Dysfunctional Relationships

Often, the basic problem is lack of COMMUNICATION or poor communications between family members, even though they live in the same household. An example of a dysfunctional family is one in which marital conflict between parents manifests itself in the aggressive behavior in school of their young child. The family may come to the attention of a school nurse because of the behavior problems of the child, which may be a symptom of the dysfunction at home. The parents may be unaware that their behavior is causing a great deal of stress for the child.

In a dysfunctional family, there is little emphasis on encouraging each child to develop AUTONOMY. An example is a family that expects its adolescent child to obey curfew rules appropriate for a younger child.

Dysfunctional families usually do not communicate constructively when they are having difficult times. For example, when a child becomes seriously ill, there may be little communication about the illness between family members, and this leads to unexpressed feelings of guilt. Alcoholism and substance abuse tends to be a characteristic of dysfunctional families, as the substance abuser cannot be depended on to fulfill expectations.

Family therapy is helpful in improving life situations for members of dysfunctional families. In therapy, family members learn to improve their communication skills and learn new coping skills to deal with everyday problems, phobias and fears, as well as major life events.

See ALCOHOLISM; AGGRESSION; COPING; FAMILY; INTIMACY; PSYCHOTHERAPIES; RELATIONSHIPS; STRESS.

dysmenorrhea   See MENSTRUATION.

dysmorphophobia   Fear of a specific bodily defect that is not noticeable to others. Several parts of the body may be involved including faces, breasts, hips, and noses. Dysmorphophobics also complain of body or limbs being too small or too large, misshapen or wrinkled, and of bad odors (imagined) coming from the mouth, underarm sweat, genitals, or the rectum. Sufferers may try to conceal the body part about which they are self-conscious— for example, wearing long hair to hide imagined floppy ears or wearing dark glasses to cover wrinkles around the eyes. Some fear looking in mirrors because they become anxious and upset when they see themselves. These disorders are categorized in DSM-IV as body dysmorphic disorders.

See also DEFORMITY, FEAR OF.

dyspareunia, fear of   Fear of painful vaginal SEXUAL INTERCOURSE. This is a common fear of some women. If they have experienced pain in the past, they may fear recurrence of the pain. The pain may be caused by a local irritation, such as from a spermicide or the material of a condom or diaphragm, or by an infection such as moniliasis (yeast) or trichomonas.

A woman who has had little experience with intercourse may feel pain when the penis enters her vagina because of an inadequately stretched hymen. Some women experience pain when the penis contacts their cervix (the neck of the uterus). This pain can be avoided by a change in position or less deep penetration. A pain that is felt deep in the pelvis may come from endometriosis, ovarian tumors or cysts, or some other condition that should be investigated and treated by a physician. Also, ANXIETY, tension, and a lack of stimulation before actual penetration may contribute to a painful experience. With sufficient foreplay (stimulation) before intercourse, the vaginal walls secrete lubricating fluid that will make intercourse more comfortable. After menopause and during breast-feeding secretions may not be sufficient, and a water-soluble jelly may be used as a lubricant. Use of such a lubricant may reduce the woman's fear of discomfort and pain.

Fears of disease and injury are associated with fear of pain during sexual intercourse; the pain also triggers fears of the UNKNOWN. Some fears can be allayed with a better understanding of human anatomy. A woman's pain during sexual intercourse also arouses fears in the male partner that he may be injuring her.

See also PSYCHOSEXUAL ANXIETIES; SEXUAL FEARS.

dysthymic disorder   A chronic emotional disturbance involving depressed mood (or irritable mood in children or adolescents) that lasts most of the day and occurs more days than not for at least two years (one year for children and adolescents). The disorder is also known as dysthymia. During periods of depressed mood, the individual may experience anxiety, poor appetite or overeating, inability to sleep or oversleeping, low energy and fatigue, low self-esteem, poor concentration or difficulty making decisions, and feelings of hopelessness. In making a diagnosis it is difficult to distinguish between dysthymia and major depression, as the two disorders share similar symptoms and differ only in duration and severity. Dysthymia usually begins in childhood, adolescence, or early adult life, with a clear onset. Impairment in social and occupational functioning is usually mild or moderate because the condition is chronic rather than severe, as depression may be. In children and adolescents, social interaction with peers and adults frequently is affected; children with depression may react negatively or shyly to praise and may respond to positive relationships with negative behaviors, such as resentment or anger. Children who have this disorder may not perform and progress well in school. Dysthymia is more common in females than males, although in children it occurs equally frequently in both sexes. It is slightly more common among first-degree biologic relatives of people who have depression than among the general population.

See also AFFECTIVE DISORDERS; DEPRESSED PARENTS, CHILDREN OF; DEPRESSION, ADOLESCENT; MOOD.

American Psychiatric Association, *Diagnostic and Statistical Manual IV* (Washington, DC: American Psychiatric Press, 2000).

dystychiphobia Fear of accidents.
See also ACCIDENTS, FEAR OF.

earthquakes, fear of Individuals who fear earthquakes fear the shaking, rolling, or sudden shock that occurs during an earthquake. They fear losing control of themselves and their environment for the few-second duration of the quake. Some fear motion and hence fear motion of the earth. Some fear the landslides that may bury areas or change mountain shapes or the fires ignited in cities by damage to gas mains, water pipes, and power lines. Some fear falling buildings. Many fear indirect damage from an earthquake, such as falling rubble.

While most earthquakes do not cause damage, fear of earthquakes is a realistic fear in many parts of the world where earthquakes occur with some frequency and have wreaked disaster in past years. Fear of earthquakes is related to fear of the UNKNOWN. Although accurate prediction of earthquakes is almost impossible, scientists do know the regions where earthquakes are most likely to occur. Individuals who have a morbid fear of earthquakes usually avoid such areas or learn to live with their fear. Builders in such areas also fear the damage that might be caused by earthquakes and incorporate certain safety features into new buildings.

See also LOSS OF CONTROL, FEAR OF; MOTION, FEAR OF.

eaten, fear of being Fear of being eaten originates early in the oral stage of development of the infant's personality. During this stage, when the infant develops the normal aim of satisfaction and pleasure through eating, and, in a more general sense, through the incorporation of objects, frustrations relating to eating or fears of this frustration occur frequently. These anxieties take the form of a fear of being eaten, because in the infant's mind, what he feels and does will also take place in the world around him. In psychoanalytic practice, it has been found that fear of being eaten may also be a disguise for castration anxiety, distorted through regression into the older fear of being eaten.

See also DEVELOPMENTAL STAGES; ORAL STAGE; PSYCHOANALYSIS.

Campbell, Robert J., *Psychiatric Dictionary* (New York: Oxford University Press, 1981).

eating disorders Eating disorders involve compulsive misuse of food to achieve some desired physical and/or mental state. They are characterized by an intense fear of being fat and disproportionate and severe weight loss and may result in ill health and psychological impairments. In some cases, eating disorders may be related to a fear of body shape, or DYSMORPHOPHOBIA.

People who have eating disorders may be experiencing anxieties in some aspect of their lives that they think will be improved by dieting in excess, often low SELF-ESTEEM and an irrational fear of obesity. When sufferers acknowledge their compulsive behavior, their stress is often expressed in feelings of DEPRESSION and a wish to commit SUICIDE. Sufferers typically hide their illness; when family, friends, or coworkers discover their illness, they try to help. Typically, people with eating disorders feel they don't deserve to be helped, and this creates a great deal of anxieties for all concerned.

Eating disorders share common addictive features with alcohol and drug abuse, but unlike alcohol and drugs, food is essential to human life, and proper use of food is a central element of recovery.

Estimates indicate that there are 8 million reported victims of eating disorders in the United States—7 million of them women (although the number of males is increasing) between the ages of 15 and 30. Eating disorders can be cured when the sufferer accepts treatment; an estimated 6 percent of all reported cases end in fatality (usually caused by an anorexia disorder).

Anorexia Nervosa

Anorexia nervosa is a syndrome of self-starvation in which people willfully restrict intake of food out of fear of becoming fat, resulting in life-threatening weight loss. Anorexics (people who suffer from anorexia nervosa) "feel fat" even when they are at normal weight or when emaciated, deny their illness, and develop an active disgust for food. Deaths from anorexia nervosa are higher than from any other psychiatric illness.

Causes of anorexia vary widely. Many anorexics are part of a close family and have special relationships with their parents. They are highly conforming, anxious to please, and may be obsessional in their habits. There is speculation that girls who refrain from eating wish to remain "thin as a boy" in an effort to escape the burdens of growing up and assuming a female sexual and marital role. Another contribution to the increase in anorexia is contemporary society's emphasis on slimness as it relates to beauty. This is particularly prevalent in the fashion industry, with its overly thin models. Most women diet at some time, particularly athletes and dancers, who seem more prone to the disorder than other women. In some cases, anorexia nervosa is a symptom of depression, personality disorder, or even schizophrenia.

Symptoms include severe weight loss, wasting (cachexia), food preoccupation and rituals, amenorrhea (cessation of the menstrual period), and hyperactivity (constant exercising to lose weight). The anorexic may suffer from tiredness and fatigue, sensitivity to cold, and complain of hair loss.

Eating disorders sometimes result in other mental health disorders as well as depression. Individuals may suffer from withdrawal, mood swings, and feelings of shame and guilt. Both anorexics and bulimics develop rituals regarding eating and exercise. They often are perfectionists in habits, such as clothes and personal appearance, and have an "all or nothing" attitude about life.

Bulimia

Bulimia is characterized by recurrent episodes of binge eating followed by self-induced vomiting, vigorous exercise, and/or laxative and diuretic abuse to prevent weight gain. Most people view vomiting as a disagreeable experience, but to a bulimic, it is a means toward a desired goal.

Another eating disorder is bulimarexia, which is characterized by features of both anorexia nervosa and bulimia. Some individuals vacillate between anorexic and bulimic behaviors. After months and perhaps years of eating sparsely, the anorexic may crave food and begin to binge, but the fear of becoming overly fat leads her/him to vomit.

Bulimics may be of normal weight, slightly underweight, or extremely thin. Bingeing and vomiting may occur as much as several times a day. In severe cases, it may lead to dehydration and potassium loss causing weakness and cramps.

A Cycle of Addiction

Behaviors of anorexics and bulimics are driven by the cycle of addiction. There is an emotional emptiness that in turn leads to the psychological pain of low self-esteem. The individual looks for a way to dull the pain using addictive agents (starvation or bingeing), which usually result in the need to purge or medical problems. Finally, suffering from guilt, shame, and self-hate, the individual goes back to a routine of starvation and/or bingeing and purging.

TRAITS ASSOCIATED WITH DEVELOPMENT OF EATING DISORDERS

Poor sense of body image
Low self-esteem
Social phobias
Unstable moods
Perfectionism
Difficulty controlling impulses

Treatment

Medical problems caused by the disorder should be diagnosed and managed first. When the medical complications are severe, an individual may be hospitalized to stabilize physical functions and monitor nutritional intake. Often small feedings are carefully spaced because the patient cannot handle very much food at one time. In some cases, antidepressant medications are begun during the hospital stay.

In the late 1990s, treatment of eating disorders cost an excess of $30,000 a month. Many patients need repeated hospitalizations and can require treatment extending two years or more. Some therapists believe that anorexia/bulimia is never cured but merely arrested. However, some behaviorists believe that weight gain indicates a cure. There are several therapies used in treating with eating disorders; these should be discussed with the individual's therapist. A major part of therapy for eating disorders involves helping the individual rethink her/his perception of body image, because often it is perceived flaws that led to the eating disorder in the first place.

Many people with eating disorders are treated on an outpatient basis. There may be weekly counseling that includes individual and group sessions for outpatients and family, marital therapy, and specialized support for eating disorders.

eating phobias Fears of eating are relatively uncommon but troublesome kinds of phobias. They may be limited to a dread of eating in the company of others, or, in more severe cases, the fears may apply to eating food under any circumstances, whether the individual is alone or not. Some who fear eating fear swallowing and choking. Some fear swallowing solid foods but are able to swallow liquids. Phobics have an exaggerated feeling of a lump in their throat and a dry mouth, which are typical phobic responses, making it more difficult to eat.

Another type of eating phobia is food aversion, which involves only certain types of foods. Some food aversions begin in childhood or adolescence.

Some individuals will frequently complain of severe anxiety mounting to panic if they are forced to eat and are able to gain relief only by vomiting or by taking large doses of cathartics in order to get the food out of their bodies. The avoidance of eating to prevent such anxiety is a true phobic mechanism. Cognitive therapists have noted that fear-inducing thoughts accompany eating to produce anxiety and purging (avoidance).

There may be some connection between fears of eating and ANOREXIA NERVOSA. Technically, anorexia nervosa is characterized by a loss of appetite, while an individual with a phobia of eating experiences actual anxiety when eating or even considering eating. Anorexia nervosa is commonly considered either a hysterical phenomenon or a psychophysiological disorder because of the widespread secondary physical changes associated with it, such as slowing of growth and cessation of menstrual periods. However, in many cases the psychological disturbance from which all else follows is a genuine and profound phobia of eating, not a true anorexia. Eating phobias are successfully treated by graded exposure, starting with liquids and moving toward increasingly solid foods.

Fear of Eating Out

Fear of eating away from home is considered a SOCIAL PHOBIA. This fear takes many forms, including fear of being watched while eating, fear of being seen or heard burping, belching, or vomiting in public after eating, or fear of food contaminated by those who prepare it. Many individuals who have AGORAPHOBIA fear eating out.

Most manifestations of the fear of eating out involve feelings of being trapped in a restaurant by (1) having to wait for one's food, (2) close proximity to others (e.g., one's spouse) about whom one has negative (often unexpressed) feelings, (3) being stared at by others while walking in and out of the restaurant, and (4) physical factors, such as sitting on the inside of a booth or in the rear of the restaurant where exiting is more difficult.

See also EATING DISORDERS; PHOBIA; SOCIAL PHOBIAS.

ecclesiaphobia Fear of the church or of organized religion.

See also CHURCHES, FEAR OF.

echo, fear of Fear of echo is related to a fear of hearing one's own voice, known as phonophobia.

eclecticism (eclectic therapy) A system of psychotherapy that selects thoughts, suggestions, and procedures of therapy from diverse schools of thought to treat phobic or anxious individuals. Eclecticism is comprehensive psychiatry and draws from the biological, chemical, medical, neural psychological, social, environmental, and cultural points of view.

ecophobia, oikophobia   See HOME SURROUNDINGS, FEAR OF.

eczema, behavior therapy for   Eczema, a skin disease characterized by an itching rash over a large part of the body, has been relieved in some individuals with BEHAVIOR THERAPY and relaxation techniques. In a research study at the University of California at San Francisco Atopic Dermatitis Outpatient Clinic, patients were asked to record the number of times they scratched each day. The following week they were asked to add a rating of the itching intensity. Next, they were asked to note the time and what they were doing or feeling just before they scratched. Finally, they recorded how good it felt each time they scratched. By examining their records in detail, patients began to see how daily life events that were associated with feelings of ANXIETY, helplessness, anger, or resentment led to increased bouts of scratching that reinforced feelings of hopelessness about their disease and themselves as they looked at their damaged skin after scratching. To lessen the damage to their skin, patients were told to use the relaxation techniques at times of severe itching, such as just before bedtime. They were also taught to pat, rub, or slap the skin instead of scratching it. At the end of the study, severity of symptoms was reduced by half. There was a 30 percent average decrease in the use of topical steroids. No patients had to go back to systemic steroids or increase antihistamine dosage, strength of topical steroids, or number of applications.

See also RELAXATION TECHNIQUES; SKIN DISEASE, FEAR OF.

EEG (electroencephalograph)   An instrument that amplifies and records small electrical discharges from the brain through electrodes placed at various points on the skull. Dysfunction within the brain can be identified by examining electrical patterns produced on a graph or a scope. The record of the brain-wave patterns that results, the electroencephalogram, is used in studies of waking activities, the stages of sleep, drowsiness, and DREAMING, and in the detection and diagnosis of brain tumors and EPILEPSY. The EEG is frequently part of the complete physical examination for individuals who have extreme ANXIETIES, repeated INSOMNIA, or severe HEADACHES.

See also DIAGNOSIS.

ego   A Freudian term describing the part of the personality that deals with the external world and practical demands. According to Freud, there are three structural parts to the psychic apparatus: the ego, id, and superego. The ego constitutes executive function and enables the individual to perceive, reason, solve problems, test reality, delay drive discharge, and adjust instinctual impulses (the id) according to the demands of reality through the individual's conscience (the superego). Most of the functions of the ego are automatic. The most important function of the ego is adaptation to reality. This is accomplished by delaying drives until acceptable behaviors are carried out, instituting defense mechanisms as safeguards against release of unacceptable impulses, and conducting executive functions such as memory, planning, thought, etc. Anxiety arises from the ego as a signal that unacceptable unconscious material is building toward conscious discharge.

Ego Defense Mechanisms

These are unconscious strategies an individual uses to protect the ego from threatening impulses and conflicts. The most common ego defenses are repression, projection, sublimation, and displacement.

Ego Integrity

The last of Erikson's first eight STAGES OF MAN. *Ego integrity* seems to mean "the serenity of old age," the looking back on one's life with completeness and satisfaction and the acceptance without fear of one's own death as natural and as part of the life cycle. Without ego integrity, the individual may look back in despair, seeing his life as a series of mistakes and missed opportunities; DEPRESSION may result.

SUMMARY OF SOME EGO DEFENSE MECHANISMS

Compensation	Covering up weakness by emphasizing desirable traits or making up for frustration in one area by gratification in another
Denial of reality	Protecting self from unpleasant reality by refusal to perceive it
Displacement	Discharging pent-up feelings, usually of hostility, on objects less dangerous than those which initially aroused the emotion
Emotional insulation	Withdrawing into passivity to protect self from being emotionally hurt
Fantasy	Gratifying frustrated desires in imaginary achievements ("daydreaming" is a common form)
Identification	Increasing feelings of worth by identifying self with another person or institution, often of illustrious standing
Introjection	Incorporating external values and standards into ego structure so individual is not at the mercy of them as external threats
Isolation	Cutting off emotional charge from hurtful situations or separating incompatible attitudes into logic-tight compartments (holding conflicting attitudes which are never thought of simultaneously or in relation to each other); also called *compartmentalization*
Projection	Placing blame for one's difficulties upon others, or attributing one's own "forbidden" desires to others
Rationalization	Attempting to prove that one's behavior is "rational" and justifiable and thus worthy of the approval of self and others
Reaction formation	Preventing dangerous desires from being expressed by endorsing opposing attitudes and types of behavior and using them as "barriers"
Regression	Retreating to earlier developmental level involving more childish responses and usually a lower level of aspiration
Repression	Pushing painful or dangerous thoughts out of consciousness, keeping them unconscious; this is considered to be the *most basic of the defense mechanisms*
Sublimation	Gratifying or working off frustrated sexual desires in substitutive nonsexual activities socially accepted by one's culture
Undoing	Atoning for, and thus counteracting, unacceptable desires or acts

From *Psychology and Life,* by Philip G. Zimbardo. Copyright © 1985, 1979 by Scott, Foresman and Company. Reprinted by permission.

See also DEATH, FEAR OF; DEFENSE MECHANISMS; DEVELOPMENTAL STAGES; ID; REALITY TESTING; SUPEREGO; SUPEREGO ANXIETY.

eidetic psychotherapy   A type of therapy that uses eidetic imagery, or mental imagery. Imagery of vivid and detailed memories is usually visual but may also be auditory and closely resembles actual perception.

See also BEHAVIOR THERAPY.

eisoptrophobia   Fear of MIRRORS.

ejaculation   The emission of semen from the penis at orgasm, usually during intercourse or masturba-tion. Ejaculation disorders are conditions in which ejaculation occurs before or very soon after penetra-tion, does not occur at all, or in which the ejaculate is forced back into the bladder. Because ejaculation disorders interfere with the completion and enjoy-ment of sexual intercourse, they produce anxieties for men as well as for their partners, who do not always know how to help and may assume some blame.

Ejaculatory difficulties are involved in some men's sexual fears. Some men fear the automatic expulsion of semen and seminal fluid through the penis resulting from involuntary and voluntary con-tractions of various muscle groups during orgasm. Some men have a variety of fears regarding ejacu-lation, including premature ejaculation, delayed ejaculation, and ejaculatory incompetence—leading to embarrassment—and perceived male-role inadequacy. They also fear impregnating and consequent responsibilities.

Early ejaculation is ejaculation occurring within 10–60 seconds after penile penetration of the vagina, also known as premature ejaculation. It is the most common sexual problem in men, often because of overstimulation or anxiety and stress about sexual performance.

Inhibited ejaculation is a rare condition in which erection is normal but ejaculation does not occur. It may be psychological or it may be a result of a complication of other disorders or drug use.

Retrograde ejaculation occurs when the valve of the base of the bladder fails to close during an ejaculation. This forces the ejaculate backward into the bladder. Retrograde ejaculation may be the result of a neurological disease or can occur from pelvic surgery, surgery on the neck of the bladder, or after a prostatectomy.

Treatment for ejaculation difficulties may begin with a visit to a physician, a urologist, or a sex therapist.

See also SEX THERAPY; SEXUAL ANXIETIES; SEXUAL FEARS; SEXUAL RESPONSE CYCLE; VIAGRA.

Electra complex   A term describing a characteristic relationship that presumably occurs between a young daughter and her father during the phallic stage of psychosexual development as described by Freud. According to this Freudian view, female children during the phallic stage develop a strong desire to possess their fathers. This feeling is sexualized and corresponds to the Oedipal feeling young boys presumably develop toward their mothers at this stage. Successful resolution requires identification with the mother or father and thus allows sexual roles as well as superego structures to develop.

See also DEVELOPMENTAL STAGES; OEDIPAL.

electricity, fear of   Fear of electricity is known as electrophobia. Some who fear electric current, or the passage of electricity along a wire or other electrical conductor, fear the power of electricity. Some fear getting an electrical shock by touching wires or objects that conduct electricity. Some fear fires caused by electricity or faulty wiring or fear being near outdoor electrical wires. Fear of electricity can be a hindrance to enjoyment of modern conveniences, as many labor-saving appliances are electric. Some choose gas appliances as an alternative. Many people with this fear wear insulated shoes and will activate or deactivate wall switches only with wooden sticks or have others do so.

electrocardiogram (EKG)   A graph consisting of a wavelike tracing that represents the electrical action of the heart muscle as it goes through a typical cycle of contraction and relaxation. The wave patterns reveal the condition of the various heart chambers and valves. The heart's electrical currents are detected by electrodes placed on the individual's chest and amplified more than 3,000 times in an electrocardiograph, an electronic machine that creates the electrocardiogram. An EKG is usually part of a complete physical examination and may be repeated at intervals for individuals who have ANXIETIES and PANIC DISORDERS. Changes in the EKG may occur as a side effect of taking certain medications and may result from long-term chronic anxiety states.

See also HEART RATE IN EMOTION.

electroconvulsive therapy (ECT)   A treatment that produces a convulsion by passing an electrical current through the brain; also known as electroshock therapy. Historically, this treatment was used for a variety of serious symptoms of mental illness. Under close medical monitoring, it is given to carefully selected patients who are unresponsive to other treatments. Anesthesia is used as well as muscle relaxants and oxygen.

ECT has been shown to affect a variety of NEUROTRANSMITTERS in the brain, including norepinephrine, serotonin, and dopamine. It is also sometimes used to treat acute mania and acute schizophrenia when other treatments have failed. The number of ECT treatments needed for each person is determined according to the therapeutic response. Individuals with depression usually require an average of six to 12 treatments; commonly, treatments are given three or four times a week, usually every other day. After a course of ECT treatments, such patients usually are maintained on an antidepressant drug or lithium to reduce the risk of relapse of the condition. ECT has a high rate of therapeutic response (80–90 percent) but may have a relapse rate of 50 percent in one year, which can be reduced to 20 percent with maintenance medication.

The treatment can be lifesaving in people who are too medically ill to tolerate medication or who are not eating or drinking (catatonic). Side effects, including memory loss, are not uncommon. Patients must give informed consent to have ECT, as in the case of any operative procedure. Some studies have shown damage to the brain as a result of ECT.

See also DEPRESSION.

electromyographic pattern analysis (EMG)   Analysis of the electromyogram (EMG)—a recording of the electrical activity of the muscles through electrodes placed in or on different muscle groups when they are relaxed or during various activities—is used in BIOFEEDBACK therapy and in diagnosis and treatment of certain diseases involving the muscles, such as muscular dystrophy and spasmodic torticollis. EMG is used in biofeedback as a measure of muscular tension for people who have anxieties.

electrophobia   Fear of electricity.
See also ELECTRICITY, FEAR OF.

eleutherophobia   Fear of freedom.

elevated places, fear of   Fear of elevated places or heights, known as acrophobia, is very common. Some fear standing on elevated places, such as mountains in a distance, while others fear just looking at them. Some fear being at the edge of an elevated place.

See also HEIGHTS, FEAR OF; HIGH OBJECTS, FEAR OF; HIGH PLACES, FEAR OF LOOKING UP AT.

elevators, fear of   Many people fear riding in elevators. Some fear that the elevator cables will break and the elevator will crash. Others fear that the elevator may get stuck between floors, that the doors will not open, or that they will starve or suffocate inside. Some who fear riding in elevators do not fear riding only a few floors and feel safe before the elevator rises above the second or third floors. Some who fear elevators also have fears of closed spaces, such as tunnels, or fears of crowds. Many who have agoraphobia also fear elevators; in both phobias there is a fear of air deprivation. Some elevator phobics fear heights. In most cases, the phobic person feels somewhat trapped in the elevator until it stops and the doors open, which usually brings relief. Crowded elevators produce even greater feelings of being trapped and fears of losing emotional control, resulting in anticipated embarrassment, humiliation, rejection, etc.

There are social as well as physical fears associated with elevators. For example, some fear "going crazy" or fainting and being socially embarrassed if there are other people present in the elevator.

Fear of elevators influences where an individual lives, works, or conducts business. It can be a disabling fear because it limits one's activities. Therapists treat elevator phobia with many techniques, of which the exposure therapies are the most effective.

See also, ACROPHOBIA; AGORAPHOBIA; BEHAVIOR MODIFICATION; CLAUSTROPHOBIA.

Beck, Aaron T. and Gary Emery, *Anxiety Disorders and Phobias* (New York: Basic Books, 1985).

elurophobia   Fear of cats.
See also CATS, FEAR OF.

emetophobia   Fear of vomiting.
See also VOMITING, FEAR OF.

emphysema   A chronic, obstructive lung disease that causes its victims to struggle for every breath they take. Because their lungs have lost much of their natural elasticity, people suffering from this disease cannot completely exhale the carbon dioxide that is trapped in their lungs. They experience extreme fear and anxiety as they fight to replace the stale air with fresh oxygen. Family members who wish to be helpful feel useless, frustrated, and fearful.

Emphysema develops over time. A chronic cough, often called a "smoker's cough," and a general shortness of breath are warning signs of emphysema. Sufferers do not realize they have it until the first signs of breathlessness appear, and by then delicate lung tissue may have been damaged excessively. Emphysema is a chronic illness; there is no cure.

Some people who have emphysema require use of a portable oxygen tank, making traveling complicated and stressful because of the need to make arrangements to replenish their supplies periodically. For those individuals, because of the constant use of oxygen, eating out in restaurants, or going to movies or concerts, is also a stressful experience for them as well as their companions.

There is no known cause for emphysema, but most cases are related to cigarette smoking. Other contributing factors are air pollution and certain dusts and fumes. The disease is not caused by a germ or a virus and it is not an infectious or contagious disease.

Easing the Anxieties and Fears of Emphysema

Physicians can prescribe medications to relieve the feeling of breathlessness that accompanies this disease. There are also medicines that help clear mucus from the lungs and that can ward off chest infections. Also, emphysema patients can be taught by physical therapists to use their abdominal, chest, and diaphragmatic muscles to help them breathe more easily.

See also BREATHING; CHRONIC ILLNESS; SMOKING.

Employee Assistance Programs (EAPs) EAPs are designed to provide employees with help for anxiety-related problems they face on or off the job. EAPs also can make referrals to experts in anxiety treatment. Having an EAP is an important employee benefit. From the employer's point of view, what-

ever EAPs can do to help reduce employee's fears and anxieties helps the business.

EAPs have been in existence since the 1950s. Most authors trace their origin to the founding of Alcoholics Anonymous in 1935. In the 1960s and 1970s the scope of EAPs began to include help for employee problems such as DEPRESSION and other mental health concerns, drug abuse, DIVORCE, and other family difficulties. In the 1980s and 1990s, these programs have been expanded to include issues such as environmental stress, corporate culture, managing rapid technological change, and retraining.

According to the Employee Assistance Professional Association (Arlington, Virginia), in the early 1990s, about one-third of the nation's workers were covered by some form of EAP and about 75 percent of the Fortune 500 companies have EAPs.

How EAPs Work

There are two types of EAPs: internal and external. The majority of EAPs use independent companies that provide EAP services under a contract with the employer.

While the programs are geared to identifying employees whose personal problems may adversely affect their job performance, they also take a proactive stance in helping employees avoid problems before they occur. For example, companies are offering their employees seminars on stress reduction, PARENTING, adolescents and drugs, exercise, health, and diet.

EAPs provide referrals to appropriate professional services for employees and their immediate families. Confidentiality is assured; most employees would not use an EAP if they thought their problems would be revealed.

Employers implement EAPs for a variety of reasons. One is the skyrocketing costs related to providing a medical benefits program; another is the huge cost attributed to down time due to employee alcohol addiction and mental illness. A four-year study of mental health care received by employees of the McDonnell Douglas Corporation estimated that the company could save $5.1 million over three years if those employees who did not seek treatment had done so. Employees who used the EAP for chemical dependency also lost 44 percent fewer work days and filed fewer medical claims than those who did not.

"empty chair"

A technique used in Gestalt theory to resolve unfinished business or unresolved feelings toward another or to help identify reactions to another (usually someone from the past). The client is asked to talk to an empty chair as though it contained the person he or she reacted to or had unresolved feelings about. The therapist might also ask the client to sit in the empty chair and then to address his or her vacated chair from the point of view of the adversary. Fritz Perls (founder of gestalt therapy) felt that fear was the underlying factor in all unresolved situations and that inhibition was a form of avoidance of the fear. The empty-chair technique is a way of confronting and overcoming fears.

empty nest syndrome

A source of anxiety experienced by many middle-aged parents whose children have grown up and left home. Typically, the syndrome seems to affect women more than men, and particularly women whose lives have focused on their children. For these women, the empty nest syndrome can be a mild form of DEPRESSION that occurs after the children have left. Such women (and men, too, to some extent) no longer feel needed and feel a void in their lives.

On the other hand, there are many middle-aged couples who view their children leaving home with a sense of relief and fulfillment for having accomplished a major life task. Many empty nesters, particularly women, return to work, take on volunteer activities in their community, enroll in classes, or engage in new hobbies for which they previously had no time.

See also MENOPAUSE.

empty rooms and empty spaces, fear of

Fear of empty rooms is known as kenophobia or cenophobia. This may be the opposite of CLAUSTROPHOBIA, in which one fears crowded rooms, closed places, or enclosed spaces.

See also AGORAPHOBIA.

enabler   See CODEPENDENCY.

enclosed spaces, fear of

Fear of enclosed spaces is known as CLAUSTROPHOBIA. Many people have this fear in elevators, small rooms, or crowded rooms, on airplanes or buses, or in other places where they cannot readily leave if they choose to do so. Some become fearful if there is no window in the room they are in, or if they cannot open a window, as on an airplane.

Some individuals are fearful of going into an enclosed space. Others may easily enter the space and feel comfortable and secure in it and later on become overwhelmed by a feeling of anxiety that something dreadful will happen while in the enclosed space. Sometimes the same individual experiences different feelings at different times. The person might perceive a "closed space" even though he or she is not enclosed. For example, left-turn lanes are often experienced as such. It should be noted that closed, tight spaces produce a natural aversive reaction that is preprogrammed in humans (and many animals) as a survival mechanism. This natural aversion can become phobic in nature under conditions of learning.

Some individuals who have fear of enclosed places also have some social phobias or agoraphobia. For example, the individual who is fearful of meeting new people, of being looked at, of being stared at, or of being critized may anticipate these fears before entering a crowded room from which there is no easy escape and thus become anxious and fearful of entering the room. Some individuals are fearful that they will do something embarrassing or unacceptable, such as faint, lose control, or look stupid, or be unacceptable because they are anxious in public and thus fear being in an enclosed place or an open place without shelter or ease of exit. Fear of enclosed places is a common anxiety symptom, but for some individuals under some circumstances it can produce a panic attack.

Some psychoanalytic points of view relate fears of enclosed places to fantasies of wishing or fearing symbiotic reunion with the mother, or peaceful sleep in the womb. There may be fantasies of being extruded or suffocated by a closing of the birth canal, or being stuck in the birth canal. The basic fear of the claustrophobe is considered by some analysts a castration anxiety. The fear may also be related to a death fear, because the individual, either consciously or unconsciously, fears that there will be no air and he or she will suffocate. Many types of therapies are used to help individuals who fear enclosed places, including behavior therapy, in which the individual learns to face the feared situations and not have a claustrophobic reaction. For some individuals, therapy for generalized anxiety will also help overcome specific fears, such as the fear of enclosed spaces.

See also AGORAPHOBIA; BEHAVIOR THERAPY; CASTRATION ANXIETY.

encounter group therapy A form of training or therapy sometimes used by support groups for individuals who have phobias. Emphasis is on experiences of individuals within the group with minimum input from the therapist-leader. Encounter groups focus on the present, or here-and-now feelings rather than past or outside problems of participants. The term "encounter group" was coined by J. L. Moreno in 1914.

endocrine system A major body system that is comprised of ductless glands that release hormones directly into the blood or lymph system. Some glands produce hormones that directly affect the body, such as thyroid hormone, adrenaline, estrogen, and insulin. Some glands produce hormones that cause the release of other hormones. For example, the hypothalamus releases hormones that cause other hormones to be released, such as growth hormone-releasing hormone (GHRH), which causes the pituitary gland to release growth hormone. The hypothalamus also stimulates the pituitary of release other hormones, such as thyrotropin-releasing hormone (TRH), which causes the pituitary to release thyroid-stimulating hormone (TSH), used by the thyroid gland. If the levels of thyroid are low, both the hypothalamus and the pituitary can detect this insufficiency and increase the secretion of TRH and TSH to stabilize the thyroid levels.

The endocrine glands include the following glands (the hormones they secrete are in parentheses)

- adrenals (adrenalin and cortisol)
- hypothalamus (thyrotropin-releasing hormone, growth hormone–releasing hormone, gonadotropin-releasing hormone, corticotrophin-releasing hormone, dopamine)
- ovaries in females (estradiol, progesterone)
- pancreas (insulin, glucagon)
- parathyroids (parathyroid hormone, also known as parathormone or PTH)
- pineal (melatonin)
- pituitary (adrenocorticotropic hormone; thyroid-stimulating hormone; luteinizing hormone; follicle-stimulating hormone; prolactin; growth hormone; pro-opiomenalnocortin)
- testicles in males (testosterone, dehydroepiandrosterone, and androstendione)
- thymus (unknown but believed to be important in the immune system of the fetus and young infant)
- thyroid (thyroid hormone)

Adrenaline, also known as epinephrine, is particularly important in times of crisis and is elevated in individuals experiencing a phobic reaction. It is also known as the fight-or-flight hormone because it enables the individual to become very alert and to better cope in the face of either real or perceived danger. Sometimes adrenaline is administered by injection to individuals on an emergency basis if they are experiencing a life-threatening allergic reaction to a drug or other substance.

Petit, Jr., William A., M.D., and Christine Adamec, *The Encyclopedia of Endocrine Diseases and Disorders.* (New York: Facts On File, Inc., 2005).

end of the world, fear of See APOCALYPSE, FEAR OF.

endogenous depression Profound sadness that may be caused by a biological malfunction, in contrast to a DEPRESSION brought on by an environmental

ENDOCRINE SYSTEM

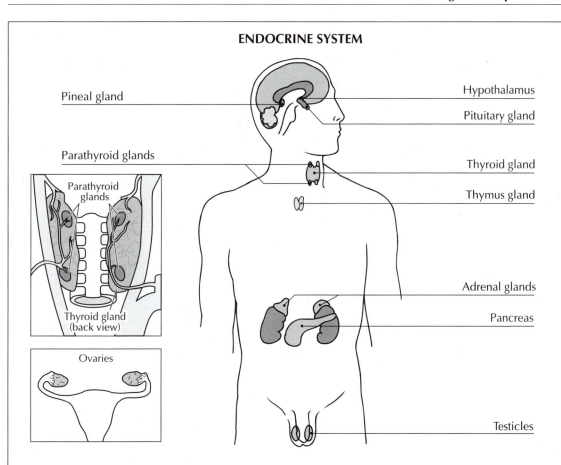

Your endocrine system is a collection of glands that produce hormones that regulate your body's growth, metabolism, and sexual development and function. The hormones are released into the bloodstream and transported to tissues and organs throughout your body. The table below describes the function of these glands.

Adrenal glands	Divided into 2 regions; secrete hormones that influence the body's metabolism, blood chemicals, and body characteristics, as well as influence the part of the nervous system that is involved in the response and defense against stress
Hypothalamus	Activates and controls the part of the nervous system that controls involuntary body functions, the hormonal system, and many body functions, such as regulating sleep and stimulating appetite
Ovaries and testicles	Secrete hormones that influence female and male characteristics, respectively
Pancreas	Secretes a hormone (insulin) that controls the use of glucose by the body
Parathyroid glands	Secrete a hormone that maintains the calcium level in the blood
Pineal body	Involved with daily biological cycles
Pituitary gland	Produces a number of different hormones that influence various other endocrine glands
Thymus gland	Plays a role in the body's immune system
Thyroid gland	Produces hormones that stimulate body heat production, bone growth, and the body's metabolism

(CREDIT: American Medical Association)

event. Endogenous depression has a more severe set of symptoms than EXOGENOUS DEPRESSION. The term endogenous (quick, "arising from within") is now passing out of use, because there is no evidence that a major depressive episode has different symptoms just because a precipitating factor was external or internal.

See also ANTIDEPRESSANTS.

endorphins   Naturally occurring endogenous opioid components produced in the pituitary and hypothalamus. They play important roles in control of emotional behaviors such as those associated with pain, ANXIETY, tension, and FEAR. Stress, both physical and psychological, seems to stimulate secretion of endorphins.

The binding sites of the endorphins are concentrated in the limbic system. A number of specific endorphins have been identified.

enetophobia   Fear of pins.

eneuresis   See BED-WETTING.

England   Fear of England, the English (British) language, and things relating to the English culture is known as Anglophobia.

enissophobia, enosiophobia   Fear of sin.
    See also SIN, FEAR OF.

enochlophobia   Fear of crowds.
    See also CROWDS, FEAR OF.

entomophobia   See INSECTS, FEAR OF.

envy   A sense that something that others have is lacking in one's life. It is an anxiety-producing emotion that people are frequently unwilling to admit to.

Envy can result from many types of situations. However, it is most often those involving friends, relatives, neighbors, or colleagues that contribute to envy. An ability to imagine or identify with an admired person's strengths is an intellectual asset that may enable individuals to progress and better themselves. However, it becomes negative when the envious person remains fixated on another person's life and does not try to better his own life in a constructive way. Low SELF-ESTEEM produces envy, which often does not improve with the attainment of material things, status symbols, or fame. Healthy self-esteem makes envy unlikely and allows for creative identification with admired traits in others.

Modern American life is full of elements that create envy. For example, the mobile quality of society de-emphasizes social class and creates feelings that all things are possible for all people. This can create stressful feelings of FRUSTRATION, failure, and envy when expectations are thwarted. Mass media, especially television, allows Americans to view "lifestyles of the rich and famous." Advertising plays on feelings of envy with situations of "keeping up with the Joneses." The "Me Decade" of the 1980s, with its narcissism and "yuppie" life-style, created a climate in which envy flourished. Faced with a wide array of consumer products made available by high technology, it is always possible for individuals to feel that someone else has more than they do.

Because feelings of envy imply that someone is in a superior position and because most religions regard envy as sinful, people develop various ways of masking or suppressing it. To avoid expressing envy, some people develop a superior and snobbish attitude and gossip, criticize, or imply that the person to be envied is really the envious one.

See also JEALOUSY.

eosophobia   Fear of dawn.
    See also DAWN, FEAR OF; LIGHT, FEAR OF.

epidemic anxiety   Acute anxiety among many members of a given community at the same time. Epidemic anxiety is also known as MASS HYSTERIA. Usually a common factor for the anxiety can be identified, and individuals usually recover without long-lasting effects.

Epidemic anxiety has occurred following chemical explosions and similar crises of public safety. In such cases people commonly report nausea, vomiting, and headaches and attribute all such symptoms (whether correctly or not) to the recent discovery.

Greist, John H., James W. Jefferson, and I. M. Marks, *Anxiety and Its Treatment: Help Is Available* (Washington, DC: American Psychiatric Press, 1986).

epidemiology   The study of mental and physical disorders and diseases in populations. Epidemiology relates the distribution of disorders (incidence and prevalence), such as anxieties and phobias, to any conceivable factor, such as time, place, or a person existing in or affecting that population. By understanding the magnitude of a disorder and the patterns of risk for the occurrence of a disorder, researchers obtain clues as to what alterations might lead to prevention of the disorder.

The study of population samples includes both treated and untreated persons to obtain a true estimate and better understanding of the disorder. However, for many disorders, only a small fraction of ill persons seek medical treatment, and those who do seek treatment may not be representative of the population with the disorders. This is particularly true of anxiety disorders.

See also INCIDENCE; PREVALENCE OF PHOBIAS AND ANXIETIES.

epilepsy, fear of   Fear of epilepsy is known as hylephobia. This is one of many specific disease phobias. Some individuals fear having epilepsy themselves; others fear viewing a person having an epileptic attack.

Fears often accompany epilepsy. For example, after a seizure, an epileptic may become phobic about going to the place where the seizure occurred. Also, the epileptic may fear the social embarrassment of having an attack in the presence of others.

See also ILLNESS PHOBIA.

epinephrine   See ADRENALINE.

epistaxiophobia   Fear of nosebleeds.
See also NOSEBLEEDS, FEAR OF.

equinophobia   See HORSES, FEAR OF.

erectile dysfunction, fear of   See SEXUAL FEARS.

eremophobia (eremiophobia and ermitophobia)   Fear of being oneself. This fear is common in a large percentage of agoraphobic individuals.
See also AGORAPHOBIA; ALONE, FEAR OF BEING; SOLITUDE, FEAR OF; STILLNESS, FEAR OF.

ergasiophobia   A fear that one's movements will disastrously affect the surrounding world. Sometimes the word ergasiophobia is used to refer to fear of surgical operations.
See also SURGICAL OPERATIONS, FEAR OF; WORK, FEAR OF.

ergophobia   Fear of work. This can be related to social anxieties, perfectionism, and fear of failure as well as anxiety over exertion and effort.

ergot   Ergot, a naturally occurring substance derived from a fungus that infests rye plants, is used in medications to treat migraine HEADACHES. It stops the headaches by constricting the blood vessels and reducing the dilation of the arteries. Many individuals find that if they take it early enough in prepain stages of an attack, they can abort their headaches or at least reduce their intensity. Many migraine-headache sufferers become less anxious about having a migraine attack when they begin prophylactic (preventive) treatment.

Erikson's psychosocial stages   See DEVELOPMENTAL STAGES.

erotophobia Fear of sexual love is known as erotophobia. The term also relates to fear of anything that arouses sexual or erotic feelings, such as thoughts, printed matter, or films.

See also DEVELOPMENTAL STAGES; SEXUAL LOVE, FEAR OF.

error, fear of Fear of errors is known as hamartophobia. Those who have this phobia may fear one of several types of errors, including memory error, which differs from forgetting; false recollection; accidents, such as while driving a car; or minor accidents, such as spilling things or dropping things. From the psychoanalytic point of view, errors stem from repression; the error reveals unconscious feelings and motives (for example, slips of the tongue). Individuals who fear making errors are often perfectionists; some are compulsive about always being right, knowing answers, and always performing correctly.

See also OBSESSIVE-COMPULSIVE DISORDER; PSYCHOANALYSIS; REPRESSION; SLIPS OF THE TONGUE, FEAR OF.

erythrophobia, erytophobia, ereuthophobia Fear of BLUSHING and fear of the color red. This fear is sometimes associated with a fear of BLOOD. Blushing is often a reaction to social attention, teasing, and emotional expressions that bring on anxiety, self-consciousness, and similar responses that one wishes to hide from others. Blushing is caused by increased blood flow to the facial area and seems to be a physiological response peculiar to some individuals. Relaxation training combined with assertiveness training are usually sufficient to treat this reaction.

See also BLOOD AND BLOOD-INJURY PHOBIA; BLUSHING, FEAR OF.

escalators, fear of Escalators, moving stairways widely used in stores and train, bus, and airline terminals, are feared by many individuals who fear CONFINEMENT, HEIGHTS, MOTION, STAIRS, or STANDING. The steps on an escalator run up or down on an endless belt, which may cause some who fear INFINITY to fear the endless motion. Some may fear acci-

dents or fear falling on escalators, but most fears are associated with feeling trapped in a social situation in which others might see one's anxiety. This is a common fear in agoraphobics. Fear of escalators is a 20th-century fear. The first escalator was installed by the Otis Elevator Company at the Paris Exposition in 1900.

See also ACCIDENTS, FEAR OF; FALLING, FEAR OF; MOTION, FEAR OF; STAIRS, FEAR OF; STANDING, FEAR OF.

escape behavior The actions a phobic person takes to remove him or herself from an aversive object a phobic object when such an object cannot be avoided. An example is running at the sight of a snake. An alternative to escape behavior would be an AVOIDANCE RESPONSE, which might involve walking around a grassy patch in which snakes may be lurking instead of walking through it. Avoidance and escape behaviors help the individual feel less fearful of a specific situation. Where avoidance or escape behavior is not possible, the phobic individual may show other signs of anxiety or fear, such as trembling hands, shaking, or stammering speech, fidgeting and squirming, or other mannerisms.

esodophobia Fear of virginity, either of losing one's own or relating to the loss of virginity in oneself or another.

See also VIRGINITY, FEAR OF.

estrogen replacement therapy See MENOPAUSE.

eternity, fear of Fear of eternity was described by Otto Fenichel (1899–1946), an Austrian psychoanalyst and disciple of Freud, as part of a group of fears "surroundings that imply the loss of the usual means of orientation," such as fear of cessation of customary routine, fear of death, fear of uniform noises, etc. The individual who has such fears is particularly afraid of a loss of control over infantile sexual and aggressive impulses and then projects onto the outside world his own fears of losing control. On the other hand, the existential therapists would point out that to experience eternity is to come into contact with our basic sense of alienation and separateness, which engenders great fear.

euphobia   Fear of hearing good news. This may also be related to the fear of gaiety, fear of laughter, or fear of success.

See also GOOD NEWS, FEAR OF; LAUGHTER, FEAR OF; SUCCESS, FEAR OF.

eurotophobia   Fear of FEMALE GENITALS.

See also PSYCHOSEXUAL ANXIETIES; SEXUAL FEARS.

eustress   A term referring to "good stress" coined by Hans Selye (1907–82), pioneer researcher in the field of stress. During eustress and dis-stress (bad stress), the body undergoes virtually the same non-specific responses to the various positive or negative stimuli acting upon it. However, Selye explained, the fact that eustress causes much less damage than dis-stress demonstrates that "how you take it" determines whether one can adapt successfully to change.

Examples of "good stress" include starting a new romance, getting married, having a baby, buying a house, getting a new job, or getting a raise at work. All these situations, as well as others, demand adaptations on the part of the individual. Both eustress and dis-stress are part of the GENERAL ADAPTATION SYNDROME (G.A.S.), which Selye described as being the controlling factor in how people cope with stresses in their lives.

Later researchers (Holmes and Rahe) included several "good stress" situations in their SOCIAL READJUSTMENT RATING SCALE, which was designed to be a predictor of ill health. Sources of good stress included marriage, marital reconciliation, retirement, pregnancy, buying a house, and outstanding personal achievement.

See also ANXIETY; COPING; DIS-STRESS; HOMEOSTASIS; LIFE CHANGE SELF-RATING SCALE.

Selye, Hans, *Stress Without Distress* (New York: Lipincott, 1974).

———, *The Stress of Life*. Rev. ed. (New York: McGraw Hill, 1978).

everything, fear of   Fear of everything is known as panphobia, panophobia, pantophobia, or pamphobia. This may be an anxiety disorder rather than a true phobia.

See also ANXIETY, BASIC; ANXIETY DISORDERS.

evil eye, fear of   Many civilizations have believed in the evil eye, a superstition that certain individuals have the ability to bring on bad luck or injury by looking at another. Belief in the evil eye may stem from the ability of the eye to change color and adapt or from the awareness most people have of being stared at or even stared awake by someone they cannot actually see.

The evil is part of witch and voodoo beliefs, which may be an intense occult projection of the feeling of jealousy. Individuals who are prone to disaster and misfortune were thought to have an involuntary evil eye. Both the gods and men were thought be be envious of anyone experiencing good fortune and to wish him ill. The evil eye could cause illness, bad luck, and damage to property and livestock. According to 16th- and 17th-century witch beliefs, the power of the evil eye came directly from a pact with Satan. Babies and children were targets for the evil eye and were sometimes disguised in ragged or inappropriate clothing to protect them. Strings of blue beads and salt carried in a pocket were also thought to protect children. The bridal veil and other marriage customs fended off the power of the evil eye on the happy occasion of a wedding. Sexual functions were thought to be particularly vulnerable to the power of the evil eye. Sexual symbols such as ornaments in the shape of a phallus and a gesture of the hand with thumb between first and second fingers were believed to be powerful protection.

Some people still believe that direct praise, compliments, and discussion of good fortune attracts the attention of the evil eye. A compliment paid in even the most veiled way, according to fearers of the evil eye, should be followed by the act of spitting, which is considered a protective measure against the jealous influence of the evil eye.

See also CROSS-CULTURAL INFLUENCES; VOODOO, FEAR OF; WITCHES AND WITCHCRAFT, FEAR OF.

Brasch, R., *Strange Customs* (New York: David McKay, 1976), pp. 127–133.

Carroll, Michael P., "On the Psychological Origins of the Evil Eye: A Kleinian View." *The Journal of Psychoanalytic Anthropology* 7, no. 2 (Spring 1984): pp. 170–187.

Dossey, Larry, "The Evil Eye." *Alternative Therapies* 4, no. 1 (January 1980): pp. 9–18.

Cavendish, Richard (ed.), *Man, Myth and Magic* (New York: Marshall Cavendish, 1983).

Galt, Anthony H., "The Evil Eye as synthetic image and its meanings on the island of Pantelleria, Italy," *American Ethnologist* 9, no. 4 (November 1982): pp. 664–681.

evocative therapy   A term used in psychotherapy to denote emphasis on evoking responses from the individual rather than guiding the individual toward some therapeutic goal. Therapists often use this approach to treat individuals who have ANXIETIES and PHOBIAS.

See also THERAPIES.

examination phobia   See TEXT ANXIETY.

excrement, fear of   See FECES, FEAR OF.

exercise, compulsion to   An irresistible and often self-abusive impulse to perform frequent and long-lasting physical exercise, which is sometimes known as *exercise dependence*. This compulsion may stem from psychological problems and anxieties similar to those found in people with EATING DISORDERS and body image issues. In addition, individuals with some eating disorders, such as anorexia nervosa or bulimia nervosa, may develop a compulsion to exercise in order to control their weight and body appearance.

Both men and women may become compulsive at exercising. Individuals in some careers are at greater risk for exercise dependence, such as actors, models, dancers, and some athletes, such as jockeys or boxers. In these career fields, an individual's weight is considered highly important.

Some experts believe that college students may be more prone than others to developing a compulsion to exercise. In one study reported in the *Journal of American College Health* on 257 students at the school of physical education and dance at the Kutztown University of Pennsylvania, the researchers found that about 22 percent of the students exercised 36 or more hours per week and they exhibited atypical exercise patterns.

The *exercise addict* spends inappropriate amounts of time each day exercising, frequently continuing to exercise even when he or she is injured and/or in severe pain. In many cases, the compulsive exerciser has no real athletic goals, but instead uses exercise to fill the emotional gaps in his or her life; for example, using exercise to replace missing or unsatisfactory relationships. Exercise also allows some individuals to feel in control, when the rest of their life may seem out of control.

The compulsive exerciser may also seek the more socially acceptable euphoria that is produced by prolonged strenuous exercise rather than turning to drugs or alcohol to produce euphoric feelings.

Compulsive exercise can also be a way for an individual to distract him or herself from feelings of anxiety, as well as a method to reduce anxiety once it occurs. Some people with anxiety reactions have been known to engage in compulsive strenuous physical exercise to the point of running or working out in the middle of the night.

Exercise dependence is not a recognized disorder by the American Psychiatric Association but it is of increasing interest to many experts. Researchers Heather Hausenblas and Danielle Symons Downs recommended in their article for *Psychology of Sport and Exercise* that exercise dependence be defined when there is a manifestation of three or more of the following behaviors

1. tolerance, or a need for increased exercise to achieve the same effect
2. withdrawal, or symptoms of anxiety or fatigue if the individual does not exercise, or exercising occurs in order to avoid withdrawal symptoms

3. intention effects—when the person exercises over a longer period than planned
4. inability to cut back on exercising
5. excessive amount of time exercising—vacations devoted to exercising
6. conflict—exercising causes forgoing important work or social activities
7. continuance—exercising when the person knows there is a physical problem that would worsen with further exercising

See also FITNESS ANXIETY.

Garman, J. G., et al., "Occurrence of Exercise Dependence in a College-Aged Population," *Journal of American College Health* 52, no. 5 (March–April 2004): pp. 221–228.

Gwinnell, Esther, M.D., and Christine Adamec, *The Encyclopedia of Addictions and Addictive Disorders.* (New York: Facts On File, Inc., 2005).

Hausenblas, Heather, and Danielle Symons Downs, "Exercise Dependence: A Systematic Review," *Psychology of Sport and Exercise* 3 (2002): pp. 89–123.

exhaustion, fear of Fear of exhaustion is known as kopophobia. Some individuals fear becoming exhausted because they fear being weak, or possibly fainting, and thus being powerless or out of control.

See also LOSS OF CONTROL, FEAR OF.

existential analysis A phase in existential psychotherapy in which the individual explores his own values, relationships, and commitments. The object of existential analysis is to develop new and more satisfying patterns of life, such as new ways of facing and coping with ANXIETIES and PHOBIAS. Existential anxiety, however, is viewed as a universal experience of humans due to their alienation.

See also EXISTENTIAL THERAPY.

existential anxiety A term that applies to a normal response to confronting one's life condition. It is differentiated from neurotic anxiety that is out of proportion to the situation, is typically out of awareness, and tends to immobilize the person. Decisions and fundamental changes in one's life produce existential anxiety, which acts as a stimulus for growth and helps to increase awareness and personal freedom.

See also EXISTENTIAL THERAPY.

existential neurosis A term that applies to a lack of an inner sense of oneself and of meaning in life. The term was popularized by Viktor Frankl (1905–97), a German-born American psychiatrist, who originated logotherapy, an existential approach that recognizes an inability to see meaning in life as a cause for anxiety, fear, and phobia.

Existential neurosis comes from a failure to experience life on one's own terms. Individuals whose lives are directed solely toward satisfying society's demands or goals without creating their own personally chosen destinies may develop existential neuroses.

See also EXISTENTIAL THERAPY.

existential therapy A form of therapy for anxieties and phobias in which treatment of the entire person is emphasized. Unlike other therapies that emphasize biology, behavior, or unconscious features, existential therapy focuses on the individual's subjective experiences, free will, and ability to be responsible for his own existence. Existential therapy is also known as humanistic-existential therapy. The therapeutic process encourages the individual to verbalize intimate thoughts, intentions, and convictions in order to reveal the deepest meaning he or she gives to his or her life. The relationship between the therapist and anxious individual becomes a continuous process of sharing, questioning, and probing inner experiences. In the therapeutic situation, there is no transference from individual to analyst, or vice versa, because each relates to the other in a genuine interpersonal expression of feelings. The therapist tries to understand the meaning of a phobic individual's conscious act, for example, as it appears currently in daily life, in the past, and in how the individual perceives that it might happen in the future.

Existential therapists assume that there are four dimensions of mental disturbances: intrapsychic disturbances, disturbed learning processes, systemic disturbances, and existential disturbances. Existentialists believe their aspect of the discipline has been neglected because of the general decline in the use of symbolic language in psychotherapy.

Existential counseling is designed to expand self-awareness and increase the client's concept of the amount of control he or she has making choices in life. Additionally, existential counselors help reduce anxiety in a client's life by helping him or her to transform anxiety from a negative to a positive energy for life.

The founder of existential therapy was Rollo May, an American psychoanalyst, who was particularly concerned with combating feelings of emptiness, cynicism, and despair by emphasizing basic human values, such as love, free will, and self-awareness.

See also ANGST; ANXIETY; EXISTENTIAL NEUROSIS; GESTALT THERAPY.

Kleinknecht, Ronald A., *The Anxious Self* (New York: Human Sciences Press, 1986).

Lande, Nathaniel, "On Existential Analysis." In *Mindstyles/Lifestyles* (Los Angeles: Price/Stern/Sloan, 1976), pp. 64–65.

exogenous depression   Profound sadness assumed to be caused by an environmental event. Many agoraphobics have this type of depression, but it recedes as the anxiety diminishes and the person becomes more functional. This term is going out of common use.

See also AGORAPHOBIA; ANTIDEPRESSANTS; DEPRESSION; ENDOGENOUS DEPRESSION.

exorcism   A fear that evil spirits in the form of demons or ghosts can gain control of the human body, places, or animals is the basis for the ritual of exorcism. Exorcism has taken different forms, ranging from a simple prayer to God for deliverance from the power of evil to an elaborate ceremony described in the Roman ritual of the Catholic church. All forms of exorcism attempt to rid the person of evil possession.

Demons, fallen angels who rebelled against God, are believed to have the ability to possess human souls; but demons are supposedly subject to the powers of religious rituals designed to drive them out of their victims. Reports of demonic possession from the past closely resemble modern cases of schizophrenia and hysteria. The dialogue between priest and evil spirit, speaking through the victim, also resembles the exchange between psychotherapist and patient and has frequently had similar results. A strong fear associated with exorcism was that the exorcist himself might become possessed by the evil spirit.

In modern times, exorcism is associated with the Catholic church, but it has an ancient history in Greek, Mesopotamian, and Jewish cultures. The New Testament records that Jesus Christ drove demons out of their victims and conferred this power on his Apostles. Early Christians spread the word of the power of Christianity by exorcising evil spirits.

According to some European witch beliefs, witches could inflict demonic possession by contaminating the victim's food with evil spirits. Apples were considered a favorite vehicle for a demon. Simulation of demonic possession was apparently used both by those who feared charges of witchcraft because of their unusual behavior and by those who wished to bring witchcraft charges. Nuns were frequent victims of demonic possession. The condition spread through convents as a type of hysteria. Descriptions of demonic possession included both mental and physical symptoms: sharp pains that made the victim cry out, vomiting, swelling, melancholy, a desire for bad food, wicked, blasphemous language or behavior, and superhuman mental or physical ability.

Interest in exorcism revived in the 1970s partly due to the success of William Blatty's novel *The Exorcist* and the film based on it. Recently, religious leaders and psychotherapists have debated the issue of whether treating devils as entities capable of controlling the human body and soul is helpful or harmful in the treatment of mental cases. The *New Catholic Encyclopedia* makes the following comment: "Exorcisms are rarely performed today, not because the Church has lost its belief in the power and activity of Satan, but because it recognizes that true cases of possession are rare. What often appeared to be possession in earlier ages is now recognized as a pathological state attributable to one or more anxiety disorders and for those the proper remedies are neurology, psychiatry or depth psychology."

See also DEMONS, FEAR OF.

experiential family therapy   An approach to family therapy that focuses on actual experiences between therapist and family and among family members during the therapy session. It is also known as symbolic-experiential family therapy. This therapy may be useful in helping families of agoraphobic individuals or those who have other anxieties or phobias. The therapy is based on existentialism and humanistic approaches and emphasizes the family's "process of becoming," through which the family can learn to use its symptoms and anxieties in constructive ways.

See also FAMILY THERAPY.

exposure therapy   (See charts that follow on pp. 226–227.) A generic term for behavior therapies that focus on altering an individual's reactions and responses to phobic behavior while gradually

---

STEPS TO PREPARE ONESELF FOR EXPOSURE TREATMENT

1. Work out exactly what you fear; do not waste time treating the wrong thing.
2. Write down the specific problems and goals you want to work on.
3. Prepare a timetable for exposure to things that frighten you. Record what happens after each exposure session. Revise your goals as you progress.
4. Determine what thoughts or body sensations bother you.
5. Plan goals for each particular session.
6. Leave enough time, possibly several hours, to reach a specific goal by the end of a session.
7. Write down the coping strategies you will use on cards to carry with you.
8. Record your achievements after every session.

---

increasing his or her exposure to the phobic situation.

Before considering exposure therapy as a possible treatment, an individual can test him or herself with the questions shown in the chart to determine if exposure treatment would be appropriate.

See also BEHAVIOR THERAPY; CATASTROPHIC ANXIETY; FLOODING; IMPLOSIVE THERAPY; SELF-HELP; SIMPLE PHOBIA. (The charts in this section have been adapted, with permission, from *Living with Fear* by Marks, Isaac M. [New York: McGraw-Hill, 1978].)

extramarital affairs   See ADULTERY; MARRIAGE.

extroversion   See INTROVERSION; PERSONALITY DISORDERS.

eyeglasses, fear of   Many infants fear people who wear eyeglasses because the glasses distort natural facial features. Most children, however, outgrow this fear as they discover that some people wear glasses and others do not. When children begin to wear glasses, they may fear breaking their glasses or they may fear ridicule and name-calling from other children. Some individuals, particularly those in middle age, fear having to wear glasses, or particularly bifocal eyeglasses, because they associate this type of eyewear with old age. Individuals who must wear glasses for comfortable vision fear losing their glasses because they feel out of control and helpless without them. Goethe (1749–1832), the German poet, novelist, and playwright, is said to have feared bespectacled people.

See also AGING, FEAR OF; CHILDHOOD FEARS; LOSS OF CONTROL.

Vierordt, Hermann, *Medizinisches aus der geschichte* (Tübingen, Germany; Laupp, 1910).

Eye Movement Desensitization and Reprocessing (EMDR)   EMDR is a technique for treating traumatic experience locked in the nervous system by skillfully combining a representation of the trauma,

EXPOSURE THERAPY DAILY RECORD

This is an example of how one can keep a record of exposure therapy tasks.

Day	Date	Session Began	Ended	The exposure task I performed was:	(0 = complete calm, 100 = absolute panic) My anxiety during the task was:	Comments, including coping tactics I used:	Name of cotherapist if any: (Co-therapist's signature that task was completed)
Sunday							
Monday							
Tuesday							
Example from an agoraphobia							
Wednesday		2:30 P.M.	4:30 P.M.	Walked to local supermarket and surrounding stores, bought food and gifts for family, had coffee at a coffee shop.	75	Felt worse in crowded stores, practiced deep-breathing exercises	R. Jones (husband)
Thursday		10:00 A.M.	11:30 A.M.	Walked to the park, sat for 1/2 hour till I felt better, took the bus downtown and back home.	70	Felt faint and giddy. Practiced imagining myself dropping dead.	R. Jones
Friday		2 P.M.	4 P.M.	Rode the bus downtown and back three times till I felt better about it.	60	Worst when bus was crowded. I did deep-breathing exercises.	R. Jones

Plan for next week: Repeat exposure exercises in the bus, park, and stores every day until my anxiety is no higher than 30. After that, start visits to my hairdresser and short car trips.

Saturday							
Sunday							
Monday							

self-evaluation, emotions, and body sensations while experiencing bilateral stimulation (eye movement or tapping sounds, etc.). This procedure has empirical support as a trauma treatment.

EMDR was developed in the early 1990s by Francine Shapiro, Ph.D., a Northern California psychologist.

eyes, fear of   Fear of eyes is known as ommatophobia or ommetaphobia.

See also BEING STARED AT, FEAR OF; DOUBLE VISION, FEAR OF; EVIL EYE, FEAR OF.

eyes, fear of opening one's   Fear of opening one's eyes is known as optophobia.

COPING TACTICS DURING EXPOSURE

1. Breathe slowly or steadily. If you find yourself breathing very rapidly, slow your breathing to about 20 breaths a minute.

2. Be aware that even though you may feel tense or even miserable for a while, things will improve. Learn to tense and relax your muscles repeatedly. Eventually you will be able to relax them more easily. Concentrate particularly on muscles you feel are tense.

3. Keep track of your thoughts. During exposure, you may find yourself thinking about your rapid heartbeat and worrying about having a heart attack. Catastrophic thoughts such as these will make you more tense. Tell yourself that this is an unreasonable thought and be assured that your therapist has repeatedly told you that your heart is fine.

4. Watch your anxiety level rise and fall. Construct a scale from one to ten, ten being the worst anxiety feeling, and give yourself ratings while you practice.

5. Here are some sentences to say to yourself:
   I feel terrible now; if I persist, I will get over this.

   I am terrified, as I was told I would be, but the anxiety will subside if I persist.

   I am embarrassed by all this, but I will get used to it.

   I must remember that dizziness, pounding heart, shaking, sweating, pressure, and pain in my chest is just anxiety. It is the body's natural fear reaction.

   I have an impulse to leave the situation. If I do, I will feel worse. If I remain until my anxiety subsides, I will feel better for the effort, and it will probably become easier as I practice.

6. During exposure, monitors give bodily reaction on the ten-point scale. Start response only when your reaction is below a 3 (some mild bodily symptoms and apprehension). Try to keep the reaction down during exposure. If the reaction reaches a 5 or 6, stop the approach and relax. Go on after your reaction is back down below 3. This retreat-approach should be used in any exposure session. If the reaction becomes strong or cannot be brought down by stopping or retreating, then discontinue exposure and return another time.

See also BEING LOOKED AT, FEAR OF; DOUBLE VISION, FEAR OF; EVIL EYE, FEAR OF.

Eysenck Personality Inventory (EPI)   Two scales to measure aspects of personality developed by German-born British psychologist Hans Jurgen Eysenck (1916–97). One is an extroversion scale; the other is the neuroticism scale known as the N scale, designed to measure the dimension of stability/instability, or trait anxiety.

See also STATE-TRAIT ANXIETY INVENTORY; TAYLOR MANIFEST ANXIETY SCALE.

Eysenck, H. J., and S. B. G. Eysenck, *Eysenck Personality Inventory* (San Diego: Education and Industrial Testing Services, 1963).

fabrics, fear of certain Fear of certain fabrics is known as textophobia. These fears may involve wools, fuzziness, satins, or silks.

See also FUZZ AVERSION.

failure, fear of Fear of failure is known as kakorraphiophobia, kakorrhaphobia, kakorrhaphiophobia, and atychiphobia. Some individuals fear failure because they lack confidence in themselves; some fear RIDICULE by others for failures. Those who fear RISK TAKING also fear failure. Many who fear failure hold excessive, rigid, or unrealistic expectations or standards for behavior.

See also CRITICISM, FEAR OF.

fainting, fear of Fear of fainting is known as asthenophobia. Fainting—an abrupt, usually brief loss of consciousness, generally associated with failure of normal blood circulation—is a PHOBIA in its own right and a symptom of other phobias. It is not unusual for otherwise normal people, including medical students and nurses, to faint from slowed heart rate at first sight of BLOOD, surgery, or INJURY. Fainting at the sight of blood may run in families, because some blood-injury phobias are thought to originate in a genetically determined, extreme AUTONOMIC response. Unlike most phobics who experience rapid heartbeat on encountering their phobic stimuli, blood-injury phobics experience a two-phase response to their phobic stimuli, consisting of rapid heartbeat at first and then a period of profound slower heartbeat to the point of fainting. Those who have an extremely slow heartbeat may develop a fear of fainting. The fainting response of blood-injury phobics is similar to that of blood donors, dental patients, and audiences of violent films.

Heart rate also slows in children seeing films of dental procedures for the first time. Children, under such circumstances, have been known to faint and then become fearful that they will faint again, causing embarrassment to themselves. Exposure by video to models of people going through dental experiences while relaxed can help such children.

See also BLOOD AND BLOOD-INJURY PHOBIA; VASOVAGAL RESPONSE.

fairies, fear of Some children develop a fear of imaginary fairies after reading about curses and wicked spells of bad fairies in stories such as "The Sleeping Beauty." However, even good fairies have habits that may disturb mortals. For example, according to folklore, fairies prize human babies and have been known to steal an unchristened infant and leave a changeling, or substitute, in its place. Some fairies only borrow human possessions, but others steal, especially if they think the victim is bad or undeserving. Appropriate treatment would probably include gradual exposure to fairy tales.

See also FAIRY TALES, FEAR OF.

fairy tales, fear of Some storybooks, fairy tales, and even nursery rhymes may lead to some childhood fears and ANXIETIES. Many fairy tales are frightening to children because they contain bad wolves, powerful giants, wicked witches, and abusive adults. For example, some FEARS are created or increased by stories such as the one about the kidnapping WITCH in "Hansel and Gretel," the ferocious wolf in "The Three Little Pigs," and the SPIDER in "Little Miss Muffet." There is some debate among psychologists about the effects of fairy tales on children. Some point out that children love fairy tales because they enjoy a certain level of fear as stimulation. Bruno Bettelheim, child psychologist, suggested that encounters with these frightening creatures and circumstances in stories that ultimately reach a happy ending actually help a child's developmental process. By experiencing frightening situations on a fantasy level, the child works out conflicts and accepts adversity in his own life. The happy ending of a fantasy promotes hopeful, positive feelings without the promise and inherent disappointments of the conclusion of a realistic story. While other experts on child development accept the value of folk and fairy tales, they point out that such stories have produced anxiety in some children and should be used with discretion and sensitivity to the individual child's reaction.

See also ANIMISM; CHILD ABUSE, FEAR OF; CHILDHOOD ANXIETIES, FEARS, AND PHOBIAS.

Bettelheim, Bruno, *The Uses of Enchantment* (New York: Knopf, 1976).

Sarafino, Edward P., *The Fears of Childhood* (New York: Human Sciences Press, 1986).

Zipes, Jack, *Breaking the Magic Spell: Radical Theories of Folk and Fairy Tales* (New York: Methuen, 1984).

faith healing   The belief that faith can cure sickness and other ills. For believers, healing is a matter of "mind over matter." For some people, belief in faith healing contributes to relief of anxieties and fears.

Historically, some faith healing takes place with the assistance of a "healer" who places hands on the individual to be healed. For example, faith healing was and still is an accepted phenomenon of Roman Catholicism, where certain saints have been thought to have healing powers received from God. The Catholic shrine at Lourdes is acknowledged to be the site of several miraculous recoveries. Native American religious practice includes rituals intended to promote healing of mental and physical ills. Faith healing is a central doctrine of Christian Scientists, who actively discourage reliance on doctors and conventional medicine. Today, there is a renewed interest in faith healing as a result of the resurgence of fundamentalist and Pentecostal religious movements. Some of the movements' ministers seem able to cure their congregants' afflictions by arousing in them a religious fervor or hysterical response.

Psychosomatic illnesses are thought to lend themselves best to the faith-healing process. To counter the claim that faith healing has succeeded where conventional medical treatments have failed, some skeptics take the position that patients resort to faith healing only when desperate. Feeling that something must work, a person gets into a state of mind in which psychosomatic symptoms disappear, or if the problem is genuinely physical, at least feels better.

Research methods are difficult to apply to faith-healing, in part because of the questionable psychosomatic aspects of many diseases. Also, many spontaneous remissions or recoveries from serious or hopeless conditions without benefit of the faith healing process have been recorded. A psychological study of individuals who had a physical stress condition relieved by faith healing showed that, while there was little indication of mental illness, they had strong DENIAL mechanisms. These denial mechanisms could keep them from recognizing continuing symptoms of their stress.

See also COMPLEMENTARY THERAPIES; CROSS-CULTURAL INFLUENCES; IMMUNE SYSTEM; MIND-BODY CONNECTIONS; PLACEBO EFFECT; PRAYER; RELIGION.

Oxman, T. E., et al., "Lack of social participation or religious strength and comfort as risk factors for death after cardiac surgery in the elderly," *Psychosomatic Medicine* 57 (1995): pp. 681–689.

Sobel, David, and Robert Ornstein, ed., "Faith Heals." *Mental Medicine Update* 4, no. 2 (1995).

falling, fear of   Fear of falling is sometimes linked to fear of HEIGHTS. For example, a phobic may be afraid of being drawn over the edge of a height, or over the edge of a platform at a train station. Some people fear falling to the extent that they cannot walk anywhere outdoors without holding on to a wall, furniture, or another person for support. Individuals who fear falling may have a distorted perception of space. Fear of falling may be related to fears of epilepsy; historically, epilepsy has been known as "falling sickness." Fear of falling may also have various psychoanalytic interpretations; for example, it might be related to the figurative sexual "falling." The fear of falling is one of the innate fears of man and usually does not completely vanish with age or therapy.

See also EPILEPSY; SPACE PHOBIA; WALKING, FEAR OF.

false statements, fear of   Fear of making false statements is known as mythophobia. This may be related to a social phobia, in that the individual fears criticism or ridicule by others, particularly if he or she unintentionally says something that is incorrect. Fear of lying, or telling something known to be untrue, may be related to a fear of being caught and punished.

See also LYING, FEAR OF; RIDICULE, FEAR OF.

families   Family and other relationships sometimes buffer the anxieties faced by individuals. However, for many people, families can also be a source of anxieties. As an example, men and women going through marital problems are especially vulnerable to the effects of relationship conflict. They may suffer from emotional consequences such as DEPRESSION and can have a compromised immune function leading to an increased rate of physical illness. CAREGIVERS who provide support for family members who are ill are another example of a highly stressed group. A decreased immune function has been observed in spouses caring for mates with ALZHEIMER'S DISEASE.

George R. Parkerson, M.D., and colleagues at Duke University Medical Center reported in the *Archives of Family Medicine* (March 1995) that individuals who see themselves as enduring high family stress are likely to have greater health problems than those reporting low family stress. Patients completed several different surveys that looked at SELF-ESTEEM, life events and changes, DEPRESSION, and family-induced stress. In addition, information on the number of physician visits, referrals to other physicians, hospitalizations, severity of illness, and cost of treatment incurred by these patients was tabulated. Results showed that family stress often had a stronger impact on health outcomes than other types of stress, such as social or financial stress. Those with high family stress scores had more frequent follow-up visits to the clinic, more referrals to specialists, more hospitalizations, a higher severity of illness, and incurred higher charges for clinical health care than those with low family stress. They also had fewer social support systems.

In evaluating family stress, researchers used the Duke Social Support and Stress Scale (DUSOCS), a 24-item questionnaire; patients indicated personal stress and/or support from each of six different types of family members and four different types of non-family members. In their report, researchers note: "It is important to remember that the study examines only the effect of family stress as perceived by the patient and does not measure family stress in terms of the family as a total system, nor does it measure perceptions of other members of the patient's family."

The Duke University researchers recommended that family physicians identify patients with high family stress and give them the special care they may require to prevent unfavorable outcomes. They suggested that questionnaires such as those used in the study can help identify patients who are at high risk of adverse health-related outcomes and who may not be recognized as such through standard medical history reports, physical exams, and medical tests.

Having patients bring family stress issues out in the open with their physicians can be useful. The researchers said that one randomized, controlled trial showed when family physicians discussed details about stressful and supportive family members with their patients after reviewing questionnaire results, patients said they felt generally better and the process helped them to improve relationships with their families.

See also COMMUNICATION; INTIMACY; RELATIONSHIPS.

Burg, M. M., and T. E. Seeman, "Families and health; the negative side of social ties." *Annals of Behavioral Medicine* 16 (1994): pp. 109–115.

Parkerson, George R., et al., "Perceived Family Stress as a Predictor of Health-Related Outcomes," *Archives of Family Medicine* 4 (March 1995).

family influence   Behaviors or attitudes learned through interaction with other members of the family. For example, parents may influence a child to be fearful of situations or objects that they fear; some fears of ANIMALS, SNAKES, DARKNESS, WATER, etc., may be learned through family influence.

Family influence also relates to how members of a particular family interact with an individual in that family. For example, the family of an agoraphobic may influence the agoraphobic member not to improve because they are providing services that enable the agoraphobic individual to remain housebound. Likewise, improvement may be facilitated by healthy family attitudes and support.

Most research on family data and fears relates to agoraphobia and blood-injury phobias. There is a higher prevalence of anxiety, panic, depressive disorders, and alcoholism among relatives of agoraphobics than those of social and simple phobics. Why agoraphobia runs in families in unclear. However, it is known that more women than men become agoraphobic, and there is an increase in alcoholism among male relatives of agoraphobics.

Blood-injury phobics have the strongest family history of all phobics. A majority of blood-injury phobics report other family members with a similar problem. This strong family history suggests that blood-injury phobia may come from a genetically determined, autonomic response. Unlike the rapid heartbeat that is the common phobic response to phobic stimuli, the heartbeat response of blood-injury phobics to their phobic stimuli is at first fast (tachycardia) and then extremely slow (bradycardia), even to the point of fainting.

See also AGORAPHOBIA; BLOOD-INJURY PHOBIA; LEARNED HELPLESSNESS; SECONDARY GAIN.

Marks, Isaac M., *Fears, Phobias and Rituals* (New York: Oxford University Press, 1987).

family neurosis   Patterns of emotionally disordered behavior within a family. An example of a family neurosis might be DEPRESSION, fear of closed places, fear of HEIGHTS, AGORAPHOBIA, or a tendency to have generalized ANXIETY DISORDERS or PANIC DISORDERS. Environmental factors are important in developing family neuroses. Some families are

more fearful than others and encourage and teach members to be fearful of the same things, on either a conscious or unconscious basis.

See also LEARNED HELPLESSNESS; NEUROSIS; SECONDARY GAIN.

family therapy   Therapy for all members of a family to help one or more phobic individuals in the family. The whole family meets as a group with the therapist and explores its relationships and processes. Psychotherapy is directed to all sources of disturbances that affect the interpersonal relationships and conflicts within the network of the individual family member's most significant and intimate relationships. The emotional relationships of the individual with his family group exert an important influence on the tendency of any one member toward the phobia. The emotional climate of family life may bind a member to a phobia, for example, by rewarding him for maintaining it, or alternately may reinforce his incentive for recovery. In family therapy, the identified patient—i.e., the phobic—is viewed as symptomatic of the family itself so that the family pattern disturbance must be the focus of the treatment and not the patient.

See also ACCEPTANCE; CLIENT-CENTERED THERAPY; SECONDARY GAIN.

fantasy   A mental image or figment of the imagination in which individuals fulfill their conscious or unconscious wishes and/or impulses. Fantasies should be differentiated from physical situations that produce PHOBIAS and FEAR reactions, although many fantasies precede anxiety and AVOIDANCE.

See also FAIRY TALES, FEAR OF.

fat, fear of being   Fear of being fat is related to a fear of gaining weight, or obesiophobia. Along with the harmful physical effects associated with obesity, such as HIGH BLOOD PRESSURE and DIABETES, fat individuals fear social discrimination. In an age in which thinness and fitness are considered desirable, fat individuals may be considered lazy and unattractive. Fear of being fat may lead to EATING DISORDERS.

See also WEIGHT GAIN, FEAR OF.

father-in-law, fear of   Fathers-in-law are some-times feared and disliked by sons-in-law because the young men resent the success of their wives' fathers and feel inadequate. A new husband may also fear a very strong father's retention of control over his daughter. A young bride may also fear her father-in-law if her husband is involved in a family-owned business. A young man entering his father's or his father-in-law's business may be expected to work long hours and meet extremely high standards of achievement to prove that he is worthy of eventually inheriting his father's or his father-in-law's position.

See also RELATIVES, FEAR OF.

fatigue, fear of   fear of fatigue is known as pono-phobia or kopophobia. Some people fear fatigue because they fear that fatigue will interfere with their control of a given situation. For example, an airline pilot will fear fatigue because it will interfere with his judgment and the safety of his passengers. Fatigue, or tiredness, is a normal reaction to physical exertion, BOREDOM, lack of rest, or emotional strain and usually results in a loss of efficiency. Fatigue may be localized and involve only certain muscles, or it may be a general feeling throughout the mind and body. Fatigue is usually a temporary state.

See also BOREDOM; CHRONIC FATIGUE SYNDROME.

fear   An emotion of uneasiness that arises as a normal response to perceived threat that may be real or imagined. Fear includes an outer behavioral expression, an inner feeling, and physiological changes. The word "fear" comes from the Old English word "faer," meaning sudden calamity or danger, and refers to justified fright.

Fear may cause any of a variety of unpleasant feelings including terror, a desire to escape, a pounding heart, muscular tenseness, trembling, DRYNESS of the throat and MOUTH, a sinking feeling in the stomach, NAUSEA, perspiration, difficulty in breathing, feeling of unreality, paralyzing WEAKNESS of the limbs, a sensation of FAINTNESS and falling, a sudden urge to URINATE or DEFECATE or a great urge to CRY.

Fear may induce certain types of behavior, such as flight, fighting, or concealment. Chronic fear in healthy people may result in FATIGUE, DEPRESSION, slowing down of mental processes, restlessness, aggression, loss of appetite, INSOMNIA, and NIGHTMARES.

Fear is a normal and useful emotion. When one faces a threat, fear often leads to rapid action, such as fighting back or removing oneself from the scene. Fear also can motivate learning and performance of socially useful responses such as careful driving or completing an examination in school.

Fears, phobias, anxieties, and PANIC, often used inappropriately as interchangeable terms, in fact have distinct meanings. Fear is considered specifically as an appropriate response to a concrete, real, knowable danger. Anxiety usually refers to a fear of uncertain origin; the individual may not know why he is afraid. A phobia is an intense, irrational fear directly associated with specific events or situations that is out of proportion to the potential danger, cannot be explained or reasoned away, is largely beyond voluntary control, and leads to avoidance of the feared situation. Panic refers to a sudden upsurge of acute, intense fear, often associated with frantic attempts to escape. Panic is extreme fear, with all the symptoms of fear intensified. Fear differs from anxiety in intensity but not quality; anxiety is a vague feeling of uneasiness or apprehension, such as anticipation of impending doom that has a relatively uncertain or unspecific source. Sometimes anxieties are related to feelings of low self-worth and anticipation of a loss of either self-esteem or the esteem of others.

There is a difference between "real fear" and "neurotic fear." An individual experiencing neurotic fear feels instinctual urges that are unacceptable to the conscious mind.

Fear can be learned by CLASSICAL, OPERANT, or vicarious conditioning.

See also ANXIETY; PANIC ATTACK; PHOBIA; RESPONSE PROPERTIES; STIMULUS PROPERTIES.

Goodwin, Donald W., *Phobia: The Facts* (Oxford: Oxford University Press, 1983).

Marks, Isaac M., *Fears and Phobias* (London: Heinemann Medical, 1969).

———, *Fears, Phobias and Rituals* (New York: Oxford University Press, 1987).

Sarafino, Edward P., *The Fears of Childhood* (New York: Human Sciences Press, 1986).

fear, enjoyment of Many people seek out and enjoy the fearful thrill of experiencing and mastering danger. Included in this category are some tightrope walkers, racing car drivers, bullfighters, certain test pilots, and mountaineers who expose themselves to extreme danger. Spectators enjoy watching dangerous sports or frightening films. Others enjoy roller coaster rides and being "scared silly."

See also SCARED STIFF.

fear, fear of Fear of fear is known as phobophobia. The fear of fear is thought to underlie agoraphobia, since the agoraphobic who fears becoming anxious in a situation and having a panic attack is afraid of fear. Fear of fear was immortalized by Franklin D. Roosevelt in his first inaugural address on March 4, 1933, when he said: "But first of all let me assert my firm belief that the only thing we have to fear is fear itself—nameless, unreasoning, unjustified terror, which paralyzes needed efforts to convert retreat into advance."

fear, guilty A term for the fear that dire consequences will befall one because of a misdeed or forbidden impulse. The term guilty fear was coined by Sandor Rado, a Hungarian-born American psychoanalyst (1870–1972). Guilty fear is related to a dread of conscience and is a prominent feature of the obsessive syndrome in which the individual represses defiant rage.

See also OBSESSIVE-COMPULSIVE DISORDER.

fear, impulse A FEAR that comes instinctively from within the individual, as contrasted with real fear, which is associated with some actual object in the environment. For example, the fear of imminent DEATH, while one is in good health, is an impulse fear, while the fear of being in a THUNDERSTORM is a reality fear.

Fear Inventory or Fear Survey Scale Tests to determine information about an individual's specific fears. Psychologists have developed tests in questionnaire form regarding fears of death, dentistry, sex, spiders, mutilation, social anxiety, test anxiety, acrophobia, agoraphobia, and other fears. These scales can be used to assess the various features associated with a feared object or situation and the various ways in which an individual might respond.

Typical scales are: Death Anxiety Scale (DAS), Spider Questionnaire (SPQ), Mutilation Questionnaire (MQ), Social Anxiety Inventory (SAI), Test Anxiety Scale (TAS), Acrophobia Questionnaire (APQ), and Agoraphobic Questionnaire Cognitions. (See also SEX ANXIETY INVENTORY; SNAKE QUESTIONNAIRE.)

The Fear Survey Scale (FSS) was developed by Joseph Wolpe (1915–97) and Peter Lang (1936–   ) as a self-report instrument to assess overall level of anxiety in a person's life, as well as particular areas of anxiety (such as social situations, injury, death, animals, etc.).

The FSS is used by clinicians as an objective measure of overall anxiety and as a measure of change with therapy. The original FSS contained over 100 items. The following is a sample of the types of items used in the scale. As can be seen, it is simple to administer and score. It utilizes a 5 point intensity scale for self-ratings.

1. Noise of vacuum cleaners
2. Open wounds
3. Being alone
4. Being in a strange place
5. Loud voices
6. Dead people
7. Speaking in public
8. Crossing streets
9. People who seem insane
10. Falling
11. Automobiles
12. Dentists
13. Being teased
14. Thunder
15. Sirens
16. Failure
17. Entering a room where other people are already seated

18. High places on land
19. Looking down from high buildings
20. Worms
21. Imaginary creatures
22. Receiving injections
23. Strangers
24. Bats
25. Journeys by train
26. Journeys by bus
27. Journeys by car
28. Feeling angry
29. People in authority
30. Flying insects
31. Seeing other people injected
32. Sudden noises
33. Dull weather
34. Crowds
35. Large open spaces
36. Cats
37. One person bullying another
38. Tough-looking people
39. Birds
40. Sight of deep water
41. Being watched working
42. Dead animals
43. Weapons
44. Crawling insects
45. Dirt
46. Sight of fighting
47. Ugly people
48. Fire
49. Sick people
50. Dogs
51. Being criticized
52. Strange shapes
53. Being in an elevator
54. Witnessing surgical operations
55. Angry people
56. Mice
57. Blood
    a. Human
    b. Animal
58. Parting from friends
59. Enclosed places
60. Prospect of a surgical operation
61. Feeling rejected by others
62. Airplanes
63. Medical odors

64. Feeling disapproved of
65. Harmless snakes
66. Cemeteries
67. Being ignored
68. Darkness
69. Premature heartbeats (missing a beat)
70. a. Nude men
    b. Nude women
71. Lightning
72. Doctors
73. People with deformities
74. Making mistakes
75. Looking foolish
76. Losing control

Kleinknecht, Ronald A., *The Anxious Self* (New York: Human Sciences Press, 1986).

fears, childhood   See CHILDHOOD ANXIETIES, FEARS, AND PHOBIAS.

fears, minor   See MINOR FEARS.

Fear Survey Schedule II   Developed by J. M. Geer after extensive factor analytic and statistical studies of the original Fear Survey Schedule. This version has a seven-point intensity scale and covers fifty-one items. Items are nouns relating to animals, social situations, injury and death, objects, noises, and other situations. Mean scores usually center around 100–108 for females and around 75–82 for males.

Geer, J. M., "The Development of a Scale to Measure Fear," *Behavioral Research and Therapy* 3 (1965), pp. 45–53.

THE GEER FEAR-SURVEY SCHEDULE II

Item
1. Sharp objects
2. Being a passenger in a car
3. Dead bodies
4. Suffocating
5. Failing a test
6. Looking foolish

7. Being a passenger in an airplane
8. Worms
9. Arguing with parents
10. Rats and mice
11. Life after death
12. Hypodermic needles
13. Being criticized
14. Meeting someone for the first time
15. Roller coasters
16. Being alone
17. Making mistakes
18. Being misunderstood
19. Death
20. Being in a fight
21. Crowded places
22. Blood
23. Heights
24. Being a leader
25. Swimming alone
26. Illness
27. Being with drunks
28. Illness or injury to loved ones
29. Being self-conscious
30. Driving a car
31. Meeting authority
32. Mental illness
33. Closed places
34. Boating
35. Spiders
36. Thunderstorms
37. Not being a success
38. God
39. Snakes
40. Cemeteries
41. Speaking before a group
42. Seeing a fight
43. Death of a loved one
44. Dark places
45. Strange dogs
46. Deep water
47. Being with a member of the opposite sex
48. Stinging insects
49. Untimely or early death
50. Losing a job
51. Auto accidents

Response Properties

Are qualities of reactions to fearful situations that help therapists differentiate fear from anxiety. In differentiating fear and anxiety, therapists consider the duration and intensity of response. If a source of threat is vague and not predictable, the response might last longer and be more pervasive, keeping the individual in a state of chronic arousal, apprehension, or anxiety. However, fear is considered a response to a more specific, predictable source, and though it would be more acute, the episode might end quickly. A more intense reaction is considered fear; less intense, anxiety.

The following table further explains differentiation between fears and anxieties.

DIFFERENTIATING FEAR AND ANXIETY		
Response Properties	Fear	Anxiety
Response components	Behavioral Cognitive Physiological	Behavioral Cognitive Physiological
Duration	Elicited by specific stimuli	Elicited by generalized stimuli
	Short duration	Long-lasting
Intensity	More intense	Less intense

See also ANXIETY; FEAR; STIMULUS PROPERTIES.

feathers, fear of   Feathers in pillows and on clothing arouse fear in certain phobic individuals. Feather phobia, which may be related to BIRD phobia, is frequently embarrassing to the sufferer who is aware of its ridiculous appearance to others. Some feather phobics are afraid to go outdoors for fear of seeing a creature with feathers, such as a bird; and some have disturbing dreams about feathers. Some who fear feathers avoid going to farms and barnyards where they may see chickens, ducks, or other fowl. Fear of feathers is probably a fear of birds or other feathered creatures.

See also BIRDS, FEAR OF; WINGED THINGS, FEAR OF.

Melville, Joy, *Phobias and Obsessions* (New York: Coward, McCann and Geoghegan, 1977).

febriphobia   See FEVER, FEAR OF.

FEAR QUESTIONNAIRE

Following is a brief, self-administered fear questionnaire (patterned after Marks's design) identifying common fear areas, particularly for agoraphobics. There are no norms on this scale, but the individual can use it for measuring progress in overcoming phobic problems.

Choose a number from the scale below to show how much you avoid each of the situations listed, because of fear or other unpleasant feelings. Then write the number you chose in the box opposite each situation.

0	1	2	3	4	5	6	7	8
Would Not Avoid It		Slightly		Definitely		Markedly		Always

1. Traveling alone by bus or train   ____
2. Walking alone in busy streets   ____
3. Going into crowded stores   ____
4. Going alone far from home   ____
5. Large open spaces   ____
6. Injections or minor surgery   ____
7. Hospitals   ____
8. Sight of blood   ____
9. Thought of injury   ____
10. Going to the dentist   ____
11. Eating or drinking with other people   ____
12. Being watched or stared at   ____
13. Talking to people in authority   ____
14. Being criticized   ____
15. Speaking or acting to an audience   ____
16. Other situations (describe, e.g., animals, thunder)   ____

GRAND TOTAL   ____

Below describe in your own words the *main* phobia you want treated (e.g., "shopping alone in a busy supermarket" or "fluttering birds"):

Isaac M. Marks, *Living with Fear* (New York: McGraw-Hill, 1978).

feces, fear of   Fear of feces is known as coprophobia. Feces—waste matter expelled from the bowels—are also known as excrement and fecal matter. This phobia may include fear of expelling one's own feces, or of coming into contact with or viewing feces. In psychoanalytic terms, withholding the feces is one of the earliest expressions of the drive for aggression and independence. Fear of fecal matter is known as scatophobia.

See also PSYCHOANALYSIS.

feedback   In therapy, information given to the individual about the nature and effects of his or her behavior. Feedback may take many forms, including direct comments, role playing, or videotape replays. Feedback affects correction and self-correction and may change or reinforce behavior. Therapists in some types of therapy offer more feedback than those in others; for example, in behavior therapy there is more feedback than in psychoanalysis.

See also BEHAVIOR THERAPY; PSYCHOANALYSIS; THERAPY.

Feldenkrais method   See BODY THERAPIES.

felinophobia   See CATS, FEAR OF.

female genitalia, fear of   Known as eurotrophobia. Female genitalia consist of the vagina, uterus, ovaries, fallopian tubes, and related structures. Those who have this fear may focus their energy on nonsexual objects that resemble or symbolize the female genitalia and may develop FETISHES (neurotic preferences) for them. Fear of female genitalia affects women and men.

See also SEXUAL FEARS.

feminophobia   See WOMEN, FEAR OF.

feng shui   A philosophy that seeks to ensure harmony and good fortune by following the Chinese art of geomancy. The practice may help relieve some anxieties and fears. Feng shui involves the proper alignment of objects with geographical features. In *Hemispheres* magazine (November 1993), John Goff translates *feng shui* as "wind and water" and defines it as "a product of a culture that honors the spirits of mountains and rivers and views the landscape as a living thing with cosmic currents."

Practiced first in Hong King, where it influenced the design of many corporate buildings, including the offices of Citicorp International and Motorola Semiconductors Hong Kong, Ltd., feng shui has

---

HOW TO USE FENG SHUI TO PREVENT ANXIETIES WHEN BUILDING OR FURNISHING A HOUSE

- Entryways and windows should be wide enough to allow light, which symbolizes the Sun and allows good energy to come in.
- Mirrors are particularly useful in cramped spaces and over furniture that does not face windows or doors because they reflect positive energy and deflect negative forces.
- Buildings near water are good because water is an element of wealth, insight, and motivation. Avoid building near tall buildings, because they block positive energy, and on cul de sacs, because negative energy has no place to escape.

---

spread to other parts of the world as well. In addition to corporate offices, there are factors that can remove anxieties from a household.

fetish   A nonsexual object or part of the body that arouses sexual interest or excitement by association or symbolization. Common fetishes are feminine undergarments, shoes, or boots. Individuals who have fetishes obtain sexual gratification from fondling, kissing, or licking the object on which they focus. A fetish may develop because of a fear of a part of the body, such as the genitalia, but most are the result of masturbation in the presence of the fetish object. Some individuals fear fetishes or fetishism. Some fetishes are associated with a childhood caretaker, such as a mother's lingerie on the clothesline, etc.

The term fetish was derived from the Portuguese word *fetico,* meaning "a charm." Alfred Binet first used the term in the psychoanalytic sense—that is, referring to an object that becomes emotionally charged and, in some cases, is the source of perverted sexual gratification—in 1888.

See also FEMALE GENITALIA, FEAR OF; SEXUAL FEARS.

fever, fear of   Fear of fever is known as febriphobia, fibriophobia, and pyrexiophobia. Individuals who fear ILLNESS may also fear fever. Some who fear fever do so because they fear a LOSS OF CONTROL over their behavior. Some fear the HALLUCINATIONS, DELUSIONS, or CONVULSIONS that may accompany high fever. Such individuals fear doing something to embarrass themselves at those times.

See also HALLUCINATIONS, FEAR OF.

fibromyalgia   A common form of arthritis that causes pain in the muscles and tendons of the body. It is sometimes called fibromyalgia syndrome or FMS. Fibromyalgia affects about 6 million people in the United States, primarily women between the ages of 20 to 45.

Fibromyalgia is an accepted clinical syndrome that may trigger considerable anxiety for the sufferer, not only because of the pain and discomfort and the loss of function, but also because of the often extreme difficulty in having this medical problem diagnosed properly. In some cases, patients are not diagnosed for years, and some are referred to psychiatrists because their physicians believe the pain is imaginary. Yet the pain of fibromyalgia is real, and studies by physicians such as Roland Staud, M.D., have demonstrated that patients with fibromyalgia experience pain faster, more acutely, and for longer periods than those who do not have fibromyalgia.

ANXIETY DISORDERS are more common among patients diagnosed with fibromyalgia than those without this disorder. According to a 2006 study based in New York in *Pain* by researchers K. G. Raphael et al., the lifetime risk of the development of anxiety disorders, especially OBSESSIVE-COMPULSIVE DISORDER and POST-TRAUMATIC STRESS DISORDER, was five times greater among women with fibromyalgia.

In another study which analyzed 2,595 cases of fibromyalgia from 1997–2002, reported in a 2006 issue of the *Journal of Clinical Rheumatology,* researchers found that the patients diagnosed with fibromyalgia were from two to seven times more likely than those without fibromyalgia to have one or more of the following conditions: anxiety, DEPRESSION, chronic fatigue, HEADACHE, IRRITABLE BOWEL SYNDROME, rheumatoid arthritis, and systemic lupus erythematosus. Other studies have demonstrated that hepatitis B and C are often associated with patients with fibromyalgia.

There are a variety of theoretical triggers for fibromyalgia, such as childhood abuse, severe injuries, and imbalances of a variety of neurochemicals and hormones of the body. Researchers continue to seek to determine causal factors.

Symptoms and Diagnostic Path

There are no laboratory tests or imaging tests to detect fibromyalgia, and physicians must diagnose patients based on their medical history and their symptoms. Physicians may order tests to rule out other disorders, such as HYPOTHYROIDISM, chronic fatigue syndrome, arthritis, and Lyme disease. Rheumatologists and other physicians use the 18 tender points system developed by the American College of Rheumatology to diagnose fibromyalgia. With this system, individuals who experience pain in at least 11 of 18 tender points are considered to have fibromyalgia. These tender points are located in different areas of the body, such as at the back of the neck, the front of the neck, the upper shoulder blades, the shoulders, the back of the elbow, the lower back, the upper leg, and the knees.

Most patients with fibromyalgia have difficulty sleeping because of their chronic pain, and a sleep disorder, as well as chronic and generalized pain, is another indicator to the physician that fibromyalgia may be present.

Treatment Options and Outlook

Nonsteroidal anti-inflammatory medications are often used, as are corticosteroids. Some patients experience improvement with prescribed transdermal skin patches placed over the painful areas, such as Lidoderm. Some ANTIDEPRESSANTS may be helpful, particularly serotonin norepinephrine reuptake inhibitors such as duloxetine (Cymbalta), which has been demonstrated to relieve pain as well as depression and anxiety. Tricyclic antidepressants may help to improve sleep because they are sedating. They are not habit forming. Some patients may need to take a prescribed sleep remedy, although it is important to not become dependent on such drugs.

Non-pharmacologic treatment emphasizes aerobic exercise, particularly water aerobics. Sports such as swimming, bicycling, and walking are encouraged. Some people find ACUPUNCTURE, BIOFEEDBACK, hypnotherapy, MASSAGE, and SUPPORT GROUPS to be helpful. Many patients, in an acute stage of their disease, worry about having bone cancer or other ominous disorders; some become very anxious. Psychotherapy can help certain individuals overcome the attendant stresses of this disorder. A proper diagnosis will also help to alleviate anxiety over the symptoms of fibromyalgia.

Risk Factors and Preventive Measures

Women of childbearing age are more prone to developing fibromyalgia than men or older women, which may be related to hormonal fluctuations, although this is unclear. There are no known preventive measures against the onset of fibromyalgia.

Cold weather, extremes of activity, fluctuation of barometric pressure, and stress often aggravate the symptoms of fibromyalgia in those with this medical problem. Although these conditions cannot be alleviated, patients can often anticipate cold weather or barometric changes and try to arrange an easier schedule on those days.

See also PAIN; PSYCHOTHERAPIES.

Arnold, L. M., et al., "A Randomized, Double-Blind, Placebo-Controlled Trial of Duloxetine in the Treatment of Women with Fibromyalgia with or without Major Depressive Disorder," *Pain* 119 (December 15, 2005): pp. 5–15.

Raphael, K. G., et al., "Psychiatric Comorbidities in a Community Sample of Women with Fibromyalgia," *Pain* 124, nos. 1–2 (May 12, 2006): pp. 117–125.

Staud, Roland, M.D., with Christine Adamec, *Fibromyalgia for Dummies.* (New York: Wiley Publishing, 2002).

Weir, P. T., et al., "The Incidence of Fibromyalgia and Its Associated Comorbidities: A Population-Based Retrospective Cohort Study Based on International Classification of Diseases, 9th Revision Codes," *Journal of Clinical Rheumatology* 12, no. 3 (June 2006): pp. 124–128.

fight or flight response   The sequence of internal activities triggered when an individual is faced with a threat. The response helps prepare the body for combat and struggle or for running away to safety. This is associated with sympathetic nervous system arousal.

filth, fear of   Fear of filth is known as mysophobia, rhyphobia, rypophobia, and rupophobia. This fear may be related to fears of CONTAMINATION and GERMS and to fears of using public toilet facilities. Some obsessive-compulsives fear filth.

See also OBSESSIVE-COMPULSIVE DISORDER.

financial anxieties   See MONEY.

fire, fear of   Fear of fire is known as arsonphobia or pyrophobia. People who are phobic about fire may avoid striking matches and attending occasions that involve cooking outdoors over a campfire. They may become obsessive about CHECKING the gas supply in their homes and making sure that there is an escape route when they are in an unfamiliar building.

Historically, fire has been a fear- and awe-inspiring symbol in the mind of man, with both divine and evil associations. The tradition of a sacred fire tended by virgins was present in early Greek, Irish, and Peruvian cultures. The pantheon of gods in most religions includes a god of fire. Fire was considered to be a test of power or purity, and in many cultures magicians and wizards demonstrated their power by walking over coals or swallowing fire. Christian saints and priests were supposedly immune to injury by fire. Trial by fire was considered a test of virginity, truthfulness, and honesty in general. Fire has also had associations with evil and the powers of darkness. The fires of hell are the fate of sinners. Burning was the method of execution for WITCHES and heretics. Smiths were held in awe and considered possible agents of the DEVIL because of their work with fire. Marsh fires in Britain once were thought to have SUPERNATURAL causes. The strange phenomenon called St. Elmo's fire, a flickering light around ships' masts, was believed to prophesy bad weather.

Psychologically, fire is associated with ANGER and aggression. For example, a "firebrand" is an agitator, a promoter of strife. When someone is angry, he is said to have smoke or steam coming out of his ears. There are many hostile fire-breathing dragons in legends and fairy tales.

Arthur Schopenhauer (1788–1860), a German philosopher, is said to have always lived on a first story because he feared fire.

Modern fears of fire have valid foundations; children playing with matches account for 75,000 fires a year in the United States, which kill about 10,000 people.

See also OBSESSIVE-COMPULSIVE DISORDER.

Cavendish, Richard, ed., *Man, Myth and Magic* (New York: Marshall Cavendish, 1983), "Fire."

Melville, Joy, *Phobias and Obsessions* (New York: Coward, McCann & Geoghegan, 1977), p. 146.

World Book, Inc., *World Book Encyclopedia* (Chicago: World Book, Inc., 1987), "Fire Prevention."

fish, fear of   Fear of fish is known as ichthyophobia. This fear may include looking at fish, imagining or seeing pictures of fish, or eating fish. Fear of being near lakes or the seashore may be related, if the bodies of water are filled with fish.

See also LAKES, FEAR OF; WATER, FEAR OF.

fitness anxiety   Individuals who have fitness anxiety have a fear of general unfitness or poor health. Fitness anxiety seems to be a result of the 1980s "fitness craze" and the rising popularity of jogging, aerobic exercise, and health clubs, as well as medical evidence that suggests that diet and exercise patterns may be significant in the prevention of heart disease and other major health hazards. Fitness anxiety can lead to obsessive behavior regarding one's own exercise habits or diet. Some individuals—for example, runners—develop compulsions to do their extra mile every day or a given number of miles every week, regardless of weather conditions or how they feel. Some individuals actually overexercise—for example, young women runners who run excessively lose weight, become very thin, and cease to menstruate.

See also EATING DISORDERS; EXERCISE, COMPULSION TO.

fixation   An obsessional preoccupation with a simple idea, impulse, or aim; sometimes known as an "idée fixe." This may occur in OBSESSIVE-COMPULSIVE DISORDER, AGORAPHOBIA, and other psychological disorders. In PSYCHOANALYSIS, a fixation is the persistence of an early stage of development or an inappropriate attachment to an early psychosexual object or mode of gratification, such as anal or oral activity. Such a fixation persists during adulthood in immature and neurotic form, interfering with other normal attachments. Smoking is sometimes interpreted as an oral fixation, hoarding as an anal-stage fixation, and anxiety as a response to unresolved Oedipal conflicts during the phallic stage.

See also FIXATION PHOBIA.

fixation phobia   Early childhood fears of a specific event or object that a person retains into adulthood without resolving. Although older people tend to fear social harm, the FEARS of children usually involve danger of some kind of physical INJURY or DEATH. Common fears include WATER, THUNDERSTORMS, DOCTORS, and BLOOD. Children usually outgrow fears related to SUPERNATURAL agents such as GHOSTS, WITCHES, CORPSES, or mysterious events, being alone in DARK or strange places, BEING LOST, being attacked by humans or animals, bodily INJURY, ILLNESS, surgical operations, PAIN, FALLING, or traffic accidents. SOCIAL PHOBIAS, such as attending parties, shaking hands, or PUBLIC SPEAKING, may also become fixation phobias.

Fixation phobias may persist into adulthood because phobic children begin to avoid their feared objects or situations at an early age, and their fears may be reinforced by the fears of their parents.

In psychoanalytic theory, a fixation is the arrest of psychosexual development at a particular stage through too much or too little gratification.

See also DEATH, FEAR OF; DEVELOPMENTAL STAGES; ILLNESS, FEAR OF; INJURY, FEAR OF; PHOBIA; PSYCHOANALYSIS; SOCIAL PHOBIA.

Beck, Aaron T., and Gary Emery, *Anxiety Disorders and Phobias* (New York: Basic Books, 1985).

flashbacks   See ANXIETY DISORDERS; POST-TRAUMATIC STRESS DISORDER.

flashing lights, fear of   Fear of flashing lights is known as selaphobia. This fear may be related in a general way to fear of light, glaring lights, or light and shadows. Some individuals fear driving at night because of flashing lights.

See also LIGHT, FEAR OF; LIGHT AND SHADOWS, FEAR OF.

flatulence, fear of   Flatulence, or the expulsion of air from the digestive tract through the mouth or anus, is a common symptom experienced by individuals who have digestive disorders or IRRITABLE BOWEL SYNDROME. Belching may be caused by unwittingly swallowing large amounts of air during rapid eating, gum chewing, or as a nervous habit. Fear of passing wind (gas), or of BELCHING, are SOCIAL PHOBIAS. The individual fears embarrassing himself or herself, making disagreeable noises, or causing unpleasant odors. Some who have this fear may avoid social situations in which they are near people or in enclosed spaces with other people, such as elevators.

See also BELCHING, FEAR OF.

flood, fear of   Fear of flood is known as antlophobia. This is one of many fears of natural disasters, which include tornadoes and hurricanes. Some who live in areas that commonly flood after a rainy season have a realistic fear of flood and many take precautions, such as stocking sandbags at the appropriate time. Only when such a FEAR is unreasonable is it considered a PHOBIA.

flooding   A technique of behavior therapy in which the individual experiences the fear-provoking object or situation in his or her imagination without being instructed to relax. The theory behind flooding is that after prolonged exposure the individual will become accustomed to imagined feared objects or situations and thus eventually fear them less. This process is thought to follow the laws of extinction or a gradual diminution with repeated exposure. Exposure to fear-producing stimuli might occur at full intensity for a minimum of two hours and usually three to four hours per session.

In World War II, a group of U.S. soldiers who were severely startled by noise and even music were hospitalized and forced to watch twelve fourteen-minute showings of increasingly loud war films. Reactions to the films gradually changed from terror to boredom, and all but one of the soldiers improved.

See also DESENSITIZATION; EXPOSURE THERAPY; IMPLOSION THERAPY.

flowers, fear of   Fear of flowers is known as anthophobia. This fear may be of a particular flower, or of a characteristic of some flowers, such as size or texture.

fluoxetine   An antidepressant drug.

See also ANTIDEPRESSANTS; DEPRESSION.

flutes, fear of   Fear of flutes is known as autophobia and aulophobia. In some societies, flutes are considered to be voices of spirits and therefore represent supernatural beings (who may have been mythological ancestors of the clan). In some cultures, flutes are made of bamboo and cane with a wooden stopper and may be decorated with hair, feathers, and shells. Their motifs may represent clan totems, either human figures or animals, especially birds. Flutes are often played during initiation or cult ceremonies. Because of their shape, for some, flutes may be phallic symbols. Individuals who fear rods or sticks may also fear flutes.

See also RODS, FEAR OF.

fluvoxamine   An antidepressant drug.

See also ANTIDEPRESSANTS; DEPRESSION.

flying, fear of   Fear of flying, known as aerophobia, represents one of the major fear categories for adults in the United States and probably throughout the world. Estimates of the number of fearful people vary, but the most comprehensive survey concluded that some 25,000,000 Americans—one of every six adults—are afraid to fly.

Flying phobia is sometimes considered a specific phobia, but it also occurs as part of the agoraphobic syndrome. People with the specific phobia

FACTORS LEADING TO FEAR OF FLYING

Fear of experiencing a panic attack on the flight

Expectation of claustrophobic feelings on the flight

Media/verbal information about dangers inherent in flying

Vicarious acquisition of the fear

Turbulent weather or expectation of bad weather

Delays in landing

Emotional reactions (e.g., grief) that are brought to the flight avoid flying because they may fear crashes or other calamities. Those who have agoraphobia fear having a panic attack and its consequences.

The fear of flying itself has two points of origin—the anticipatory situation and the flying situation itself. Anticipatory anxiety occurs because a commitment has been made to fly (a reservation has been made, ticket purchased, people informed of trip, etc.). Anticipatory anxiety usually is experienced as feelings of dread, rapid pulse, total body sensations (tension, warmth, etc.), and fear-inducing images and thoughts. Interestingly, the anticipatory fear is usually not of the airplane itself but of uncontrollable outcomes such as fear of losing control of oneself in the airplane and going crazy or embarrassing oneself in public; fear of separation from loved ones, fear of death; fears of relinquishing control to someone else; thoughts of falling from the sky and dying in a crash; and so on. Fear in the plane itself may encompass many of the anticipatory fears just described but also usually involves fears of being enclosed, fears of being alone or away from others one depends on, feeling trapped and unable to leave at will, fears of social rejection due to the reaction, fear of the fear sensations, and sometimes feelings about the place or person the individual is leaving or the place or person the individual may be seeing at the destination.

News reports of air crashes, stories and television and movie depictions can also provide stimuli for fear thoughts and reactions. It has also been pointed out that much of the common language used in the air-travel industry has a fatalistic and fear engendering ring, such as "terminal," "final boarding," "final approach," "departure lounge," and so on; the fears engendered by terminology may be supplemented by insurance desks, oxygen masks, crash procedures, and a number of reminders of possible adverse consequences to flying. Many of these factors are external cues for anxiety while thoughts and sensations represent internal triggers to anxiety.

Treatment for the fear of flying has varied from traditional therapies to hypnosis, flooding, and exposure therapies. The last provide the best long-term success rate at about 75 percent to 80 percent. A "cue-controlled" relaxation procedure in which the phobic learns to produce relaxation on cue seems to offer promise as an effective technique. Success, of course, involves more than just being able to fly. The more rigorous criterion involves flying with progressively increased ease and comfort over a long-term series of trials. Unfortunately, there are very few experimental studies to date that demonstrate comparative therapy effects.

The most commonly used drug for the fear of flying is probably alcohol. Unfortunately, while alcohol reduces autonomic arousal, it tends to produce anxiety-like sensations (such as dizziness, loss of balance, mental confusion, lack of control of perceptual-motor functions, and so on), which, in turn, can trigger an anxiety response. PROPRANOLOL and ALPRAZOLAM are two drugs commonly used for fear of flying. They are both fast-acting and produce relatively few side effects. Triazolam has also been used on a more experimental basis.

Efforts to identify personality qualities associated with the fear of flying have not been fruitful. Interestingly, family trauma associated with flying (such as loss of or injury to a family member—even a distant one—in an aircraft accident) is a significant predictor of phobic reaction. This would support a modeling theory of acquisition. Also, multiphobics or individuals suffering from panic disorders have a higher incidence of aerophobia than uniphobics and seem to be much more difficult to treat than the latter.

Flying Fear in Aircrew

Flying phobia disables aircrew members as well as some individuals in the public. Fear of flying is a major cause of airline and air force personnel being grounded. Flying phobia may come on gradually along with irritability and insomnia. Some who become fearful of flying report more childhood and other adulthood phobias before the fear of flying began and more flying accidents in their families. Some flying phobics also have more marital or sexual problems than those in the general population and are more neurotic and introverted than aircrew members who do not fear flying.

Experimental comparison studies of phobic and nonphobic aircrews reveals that galvanic skin responsibility (GSR), history of childhood anxiety and phobias, worries about spouse and children,

---

TIPS ON HOW TO FLY MORE COMFORTABLY

1. Make a commitment to fly when you choose to do so. Don't agree to fly with the idea you will back out. See flying as an opportunity for you to become less fearful.
2. Prepare yourself far in advance. Practice relaxation so you build skills in calming yourself. This will not prevent you from becoming anxious, but it will lessen the intensity, allow you to recover faster, and give you some control over the situation. Visualize yourself flying comfortably (as you would like to be able to fly) when you are relaxed.
3. Practice some desensitization. For example, go to the airport to relax yourself in that environment. Watch the planes take off and land and relax yourself. Imagine being comfortable in an airplane that you are watching.
4. Take things with you to occupy yourself when flying. Also, make a tape for relaxation and to remind yourself of thoughts and ideas that will help you cope on the plane.
5. Remember, the fear will not go away without practice, preparation, and continued flying on a regular basis.

---

and family traumas (loss of life) associated with flying were 85 percent predictive of groupings.

Fear of flying has not been noted as a problem in the 8 percent of aircrew who survive ejection from an aircraft despite injuries. Many have had continuing emotional reactions including FEAR, ANXIETY, anger, disgust, or altered motivation. Some aircrew members who become agoraphobic responded well to some form of guided exposure. Behavior therapies are demonstrably effective in aircrews and pilots.

Some members of the military suffer a FEAR OF FLYING as a symptom of POST-TRAUMATIC STRESS DISORDER.

See also AGORAPHOBIA; ANXIETY DISORDERS; CLAUSTROPHOBIA; CONTROL; EXPOSURE THERAPY.

Beckham, Jean C., Scott R. Vrana, Jack G. May et al., "Emotional Processing and Fear Measurement Synchrony As Indicators of Treatment Outcome in Fear of Flying," *J. Behav. Ther & Exp. Pychiatr* 21, no. 3 (1990): pp. 153–162.

McCarthy, Geoffrey W., and Kenneth D. Craig, "Flying Therapy for Flying Phobia." *Aviation, Space, and Environmental Medicine* 66, no. 12 (December 1995).

McNally, Richard J., "Fear of Flying in Agoraphobia and Simple Phobia: Distinguishing Features." *Journal of Anxiety Disorders* 6 (1992): pp. 319–324.

Ost, Lars-Goran, Mats Brandberg, and Thomas Alm, "One Versus Five Sessions of Exposure in the Treatment of Flying Phobia," *Behav. Res. Ther.* 35, no. 11 (1997): pp. 987–996.

Wilhelm, Frank H., and Walton T. Roth, "Clinical Characteristics of Flight Phobia." *Journal of Anxiety Disorders* 11, no. 3 (1997): pp. 241–261.

flying things, fear of   Some people fear flying things, such as birds, flying insects, bats, or butterflies, because such creatures fly at them unpredictably, scare them with sudden motion, and may get in their hair. Those who fear flying things may keep their windows closed tightly and rarely venture outdoors. They also avoid enclosed spaces in which they might become trapped with a flying thing, such as a bat in a barn or belfry. Many people have overcome these fears with exposure therapy.

See also BATS, FEAR OF; BIRDS, FEAR OF; EXPOSURE THERAPY; WINGED THINGS, FEAR OF.

fog, fear of   Fear of fog is known as homichlophobia and nebulaphobia. Fog is frightening because it stimulates near-blindness, distorts shapes, and produces a closed-in, claustrophobic sensation that makes an individual feel a LOSS OF CONTROL over his environment. An object or person can be invisible very close at hand and then appear out of the fog in a startling manner. Fog is associated with confusion and lack of clarity; foggy thinking and language are muddled and imprecise.

Fog is frequently used in suspenseful scenes in horror or mystery films because of its power to inspire fear and apprehension. Fog patches that appear and move suddenly cause particular fear and an impending sense of danger.

See also AIR POLLUTION, FEAR OF.

folk healers   Many individuals around the world consult folk healers for anxiety problems. Before the advent of formalized medical systems, many societies devised ways to cope with fear and phobias. These include use of magic and charms and invocation of divine intervention. Studies during the 1960s indicated that exorcism and antiwitch measures were still prevalent in many Far Eastern cultures. Demonological and astrological remedies were (and still are) prescribed along with recently developed drugs to relieve anxieties. Medicine men are still used extensively by Indians in some societies today. Additionally, witch doctors, healers, and medicine men are still common in Third World countries.

See also DEPRESSION ACROSS CULTURES; WITCHES AND WITCHCRAFT, FEAR OF.

food fears   Fear of food, or certain foods, is known as sitophobia, sitiophobia, and cibophobia. Some individuals fear eating certain foods, such as meat. For some, the fear is related to religious TABOOS. For example, many Hindus are vegetarian, and Muslims and Jews are forbidden to eat pork. If a religious individual eats a forbidden food by mistake or coercion, he or she may feel various reactions and may vomit or feel nauseous for days.

Food Aversions

Many people strongly dislike certain foods, often because they associate them with nausea and vomiting. Most food aversions are taste aversions, but individuals may also dislike its sight, smell, or symbolic aspects. Many people avoid new foods. Individuals decide which foods are acceptable based on cultural and individual rearing patterns. Some, who mistakenly eat a taboo food, may become terrified of imagined consequences.

See also EATING, FEAR OF; NAUSEA; SWALLOWING, FEAR OF; TABOOS.

foreigners, fear of   Fear of foreigners or strangers is known as zenophobia or xenophobia. Many who fear novelty, newness, or anything different may also fear foreigners.

See also NEWNESS, FEAR OF; NOVELTY, FEAR OF; STRANGERS, FEAR OF.

forests, fear of   Fear of forests is known as hylophobia, hylephobia, and xylophobia. Fear of forests may be related to fears of trees or of landscapes.

See also LANDSCAPES, FEAR OF; TREES, FEAR OF.

forgetting   An inability to retrieve stored long- or short-term memories. It is a common occurrence and a source of anxiety for many people. Most people forget short-term as well as long-term memories, particularly the elderly, who experience memory loss as they grow older. But forgetting is not just a sign of old age. Many people consciously block out stressful memories, and many are simply forgetful. They may forget recently made appointments, what their boss told them earlier in the day, or occurrences that happened in childhood.

Scientific studies have concentrated primarily on two factors: inhibition and loss of retrieval clues. Inhibition is the theory that similar kinds of learning, either before or after the event to be remembered, interfere with later recall of that event. Loss of retrieval clues is based on the theory that recall is easier when the individual is dealing with familiar people, things, and situations. Other theories hold that individuals have "selective" memories, and may forget events or situations previously encountered that were unpleasant, stressful, or even traumatic. This concept is related to repression, which suggests that forgetting is a COPING mechanism.

Many individuals have fears of developing ALZHEIMER'S DISEASE when they begin to experience symptoms of forgetting.

See also FLASHBACKS; MEMORY; POST-TRAUMATIC STRESS DISORDER.

Framingham Type A scale   See CORONARY-PRONE TYPE A BEHAVIOR.

Francophobia   Fear of France and things relating to the French culture. Also known as Gallophobia. Often such fears relate to hearing the spoken language.

See also FOREIGNERS, FEAR OF; STRANGERS, FEAR OF.

free association A therapeutic technique in which the individual is encouraged to relax conscious control over his or her thoughts and to say anything and everything that comes to mind. This technique may be useful in associating past events, feelings, and attitudes with phobic behavior. Free association is a key procedure in PSYCHOANALYSIS. The assumption is that over time, hitherto repressed material will come forth for examination by the ANALYSAND and the analyst.

freedom, fear of Fear of freedom is known as eleutherophobia. Such fears were noted after the Civil War in the United States when many former slaves returned to work for their masters because they did not want (or were not able) to be free. Similarly, convicts released from prison will sometimes commit another crime in order to return. This phenomenon is also unfortunately associated with "treatment" of the mentally ill in hospitals where they quickly become "institutionalized" by regimes that enforce compliance, passivity, and noninteraction.

free-floating anxiety Continual ANXIETY not easily attributable to any specific STIMULI or reasonable danger. This was a Freudian term used in the first diagnostic system. The current preferred terminology is GENERALIZED ANXIETY, indicating an anxiety state that persists through a person's daily activities (perhaps varying in intensity at different times or locations).

See also FEAR; PHOBIA.

friends Friendships are unique among human RELATIONSHIPS. While individuals have little or no choice in family or neighbors, they can choose their friends. Some friendships evolve from shared interests or values, some simply from a shared history, and some from compatible personalities. Qualities most appreciated in friends include loyalty, trust, and an ability to keep a confidence. People want to feel that they can rely on their friends and have open and honest dealings during good as well as anxious and stressful times.

When friends are supportive, they help relieve anxieties during periods of turmoil or crisis. Individuals who experience DEPRESSION often report a lack of friends, although having a wide circle of friends is not a preventive factor for depression. Some reports have indicated that individuals who have many friends may be healthier and actually live longer than those who do not.

Friends can also be sources of anxiety, because they may challenge or be challenged by other relationships in the individual's life. For example, a friendship may be broken or changed when a friend marries. A closer friend may be unsettling to a spouse or lover. Friends who do not meet with parents' approval can be a source of family conflict. Friends who decide to share housing or enter into a business partnership sometimes discover undesirable facets of the other person's personality that could be ignored when the relationship was less formal. In the WORKPLACE, a friendship may dissolve when two people are vying for the same promotion.

A 1990 Gallup Poll reported that the typical American places much importance on friendship. It also indicated some frustrations about the time and flexibility needed to form friendships. The survey showed that women and men approach friendship quite differently. Women tended to form more intimate relationships with other women than men with men. One-on-one activities that promote conversation are more popular with women, whereas men are more likely to get together in groups for sports, cards, or other such activities. Men rely on their wives for emotional support, but many women, even those who are married, often rely on women friends. Women are more likely than men to have a best friend of the same sex, but a third of the men surveyed said a woman was their best friend.

People make friends in many ways. In the Gallup report, 51 percent of the 18- to 29-year-olds made most of their friends at school. Of the 30- to 49-year-olds, 51 percent said they made most of their friends through work. From the age of 50, friends came from a greater variety of sources, including church, work, clubs, or other organizations.

When participants were asked about arguments with friends, those under age 30 reported more disagreements. Friendship evidently becomes more tranquil with age, possibly because friends settle their differences and learn to recognize sore spots, or, possibly, because age enables people to recognize and discard difficult and stressful relationships.

See also INTIMACY; RELATIONSHIPS.

frigidity   A woman's inability to obtain satisfaction (usually orgasm) during SEXUAL INTERCOURSE. This may result from a lack of adequate stimulation or a misunderstanding between the partners concerning sexual behavior and wishes. Cultural rejection of certain practices may also play a part. Freudian psychoanalysts attribute frigidity to many sources, including aggressive inhibition, ill-managed parental love, penis envy, and imperfect transfer of capacity for stimulation from the clitoris to the vagina. Modern sexual therapists reject Freud's theory of two types of orgasms, associated respectively with the vagina and the clitoris, as unproven, and modern sex-therapy treatments for frigidity are behavioral in nature.

See also PSYCHOSEXUAL ANXIETY; SEXUAL FEARS.

frigophobia   Fear of cold and cold things.
See also COLD, FEAR OF.

frogs, fear of   Fear of frogs is known as batrachophobia. This fear may be related to fears of other reptiles, and possibly to slimy things (often snakes). Frogs may be considered any of a number of tailless, chiefly aquatic amphibians. They usually have a smooth, moist skin, webbed feet, and long hind legs adapted for leaping.

See also SLIMY THINGS, FEAR OF; TOADS, FEAR OF.

frost, fear of   Fear of frost is known as pagophobia. Individuals who fear cold things, or fear ice, may also fear frost.

See also COLD, FEAR OF; ICE, FEAR OF.

frustration   Interference with an individual's impulses or desired actions by internal or external forces. Internal forces include inhibitions and anxieties, and external forces can be parents, teachers, friends, as well as social conventions. Deep feelings of discontent and tension arise because of unresolved problems, unfulfilled needs, or roadblocks to personal goals. Regardless of the cause, frustration causes anxiety for most people.

Modern life is filled with frustrations from birth to old age. Crying babies may be frustrated because of hunger; school-age children may be frustrated by high expectations of their parents; parents may be frustrated by their jobs; and the elderly may be frustrated by their increasing lack of independence.

People who constantly feel anxious because of frustrations respond in many ways. A person who is mentally healthy usually deals with frustration in an acceptable way, sometimes with HUMOR. Others react with ANGER, HOSTILITY, AGGRESSION, or DEPRESSION, while still others become withdrawn and passive. Many children and adults who are constantly frustrated show regressive behavior—resorting to childlike actions, particularly aggression or depression—and may become unable to cope with problems on their own.

See also CONTROL; COPING; GENERAL ADAPTATION SYNDROME; STRESS MANAGEMENT.

functional approach   A model of human behavior that achieves prediction and control by analyzing the relationship or function of behavior, its antecedents and consequences, in the environment.

fur, fear of   Fear of touching an animal's fur is known as doraphobia. This fear may be related to a fear of textures or an aversion to fuzz.

See also FABRICS, FEAR OF CERTAIN; FUZZ AVERSION; TEXTURES, FEAR OF.

fuzz aversion   Some individuals do not like to touch certain textures, such as new tennis balls, the skin of a kiwi fruit, or a fuzzy sweater. They tend to avoid fabrics that cause fuzz.

See also FABRICS, FEAR OF CERTAIN; TEXTURES, FEAR OF.

GABA   See GAMMA-AMINO BUTYRIC ACID (GABA).

gagging, hypersensitive   The feeling that one will gag or choke is often a symptom of anxiety. A fear of gagging is related to the feeling of a lump in the throat that one cannot seem to swallow. Those who are hypersensitive gaggers cannot tolerate foreign objects in their mouths, such as those used during dental treatment. In some cases, individuals may gag, retch, or vomit, if they even hear or think about dentistry or smell an odor associated with dental procedures.

Gagging is a normal protective reflex for the oropharynx; the sensitivity and trigger area is greater in some individuals than in others. In mild cases, gagging can be triggered just by touching near the back of the mouth with the tongue or being touched by a dental instrument. In more severe cases, the trigger can be touching the front of the mouth, the face and the front of the neck, certain smells, or sights associated with unpleasant oral experiences, such as dentistry, or with becoming ill due to certain foods.

Some hypersensitive gaggers swallow with their teeth clenched and thus have difficulty during dental procedures. Such individuals have particular difficulty in swallowing with their teeth apart.

There are several ways that individuals who experience gagging can be helped. General relaxation techniques are beneficial. Communicating one's fears to the dentist before a procedure is important. Use of a rating scale, on which the patient indicates what types of procedures are likeliest to induce the most gagging, will improve communications between patient and dentist. During dental procedures, hypersensitive gaggers can be taught to signal (with a raised hand) whenever gagging is about to occur.

Hypersensitive gaggers can learn to modify their swallowing pattern—for example, swallowing with the teeth slightly apart and the tongue further back in the mouth. When sharp teeth make the tongue hypersensitive, the teeth can be smoothed down somewhat. Some dentists give anxious patients homework assignments, such as learning to hold buttons under the tongue and rolling them around in the mouth, so they become accustomed to having foreign objects in their mouth without gagging.

See also DENTAL FEARS; SWALLOWING, FEAR OF; VOMITING, FEAR OF.

gaiety, fear of   Fear of gaiety is known as cherophobia.

galeophobia   Fear of cats.
See also CATS, FEAR OF.

Gallophobia   Fear of France, the French language, and things relating to the French culture is known as Gallophobia.
See also FRANCOPHOBIA.

galvanic skin response (GSR)   Changes in resistance in the skin to psychological stimulation as measured by an electronic device. Emotional arousal (positive and negative) generally leads to increased sweat gland activity, which, in turn, lowers electrical resistance. Electrodermal responses are taken by pairing a small (imperceptible) electrical current between two electrodes on the skin. Increases in conductance (lowered resistance) are thought to reflect increased autonomic (emotional) activity. The sweat glands are activated by SYMPA-THETIC NERVOUS SYSTEM activity, and therefore the GSR measures reflect changes in the sympathetic system.

gambling, fear of; compulsion   Individuals who fear gambling usually prefer secure situations to situations involving risks. They may be fear-ful of losing or making errors, or fearful of what they regard as sin or wrongdoing. They may not feel comfortable when they relinquish a certain amount of control over their circumstances, which is usually involved in gambling. Individuals who feel that they are compulsive gamblers, unable to stop once they get started, may actually fear gam-bling because of what they perceive as its control over them and the ensuing detrimental effects on their lives. Those who have had bad experiences with gambling may fear it more than those who have never gambled before.

See also RISK TAKING, FEAR OF.

gamma-amino butyric acid (GABA)   A neurotrans-mitter in the brain that relates to ANXIETY. ALPRA-ZOLAM, a BENZODIAZEPINE (popularly known as Xanax), binds to the GABA receptors in the brain. (A drug or NEUROTRANSMITTER "binds" to chemical receptors that are shaped to receive and use it rather than other chemicals.) It is known that when taken in therapeutic doses, both Valium (which is not effective in treating panic attacks) and alprazolam change the shape of the receptor molecule (GABA) they share. The chemical interaction between alprazolam and the diazepam receptor changes the metabolism of GABA, which in turn produces a series of changes in the biochemistry of the cell and thus lessens anxiety. Researchers speculate that PANIC DISORDER may be a deficiency disease and may result when a hormone or neurotransmitter that usually regulates anxiety is missing or deficient in some way.

gamophobia   Fear of marriage is known as gamo-phobia or gametophobia.

See also MARRIAGE, FEAR OF.

garlic, fear of   Fear of garlic is known as allium-phobia. This fear may extend to a variety of plants characterized by their pungent odor, including the onion, leek, chive, and shallot.

See also ODORS, FEAR OF.

gastrointestinal complaints   Abdominal discom-fort, cramping, DIARRHEA, urgency to defecate, FEAR OF LOSING CONTROL, CONSTIPATION, and NAU-SEA are common complaints of many individuals who have ANXIETY DISORDERS, PANIC DISORDERS, and DEPRESSION. Many individuals seek help for gastrointestinal complaints before seeking treat-ment for their anxieties. In many cases, the gastrointestinal complaints are relieved with anti-anxiety therapy.

See also IRRITABLE BOWEL SYNDROME.

gatophobia   Fear of cats.

See also CATS, FEAR OF.

geliophobia   Fear of laughter. This fear may be related to a fear of gaiety (cherophobia).

See also GAIETY, FEAR OF; LAUGHTER, FEAR OF.

gender identity and gender identity disorder   An individual's sense of "maleness" or "femaleness," and an acceptance and awareness of one's biologi-cal sex. Gender identity disorder is a type of psy-chosexual disorder in which an individual's gender identity is not congruent with his or her anatomical sex. When an individual believes that he or she is a man or woman in the body of the other gender, anxieties naturally result. If an individual has inter-nal conflicts regarding his or her gender identity and does not accept his or her biological designa-tion, frustration and anxieties may develop, lead-ing the individual into practices that may include "cross dressing" and taking on the role of the other gender.

Some individuals who have these feelings relieve their anxieties by having a sex-change operation, also called "reassignment" surgery.

See also GENDER ROLE; SEXUAL FEARS.

gender role The set of behaviors and attitudes that are socially associated with being male or female. These attitudes may be expressed to varying degrees by the individual. Historically, in Western cultures, gender role for many women was passive and submissive, which led to many ANXIETIES and frustrations, until the "women's liberation" movement and "sexual revolution" in Westernized countries during the latter half of the 20th century. As a result of many societal changes, gender roles have also changed significantly. For example, child care is no longer exclusively the woman's role, and earning the larger part of the family income is no longer exclusively the man's role. However, changes in gender roles have led to many contemporary anxieties, such as women's feelings of conflict between motherhood and career and men's fears of inferiority when the wife advances rapidly in her career and outearns the husband.

general adaptation syndrome (G.A.S.) A term we now know as *stress;* it was coined by Hans Selye (1907–82), an Austrian-born Canadian endocrinologist and physiological researcher in his landmark book, *The Stress of Life* (1956). The G.A.S. is the manifestation of stress in the whole body as it develops over time. It is through the G.A.S. that various internal organs, especially the endocrine glands and the nervous system, help individuals adjust to constant changes occurring in and around them and "navigate a steady course toward whatever they consider a worthwhile goal."

Dr. Selye was a pioneer in an area that has continued to look at stress as a threat to wellness. The secret of health, he contended, was in successful adjustment to ever-changing conditions. Life, he said, is largely a process of adaptation to the circumstances in which we exist. He viewed many nervous and emotional disturbances, such as high blood pressure and some cardiovascular problems, gastric and duodenal ulcers, and certain types of allergic problems as essentially diseases of adaptation.

Selye called his concept the *General Adaptation Syndrome* because it is produced only by agents that have a *general* effect on large portions of the body. He called it *adaptive* because it stimulates DEFENSE

MECHANISMS. He used the term *syndrome* because individual manifestations are coordinated and interdependent on each other.

There are three stages in the G.A.S., Selye said. Individuals go through the stages many times each day as well as throughout life. Whatever demands are made on us, we progress through the sequence. The first is an alarm reaction, or the bodily expression of a generalized call for our defensive forces. We experience surprise and anxiety because of our inexperience in dealing with a new situation. The second stage is resistance, when we have learned to cope with the new situation efficiently. The third stage is exhaustion, or a depletion of our energy reserves, which leads to fatigue. Adaptability, Selye continued, was a finite amount of vitality (thought of as capital), with which we are born. We can draw from it throughout life, but cannot add to it.

See also COPING; DIS-STRESS; EUSTRESS; HARDINESS; HOMEOSTASIS; PSYCHONEUROIMMUNOLOGY; STRESS.

Selye, Hans, *The Stress of Life* (New York: McGraw Hill, 1956).
———, *Stress without Distress* (Philadelphia: J. B. Lippincott, 1974).

generalized anxiety disorder (GAD) One commonly occurring form of ANXIETY DISORDER. Generalized anxiety disorder (GAD) is a psychiatric problem that is experienced by 6.8 million adults ages 18 and older in the United States in any given year, or 3.1 percent of the population. The one-year prevalence of GAD in the population is about 3 percent. Children with GAD are said to have *overanxious disorder of childhood.*

According to the National Institute of Mental Health (NIMH), the onset of GAD may occur at any age, but the median age of onset is 31 years. It should also be noted that many individuals with GAD have other psychiatric disorders, such as other forms of anxiety disorders or DEPRESSION, as well as issues with substance abuse or dependence.

GAD can be extremely debilitating and impairs individuals on the job and at home. The person with GAD may feel overwhelmed and even paralyzed with anxiety and indecision. In addition, the person may feel stupid or ridiculous because he or she is aware that the excessive worry is unreasonable; however, they are unable to talk themselves out of it without professional assistance.

Symptoms and Diagnostic Path

Continued and unrealistic worry over at least several everyday problems that has lasted for six months or longer is a symptom of GAD. The individual with GAD may feel a sense of impending doom most of the time, even when he or she is very aware that this feeling is irrational and excessive. Low to moderate levels of long-lasting, chronic anxiety occur.

Some physical symptoms and signs that often accompany GAD may include the following

- insomnia
- headaches
- lightheadedness or even brief periods of unconsciousness
- excessive sweating
- feeling out of breath (some individuals may fear that they are having a heart attack)
- muscle aches
- frequent urination
- difficulty swallowing

These symptoms and signs usually occur both at home and at work.

Most people with GAD are diagnosed by their family doctor or by a psychologist or a psychiatrist. Other possible medical problems such as hyperthyroidism should be ruled out before the diagnosis of GAD is made, because individuals with hyperthyroidism may exhibit many of the same symptoms that are found among those with GAD. The diagnosis of GAD often occurs only after many years of suffering with the disorder.

Treatment Options and Outlook

Antianxiety medications, known as BENZODIAZEPINES, are often used to treat GAD, including such drugs as CLONAZEPAM (Klonopin) and ALPROZOLAM (Xanax). Buspirone (Buspar) is an antianxiety medication that is sometimes used to treat GAD. It is not a benzodiazepine medication, but it is an approved drug for the treatment of anxiety.

Sometimes ANTIDEPRESSANTS are used to treat anxiety disorders such as GAD, such as venlafaxine (Effexor), a reuptake serotonin norepinephrine inhibitor (SNRI). In some cases, older medications such as tricyclic antidepressants may be used to treat GAD. Imipramine (Tofranil) is a tricyclic medication which is sometimes used to treat GAD, according to the NIMH.

BUPROPION (Wellbutrin), a dopamine reuptake inhibitor that is neither an SSRI or an SNRI, is also sometimes used to treat GAD. The medication is usually prescribed at the lowest dosage level and titrated upward as needed. A combination of medications may be needed to bring the individual's anxiety within tolerable levels. If individuals are prescribed medications for their anxiety, they should not suddenly stop taking the drugs without checking first with their physician.

Psychotherapy, particularly cognitive-behavioral therapy, helps patients with GAD to learn to identify their irrational thoughts and to challenge them, replacing them with more realistic thoughts. Some patients also find relief by joining support groups of fellow sufferers of anxiety disorders.

Most patients with GAD need a combination treatment of both cognitive behavioral therapy and medication.

Risk Factors and Preventive Measures

Women are more likely than men to have GAD: females have about twice the risk of developing GAD, according to the NIMH. In addition, those with a family history of anxiety disorders, particularly GAD, have an increased risk for the development of this disorder. There are no known means of preventing the development of GAD.

Beck, Aaron T., M.D., and Gary Emery, *Anxiety Disorders and Phobias: A Cognitive Perspective* (New York: Basic Books, 2005).

"generational anxiety" See "SANDWICH GENERATION."

generation gap See BABY BOOMERS; COMMUNICATION; INTERGENERATIONAL CONFLICTS; LISTENING.

geniophobia   Fear of chins.
See also CHINS, FEAR OF.

genital fears   Fear of the female genital organs is known as *kolpophobia* or *eurotophobia*. Fear of the male genital organs is known as *phallophobia*.
See also FEMALE GENITALS, FEAR OF; SEXUAL FEARS.

genital stage   The final stage of psychosexual development, also known as genital phase. According to psychoanalytic theory, the genital stage follows the oral and anal phases and is reached during adolescence, when sexual relationships with another becomes the major aim of sexual interest. In some cases, when appropriate transitions from other stages of development do not occur, the individual may develop phobias and anxieties that interfere with later sexual relationships and adjustments to marriage. The goal of psychoanalysis is to help the individual reach his or her genital potential.
See also STAGES OF DEVELOPMENT.

genophobia   Fear of sexual intercourse.
See also PSYCHOSEXUAL ANXIETIES; SEXUAL FEARS; SEXUAL INTERCOURSE, FEAR OF.

genuphobia   See KNEES, FEAR OF.

geophagia   See CROSS-CULTURAL INFLUENCES.

gephyrophobia   Fear of bridges.
See also BRIDGES, FEAR OF.

gerascophobia   Fear of growing old.
See also AGING, FEAR OF; OLD, FEAR OF GROWING; RETIREMENT, FEAR OF; WRINKLES, FEAR OF.

Germanophobia   Fear of Germany, German language, and things relating to the German culture. This fear may relate to fear of hearing the German language.

germs, fear of   Fear of germs is known as bacillophobia or mikrophobia. The term germs commonly refers to any microorganism that can cause DISEASE. Germs, although a nonspecific term, for the purpose of causing anxieties and phobias, can include the many types of bacteria, molds, yeasts, and viruses. Fears of germs can lead to other behaviors, such as OBSESSIVE-COMPULSIVE DISORDER, in which an individual may constantly wash his hands, or specific disease phobias, such as TUBERCULOPHOBIA.

geropsychiatry   See PSYCHOTHERAPIES.

gestalt psychology   The study of the formation and function of patterns or configurations in human mental processes. *Gestalt* is the German word for configuration or pattern. In English, the word signifies "a unified whole, picture, or person with specific characteristics that cannot be grasped simply by noting its various parts." Gestalt psychology and therapy was best defined around 1950 by Dr. Frederick Perls (see GESTALT THERAPY). Gestalt psychology emphasizes the whole of experience, which consisted of more than the sum of its parts. For example, in a classic experiment, Edward Kohler describes a monkey given a stick who suddenly ("ah-hah" or insight) realizes that it can be used to pull some desired bananas to him that are out of reach. The whole (use of the stick for this particular purpose) was a configuration that was more than its parts.

gestalt therapy   A type of psychotherapy; one of many therapies useful in treating individuals who have phobias and anxieties. Gestalt therapy emphasizes treatment of the person as a whole, including biological aspects and their organic functioning, perceptions, and interrelationships with the outside world. Gestalt therapy focuses on the sensory awareness of the individual's here-and-now experiences, rather than on past recollections or future expectations; it can be used in individual or group therapy settings. Gestalt therapy uses role-playing, acting out anger or fright, reliving traumatic experiences, and other techniques such as the "empty chair" to elicit spontaneous feelings and self-aware-ness, promote personality growth, and help the individual develop his full potential. Gestalt therapy was developed by Frederick S. PERLS, a German-born American psychotherapist (1893–1970).

See also "EMPTY CHAIR;" GESTALT PSYCHOLOGY; HERE-AND-NOW APPROACH.

geumaphobia, geumophobia, geumatophobia Fear of taste.

See also TASTE, FEAR OF.

ghosts, fear of   Fear of ghosts is known as phas-mophobia or daemonophobia. A ghost may be the spirit of a dead person that haunts living persons or former habitats, or it may be a returning or haunt-ing memory or·image.

The fear of ghosts may have been planted in the minds of primitive man because of concern about the afterlife of deceased relatives. Dead ances-tors, who were worshipped in many early cultures as gods or near-gods, were thought to be easily angered. Gifts and ceremonies were necessary to sustain their goodwill and decrease hostilities the dead were believed to bear toward the living.

Belief in and fear of ghosts was furthered by desires for a pleasant afterlife, a heaven or Ely-sian fields, accessible to some but not all spirits. Criminals and witches were condemned to walk the earth rather than enter a restful existence after death. The spirits of murder victims or individuals who had been buried improperly could not rest in peace until the wrong had been righted. Burial cus-toms and rituals indicate a desire to keep the spirits of the dead away from the living.

See also DEMONS, FEAR OF; WITCHES, FEAR OF.

girls, fear of   Fear of girls (or young girls) is known as parthenophobia. The word is derived from the Greek word *parthenos,* or virgin. Some individuals might have a phobia about young girls because of the survival of a Victorian attitude that children, especially little girls, are pure and vulnerable to corruption by adults. Fear of girls may also be an extension of men's fear of women.

See also CHILDREN, FEAR OF; OPPOSITE SEX, FEAR OF; SEXUAL FEARS; VIRGINS, FEAR OF; WOMEN, FEAR OF.

Cable, Mary, *The Little Darlings* (New York: Scribner, 1975).

glaring lights, fear of   Fear of glaring lights is known as photoaugiophobia. Individuals who have this fear may fear being in the spotlight or fear that others are watching them. They may also fear dam-age to their eyes. Such individuals usually avoid night driving.

glass, fear of   Fear of glass is known as crystallo-phobia, hyalophobia, hyelophobia, and nelopho-bia. Some people fear the fragility of glass and fear being injured or cut by broken glass. Others fear their reflections in glass.

See also MIRRORS, FEAR OF.

glass ceiling   Refers to an invisible barrier that keeps many working women from rising to the top of their field despite good qualifications, experience, and hard work. For many, this frustration leads to anxiety and, in many cases, DEPRESSION.

There are many variations to the effects of the glass ceiling. For example, men may be brought from outside the organization to fill in high-level posts while qualified women already in the organi-zation are passed over. Women also are often kept on the periphery of the decision-making process.

Teasing and harassment of women may discour-age them from seeking a promotion. Women in lower-level positions are sometimes given respon-sible, demanding work that is not reflected in their job titles or salaries. As women attempt to prog-ress in an organization, they may find that perfor-mance standards are higher for them than for men. Women may also be inhibited by assumptions that a "feminine" management style is more passive and nurturing toward fellow workers and less goal-ori-ented and driven.

Women who do break the glass ceiling frequently credit the influence of a mentor, spouse, or parent. Some women avoid the glass ceiling by striking out on their own.

See also SEXUAL HARASSMENT.

global warming   The idea that human activities can rapidly change the Earth's climate is a cause for concern and anxiety for people all over the world.

Global warming is not a new concept. Jean Fourier, a French physicist, was the first to understand the "greenhouse" effect. In 1824 he suggested that the Earth stays warm at night because its atmosphere traps Sun-warmed gases in the same way a greenhouse holds heated air. In 1892, Svante Arrhenius, a Swedish physical chemist, predicted that if levels of carbon dioxide in the atmosphere doubled, the average temperature of the Earth would rise between 1.5 and 4 degrees Celsius, close to the prediction many climatologists share today.

Activists continue concern and debate over threats to the ecology of the world, such as cutting down rain forests and depleting water supplies. Recent studies indicate that global warming is largely a product of human behavior.

globus hystericus   The feeling that one has a lump or mass in the throat when nothing is there. The individual usually experiences difficulty in swallowing. This can be a symptom of anxiety arousal.

See also LUMP IN THE THROAT; SWALLOWING, FEAR OF.

glossophobia   Fear of speaking in public or of trying to speak.

See also SOCIAL PHOBIA.

goal   The object or end toward which therapy for anxieties or phobia is aimed. In different types of therapy there are different types of goals. For example, in BEHAVIOR THERAPY, a goal for an individual who has a specific phobia might be to face the phobic item or situation without fear. In PSYCHOANALYSIS, the treatment goal is to make unconscious material conscious. In FAMILY THERAPY, the goal is to restructure the family system and bring about a better-functioning family group. Goals should be specific, measurable, and attainable. There may be many goals for one individual, and goals may change during the course of therapy. For example, an elevator phobic's first

goal might be to face an elevator without fear. A later goal would be to enter the elevator, and then to ride up in it.

See also GOAL ATTAINMENT SCALING [GAS].

goblins, fear of   Some people fear the small, grotesque spirits known as goblins, considered by some to be a type of fairy. Goblins are at worst malicious and at best mischievious. They often live in the woods but come into homes to play their tricks. James Whitcomb Riley's poem for children, "Little Orphan Annie," plays on the fears that many children have of goblins and uses these fears to discipline children with the recurring threat, "The gobble-uns'll git you ef you don't watch out!"

> You better mind yer parents, and yer teachers
> fond an' dear. . .
> Er the Gobble-uns'll get you
> Ef you don't watch out

The poem is frightening to many young children who are not ready to distinguish creatures in their imagination from those in reality.

See also ANXIETY DISORDERS OF CHILDHOOD; CHILDHOOD ANXIETIES, FEARS, AND PHOBIAS.

Riley, James Whitcomb, *The Gobble-uns* . . . (Philadelphia: Lippincott, 1975).

God, fear of   Fear of God is known as theophobia. God as a concept has been both a producer and reducer of fear and anxiety. The mysteriousness and power of God inspires a sense of awe, which is in part fear. Part of many worship rituals are acts of self-abasement; such acts include the lowered eyes, bowed head, and clasped hands, a kneeling or prostrate position, and silence. However, the act of prayer, common to most religions, is, in the end, a reducer of anxiety. In its more primitive form, prayer is a way of asking for help or for some particular desired object or event, rather than facing the reality of luck, chance, and one's own limitations. In a more mystical, meditative form, prayer is a tension-relieving escape, a chance to be in contact with a higher power outside of time and ordinary events.

Acts of propitiation and sacrifice in many religions are indications of the fearful aspect of God. In many religions, dead ancestors were thought to be lower gods who could intercede with higher powers, and in some beliefs they were the sole gods. These spirits, also the enforcers of social taboos, required constant recognition in the form of ceremonies and gifts. Sacrifices and offerings are also common in religions that do not involve ancestor worship. Food, animals, and, in some religions, human lives have all been offered to the higher powers. For example, Aztec Indians believed that the sun would not rise and move across the sky without daily human sacrifice. Sacrifice seems to have performed some psychological functions more positive than alleviation of fear. The sacrificial victim was considered a messenger to the gods and, at least in some cases, went willingly. The ritual gave the worshiper a satisfying sense of being in touch with God and of vicariously sacrificing himself.

The Western concept of God is far more personal and potentially judgmental than that of Eastern religions, whose moving force is thought of in abstract terms of unity and harmony and, in some Eastern systems of belief, the indescribable. The Judeo-Christian God's role as a loving but judgmental power, a God whose acts are evident in the unfolding of history, who can in fact part the Red Sea for his chosen people, offers tremendous possibilities for emotional response, including fear. In the Christian tradition, juxtaposed to the fearful idea that God can and does punish sins is the belief that God sent His son Jesus to die for man's sins and that through belief in Him everlasting life is attainable. Classical and medieval Christian thinking recognized the power of God, but also that of luck and chance in men's affairs. With the Reformation, a new line of thinking developed: a belief that all actions were a working out of God's will, but admitting that God's ways were nonetheless inscrutable. This would seem to offer a soothing release from anxiety and responsibility, a sense that one's life was in God's hands, but many men and women of that period fell into endless worrisome speculation. When a calamity befell them, they wondered whether God was testing them or punishing them. Some even felt that when life was going well, it was a sign that God had lost interest in their personal situation. Although elements of belief in God's providence continue today, as a rigid set of ideas it became intolerable and dissolved into 18th-century rationalism.

Modern man retains a strong consciousness of the emotion of guilt but has lost the sense of God as a judge or inflictor of punishment. Secular institutions and disciplines now bear a large part of the responsibility for alleviating human suffering and controlling antisocial behavior. Twentieth-century philosophers' speculation that God may be dead has dealt the ultimate blow to God as a source of fear, punishment, or help. On the other hand, there are still those individuals who know that "we are the fulfillment of God; that we are that place in consciousness when God shines through, the realization that every individual is the presence of God."

Goldstein, Joel, *The Infinite Way* (San Gabriel, CA: Willing, 1947).

Hill, Douglas and Pat Williams, *The Supernatural* (New York: Hawthorne, 1965), pp. 28–68.

Sandmel, Samuel, *A Little Book on Religion (For People Who Are Not Religious)* (Chambersburg, PA: Wilson Books, 1975), pp. 46–54.

Spinks, G. Stephens, *Psychology and Religion* (Boston: Beacon Press, 1963), pp. 1–13, 31–46, 117–146.

Thomas, Keith, *Religion and the Decline of Magic* (New York: Scribner, 1971), pp. 51–112.

going crazy, fear of Many individuals who have ANXIETIES, FEARS, PHOBIAS, and PANIC ATTACKS at times fear that they are going crazy. Their misinterpretation of their situation may be heightened if they do not have any support and understanding from relatives and friends, or particularly if those close to them suggest that the phobic's feelings are "all in the mind." When individuals fear "going crazy," usually they are referring to a severe mental disorder known as SCHIZOPHRENIA. However, most individuals who have phobias, anxieties, panic attacks, depression, and OBSESSIVE-COMPULSIVE DISORDERS are not schizophrenic, and when an individual understands the nature of his or her psychological problem, he or she will have less fear of going crazy. Schizophrenia is a major mental disorder characterized by such severe symptoms as disjointed thoughts and speech, sometimes extending to babbling, delusions, or strange beliefs (for example, that one is receiving messages from outer space), and hallucinations (for example, hearing voices). Schizophrenia usually begins gradually and not suddenly (such as during a panic attack). Schizophrenia is often genetic, and in some people, no amount of anxieties or stress will cause the disorder. People who become schizophrenic usually will show some mild symptoms for most of their lives, such as unusual or bizarre thoughts or speech. Schizophrenia usually first appears in the late teens to early twenties. Individuals who are in therapy for their fears, phobias, and anxieties can be fairly certain that they are not likely to become schizophrenic, for they would have been so diagnosed during examination, interviews, and testing. At a more symbolic level, the fear of going crazy is a fear of becoming disconnected from reality and other people and living in an isolated or alienated state. The fear of going crazy often accompanies panic attacks since they are so intense and debilitating.

going to bed, fear of Fear of going to bed, being in bed, or beds in general is known as clinophobia. Such fears may be related to fear of not waking up or fear of dying during sleep.

See also BED, FEAR OF; WAKING UP, NOT, FEAR OF.

gold, fear of Fear of gold is known as aurophobia. Such fears may relate to fears of success and wealth, fear of shiny things, or fear of textures.

gonorrhea See SEXUALLY TRANSMITTED DISEASES.

good news, fear of hearing Fear of hearing good news is known as euphobia. Those who have this fear may fear that the good news will not last, that they do not deserve to have good fortune, or that they should have some guilt about the news. Some who fear good news fear that bad news may follow; some fear success. Fear of good news may be related to a fear of gaiety or happiness.

See also SUCCESS, FEAR OF.

graphophobia Fear of handwriting or writing.

See also WRITING, FEAR OF.

graves, fear of Fear of graves is known as taphophobia. Those who fear graves also usually fear cemeteries, funerals, and other rituals associated with death, and they may also fear death itself. The source of the fear may be some aspect of "contagion" in the atmosphere around graves. Some individuals who become very anxious avoid going to funerals for this reason, and some will go to the funeral service (if it is held in a place other than the cemetery or burial area), but they will not go near the gravesite. Some individuals avoid walking past cemeteries when funerals are going on, and some avoid cemeteries at all times, even to the extent of driving out of the way to avoid passing one.

See also CEMETERIES, FEAR OF; DEATH, FEAR OF.

gravity, fear of Fear of gravity is known as barophobia. This fear is related to fear of perceivable changes in air pressure.

grief reaction and grief resolution The feeling of loss and anxiety an individual experiences when a crucial bond is disrupted. Depression often follows. There is a higher death and illness risk for individuals for a year after they lose a spouse. Through the exposure approach of guided mourning the bereaved may be led to reduce avoidance of cues reminiscent of the deceased.

Grief is a type of suffering, a symptom of bereavement and loss, experienced physically, emotionally, and psychologically. Grief may be synonymous with sorrow, or the emotion that accompanies mourning. Individuals who experience grief may have sensations characteristic of emotional disorders such as ANXIETIES, INSOMNIA, DEPRESSION, loss of appetite, and preoccupation with the lost party. As a result of a classic study following the 1942

Cocoanut Grove nightclub fire in Boston, five normal stages of grief reaction were defined as: initial shock, intense sadness, withdrawal from the environment, protest of the loss, and finally, a gradual resolution of the loss. Elisabeth Kübler-Ross identified the stages of emotion experienced after the death of a loved one as: denial, anger, bargaining, depression, and acceptance. Most grieving persons will experience these or similar stages. All stages of mourning are a normal and necessary component to grief resolution.

See also STRESS MANAGEMENT.

Kübler-Ross, E., *On Death and Dying* (New York: Macmillan, 1971).

group therapy   See PSYCHOTHERAPIES.

growing old, fear of   Fear of growing old is known as gerascophobia. This is a fear shared by many middle-aged people who fear being alone as they get older, deteriorating physically and mentally, and becoming out of control and a burden to their children or others for care and possibly support. Some fear losing their memory, while others fear losing control of bodily functions and being embarrassed by their dependence on others. Many fear the financial costs of care in a nursing home, if that type of care should be needed. More specific fears related to growing old are fear of Alzheimer's disease, FEAR OF CATARACT EXTRACTION, fear of HEART ATTACK, and certain disease phobias, such as fear of diabetes, which is more prevalent in older people.

See also AGING, FEAR OF.

GSR   See GALVANIC SKIN RESPONSE.

guided imagery   A technique to help an individual generate vivid mental images that may help reduce anxieties and enhance relaxation responses. It creates positive mental pictures and promotes the relaxation necessary for a healing process. The individual pictures an image, such as a calm, serene lake with sailboats slowly moving along, breathes in

a relaxed manner, and becomes more relaxed. The individual gradually learns to notice every detail of the imagined scene and how the sense of relaxation deepens with this self-talk. He or she learns, too, that this sense of calm can be created at any time by BREATHING and imagining the positive vision.

Some case studies and clinical reports suggest that the guided imagery technique may be helpful in the treatment of CHRONIC PAIN, ALLERGIES, hypertension, autoimmune diseases, and stress-related gastrointestinal, reproductive, and urinary symptoms. In addition to direct effects, imagery may augment the effectiveness of medical treatments and help people tolerate discomforts and side effects of some medications or invasive procedures.

Imagery has qualities that make it valuable in mind/body medicine and healing; it can bring about physiological changes, provide psychological insights, and enhance emotional awareness. Use of imagery, in some cases, changes the need for medication. Depending on an individual's medical condition, imagery is best used under the supervision of a physician in conjunction with holistic medicine.

Guided imagery can be used alone or together with other relaxation techniques. It is often used in conjunction with HYPNOSIS, although the two techniques are distinct. While hypnosis serves to induce a special state of mind, imagery consists of a focused, intentional mental activity.

See also COMPLEMENTARY THERAPIES; IMMUNE SYSTEM; IRRITABLE BOWEL SYNDROME; RELAXATION; STRESS.

Goleman, Daniel, and Joel Gurin, eds., *Mind Body Medicine: How to Use Your Mind for Better Health* (Yonkers, N.Y.: Consumer Reports Books, 1993).

guilt   An emotional fear response to a perceived or actual failure to meet expectations of self or others. Guilt causes fear and anxieties for many people and can be destructive if carried to an extreme. It can destroy people's sense of SELF-ESTEEM and feeling of capability. However, these feelings can also be constructive when the affected begin to understand their sources of guilt and learn to cope with this very common aspect of the human condition.

Depending on their conscience, some individuals can steal or commit other serious crimes and not feel any guilt, while others will suffer stressful guilt feelings over relatively minor infractions that occur throughout their lives. For example, some individuals may experience guilt feelings for not remembering the birthday of a parent or spouse. Middle-aged adults may experience guilt feelings when dealing with their aging parents. Some individuals who are bereaved over a death of a loved one may feel some guilt about not having done enough for the person when they were alive. Parents of infants who die of SUDDEN INFANT DEATH SYNDROME (SIDS) suffer stress because of feelings of guilt over not preventing the death of their child. Spouses and relatives of people who commit suicide may have guilt feelings for years wondering if they could have prevented the death.

Along with guilt, an individual anticipates punishment; when he or she projects guilt onto others, he or she also anticipates their punishment. Some individuals believe, possibly unconsciously, that they have "sinned," and they fear God will attack and punish them. Guilt keeps individuals trapped because they blame themselves or others. Severe or abnormal guilt feelings may result in DEPRESSION and/or chronic ANXIETIES. Individuals who have obsessive-compulsive neuroses often feel the need to scrutinize their conduct and may have a compulsion to confess to therapists or clergypersons. Some individuals commit suicide out of profound guilt feelings over events for which death seems to be the only appropriate restitution. Guilt is a way to hold onto the past, to produce self-condemnation that keeps the individual under the control of his or her ego and supports a view that he or she is unlovable.

For some individuals, mental health counseling or participation in an appropriate support group can help relieve some of these uncomfortable feelings of guilt.

See also COPING; DEPRESSION; OBSESSIVE-COMPULSIVE DISORDER.

gymnophobia   Fear of naked bodies.
See also NAKED BODY, FEAR OF; NUDITY, FEAR OF.

gynephobia   Fear of women.
See also WOMEN, FEAR OF.

habits and habit strength   Learned responses that one performs automatically and frequently. They may be useful—as knowing how to use a computer keyboard, taking a shower in the morning, or always leaving a key in a certain place. Habits can also be responses to anxiety-producing situations, such as scratching the head, NAIL BITING, hair pulling, or reaching for a cigarette. These unwanted or undesirable habits, if continued, can contribute to a person's anxiety levels.

The strength of a habitual response (such as fear) depends on the number and extent of reinforcements and the intervals between stimulus and response and response and reinforcement. The term *habit strength* was coined by Clark Leonard Hull (1884–1952), an American psychologist. Habit strength is the central concept in Hull's theory of learning. He believed that habit strength accumulates as a direct function of the number of reinforced stimulus-response occurrences.

Habits can include certain repetitive and ritual behaviors, such as those practiced by sufferers of OBSESSIVE-COMPULSIVE DISORDER. These habits that usually cause the individual stress can be changed by BEHAVIOR THERAPY, psychotherapy, and the substitution of more constructive habits. RELAXATION therapy, GUIDED IMAGERY, HYPNOSIS, and BIOFEEDBACK may also be helpful techniques to overcome these habits.

See also ANXIETY DISORDERS; HYPNOSIS.

Ouellette, Judith A., and Wendy Wood, "Habit and intention in everyday life: The multiple process by which past behavior predicts future behavior," *Psychological Bulletin* 124, no. 1 (July 1998): pp. 54–74.

hadephobia   See HELL, FEAR OF.

hagiophobia   Fear of holy things.
See also HOLY THINGS, FEAR OF.

hair fears   Fear of hair is known as *trichophobia* or *chaetophobia*. The most frequently occurring fear regarding hair is baldness, or loss of hair. Also, some individuals fear having the hair on their head touched, pulled, brushed, combed, or washed. Some fear that they will grow bald unless their hair is untouched. Other individuals fear the sight of a hair on clothing (their own or the hair of others), on the table, or on a sink. Some fear or are averse to body hair on themselves or on others. Some fear white or gray hair on themselves or others. As with many fears, hair fear is a conditioned response or a generalized response.

Some fear unusual hair conditions, one of which is called trichorrhexis, in which the hair shaft may alter, bulge and narrow; the hair tends to split at regular intervals. The cause of this condition is not known and there is no cure for it. Some people fear having too oily or too dry hair.

Some hair-related problems involve the scalp. Such conditions include dandruff, psoriasis, seborrheic dermatitis, inflammation of the hair follicles (folliculitis), ringworm, and other infections. Some fear these conditions because particularly in the case of dandruff, they are socially noticeable. An individual who has any tendency toward social phobia may use dandruff as an excuse to avoid social situations.

Fear of Hair Loss
Hair loss refers to hair falling out, extremely thinning hair, and baldness. Hair loss makes many people anxious because they associate a full head of hair with SELF-ESTEEM and BODY IMAGE. For many,

hair loss is also symbolic of aging. Sufferers of hair loss may resort to various, sometimes dubious, treatments to encourage new hair to grow.

Hair loss is common; nearly two out of three men develop some form of balding. An even higher percentage of men and women have some form of hair loss during their lives. With appropriate diagnosis, many people suffering from hair loss can be helped. Diagnosis is the first step. Hair loss can be due to many different causes, such as pregnancy, high fever, severe infection, or severe flu. It may also be due to thyroid disease, inadequate protein in the diet, certain prescription drugs and cancer treatment drugs, birth control pills, low serum iron, major surgery, chronic illness, or ringworm of the scalp. Some forms of hair loss will regrow. Individuals undergoing chemotherapy experience hair loss; expectations are that it will grow back some time after completion of chemotherapy. Other forms can be treated successfully by dermatologists.

About 90 percent of a person's scalp hair is continually growing. Shedding 50 to 100 hairs a day is considered normal. When a hair is shed, it is replaced by a new hair from the same follicle located just below the skin surface. Scalp hair grows about a half-inch a month. As people age, their rate of hair growth slows down, and thinning hair may be noticeable.

Body Dysmorphic Disorder

Dysmorphobia is characterized by preoccupation with imagined defects in appearance. Commonly, facial flaws, shapes of the nose, mouth, wrinkles, and facial and/or body hair are the focus of this disorder. Dysmorphobia involves preoccupation and aversion but is technically not a phobia because panic-anxiety and phobic avoidance are not present. This is a diagnostic category in the *Diagnostic and Statistical Manual of Mental Disorders* (4th ed.)

Fear of Having a Haircut

Fear of having a haircut arises from a number of causes, including a fear of sitting confined in the barber or beautician's chair, a feeling of being out of control while the barber or beautician is working with a scissors or razor, or a fear of injury from these implements. Some fear being seen by others while they are having a haircut or fear being judged and compared unfavorably with others as they sit on the chair. Fear of having a haircut is related to many phobias, including agoraphobia, social phobia, and fear of blood and injury. Arthur Schopenhauer (1788–1860), a German philosopher, is said to have feared his hairdresser.

Hair Pulling

Hair pulling, known as *trichotillomania,* is a habit that involves pulling hair out of the scalp and sometimes out of eyebrows, eyelashes, and body; men may pull out beard and mustache hairs. For many people, hair pulling is a mechanism for COPING with ANXIETIES They do it when they are feeling nervous or tense, or it is a compulsion.

Some individuals pull hair in front of others, but most often the activity is pursued in secret. The hairs are carefully hidden or disposed of. The hairless areas have distinctive features and help distinguish trichotillomania from other forms of hair losses and disease. The patches are irregular in outline, not sharply defined, and the hair loss is never complete. Many of the hairs will break off rather than be completely pulled out, so that variable amounts of stubble remain. There are usually no signs of inflammation, and the scalp elsewhere is normal.

The habit can be treated with BEHAVIOR THERAPY or other forms of PSYCHOTHERAPIES.

See also AGORAPHOBIA; ANXIETY DISORDERS; BALD, BECOMING, FEAR OF; BARBER'S CHAIR SYNDROME; BARBERSHOPS, FEAR OF; BLOOD PHOBIA; HYPNOSIS; INJURY PHOBIA; OBSESSIVE-COMPULSIVE DISORDER; SOCIAL PHOBIA.

Soriano, Jennifer L., Richard L. O'Sullivan, Lee Baer, et al., "Trichotillomania and self-esteem: A survey of 62 female hair pullers," *Journal of Clinical Psychiatry* 57, no. 2 (February 1996): pp. 77–82.

Stanley, Melina A., Joy K. Breckenridge, Alan C. Swann, et al., "Fluvoxamine treatment of trichotillomania." *Journal of Clinical Psychopharmacology* 17, no. 4 (August 1997): pp. 278–283.

Hakomi A form of body-centered psychotherapy based on principles that seek to guide individuals toward harmony with themselves and others.

It promotes a state of awareness in which spontaneous and often nonverbal information becomes available and from which basic and unconscious beliefs stem and direct the lives of practitioners. Many people use Hakomi as a way of preventing the harmful effects of anxieties.

Trained to look at nuances of voice and body language, posture, and gesture, Hakomi therapists help individuals to study these avenues to unexpressed feelings and past trauma and gain release from the past. Hakomi teaches participants how to observe themselves from a step away (witnessing) as well as from inside their present experience. Individuals learn to have a choice in responses. Through the use of witnessing, unwanted defenses can be studied and willingly yielded.

Hakomi is a blend of many philosophies and ideologies, including Eastern philosophy; Western psychology; Taoism; Feldenkrais; Reichian, Rolfing and other structural bodywork therapies; Ericksonian hypnosis; focusing, and neurolinguistic programming.

See also COMPLEMENTARY THERAPIES; BODY THERAPIES.

Halloween, fear of The celebration of Halloween has its origins in fear and death. On the night of the end of the summer Druid festival called Samhain, bonfires were kindled on the hills in the British Isles to frighten away witches and the spirits of the dead who were thought to wander free on that night. A Roman holiday that honored the dead, Feralia, was Christianized by Pope Boniface IV to honor saints and martyrs and to serve as a day of prayers of intercession for dead souls who had not been thoroughly purified. In Great Britain, the observations merged into a day called Halligan or All Hallows, and the night before became All Hallows Eve or Halloween.

The American custom of trick-or-treating on Halloween is threatened during the latter part of the 20th century by very real modern fears. Urban crime has made children less likely to be allowed out and adults less willing to open their doors. A rash of incidents of treats adulterated with objects such as pins and razor blades has added still another fear to the celebration of Halloween.

See also CRIME, URBAN, FEAR OF; WITCHES AND WITCHCRAFT, FEAR OF.

hallucinations The sensory experience of seeing, hearing, smelling, tasting, or feeling something that is not present. Hallucinations are major sources of anxiety and even panic because these perceptions cannot be reinforced by anyone else (since they are false), yet the individual is convinced that the experiences are real. In most cases, the person who is hallucinating cannot be convinced by others that these sensory perceptions are false. As a result, hallucinations are highly disturbing to sufferers, and they are also distressing to others who are trying to understand what the individual is feeling and find a way to offer assistance. Individuals who are hallucinating may behave in an aggressive or fearful manner, depending on the type of hallucination and the individual.

Hallucinations sometimes occur as a reaction to certain medications, to high fever, and to serious illnesses. They also occur in some severe mental disorders such as schizophrenia. Individuals who abuse illegal drugs may experience hallucinations, such as those who abuse cocaine or methamphetamine. Hallucinogenic drugs often induce hallucinations, including such drugs as d-lysergic acid (LSD), phencyclidine, or methylenedioxymethamphetamine (MDMA)/Ecstasy.

Reactions to Hallucinogens

Hallucinogens are drugs and agents that produce profound distortions to the senses of sight, sound, smell, and touch, as well as the senses of direction, time, and distance. Although some individuals may resort to hallucinogens for relief from their anxieties, there are no acceptable medical uses for hallucinogens.

Some individuals reportedly experience a euphoric high that is associated with the use of hallucinogens, which may last as long as eight hours. However, there are aftereffects to the use of hallucinogens, including acute anxiety, restlessness, and sleeplessness. Even years after the hallucinogenic drug is eliminated from the body, the user may experience *flashbacks,* which are fragmentary recurrences of hallucinogenic effects.

See also ADDICTIONS.

Gwinnell, Esther, M.D., and Christine Adamec, *The Encyclopedia of Drug Abuse* (New York: Facts On File, Inc., 2008).

hamartophobia A fear of committing an error or sin. The word is derived from the Greek work *hamartia,* meaning "sin." Another word for fear of sin or error is enosiophobia.

See also SIN, FEAR OF.

handwringing Handwringing is usually a symptom of anxiety and uncertainty. Individuals who constantly wring their hands may have difficulty in making decisions and seem to be expressing physically a worry or concern that they do not express verbally. For many, wringing the hands as though they were constantly washing them or squeezing out a cloth may become an unconscious habit. Some individuals start wringing their hands when faced with a stressful situation, while others may do it at any time. Handwringers tend to be worriers and consider all possibilities of a situation before taking any action. Such individuals are often meticulous about what they do, sometimes to the point of being compulsive.

See also ANXIETY; NERVOUS; OBSESSIVE-COMPULSIVE DISORDER.

hangover The physical and emotional condition caused by and following excessive intake of alcoholic beverages. Symptoms of hangover include anxiety, uneasiness, HEADACHE, fatigue, NAUSEA, thirst, sweating, and fatigue. These symptoms usually occur several hours after drinking the ALCOHOL. A headache occurs because alcohol causes the arteries in the scalp to stretch. Also, TYRAMINE and HISTAMINE, chemicals in such alcoholic beverages as red wine and brandy, get into the blood, leading to the throbbing pain on one side of the head. Often with the headache comes extreme sensitivity to light and noise (photophobia and phonophobia) and increased vulnerability to anxiety and panic.

The nausea and stomachache that are part of some hangovers result from irritation of the lining of the stomach by alcohol.

SELF-HELPS FOR TREATING A HANGOVER AND RELATED ANXIETIES

1. Take aspirin or buffered aspirin, or ibuprofen; if the stomach is upset, take acetaminophen.
2. Drink fluids (nonalcoholic). Fruit juices are best because they contain sugar, which may help headaches. Coffee may help at first because of its caffeine content, but after a while the throbbing may get worse as the caffeine leaves the body and a rebound effect takes hold.
3. Wearing a sweatband (not too tight) helps some people because it helps compress some stretched-out scalp arteries. Rubbing one's temples can accomplish the same result. Cold compresses applied to the painful side of the head also may help shrink those arteries.
4. Breathe deeply. Taking in more air, especially fresh air, increases the oxygen level of the blood, which also helps relieve the pain. This may be one reason that a brisk walk often relieves a hangover.
5. Hangovers usually end in 12 to 24 hours without medical help.

(Dr. Daniel B. Hier, chairman, Dept. of Neurology, Michael Reese Hospital and Medical Center, Chicago, Illinois.)

See also ALCOHOLISM; LIGHT, FEAR OF; NOISE, FEAR OF.

haphephobia A fear of being touched. Other words for this phobia are haptephobia and aphephobia.

See also BEING TOUCHED, FEAR OF.

happiness, fear of Fear of happiness, or fear of gaiety, is known as cherophobia. This fear may be related to a fear of hearing good news, or even a fear of success.

See also GOOD NEWS, FEAR OF; SUCCESS, FEAR OF.

harassment See SEXUAL HARASSMENT.

hardiness A term coined by Salvatore Maddi, Ph.D., a University of Chicago psychologist, relating to anxiety-buffering characteristics of people who stay healthy. Some experts use the term *resilience* to connote the same concept. People with hardiness are able to withstand significant levels of stress without becoming ill; those who are more helpless than hardy develop more illnesses, both mental and physical.

In working with executives at a major American employer, Dr. Maddi and colleagues determined three techniques that can augment hardiness as well as happiness and health.

Focusing is a technique developed by Eugene Gendlin, an American psychologist. It is a way of recognizing signals from one's body that something is wrong, such as tension in the neck or a mild headache. With stress, these conditions worsen. Maddi suggests mentally reviewing where things are not feeling just right and reviewing situations that might be stressful. Focusing increases one's sense of CONTROL over stress and enables one to make changes.

Reconstructing stressful situations.   This is a technique in which you think about a recent stressful episode and write down three ways it might have gone better and three ways it might have gone worse. If you can't think of what you could have done differently, focus on a person you know who deals with stress well and what he or she would have done. Realize that things did not go as badly as they could have. Also, realize that you can think of ways to cope better with the same situation.

Self-improvement.   In this technique, you know there are some situations you cannot control; you cannot avoid some situations, such as a serious illness or illness of a member of your family. To regain your sense of control and achieve more effective COPING, choose a new task to master, such as learning how to swim or dance, or develop a new hobby.

Suzanne Kobasa, a City University of New York psychologist, also used the term *hardiness* to identify and measure a style of psychological coping. Some of the characteristics people with hardiness exhibited included viewing life's demands as challenges rather than threats, responding with excitement and energy to change, and having a commitment to something they felt was meaningful, such as their work, community, and family. A third trait was a sense of being in control. Having the right information and being able to make decisions can make an important difference in coping with stress.

Issue of Control in Hardiness

A study reported in the *Journal of Personal and Social Psychology* (April 1995) detailed how 276 Israeli recruits completed questionnaires on hardiness, mental health, and ways of coping at the beginning and end of a demanding, four-month combat training period. Two components of hardiness, commitment and control, measured at the beginning of the training, predicted mental health at the end of the training. Commitment improved mental health by reducing the appraisal of threat. Control improved mental health by reducing appraisal of threat and by increasing the use of problem-solving and support-seeking strategies.

See also GENERAL ADAPTATION SYNDROME; LEARNED HELPLESSNESS; STRESS.

Floria, V., et al., "Does hardiness contribute to mental health during a stressful real-life situation? The roles of appraisal and coping," *Journal of Personal and Social Psychology* 68 (April 1995): pp. 687–695.

Goleman, Daniel, and Joel Gurin, eds., *Mind Body Medicine: How to use your mind for better health* (Yonkers, NY: Consumer Reports Books, 1993).

Padus, Emrika, ed., *The Complete Guide to your Emotions and your Health* (Emmaus, PA: Rodale Press, 1992).

harpaxophobia   A fear of becoming a victim of robbers.

See also ROBBERS, FEAR OF.

"having it all"   An expression that became popular during the 1980s. It refers to career women who follow their chosen business or profession, get married, and raise a family. For many, this has become a satisfying way of life, but for others it has led to many anxieties and frustrations. Some women feel that they are not giving adequate attention to their marriage and children, are constantly tired, and feel some guilt over having their children in day-care centers.

Nevertheless, an increasing number of women do opt to enter business and the professions. Those who are most successful say it is due to the help and understanding of their spouse, as well as adequate day care.

See also MARRIAGE; WORKING MOTHERS.

headaches   Headaches, one of the most frequent complaints of individuals who visit physician's offices, are also reported by many who visit therapists for ANXIETY DISORDERS and sleep disorders. Headaches cause anxieties and stress not only to the sufferer but also to family members who are affected by the sufferer's recurring discomfort. Anxiety, in turn, can cause headaches.

Causes of headaches are not entirely understood. However, heredity is considered important; as many as 75 percent of migraine sufferers come from families in which other members have the same disorder. ANXIETIES, STRESS, diet, and environmental pollutants (including cigarette smoke) are also thought to contribute to headaches.

Anxiety sufferers complain of a variety of headaches, including migraine, cluster, and muscle contraction (tension) headaches.

Migraine Headaches

The word migraine was derived from the Greek word *hemicrania,* meaning half a head. This kind of headache is called migraine because in many cases, pain is limited to one side of the head. At times it may shift from side to side, and sometimes it may hurt on both sides. Migraine headaches usually recur, causing the sufferer the anxiety of not knowing when an attack will occur, and the fear that an attack will come at a critical time, such as before an important examination, performance, or interview.

Estimates indicate that between 25 and 30 million Americans have migraine headaches. Sometimes the headaches start in childhood, and most begin before the age of 30. Migraine headaches seem to decrease as people age. About six out of every 10 migraine sufferers are women.

Migraine headaches often begin around stressful times, such as during puberty, at the time of a school or job change, around the time of a divorce or death of a mate, or during menopause. In diagnosing a headache, a physician will inquire about stresses in the individual's life, demands on the person's time, and how the individual copes with his or her own anxieties and stresses.

Migraine headaches are vascular; the headache results from distention and dilation of blood vessels of the scalp. Some individuals who have migraines report nausea and vomiting during a migraine attack. Generally, an attack begins with a warning, known as an AURA. This may include some kind of visual disturbance, such as blurring or wavy lines resembling heat waves, or a hearing disturbance. Sometimes this disturbance lasts for 10 to 15 minutes. In some cases, hands, face, arms, or legs feel numb or may twitch. The sufferer may be extremely sensitive to light and sound. When the headache pain begins, it may be aggravated by sudden movement of the head, vomiting, sneezing, or coughing. There may be chills or sweating. Sleep usually provides relief, and many migraine sufferers become sleepy during an attack and go to sleep. The entire attack, including the warning period, pain, and sleep, may last from several hours to several days, leaving the person exhausted afterward.

There are many variations of the headache; only 25 percent of migraine sufferers have classic attacks.

Heredity and personality   Migraine headaches, which often occur in members of the same family, may result from a predisposing genetic biochemical abnormality. Additionally, personality traits may play a role in determining who gets migraine headaches. While there is no typical migraine personality, many migraine sufferers have characteristics of perfectionism and compulsion.

Stress and anxieties as a cause   Emotional tension and stress may lead to migraine attacks, because under extreme stress the arteries of the head and those reaching the brain draw tightly together and restrict the flow of blood. This in turn may result in a shortage of oxygen to the brain. When blood vessels dilate or stretch, a greater amount of blood passes through, putting more pressure on the pain-sensitive nerves in and close to the walls of the arteries. The tension on the wall of a blood vessel depends on the pressure of the blood within it as well as the diameter of the vessel itself. The wider the vessel, the greater the tension produced.

Foods and alcohol   Foods and alcohol can make a difference in the frequency and severity of migraine headaches for certain susceptible individuals. Some foods may provoke a headache because they contain substances that affect the constriction or expansion of blood vessels. One of these substances is tyramine, which is found in aged cheeses, chicken livers, and

---

FOODS TO BE AVOIDED BY MIGRAINE SUFFERERS

- Ripened cheeses: Cheddar, Emmentaler, Gruyère, Stilton, Brie, and Camembert (American, cottage, cream, and Velveeta cheeses are permitted)
- Herring
- Chocolate
- Vinegar (except white vinegar)
- Anything fermented, pickled, or marinated
- Sour cream, yogurt
- Nuts, peanut butter, seeds: sunflower, sesame, pumpkin, etc.
- Hot fresh breads, raised coffee cakes, and raised doughnuts. (These are permitted if they are allowed to cool. Toast is permitted.)
- Pods of broad beans: lima, navy, pinto, garbanzo, and pea pods
- Any foods containing large amounts of monosodium glutamate (Oriental foods)
- Onions
- Canned figs
- Citrus foods (No more than one serving per day: one orange, one grapefruit, one glass of orange juice)
- Bananas (No more than one-half banana per day)
- Raisins
- Papayas
- Excessive tea, coffee, and cola beverages (No more than 2 cups total per day)
- Avocado
- Fermented sausage (Processed meats such as ham, hotdogs, bologna, salami, pepperoni, and summer sausage)
- Chicken livers
- All alcoholic beverages (if possible). If you must drink, limit yourself to two normal-sized drinks selected from among Haute Sauterne, Riesling, scotch, or vodka.

---

a variety of other foods. Another is sodium nitrite, a preservative used in ham, hot dogs, and many other sausages. Only about 30 percent of people who have migraine headaches experience this reaction to certain foods. However, some migraine researchers have recommended that all migraine sufferers avoid these foods (see chart at left).

Hormonal effects   Hormones play a role in causing migraine headaches. Many women who have migraine headaches report that attacks come around the time of their menstrual periods, and some have headaches before, during, or at the end of their periods. Some women have migraine headaches during the first months of pregnancy. Some women have them around MENOPAUSE (when menstrual periods cease). Many women who suffer from migraine headaches have found that use of oral contraceptives and hormonal therapies increases the severity and frequency of headaches.

Other causes   Some people have headaches as a result of HYPOGLYCEMIA (too little sugar in the blood). Oversleeping and missing a meal can cause hypoglycemia in some individuals. This condition occurs during insulin shock, when the sugar content of the blood is reduced by insulin or by other means, or after fasting. Hypoglycemia causes dilation of the blood vessels of the head and the resulting pain.

Historical notes   Migraine headaches were known to affect such historical figures as Julius Caesar, Joan of Arc, Thomas Jefferson, Ulysses S. Grant, and Sigmund Freud.

Cluster Headaches

Cluster headaches are so called because they occur in repeated groups. The painful episodes may be as short as 30 minutes and usually are not longer than three or four hours. Sometimes attacks occur every day for several weeks or even months. In many cases there is a remission period with no headaches, and then they may start again. There may be several episodes within a 24-hour period, sometimes regularly at the same time each day. The early-morning hours and one or two hours after going to bed are times when these headaches frequently occur.

The cluster headache pain is intense and is more of a steady, boring pain than the pulsating, throbbing migraine headache. The pain is usually on one side and behind the eyes. It usually reaches its peak of intensity soon after the attack begins. Pain in the eye, nasal congestion, and a runny nose may accompany these headaches.

In a general way, people who have cluster headaches are likely to be smokers and to drink more alcohol than the average population, are conscientious, responsible, self-sufficient, tense, anxious, frustrated, and aggressive. Cluster headaches occur eight to 10 times more frequently in men than in women and usually begin in the early twenties.

Cluster headaches differ from migraines in the duration of the attacks, the character of the pain, biochemical changes, and according to the sex of the sufferer, although the pain of both occurs because of changes in the blood vessels. They are similar in that both usually cause pain on one side and may result from use of vasoactive drugs, certain foods or beverages, emotional stress, and possibly hormonal and biochemical changes in the body. Medications that are effective for migraine are usually also effective for cluster headaches.

While the person with a migraine headache will want to lie down in a dark, quiet room and feels overly sensitive to light, noise, or odors, the cluster sufferer may want to become physically active, pace about, or take a walk because the intensity of the pain may prevent him or her from lying down or sitting still.

Muscle-Contraction (Tension) Headaches

Tension or muscle-contractions headaches may be the most frequently occurring type. Most tension headaches are associated with anxiety, depression, or unresolved conflicts, rather than a disease condition. Such headaches may begin during a period of stress, such as a family crisis, or a period of fatigue. They often go away after the stressful stimulus disappears or is resolved. Many people with these headaches have SLEEP DISORDERS in the form of frequent and early awakening, which may also be related to tension and stressful life situations. Some people with muscle-contraction headaches have a depressive illness that contributes to the headaches.

Tension headaches are often associated with contraction of the head and neck muscles. In many cases, such headaches are not severe and do not last long, but in other cases, scalp-muscle-contraction headaches may be incapacitating. Individuals who have these headaches describe them as tight, pressing, squeezing, or aching sensations.

Some individuals have chronic muscle-contraction headaches in which the pain is constant for weeks or longer, and at times there may be feelings of jabbing, stabbing, or piercing. Some sufferers of muscle-contraction headaches also have an associated vascular headache, which is aggravated by jarring of the head due to coughing, sneezing, or bending over.

More women than men have tension headaches, and these headaches often run in families.

Other Forms of Headache

Traction headaches   The term traction headache applies to many nonspecific headaches that are secondary to a variety of diseases including brain tumors and strokes. An inflammation of the pain-sensitive structures inside and outside the skull may be the cause.

Mixed headaches   Combined or tension-vascular headaches have features of both vascular head pain and muscle-contraction head and neck pain. Some aspects of vascular headaches, such as throbbing pain on one side of the head, nausea, and vomiting, may be present along with the features of tension headache, such as a dull, constant, aching pain or tightness around the head and neck. There may also be tenderness of the scalp or neck.

Caffeine headaches   Individuals who drink too much caffeine in coffee, tea, and soft drinks sometimes have headaches from the caffeine. Excessive coffee drinking can bring on a group of symptoms including headache, sleeping problems, upset stomach, shortness of breath, and shaky hands. Eliminating coffee may eliminate these symptoms for some individuals. However, some people who drink large quantities of coffee and stop abruptly may suffer caffeine withdrawal symptoms, including headache, irritability, depression, and sometimes nausea. Those who want to cut down on the amount of coffee they drink can mix increasing amounts of decaffeinated coffee into their usual brew.

Hangover headaches   A headache is one of the uncomfortable symptoms of an excessive consumption of alcohol. Alcohol causes the headache by making blood vessels swell, brings on nausea by irritating the digestive system, and leads to dehydration by causing excessive urination.

Headaches in depression Headaches frequently occur during DEPRESSION. Certain ANTIDEPRESSANT medications provide relief from headaches arising from nonorganic causes. Among these are AMITRIPTYLINE HYDROCHLORIDE, IMIPRAMINE HYDROCHLORIDE, DESIPRAMINE HYDROCHLORIDE, NORTRIPTYLINE HYDROCHLORIDE, PROTRIPTYLINE HYDROCHLORIDE, DOXEPIN, MAPROTILINE, TRAZODONE, and AMOXAPINE.

Some headache specialists recommend MONAMINE OXIDASE INHIBITORS (MAOIs) such as PHENELZINE SULFATE as mood elevators for people who have depression. These drugs also help control severe migraine pain in some individuals. However, individuals taking the MAOIs must avoid eating certain foods that contain TYRAMINE (see chart on p. 214). Dangerous side effects of the MAOIs include HIGH BLOOD PRESSURE.

Treatment Options and Outlook

Before one takes any medication for headaches, one should be properly diagnosed. Medications that help tension headaches will not help severe migraine headaches, and drugs targeted to relieve migraine headaches may not help any other type. Also, it is important that one does not overmedicate for headaches and bring on other side effects from medications. For many, aspirin or acetaminophen is enough to relieve a headache. Two aspirin tablets every three to four hours may provide some relief for tension headaches. Aspirin relieves pain and reduces inflammation by interfering with substances in the blood that cause them. However, aspirin probably will not have much effect on the persistent pain of migraine or the deep pain of other types of recurring headaches. For many individuals, aspirin can be harmful and cause upset stomach, ulcers, and internal bleeding. Some people are allergic to aspirin and should use an aspirin substitute instead.

Medication for migraine or vascular headaches is directed toward changing the response of the vascular system to stimuli such as stress, hormonal changes, or noise. Such medications interfere with the dilation reaction of the blood vessels. The most popular medication is ergot, a naturally occurring substance that constricts blood vessels and reduces the dilation of arteries, thus stopping the headaches. Ergot is sometimes given by injection, orally, rectally, or by inhalation. Many individuals find that if they take the ergot medication early enough in prepain stages of an attack, they can abort their headaches, or at least reduce their intensity. Persons who are nauseated and vomiting usually take the drug by some means other than orally. In some cases, a SEDATIVE, such as a BARBITURATE, is given along with the ergot to help relax the individual and make him or her more receptive to the action of the ergot.

Vascular headaches are sometimes treated with prophylactic (preventive) measures. Propranolol is the drug of choice for prevention of migraine in carefully selected patients. Propranolol is a vasoconstrictor that can be taken daily for as long as six months. This drug may slow down the vascular changes that occur during the migraine attack. It is frequently prescribed for some individuals who have headaches more than once each week. This drug is helpful for migraine-headache sufferers who have severe high blood pressure, angina pectoris, or conditions for which ergot preparations are contraindicated. In such situations, propranolol relieves the headache as well as the coexisting disorder. Another advantage of propranolol over ergot medications is that discontinuance of propranolol does not cause rebound headaches.

Other drugs commonly prescribed for migraine are cyproheptadine and methysergide.

Medications for tension or muscle-contraction headaches are directed toward relieving muscular activity and spasm. In some cases, injection with anesthetics and corticosteroids is helpful. ANALGESICS (pain relievers) commonly used are aspirin dextropropoxyphene and ethoheptazine. Sometimes a sedative is prescribed along with these medications.

Medications for cluster headaches include methysergide, ergotamine tartrate, and corticosteroids. LITHIUM is also effective for some in controlling chronic cluster headache. However, lithium has multiple possible side effects on the nervous system and kidneys, and its use should be carefully monitored.

Medication for traction or inflammatory headaches usually involves specific treatment for the associated underlying disease and may require consultations with other medical specialists such as neurologists, ophthalmologists (eye specialists), and otolaryngologists (eye, ear, nose, and throat specialists). Treatment may range from surgery to ANTICONVULSANTS, depending on the specific cause.

Nonpharmacological Treatments

In addition to medication, there are many other techniques used to treat headaches, particularly those associated with reducing ANXIETIES and STRESS.

Biofeedback   This is a method of treating tension headaches that involves teaching a person to control certain body functions through thought and willpower with the use of machines that indicate how a part of the body is responding to stress. Sensors are attached to the patient's forehead (frontalus muscle) to measure muscle tension, and responses are relayed to an amplifier that produces sounds. While the person is tense, the sounds are loud and harsh. As the person concentrates on relaxing the sounds begin to purr quietly or cease altogether. When the tension disappears, so does the headache.

Meditation   MEDITATION, or TRANSCENDENTAL MEDITATION, is a method for inward contemplation that proponents say helps people relax and relieve their anxieties, and in turn relieve some headaches. As the mind slows down during meditation so do other organs in the body. The heart rate decreases, and breathing becomes quieter. Muscle tensions are relaxed. The goal of meditation is productive rest followed by productive activity. While meditation can relieve headache pain for some people, for many it works as an adjunct to pharmacological therapy, helping the headache sufferer to be more receptive to the effects of medication.

Other therapies   HYPNOSIS is rarely used to treat headaches. However, hypnosis is sometimes used as a beginning for additional psychotherapy on an individual or group basis. ACUPUNCTURE, although controversial, has been successfully used to treat some individuals with headaches. The modern interpretation of why acupuncture works is that the needle insertions somehow stimulate the body to secrete ENDORPHINS, naturally occurring hormonelike substances that kill pain. ACUPRESSURE is a technique that involves pressing acupuncture points with the finger. This can be done oneself or by another lay person.

headaches, sexually related   Some individuals have HEADACHES related to sexual activity, leading to ANXIETIES and discomfort. Such persons do not use the headache to avoid sexual activity but actually do endure discomfort before, during, or after sexual intercourse. Nevertheless, the headaches become involved in a cycle of anxiety and apprehension. Sex-related headaches may include three types: muscle-contraction (tension) headaches, benign orgasmic headaches, and malignant coital headaches. Muscle-contraction headaches cause dull, aching pains on both sides of the head and are relatively brief. More men than women experience these, because many couples use positions during intercourse in which the man is more active, typically above his partner with his head and neck unsupported. In women, muscle contraction headaches can be influenced by premenstrual hormonal changes.

Benign orgasmic headaches are intense, short headaches associated with rises in BLOOD PRESSURE during sexual arousal and ORGASM. These headaches usually occur in individuals who also suffer from migraine headaches. They may be brought on by ALCOHOL and/or certain medications.

Malignant coital headaches are caused by fluid escaping through a defect in a person's spinal-cord sheath that widens during sexual intercourse. Some individuals have these headaches only while participating in sexual activity when standing and/or sitting, but not when reclining.

Sex-related headaches are associated more often with extramarital sexual relations than with intercourse between married partners. The anxiety and guilt caused by having a sexual relationship with someone other than a spouse may be the most significant reason for these headaches.

headaches in children   Headaches in children have been studied separately from adult headaches and often have their own unique set of causes. Children's HEADACHES cause the children themselves and their parents STRESS and ANXIETY. Some children's headaches are in themselves symptomatic of some anxiety conditions, but many headaches have other causes and are just as distressing. By age 15, 5.3 percent of youngsters have migraine headaches, and 5.4 percent have infrequent headaches. U.S. children lost 1.3 million days of school during 1986 because of headaches.

Youngsters have four basic types of headaches: acute, acute recurrent, chronic progressive, and chronic nonprogressive. An acute headache is one single severe headache and may be caused by general infections or infection of the CENTRAL NERVOUS SYSTEM, sinuses, teeth, HIGH BLOOD PRESSURE, or a blow to the head. An acute recurrent headache is a severe headache that returns after pain-free days or months. Migraine headaches fall into this pattern. Some youngsters who have classic migraine headaches report accompanying visual phenomena, such as shimmery lights or halos around objects, and sometimes nausea and vomiting. Chronic progressive headaches are those that increase in severity and frequency over time. These are often caused by a physical problem and should be investigated by a physician.

Chronic nonprogressive headaches are headaches that come and go but do not get worse. These are sometimes referred to as functional headaches because they may have no physical cause. They may be brought on by muscle contractions due to anxieties such as stress at school. A physical cause for this kind of headache may be chronic sinus infection.

Additionally, some children have headaches resulting from dental infections or jaw problems.

Bruckheim, Allan, "Don't Worry Too Much without Good Reason; Children Do Get Headaches," Chicago Tribune, September 1, 1987.

healing touch   See THERAPEUTIC TOUCH.

hearing loss   See DEAFNESS.

heart attack, anxiety following   Individuals who have a heart attack (myocardial infarction) are likely to have some anxiety afterward. In the United States alone, over half a million people suffer heart attacks each year, making anxiety following a heart attack a fairly common occurrence. As many as one third of these people may require some psychotherapeutic help to relieve emotional stress.

The anxiety that individuals experience during and after a heart attack often follows a pattern. Upon initial symptoms of a heart attack, a person may, although recognizing the symptoms, deny them. Unfortunately, such denial often delays life-saving medical treatment. Educating individuals known to have coronary-artery disease, as well as educating their friends and family, is an important step toward getting heart-attack victims to seek prompt medical attention.

Once in the emergency ward, a heart-attack victim often experiences much confusion, as well as fear and anxiety. At this point, treatment to minimize these feelings may be limited to a medical explanation of what is happening, plus medications to relieve physical pain. Four emotional responses are fairly common after a person has been admitted to a coronary-care unit: 1) anxiety, 2) denial, 3) depression, and 4) coping. Initially, the person is anxious and fearful of DEATH, the UNKNOWN, and PAIN. As he or she begins to feel better the individual may resort to denial, often even requesting to leave the hospital. Shortly thereafter, the individual realizes the implications of the heart attack and shows signs of depression. Following this, usually by about the fifth day in the hospital, the person is more secure and begins to return to methods of coping typical of persons who have coronary-prone (often referred to as "type A") behavior. Both drugs and nonpharmacologic treatment are often used to relieve anxiety and depression at this point for heart-attack victims. Anxiety, especially if left untreated, can bring about serious arrhythmias (variations in heartbeat). Most commonly, when medication is prescribed for anxiety or depression, it is in the form of a BENZODIAZEPINE, such as ALPRAZOLAM (Xanax). Psychotherapeutic intervention or counseling may be used to help people adapt to new requirements in lifestyle such as diet, giving up smoking, and management of STRESS resulting from type A behavior. Sexual counseling may also be of help to the heart-attack victim and spouse who have anxieties about resuming sexual activity.

See also CORONARY-BYPASS ANXIETY, POSTOPERATIVE.

heart attack, fear of   Fear of heart attack is known as anginophobia. Heart attack is the common term for a coronary occlusion. In a heart attack, one of the coronary arteries becomes blocked. The condition may or may not result in a myocardial infarction (heart attack), depending on the extent of the damage to the surrounding muscle.

See also HIGH BLOOD PRESSURE, FEAR OF.

heartburn   A burning sensation in the upper part of the abdomen or under the breastbone. It is a cause of anxiety for many people who may fear that it is related to heart disease. Heartburn is also a symptom of STRESS, because it can be brought on by nervousness or overeating. The burning sensation is actually associated with the esophagus, a muscular tube that connects the throat with the stomach. The tube passes behind the breastbone alongside the heart, which is why irritation or inflammation here is known as *heart*burn.

Heartburn and distress in the digestive tract is frequently a response to emotional stress or anxieties. Tense, nervous people who worry about their jobs and family problems often complain of "acid indigestion" and heartburn. The list of foods that disagree with heartburn sufferers includes just about anything a person would want to eat. When things go smoothly for these people, everything agrees with them. When they are upset or frustrated, nothing does. Heartburn usually starts slowly, about an hour or so after a heavy or spicy meal is eaten. The pain can sometimes be quite intense and may last a few hours.

Coping with Heartburn

In some cases, the pain is due to irritation (esophagitis) from hydrochloric acid in the stomach juice that has backed up into the esophagus, relaxation of the valve between the stomach and the esophagus is one cause of esophagitis. Hiatus hernia, in which part of the stomach slips up into the chest, is

---

TIPS FOR RELIEVING THE ANXIETY OF HEARTBURN

- Avoid certain foods that are spicy, acidic, tomato-based, or fatty, such as sausages, chocolate, tomatoes, and citrus fruits.
- Avoid alcohol, tea, colas, and coffee, even decaffeinated.
- Eat moderate amounts of food to avoid overfilling your stomach.
- Stop or at least cut back on smoking.
- Don't try to exercise immediately after eating or before lying down.
- Elevate the head of your bed or use extra pillows to raise the level of your head above your feet.
- Avoid tight belts and other restrictive clothing.
- Learn relaxation techniques.
- If none of these help, see your doctor.

---

another. This type of heartburn is often brought on by lying down, especially after overeating. It may be helped by raising the head of the bed, by avoiding certain foods, especially sweets, and by a low-fat, low-calorie diet.

People whose heartburn is brought on by stress and emotional factors may not have abnormal amounts of hydrochloric acid in their stomachs. They are probably oversensitive to normal acidity, just as they may overreact to the ordinary stressors of daily life. Adequate rest and RELAXATION and occasional use of antacids may be helpful. Individuals who suffer frequent heartburn should be checked by a physician. If there are no medical problems, a change in mental attitude toward the stressors in the individual's life should be considered. Relaxation training and medication may be helpful.

See also COMPLEMENTARY THERAPIES; INDIGESTION; MEDITATION; ULCERS.

heart disease, fear of   Fear of heart disease is known as cardiophobia. This may be a fear of any disorder or defect that interferes with normal functioning of the heart. Heart disease covers congenital defects, damage caused by diseases such as rheumatic fever or syphilis, or an atherosclerotic condition (hardening of the arteries), angina pectoris, or coronary occlusion.

See also CHOLESTEROL, FEAR OF; HIGH BLOOD PRESSURE, FEAR OF.

Fleet, Richard P., and Bernard D. Beitman, "Cardiovascular death from panic disorder and panic-like anxiety: A critical review of the literature," *Journal of Psychosomatic Research* 44, no. 1 (January 1998): pp. 71–80.

heart rate in emotion   Strong emotion, such as fear or anxiety, can increase the rate of the heartbeat through sympathetic impulses (arousal system). Parasympathetic reflexes (calming system) resulting from increased blood pressure during emotion also can alter the heart rate. A strong parasympathetic reflex can slow the heart rate to a point at which it may appear on the verge of stopping. While most phobic individuals experience rapid heartbeat when exposed to their phobic stimulus, those who fear blood often experience a slower heartbeat.

See also BLOOD AND BLOOD INJURY PHOBIA; SYMPATHETIC NERVOUS SYSTEM.

heat, fear of   Fear of heat is known as thermophobia. Some individuals fear hot weather, hot rooms, central heating, hot water, or being hot. They take measures to avoid heat, such as living in a colder climate, staying in air-conditioned places during hot spells, and wearing cool clothing.

heaven, fear of   Fear of heaven is known as uranophobia or ouranophobia. Some people fear the idea that they will be judged after life and assigned either the rewards of heaven or the punishment of HELL. Religious skeptics and radical thinkers object on social and ethical grounds to what they consider to be the carrot-in-front-of-the-donkey aspect of a belief in heaven. The prospect of heaven serves as a disciplinary element to promote good behavior and to encourage the feeling that inequities and injustices must be suffered patiently and passively in this life to earn a reward in the next. Some object to the pleasurable, delightful quality of heaven on the grounds that this image of paradise appeals to man's baser, more hedonistic qualities.

See also HELL, FEAR OF.

hedonophobia   Fear of feeling pleasure. (This term is also used to mean fear of travel.)

See also PLEASURE, FEAR OF.

heights, fear of   Fear of heights is known as acrophobia, altophobia, hypsophobia, and hypsiphobia. It is a very common phobia, especially in its milder forms. Those who have phobias of heights emphasize that their visual space is important. They will not be able to go down a flight of stairs if they can see the open stairwell. They will be frightened looking out of a high window that stretches from floor to ceiling, but not if the window's bottom is at or covered to waist level or higher. They have difficulty crossing bridges on foot because of the proximity of the edge but may be able to cross in a car. Sometimes fear of heights is related to an acute fear of falling (which is innate). Babies usually begin to be wary of heights some time after starting to crawl. Walking, like crawling, also enhances their fear of heights. The fear of heights is considered a "prepared" fear common to most humans.

Fear of heights, classified as a simple phobia, is not usually associated with other psychiatric symptoms or disorders, such as depression. The heights-phobic person is no more or less anxious than anyone else until exposed to heights, but then he or she becomes overwhelmingly uncomfortable and fearful, sometimes having symptoms associated with a panic attack, such as palpitations, sweating, dizziness, and difficulty breathing. A person who fears heights can also fear just thinking about the possibility that he might be confronted with his phobic stimulus.

Fear of heights is sometimes associated with a fear of airplanes and flying, although the height is only one element in the complex reaction that leads to fear of flying in an airplane. Fear of heights is sometimes involved in many related fears, such as bicycles, skiing, amusement rides, tall buildings, stairs, bridges, and freeways.

See also FALLING, FEAR OF; FLYING, FEAR OF; HIGH OBJECTS, FEAR OF; HIGH PLACES, FEAR OF LOOKING UP AT; PHOBIA; SIMPLE PHOBIAS.

Marks, Isaac M., *Fears, Phobias and Rituals* (New York: Oxford University Press, 1987), p. 130.

Menzies, Ross G., and J. Christopher Clarke, "The Etiology of Fear of Heights and Its Relationship to Severity and Individual Response Patterns," *Behavior Research Therapy* 31, no. 4 (1993): pp. 355–365.

heliophobia   Fear of sunlight. Also known as phengophobia.
See also SUNLIGHT, FEAR OF.

hell, fear of   Fear of hell is known as hadephobia, stigiophobia, and stygiophobia. Individuals have feared hell for thousands of years before Christianity. Egyptian writings contain some indication of a belief in judgment and punishment after death. The early Greeks believed in an afterlife that was a shadowy realm where almost all of the dead were fated to go, and Plato's writings of the fourth century B.C. indicate a growing fear of punishment after death. The original Jewish concept of the afterlife was Sheol, a dark place removed from God that was everyone's fate after death. Gradually the concept of punishment for a sinful life after death began to enter Judaism, partly to rationalize inequities in this life and partly because Jews wished to think of their oppressors as suffering after death. At this point the image of writhing in flames became part of the fearful description of punishment in the underworld. Gehenna, the term for the place of torment in Judaism, was adapted from the name of the flaming rubbish dump of Jerusalem. Later, Christians produced elaborate descriptions of hell in art and literature as well as religious writings, and these increased fears of hell. The addition of the Devil and his orders of demons as residents of hell provided a rationalization for the theological dilemma of explaining the presence of evil in a world ruled by a loving God.

The fire-and-brimstone image of hell has decreased in the 20th century. More common fears are either of annihilation after death or that God's mercy will extend to all regardless of their conduct in life on earth.
See also HEAVEN, FEAR OF.

Cavendish, Richard, ed., "Hell." In *Man, Myth and Magic* (New York: Marshall Cavendish, 1983).

Thouless, Robert H., *An Introduction to the Psychology of Religion* (Cambridge: Cambridge University Press, 1971).

Hellenologophobia   Fear of Greek terms or of complex scientific or pseudoscientific terminology.

helminthophobia   Fear of worms.
See also WORMS, FEAR OF.

helplessness   An experience of fear and indecision and a sense of not being able to personally influence the external world. Freud used the term "psychic helplessness" to describe the experience during the birth process when respiratory and other physiological changes occur; he believed that this psychic helplessness state led to later anxieties. Freud also believed that the baby's helplessness and dependence on the mother created frustration, which in turn led to an inability to cope with later tension. During the 1970s, Martin Seligman developed the concept and coined the term "learned helplessness" to describe an individual's dependence on another. Many phobic individuals have characteristics of learned helplessness, particularly agoraphobics, who cannot go away from home without someone accompanying them.
See also AGORAPHOBIA; LEARNED HELPLESSNESS.

help lines   See HOT LINES; SELF-HELP GROUPS; SUPPORT GROUPS.

hematophobia   Fear of blood or the sight of blood. Also known as hemophobia.
See also BLOOD AND BLOOD-INJURY PHOBIA; ERYTHROPHOBIA.

hemophobia   See HEMATOPHOBIA.

hemorrhoids   Enlarged veins at the lowest part of the intestine. Hemorrhoids may be painful or bleed, causing anxieties for the sufferer. The word literally means a "blood" (*hemo*) "flow" (*rhoid*), describing one of the characteristics of the disease, bleeding from the anus. "Piles" is a lay term for hemorrhoids.

Hemorrhoids also produce anxiety because in many cases their cause cannot be determined. CONSTIPATION, straining while defecating, sitting for long periods, and infections can aggravate the condition once it starts. The disorder usually is mild, but if neglected, may result in annoying or painful complications, such as itching, protrusion outside the anus or fissures in the anus, and possibly secondary infection.

Treatment consists of warm sitz baths, soothing ointments, antibiotics for infection, measures such as laxatives or stool softeners to relieve constipation, and a diet of digestible foods. Any bleeding from the anus should be investigated by a physician.

See also IRRITABLE BOWEL SYNDROME.

herbal medicine Herbal medicine (herbalism) involves use of a plant or a plant part valued for its medicinal, savory, or aromatic qualities. Herbalism gained popularity in the United States toward the end of the 20th century. Estimates are that Americans spend more than $1 billion on herbal remedies in a year; many people seek these alternative remedies to relieve anxieties.

Herbal medications are deeply rooted in most FOLK MEDICINE traditions and have played an impor-

---

USE OF HERBAL REMEDIES FOR RELIEVING ANXIETIES

- See a physician first for serious conditions. Do not attempt to self-medicate.
- Consider the sources of your products; select reputable brands.
- Choose reliable forms—such as tinctures or freeze-dried—as powdered forms may lose potency upon exposure to air.
- Overdosing can have harmful effects. Take recommended dosages at suggested intervals.
- Watch for reactions; if unwanted reactions occur, stop the medication.

---

tant role in the evolution of modern medicine and pharmacology. For example, when the Pilgrims landed in Plymouth in 1620, they set up herb gardens that contained the medicinal varieties brought from the Old World. The settlers soon discovered that the Native Americans had their own healing plants, including cascara sagrada and goldenseal. According to the World Health Organization, 80 percent of the earth's population uses some form of herbal therapy.

Many contemporary medications are based on specific herbs but are manufactured from synthetic substances believed to be more effective than the natural herbs. Still, herbal therapies remain a major component of Ayurvedic, homeopathic, and other alternative approaches.

Herbal products are marketed in the United States as foods and are permitted by the Food and Drug Administration provided that the products do not make any therapeutic claims. Herbal products are sold "over-the-counter" and are not subject to the same safety and efficacy standards that apply to over-the-counter medications. Herbal packaging labels rarely contain guidelines regarding indications for proper use. As with any medication, herbal remedies are best used under the guidance of a knowledgeable individual, in this case, an herbalist.

See also AYURVEDA; COMPLEMENTARY THERAPIES; HOMEOPATHY.

Chevallier, Andrew, *The Encyclopedia of Medicinal Plants* (New York: Houghton Mifflin, 1996).

Kligler, Benjamin, "Herbal Medicines and the Family Physician," *American Family Physician* 58, no. 5 (October 1, 1998).

National Women's Health Report, "Alternative Therapies and Women's Health," National Women's Health Resource Center, Washington, DC: May/June, 1995.

Schar, Douglas, *The Backyard Medicine Chest: An Herbal Primer* (Washington, DC: Elliott & Clark Publishers, 1995).

Zink, Therese, and Jodi Chaffrin, "Herbal 'Health' Products: What Family Physicians Need to Know," *American Family Physician* 58, no. 5 (October 1, 1998), pp. 1133–1140.

heredity, fear of Fear of heredity or of transmitted characteristics is known as patroiophobia. Some individuals fear the transmission of genetic characteristics to descendants. Heredity depends upon the character of genes contained in the chromosomes of cells, and upon the particular genetic code contained in the DNA of which the chromosomes are composed. This is a common fear, and many people fear that their children will inherit deformities or mental disorders that have been present in their family.

heresyphobia (heresophobia)   A fear of challenges to official doctrine, or a fear of radical deviation.

Spears, Richard, *Slang and Euphemism* (New York: Jonathan David, 1981).

herpes simplex virus   HSV can cause blisterlike sores almost anywhere on a person's skin. It usually occurs around the mouth and nose or the buttocks and genitals. Herpes is a name used for some 50 related viruses. Herpes simplex is related to the risk for infectious mononucleosis, chicken pox, and shingles (varicella zoster virus). HSV infections can produce anxieties because they can reappear without any predictability; also, the sores may be painful and embarrassing.

Two Types of HSV

Type 1.   Studies show that most people get Type 1, which affects the lips, mouth, nose, chin, or cheeks during infancy or childhood. It is transmitted by close contact with family members or friends who carry the virus. It can be transmitted by kissing, or by using the same eating utensils and towels. A rash or cold sores on the mouth and gums appear shortly after exposure. Symptoms may be barely noticeable or may need medical attention for relief of pain.

Type 2.   Type 2, which includes genital herpes, one of the many diseases caused by the herpes virus, most often appears following sexual contact with an infected person. It has reached epidemic numbers, affecting anywhere between 5 million to 20 million persons in the United States, or up to 20 percent of all sexually active adults. Genital herpes, although relatively uncommon in the United States until the late 1960s, may be the most common sexually transmitted disease in the late 1990s. The chronicity of the disease and the fact that no cure exists is a source of significant stress in the lives of its sufferers. Stress and anxiety associated with having this SEXUALLY TRANSMITTED DISEASE can be reduced with education, counseling, and supportive physical care.

Herpes is particularly stressful because once the virus invades the body, it remains for life, although it may be dormant most of the time. In different individuals, episodes recur with more or less frequency.

Although genital herpes is not usually a medically serious disease, it can lead to DEPRESSION and other emotional conditions. Many victims tend to resent the sex partner from whom they contracted the disease, often leading to divorce or the breaking up of a relationship. Others consider themselves damaged for life, fearing that they are unfit for marriage or a lasting relationship.

The disease is most commonly spread by direct contact, meaning that to get herpes, uninfected skin must come in contact with an active herpes sore. However, the virus may be shed without noticeable symptoms and may thus be transmitted. As herpes sores may be hidden in the internal parts of the female genitalia or may not be painful, one victim may unwittingly infect another.

Symptoms and Diagnostic Path

Once the herpes virus has entered the skin, it multiplies rapidly. First symptoms are usually itching or a tingling sensation, followed by the eruption of unusually painful sores or blisters. Typically, in the first attack, the sores appear two days to two weeks after exposure and last two to three weeks. Subsequent attacks, which may occur in a few weeks or not for years, generally last about five days. When an attack subsides, the virus lies dormant and travels along the nerve fibers until it reaches a resting place.

In rare cases, the herpes virus may travel to the brain and cause a serious, often fatal, form of encephalitis. More commonly, herpes may infect the cornea of the eye, if untreated, the infection can lead to visual damage and even blindness. None of these complications, however, is as common as periodic recurrences at the original site of infection.

A serious complication of genital herpes affects infants born to women who have active infections at the time of birth. Some infants who contract disseminated herpes infections die, and half of those who survive may suffer brain damage or blindness. Many doctors recommend that the baby be delivered by cesarean section if the mother has an active infection near the time of delivery.

Treatment Options and Outlook

There is no way to rid the body of the herpes virus. However, antiviral agents developed during the 1990s shorten the duration of an active infection, relieve discomfort, and speed healing. By halting the virus from reproducing itself and spreading to other cells, these agents stop the formation of new herpes blisters and help existing sores heal faster.

Many herpes sufferers learn to recognize patterns of recurrence and factors which trigger subsequent episodes. RELAXATION techniques to reduce stress are indicated if stress is a factor in recurrent disease. There are a number of herpes counseling centers and groups throughout the country to lend support and help to victims of the disease.

Risk Factors and Preventive Measures

The most effective way of preventing genital herpes is avoiding all sexual contact with an infected person. Use of a condom and spermicidal agent will reduce the risk, but this is not absolutely foolproof, particularly when the lesions are on the skin of the perineum and not on the penis or in the vagina.

Lutgendorf, Susa K., Michael H. Antoni, Gail Ironson, et al., "Cognitive-behavioral stress management decreases dysphoric mood and herpes simplex virus-Type 2 antibody titers in symptomatic HIV-seropositive gay men," *Journal of Consulting and Clinical Psychology* 65, no. 1 (February 1997): pp. 31–43.

Nourse, Alan Edward, *Herpes* (New York: Franklin Watts, 1985).

Sacks, Stephen L., *The Truth About Herpes*. 3d ed. (Seattle: G. Soules, 1988).

herpetophobia   Fear of snakes and reptiles. There is some evidence that humans have an innate aversion to or fear of snakes. Some of this comes from studies of animals (such as chimpanzees, who demonstrate a natural aversion to snakes) and some from epidemiological studies, which show that ninety-five percent of snake phobics have never had direct contact with a snake. This innate tendency, probably coupled with vicarious learning (e.g., stories about the danger or voracity of snakes), can lead to development of an intense anxiety response. Furthermore, since contact with snakes is relatively easy to avoid, new learning and desensitization does not take place, and the fear consequently persists and intensifies.

See also SNAKES, FEAR OF.

heterophobia   Fear of the opposite sex, considered by some psychoanalysts and learning theorists to be a partial explanation of some homosexual behavior.

heterosexuality, fear of   Fear of sexual behavior, impulses, and desires in which the object is a person of the opposite sex.

See also SEXUAL FEARS.

hex, fear of   Some individuals fear the hex, a curse or an evil spell meant to kill or harm its victim. Voodoo and witchcraft both contain this frightening idea. Hex comes from the German word for witch, *die hexe*. The Pennsylvania Dutch paint brightly colored hex signs on their barns to keep away evil spirits.

See also VOODOO, FEARS IN.

Brasch, R., *Strange Customs* (New York: David McKay, 1976).

hierarchy of needs   Some theorists believe that human behavior is motivated by a series of needs that can be arranged in a hierarchical order, beginning with the basic physiological needs, such as food and water; progressing to safety needs, such as protection against danger, social or love needs; esteem or ego needs; and self-actualization. Anxiety and fear can result from incomplete attainment of these levels. The originator of this theory was

Abraham Harold Maslow (1908–70), an American psychologist known as a leader of the human-potential movement because of his emphasis on self-fulfillment.

hierophobia   Fear of religious objects.
See also RELIGIOUS OBJECTS, FEAR OF.

high blood pressure, fear of   The fear of having high blood pressure, also known as hypertension, is closely linked with the fear of heart disease. This fear manifests itself with excessive preoccupation with blood pressure. Many fearful individuals are compulsive about having their blood pressure taken frequently and may have equipment for taking their own blood pressure at home in between visits to a physician. The term blood pressure, as used in medicine, refers to the force of one's blood against the walls of the arteries, created by the heart as it pumps blood through the body. As the heart pumps or beats the pressure increases. As the heart relaxes between beats the pressure decreases. High blood pressure is the condition in which blood pressure rises too high and stays there. High blood pressure occurs during anxiety and panic attacks but may become reduced after the panic attack subsides. If it does not, the individual should seek help from a physician.
See also CHOLESTEROL, FEAR OF; HEART ATTACK, FEAR OF; HEART DISEASE, FEAR OF; "WHITE COAT HYPERTENSION."

high objects, fear of   Fear of high objects is known as batophobia. This fear may be related to acrophobia (fear of high places) or to the fear of LOOKING UP AT HIGH PLACES (anablepophobia). Individuals who are fearful of high objects may ask others to reach items from high cabinet shelves, will not climb ladders, and will avoid selecting items from the top shelves in grocery stores.
See also HIGH PLACES, FEAR OF LOOKING UP AT.

high places, fear of looking up at   Fear of looking up at high places is known as anablepophobia. Individuals with this fear avoid looking up at the tops of tall buildings in cities and at the tops of mountains while in the country. This fear may be related to a fear of heights (acrophobia) or a fear of high objects (batophobia).
See also HEIGHTS, FEAR OF.

hippophobia   Fear of horses.
See also HORSES, FEAR OF.

hippopotomonstrosesquippedaliophobia   Fear of long words.

hives   Hives are pink swellings called "wheals" that occur in groups on any part of the skin. They cause anxieties for the sufferer because as they are forming, they usually are very itchy and may also burn or sting. Until they are diagnosed, the sufferer may be bewildered about the cause and about possibilities for relief. Hives usually go away within a few days to a few weeks. Occasionally, a person will continue to have hives for many years. About 10–20 percent of the population will have at least one episode in their lifetime.

Hives are produced by blood plasma leaking through tiny gaps between the cells lining small blood vessels in the skin. Histamine, a natural chemical, is released from cells called "mast cells," which lie along the blood vessels in the skin. Many different things, including allergic reactions, chemicals in food, or medications, can cause a histamine release. Sometimes it is impossible to find out why histamine is being released and hives are forming.

The most common foods that cause hives are nuts, chocolate, fish, tomatoes, eggs, fresh berries, and milk. Fresh foods cause hives more often than cooked foods; food additives and preservatives may also be responsible. Hives may appear within minutes or up to two hours after eating, depending on where the food is absorbed in the digestive tract.

Almost any prescription or over-the-counter medication can cause hives. Some of these drugs include antibiotics (especially penicillin), pain medications, sedatives, tranquilizers, and diuretics. Antacids, vitamins, eye and ear drops, laxatives, vaginal douches, or any other nonprescription item can be a potential cause of hives.

Many infections can cause hives. Viral upper respiratory tract infections are a common cause in children. Other viruses, including hepatitis B, may also be a cause, as well as a number of bacterial and fungal infections.

Some people develop hives from sunlight, cold, pressure, vibration, or EXERCISE. Hives due to sunlight are called "solar urticaria." This is a rare disorder in which hives come up within minutes of sun exposure on exposed areas and fade within one to two hours. Reaction to the cold is more common. Hives appear when the skin is warmed after exposure to cold. If the exposure to cold is over large areas of the body, large amounts of histamine may be released which can produce sneezing, flushing, generalized hives, and fainting. A simple test for this type of hives can be done by applying an ice cube to the skin.

Symptoms and Diagnostic Path

When hives form around the eyes, lips, or genitals, the tissue may swell excessively. Although frightening in appearance, the swelling usually goes away in less than 24 hours. Dermatologists may use the term *angioedema* to describe this type of swelling, which is also used to describe very deep large hives on other areas of the body.

In the commonest kind of hives, each individual wheal lasts a few hours before fading away, leaving no trace. New hives may continue to develop as old areas fade. They can vary in size from as small as a pencil eraser to as large as a dinner plate and may join together to form larger swellings.

Treatment Options and Outlook

Diagnosis depends on each individual's medical history and a thorough examination by a dermatologist. The best treatment for hives is to find the cause and then eliminate it, which is not always an easy task. While investigating the cause of hives, or when a cause cannot be found, dermatologists often prescribe antihistamines to provide some relief to the sufferer. Antihistamines work best if taken on a regular schedule to prevent hives from forming.

In cases of severe hives, an injection of epinephrine (adrenaline) or a cortisone preparation, may bring relief.

See also ALLERGIES.

HIV positive See ACQUIRED IMMUNODEFICIENCY SYNDROME; HUMAN IMMUNODEFICIENCY VIRUS.

hoarding A variant of OBSESSIVE-COMPULSIVE DISORDER. Compulsive hoarding may be a fear of not having enough. Some individuals fear throwing anything away and even store trash and old newspapers. They may store valueless papers from the past or buy vast quantities of food and other supplies when there are no predictable shortages. Such individuals become very anxious if others attempt to remove any of the saved or stored items.

See also RITUALS.

hobbies Activities people engage in because they want to, not because they must for economic reasons. They are sources of satisfaction, RELAXATION, and relief from the stresses of everyday life for many people. Some people who look forward to RETIREMENT do so because they will have more time for hobbies. Choosing hobbies is up to each individual, although in many cases they bring people with common interests together. For many people, collecting antiques or other collectibles is a hobby.

According to Allen Elkin, Ph.D., Director, Stress Management and Counseling Center, New York City, "people who derive most of their identity from their profession are going to need other sources of SELF-ESTEEM when they leave that profession behind." People who have hobbies usually have a consuming interest in their chosen activity. Many former workaholics find satisfaction in a hobby that forces them to concentrate and be patient, such as building a model train, bird watching, or producing clay sculptures.

Winston Churchill is said to have commented on hobbies: "The cultivation of a hobby and new forms of interest is a policy of first importance . . . to be happy and really safe, one ought to have at least two or three hobbies." Churchill, who painted, wrote the book *Painting as a Pastime.*

Godbey, Geoffrey, and John Robinson, *Time for Life: The Surprising Ways Americans Use Their Time* (University Park, Penn.: Pennsylvania State University Press, 1997).

Kanfer, Stefan, "The Art of Having Fun." *Modern Maturity,* October 1995.

hobgoblin   An object that inspires superstitious fear.

See also SUPERNATURAL, FEAR OF.

hobophobia   Fear of bums or beggars.

hodophobia   Fear of travel.

See also TRAVEL, FEAR OF.

holiday anxieties and depression   Many individuals experience DEPRESSION during periods of the year in which holidays occur or on holidays themselves. These can be times filled with anxieties, particularly for some single and widowed individuals who may feel alone and lonely and see the rest of the world in a celebratory mood surrounded by families. The anticipation of holidays induces some people to drink, eat, or smoke more.

The anxieties associated with holiday depression often occur when individuals have been uprooted from their families and relocated elsewhere for employment or other reasons. The stresses of moving and relocation are compounded by loneliness. Some individuals who are not separated from their families experience mood shifts out of nostalgia for lost loved ones or for earlier times in their lives.

Avoiding Holiday Depression

People who know that they will be alone on holidays and will feel stressed can avoid their holiday depressive episodes by planning ahead. They can take a trip to an interesting place, engage in some enjoyable activity with a group, or invite other people without families to share holiday activities together. Other individuals who know they will be alone on holidays may volunteer their services to hospitals or shelters for the homeless. Feeling that they will be helpful to others is a way of combating the stressful feelings associated with these times.

Usually the depressed mood brought about by holidays under such circumstances goes away after

COPING WITH HOLIDAY ANXIETIES AND DEPRESSION

- Have realistic expectations so that you will not place too many demands on yourself. Be assertive and learn to say no when you want to.
- Consider your support system. If you don't have one, devote some time and energy to developing a support system by reaching out to others.
- Identify your major annoyances at this time of year. Be aware of when they happen and plan to have alternative responses if you usually become anxious or depressed.

the holiday season. However, when the depressive mood does not improve as the holidays pass, individuals should seek professional help.

See also AFFECTIVE DISORDERS; DEPRESSION; SEASONAL DISORDER.

holistic medicine   Holistic medicine involves a shift in belief systems from the dualistic mind/body split toward a view of mind, body, and spirit as being closely connected. It has come to mean a specific way of thinking and practicing the art and science of medicine and for dealing with illness as well as relieving stress. Practitioners of holistic medicine view the individual as a totality, rather than as a headache to be relieved or a backache to be cured.

See also AYURVEDA; COMPLEMENTARY THERAPIES; HERBAL MEDICINE; HOMEOPATHY; MIND/BODY CONNECTIONS; PSYCHONEUROIMMUNOLOGY.

holy things, fear of   Fear of holy things or religious objects is known as hagiophobia or hierophobia.

See also RELIGIOUS OBJECTS, FEAR OF.

home, fear of returning   Fear of returning home is known as nostophobia. Some adults fear returning to their childhood home because they are afraid that things will not be as they were, that their parents or other family members may not be there, or that they may not be accepted or welcomed. Some individuals prefer to remember their home as it was in their childhood and have a fear of returning in later years. Sometimes home is associated with conflict with a spouse or other family member, and anxiety occurs in anticipation of returning.

homelessness Anxieties and fears of homeless people range from solving everyday practical problems, such as finding shelter and enough food, to serious disorders, such as substance abuse, DEPRESSION, and schizophrenia. The stresses of physical as well as mental health problems are intensified by homelessness and, conversely, homelessness precipitates health problems. Because of the nature of the population, it is difficult to assess the numbers of homeless people and their characteristic stressors.

The difficulties in providing medical and mental health care for the homeless are related in part to the reluctance of some homeless people to present themselves for care, as well as insufficiencies of community health centers. Many of the psychiatrically impaired homeless avoid contact with the health care system. Community mobile outreach services are an important way to help these individuals obtain food, clothing, and medical and mental health care.

For many of the poor and homeless populations, emergency department physicians are their source of primary care. These physicians often provide care for families that are in dire financial shape, the elderly, victims of rape and domestic violence, and drug abusers.

A survey of homeless adults living in beach areas near Los Angeles revealed a high rate of prior psychiatric hospitalization. The survey covered 529 people who had spent the previous night outdoors, in a shelter, in a hotel, or in the home of a relative with whom they did not expect to stay very long. Sixty-four percent of the people interviewed were white; 73 percent were men. They had been homeless for an average of two years. Altogether, 44 percent had been in hospitals for psychiatric reasons, including ALCOHOLISM and drug dependence. Twenty-one percent had made an outpatient visit for a mental or emotional problem within the past year. Forty-one percent had never used mental health services.

The worst symptoms were noted in the hospitalized group. There were more SUICIDE attempts, more

daily drinking and delirium tremens. Seventy-six percent of the hospitalized group and 48 percent of the others had been arrested. People who had been hospitalized were more likely to be living in shelters. The 41 percent who had never used mental health services had been homeless about half as long as the rest and were least likely to be sleeping outdoors. Surprisingly, they scored at the same level as the general population on a questionnaire evaluating well-being.

According to mental health professionals, to address the complex needs of those categorized as homeless persons requires a multidisciplinary approach. Social services are needed for short-term and long-term food, housing, and entitlement services. Networks should be developed to enable access for those people to specialty medical services, emergency food pantries, transportation, overnight shelter, and respite care for children while the parent negotiates the systems. Churches often provide for emergency needs and long-term support. Legal services are needed to advocate for rights and entitlements. Children who are homeless require interaction with school systems, health care providers, day-care centers, and, often, child protective services to promote health and prevent further illness or trauma.

Kahn, Ada P., and Jan Fawcett, *The Encyclopedia of Mental Health,* 2nd ed. (New York: Facts On File, 2001).
McFarland, Gertrude K., and Mary Durand Thomas, *Psychiatric Mental Health Nursing* (Philadelphia: Lippincott, 1991).

homeopathy Homeopathy is a system of healing based on assisting the body to heal itself and using the least amount of medication possible. Many people use homeopathic remedies to prevent, reduce, and alleviate stress. Homeopathy is considered a COMPLEMENTARY THERAPY.

Homeopathy uses medicines made from plants, minerals, animals, animal substances, and chemicals. Whereas some conventional medications suppress symptoms and the body's immune response, and occasionally unfortunate reactions to drugs or drug interactions occur, homeopathic practitioners prescribe only one medication at a time and claim that these rarely, if ever, produce unwanted side effects. Homeopathic medicines are made in accordance with processes described in the *Homeopathic Pharmacopoeia of the United States.*

A person-oriented, rather than disease-oriented, system, homeopathic practitioners treat patients based on their symptoms rather than relying solely on diagnostic techniques. Homeopathic practitioners seek to find *causes* of diseases as well as treat symptoms; this is often done in a holistic way by talking extensively with the patient to obtain a complete health and psychosocial history. In this regard, homeopathy has a characteristic in common with the Chinese belief that the best doctors do not use medicine; they heal by giving guidance for healthful living.

Homeopathy is used for a wide variety of chronic and acute problems. These include (but are not limited to) ANXIETIES, ALLERGIES, digestive problems, gynecological conditions, and skin diseases. Many homeopathic remedies can be self-prescribed and purchased over the counter. However, as with any medication, it is prudent to consult a knowledgeable practitioner. Such individuals can be located through reputable local homeopathic pharmacies or the National Center of Homeopathy, Alexandria, Virginia, or the International Foundation for Homeopathy, Seattle.

Historical Background of Homeopathy

The history of homeopathy goes back about 250 years. Samuel Hahneman, M.D., a German physician, noted that Peruvian bark cured malaria. To test his theory that the bark might *cause* as well as *cure* malaria, he ingested small amounts of the bark and developed symptoms of malaria. He termed this effect a "proving" of symptoms. Another example of a "proving" of symptoms is that poisons in large doses are fatal; moderate doses can cause symptoms, but small doses can stimulate the body toward reduction of symptoms. Homeopathy is based on the law of similars, or "let like cure like." What has the power to cause also has the power to cure.

A parallel in Western medicine are the vaccines and allergy shots that contain tiny amounts of killed virus, or allergens, which stimulate the body's immune system and prepare it for actual challenge.

The practice of homeopathy came to the United States in the early 1800s. By the mid-1800s, several medical colleges, including the New England Female Medical College, taught homeopathy. Around 1900, there were 22 homeopathic medical colleges, and one out of five doctors used homeopathy. However, by 1920, only 15 colleges remained. The decline in use of homeopathy in the United States came along with medical science's increasing view of the body as a mechanistic device, the advent of medical specialization, development of other prescription drugs and medicinal technology, and opposition by the American Medical Association.

The American Foundation for Homeopathy began teaching homeopathy as a postgraduate course for doctors in 1922. Today, courses are offered by the National Center for Homeopathy.

In recent years, interest in homeopathy has increased along with widening interest in HOLISTIC MEDICINE and COMPLEMENTARY THERAPIES. Homeopathy may appeal to many people because only natural substances are used as medications. Remedies include substances that can be dissolved in a liquid medium; metals and salts are not dissolvable. Remedies are ground together 10 times for 10 minutes. Subatomic energy is released. For an inexplicable reason, once diluted beyond the 12th dilution, nothing is found under a microscope. Also, because medications are so diluted, possibilities of side effects are reduced.

Some homeopathic practitioners in the United States also use other adjunctive therapies, such as spinal manipulation and nutritional counseling.

The largest use of homeopathic medications is in India. It is also popular in France and England and becoming popular in Australia and Germany. In Switzerland and Germany, homeopathic practitioners work under the direction of doctors of medicine. According to Dr. Sujatha Pillai, a practitioner at Ehrhart & Karl, Chicago, 32 percent of family physicians in France prescribe homeopathic medicines. A survey in the *British Medical Journal* (June 7, 1986, pp. 1,498–1,500) indicated that 42 percent of British physicians refer patients to homeopathic doctors. According to *Everybody's Guide to Homeopathic Medicines* (1991), members of the British royal family use homeopathic medicines, Queen Elizabeth is the patron of the Royal London

Homeopathic Hospital and the British Homeopathic Association.

Researchers have reported the efficacy of homeopathic medications. For example, one study reported in *Lancet* (1986) compared hay fever patients taking homeopathic preparations with those taking a placebo. The study showed that those who received the homeopathic medicine had six times fewer symptoms than those who received the placebo. Studies have been reported using homeopathic remedies for arthritis, fibromyalgia, and influenza.

Another Homeopathic Technique: Bach Flower Remedies

Bach flower remedies are named for Edward Bach (1886–1936), a British bacteriologist and homeopath. Flower remedies are a branch of homeopathic medicine, and said to be useful in acute situations. Bach developed a system of 38 flower remedies for 38 different emotional states, based only on a person's psychological symptoms. Unlike other homeopathic medicines, Bach remedies are sometimes prescribed several at a time.

Cummings, Stephen, and Dana Ullman, *Everybody's Guide to Homeopathic Medicines* (New York: Jeremy Tarcher/ Perigree Books, 1991).

Davidson, Jonathan R. T., and Susan Gaylord, "Homeopathic and Psychiatric Perspectives on Grief," *Alternative Therapies* 4, no. 5 (September 1998): pp. 30–35.

Merz, Beverly, ed., "Complementary Therapies: Homeopathy." *Harvard Women's Health Watch* 4, no. 5 (January 1997).

Thomas, Patricia, ed., "Homeopathy: Is Less Really More?" *Harvard Health Letter* 20, no. 7 (May 1995).

homeostasis   Homeostasis is the body's tendency to maintain a steady state, despite stressful external changes. The physical properties and chemical composition of body fluids and tissues tend to remain remarkably constant. However, when our self-regulating powers fail, often because of repeated anxieties, the individual's health is threatened.

In the late 19th century, Claude Bernard, a French physiologist at the College de France in Paris, taught that one of the most characteristic features of all living beings is their ability to maintain the constancy of their internal milieu, despite changes in the surroundings. Subsequently, Walter B. Cannon, a Harvard physiologist, named this power to maintain constancy *homeostasis,* which can be translated as physiological "staying power" or "self-preservation."

Coping with anxieties, stress, and disease involves a fight to maintain the homeostatic balance of our tissues, despite damage. Hans Selye, the Austrian-born Canadian pioneer in stress research, discussed the concept of homeostasis in his landmark works, *The Stress of Life* (1956) and *Stress without Distress* (1978). He said that the nervous system and the endocrine system play particularly important parts in maintaining resistance during stress. They help to keep the structure and function of the body steady, despite exposure to stress-producing or stressor agents, such as nervous tension, wounds, infections, or poisons. He explained this steady state as homeostasis.

See also COPING; GENERAL ADAPTATION SYNDROME; MIND/BODY CONNECTIONS; STRESS; STRESS MANAGEMENT.

Selye, Hans, *Stress Without Distress* (New York: Lippincott, 1974).

———, *The Stress of Life* Rev. ed. (New York: McGraw Hill, 1978).

homesickness   Homesickness (not really a sickness) happens when people are away from familiar surroundings and persons to whom they feel close. Many people have experienced the anxieties associated with homesickness as children while away at camp or visiting friends or relatives; soldiers experience it while stationed in distant lands. Homesickness may involve feelings of loneliness and confusion with the unfamiliar. How individuals adapt to such situations depends on their personal COPING skills and ability to adapt. If homesickness persists, it may lead to symptoms of mild DEPRESSION. However, in most cases of homesickness, relief occurs when the sufferer returns to the familiar or when he or she adapts to the new situation.

See also ACCULTURATION; GENERAL ADAPTATION SYNDROME; INTIMACY; MIGRATION; RELATIONSHIPS.

Van Tilburg, Miranda A., and A. Vingerhoets, et al., "Homesickness: A review of the literature." *Psychological Medicine* 26, no. 5 (1996): pp. 899–912.

home surroundings, fear of Fear of home surroundings is known as oikophobia or ecophobia and includes fear of household appliances, equipment, electricity, bathtubs, household chemicals, and other common objects in the home.

homichlophobia Fear of fog.
See also FOG, FEAR OF.

homophobia Fear of homosexuality or becoming a homosexual.
See also HETEROPHOBIA.

homosexuality Sexual activity between members of the same sex, ranging from sexual fantasies and feelings through kissing and mutual masturbation, to genital, oral, or anal contact. The individual who practices homosexuality, if a man, is termed a *homosexual;* a female homosexual is referred to as a *lesbian.* Both men and women homosexuals are sometimes referred to as *gay.* Fear of or prejudice against homosexuals is known as *homophobia* and is a source of stress to many in the general community.

Historically, attitudes about homosexuality have evolved. Homosexuals in the United States have faced the stresses of social discrimination. In 1979, the U.S. Surgeon General ordered that homosexuality not be classified as a mental disease and defect. The gay liberation movement of the 1970s brought about open discussions of homosexuality and human rights. During the 1980s, homosexual activists increased public acceptance of homosexuality.

The term *homosexuality* was popularized during the 1980s. During the 19th century, other terms were proposed, including *homoerotic,* (aroused by the same sex) and *homophile* (lover of the same sex). Cunnilingus between two women was called *sapphism* after the ancient Greek poet Sappho, and lesbianism was named for the Greek island of Lesbos where Sappho lived.

Homosexual Panic

Homosexual panic (Kempf's disease) is a PANIC ATTACK that develops from a fear or delusion that one will be sexually assaulted by an individual of the same sex. The term, coined by American psychiatrist Edward Kempf (1885–1971) in 1920, also applies to the fear that one is thought to be homosexual. This feeling occurs more often in males than females.

There may be DEPRESSION, conscious GUILT over homosexual activity, agitation, HALLUCINATIONS, and thoughts of SUICIDE. This type of panic attack may develop after many varied life circumstances, such as a loss or separation from an individual of the same sex to whom one is emotionally attached, or after failure in sexual performance, illness, or extreme fatigue.

See also GENDER ROLE; LESBIANISM; SEXUAL DIFFICULTIES.

Kite, Mary E., and Kay Deaux, "Gender Belief Systems: Homosexuality and the Implicit Inversion Theory." *Psychology of Women Quarterly* 11 (1987): pp. 83–96.

Marcus, Eric, *Is There a Choice? Answers to 300 of the Most Frequently Asked Questions About Gays and Lesbians* (San Francisco: Harper, 1993).

National Museum & Archive of Lesbian and Gay History, *The Gay Almanac* (New York: Berkley Books, 1996).

hopelessness Hopelessness is a state of mind characterized by a feeling that the stresses of life are insoluble. The hopeless may see limited or no available desirable alternatives to their problems and may experience emptiness, pessimism, and the sensation of being overwhelmed. Nothing matters, and they "give up."

Hopelessness is a symptom of DEPRESSION. A hopeless person is often passive and lacks initiative. Such an individual may not be able to reach a desired goal, accepts the futility of planning to meet goals, has negative expectations of the future, perceives a personal loss of CONTROL, and sees "no way out." Successful treatment of depression with medication and certain types of psychotherapy can reverse this profound state of hopelessness.

The stress of extreme feelings of hopelessness may lead to ADDICTION or SUICIDE. Hopelessness sometimes results from false or unrealistic expectations.

For example, hopeless people may feel that they should be able to accomplish anything and everything and they descend into despair when they fail. Some individuals with depression feel that nothing they do will work out and that they are powerless.

Some people who are stressed may tend to magnify obstacles to the extent that they appear insurmountable. Still another type of magnification results in despair, when other people and events are idealized.

The stress of hopelessness may also result from a sense of being trapped in a negative set of circumstances from which there is no escape. When presented with a task that must be performed but which seems to be impossible, a sense of FRUSTRATION and futility leads to hopelessness.

Hopelessness is also usually related to despair. There is research that children growing up in this era experience high levels of despair and hopelessness about cruelty and violence in the world and potential for human-made disasters such as a nuclear holocaust.

The anxiety associated with confusion also leads to a sense of hopelessness, as confusion contributes to people's feelings of loss of control. It is important to understand that hopelessness is a subjective state, related to the way they perceive their prospects as potentially reversible.

See also COPING; DEPRESSION; OPTIMISM; PERFECTION; PESSIMISM.

Kahn, Ada P., and Jan Fawcett, *The Encyclopedia of Mental Health,* 2nd ed. (New York: Facts On File, 2001).

hoplophobia   Fear of firearms.

hormephobia   Fear of shock.
See also SHOCK, FEAR OF.

hormone replacement therapy   See MENOPAUSE.

hormones   Hormones are substances produced and secreted by the endocrine glands. Hormones are chemically classified as steroids or proteins (or derivatives of proteins). Hormones are transported in the blood to various sites of action. They influence physiology as well as behavior. To have a sustained effect, hormones must be secreted continuously in precisely controlled quantities. In some glands, secretion is brought about by the nervous system; in others, it is stimulated by other hormones.

The brain has an important influence on hormonal activity. This occurs primarily through the pituitary gland, which is situated at the base of the brain just below the hypothalamus, to which it is neurally connected.

There are two basic kinds of hormones. One may be considered as "local" hormones, which have their effects close to the point of release. The second are "general" hormones, which enter extracellular fluids and may exert effects throughout the body. Hormonal effects can be immediate, occurring within fractions of seconds, or gradual, taking days to get started and continuing for months.

When local hormones—for example, adrenaline—are released and act upon nerve endings, their effect is almost instantaneous. When an individual is frightened, FEAR causes the release of the hormone adrenaline. The heart begins to pound, hands tremble, and the stomach constricts.

General hormones are secreted by a number of endocrine glands and then transmitted throughout the body, causing many physiological effects, often at distant points. Some general hormones affect nearly all cells in the body. These include growth hormone from the pituitary gland and thyroid hormone from the thyroid gland.

Other general hormones are more specific, acting at various points. For example, corticotropin is released by the pituitary gland and acts on the adrenal gland. When one secretion acts on a particular site, the site is called the target tissue or target organ.

Hormones are responsible for the development of secondary sex characteristics in males and females, and for the onset of menstruation and menopause in women. Hormones play a role in PREMENSTRUAL SYNDROME and may be responsible for some of the anxieties women experience at this time. Specifically, estrogen and progesterone, secreted by the ovaries, exert control over menstruation, ovulation, conception, and menopause.

Vasopressin, another hormone secreted by the posterior pituitary, affects the kidney and blood pressure.

See also ADRENALINE; BIOLOGICAL BASIS FOR ANXIETY.

horses, fear of Fear of horses is known as equinophobia or hippophobia. In some individuals, fear of horses may result from incidents such as being kicked or thrown by a horse or simply by the sight of a powerful horse rearing up. Like other animal phobias, fear of horses is most likely to develop in the preschool and early school years. One of Sigmund Freud's most famous cases, LITTLE HANS, involved a five-year-old boy's fear of horses, which Freud interpreted as a fear of his father. Behavioral psychiatrist Joseph Wolpe was able to show, however, that learning theory provided a more powerful explanation of the etiology of this fear and subsequent remission.

An obsessive feeling about horses is the subject of Peter Shaffer's play *Equus.* Filled with shame because horses (to whom he attributes divine qualities) have watched his first sexual encounter, a young man blinds them with a spike. The drama, based on an actual incident, follows the relationship between the boy and his psychiatrist as they piece together the reasons for the boy's attack on the horses.

See also ANIMALS, FEAR OF; CHILDHOOD ANXIETIES, FEARS, AND PHOBIAS.

Melville, Joy, *Phobias and Obsessions* (New York: Coward, McCann & Geoghegan, 1977).

hospitals, fear of Fear of hospitals is known as nosocomephobia. Some people fear hospitals because they fear contamination by germs, which they believe are prevalent around hospitals. Some who fear hospitals fear being ill, having pain, and being out of control of their lives. Some who fear hospitals may also fear doctors, nurses, and other health-care providers; they may also fear injury and seeing their own blood or the blood of others. Some people become anxious on seeing individuals who are ill or recovering from surgery.

Many who fear visiting others in hospitals are fearful about their own death. Visiting a hospital, where a certain number of patients die every day, reminds the anxious individual of his or her own mortality. Visiting an ill person makes many individuals anxious because as the visitor, one does not know what to talk about and is afraid to ask about the patient's condition for fear of hearing about pain and suffering.

Another fear of hospitals stems from their impersonal aspects. Many individuals fear being a patient in a hospital for this reason. Patients become known by their injuries or their conditions rather than their names. Strangers must provide very personal care and invade what many individuals view as personal bodily privacy.

Also, some individuals fear hospitals for a practical reason: costs. Hospital costs have escalated astronomically, and a relatively short stay can result in high charges. For those whose costs are not paid for by insurance or a health plan, such as the British National Health insurance, concern about paying hospital costs may also represent a fear of poverty.

Fears of hospitals can be overcome, to some extent, by visiting a local hospital while feeling well, taking a guided tour, and developing a better understanding of what services various hospitals provide for the community. Systematic desensitization also may be helpful.

Hospitalization and Anxieties

Anxieties begin with the need for a second medical opinion, which, unless there is an emergency, is often a requirement of medical insurers before commitment to a hospital can be made. Stress then follows patients to the hospital registration desk, where the approach of many admissions personnel to gather patient information does little to make them feel comfortable.

Loss of privacy, another key source of anxiety, begins at the very moment patients exchange their clothes for hospital gowns and settle down in rooms shared with at least one or more strangers who may be a great deal more or less sick than they. It is further compounded by the number of visitors they or their roommates may have—people who talk loudly as they spill into all corners and all sides of what can be too-small hospital rooms. In teaching hospitals, the stress continues to prevail when doctors and interns gather around patients' beds to discuss clinical aspects of their illnesses, sometimes as if the patients didn't exist or at least were not right there in the bed.

Anxieties escalate when loss of privacy combines with the loss of CONTROL patients experience as they are thrown into the uneven rhythm of the hospital routine—being aroused at early hours for medication before a change in shifts occurs, moving on stretchers or in wheelchairs from one end of the hospital to another, waiting in drafty corridors for countless tests and X rays, buzzing for nursing assistance that never comes, having unappealing meals served at hours when they are often least hungry, and facing constantly changing caretakers and variations in the delivery of care. The most serious sources of hospitalization stress is being in pain and having to rely on others for help in controlling that pain. A device that allows patients to control the intake of pain medication when they need it has alleviated this problem for some.

Today, patients waiting to receive various transplants—heart, lungs, kidney, and liver—experience additional anxieties regarding when or whether they will come too late. The lists of those needing transplants far exceeds their availability, and for some there is little likelihood of a match. Questions also arise concerning the criteria for the lists and for those who are given priority. An example of that arose in 1995, when baseball star Mickey Mantle received a transplant a short time after a diagnosis was made.

Anxieties follow all patients out of the recovery room—with regulations concerning how long their hospital stays can be. In 1995, length of hospital stays became a major issue in connection with childbirth. It was felt by some that first-time mothers were being sent home too soon and were often both mentally and physically unprepared to take care of a baby. For other mothers, the stress of taking care of older children while attending to the responsibilities of a newborn was increased.

Shortened hospital stays have increased the anxiety of most patients. Much of the time needed for rehabilitation and recovery now is spent outside of the hospital, which places the burden of care on patients' families. For those without families, other means of home care must be found and questions of how they can meet the costs of this care arise.

Lastly, there is the stress on the family and friends related to hospitalization of the terminally ill—ethical questions relating to withdrawal of nourishment and treatment, particularly when there are no instructions from the patient.

See also ACCESS TO CARE: AUTONOMY; CONTROL; DEATH; END OF LIFE CARE; PAIN; PERSONAL SPACE.

hostages Hostages are captives who are subjected to the extreme anxieties of isolation, confinement, and sometimes mental and physical torture. Captors frequently keep hostages in a state of uncertainty about their fate. Hostages may be held in a foreign country or locally for any number of purposes.

The sensory deprivation inflicted on hostages may produce HALLUCINATIONS. Some hostages become paranoid, depressed, and feel abandoned by their country and families.

Readjustment to normal life after release, though welcome, is sometimes stressful for ex-hostages. Many experience nightmares, insomnia, bouts with abnormal fears, DEPRESSION, and feelings of rage and helplessness for some time. Mental health professionals are gaining an understanding of the state of mind of former hostages through experience. Current thinking is that a regulated "decompression period" helps former hostages adjust to normal life and to being back with their families.

Following the Persian Gulf War during 1991, several hostages were released after long years of captivity. Richard Rahe, M.D., director of the Nevada Stress Center at the University of Nevada School of Medicine, and a former navy psychiatrist with extensive experience working with hostages and disaster victims, in an interview with *Psychiatric News*, said that how the individuals behaved before, during, and after the hostage experience can aid in predicting who might have difficulties upon reentry.

"People who do well have done well in the past with stress. They have had adequate-to-good childhoods. They did well in captivity. They passed through depression, and found themselves through helping others. They turned the experience into a positive one, by reviewing their lives, making positive changes."

Rahe also said that survivor GUILT is common, as are recriminations about the way they might have behaved in captivity. Many former hostages are angry toward their families or the government for not doing enough to help them. At greatest risk of developing full-blown POST-TRAUMATIC STRESS DISORDER are those people who already had symptoms before being taken hostage and those without a good support system.

Elmore Rigamer, M.D., chief psychiatrist, United States State Department, quoted in *Psychiatric News* (January 4, 1991) regarding the "keys to staving off deterioration" in a hostage situation, commented that "mastery" and "connectedness" are the keys to overcoming psychological hurdles associated with having been a hostage. Mastery (a sense of CONTROL) and connectedness (feeling accurately informed) are both important for hostages and their families. "The ones who were able to take control of themselves will do wonderfully. The more feeling of loss of control, the worse."

Dr. Rigamer emphasized the psychological value of relaying information to hostages and families during and after the crisis. During the crisis he spent as much time as he could on the telephone with State Department hostages in Baghdad and Kuwait and their families back home, clearing up rumors and giving out information.

In *Psychiatric News* (January 4, 1991), Thomas M. Haizlip, M.D., University of North Carolina, outlined seven stages of mastery applicable to both the hostages and their families:

1. Discriminating between good and bad forces
2. Coping by knowing what to do if it ever happens again
3. Putting your life back in order
4. Dealing with survivor guilt (having left some people and worldly goods behind)
5. Realizing that healthy people are willing to take advantage of a two-to-three week "window" after the experience, when willingness to talk is greatest
6. Hooking up any symptoms with the event, rather than further repressing them
7. Recognizing that many people do not want help because they feel they themselves are important dispensers of help

Many of these stages are also applicable after other life traumas, such as domestic violence, witnessing, or being a victim of a crime.

See also AUTONOMY; BRAINWASHING.

Haizlip, Thomas M., "Hostages," *Psychiatric News,* January 4, 1991, p. 18.

Kahn, Ada P., and Jan Fawcett, *The Encyclopedia of Mental Health,* 2nd ed. (New York: Facts On File, 2001).

hostility   Hostility is a persistent attitude of deep resentment and intense ANGER. It may be the result of stressful situations or may also cause stress for the individual. The hostile person may have an urge to retaliate against a person or situation. During some situations of intense FRUSTRATION, deprivation, or discrimination, feelings of hostility may be a normal reaction. However, hostile attitudes also may occur during ANXIETY attacks, in OBSESSIVE-COMPULSIVE DISORDER, or DEPRESSION. Some people who have antisocial personalities frequently have hostile attitudes.

At best, hostile people are simply grouchy. At worst, they are consumed by hatred. A hostile person may have a tense-looking face and body. They are easily excitable. They seem to have a chip on their shoulders and a bitterness toward the world. They may be sarcastic and moody and respond aggressively when challenged.

For many individuals, the stresses of hostilities can be worked out through EXERCISE, better COMMUNICATION skills, BEHAVIOR THERAPY, use of MEDITATION and RELAXATION, and psychotherapy.

See also AGGRESSION; PERSONALITY; PSYCHOTHERAPIES; TYPE A PERSONALITY.

Friedman, Howard S., *The Self-Healing Personality* (New York: Henry Holt, 1991).

hot flashes, fear of   Many women after age forty begin to fear having hot flashes. Some have anxieties about hot flashes as a symptom of menopause, or the cessation of their menstrual periods. Hot flashes may be one of the first menopausal symptoms a woman notices, even before her periods stop. They may continue after she no longer menstruates.

Some women have hot flashes several times a day, once a week, or less frequently. Different women find different things fearful about hot flashes. Some fear the embarrassment of knowing that what they are feeling is visible to others. Some fear being in social gatherings or at work when they break out in a sweat; some fear ruining their clothes because of perspiration. Some fear the sudden onset of perspiration, feeling clammy, or breaking out in a cold sweat at a critical time, such as when they have a business meeting or have to make a public presentation. Some fear wakeful nights due to hot flashes and the tiredness and irritability that occurs the next day. Many women fear that when they visit doctors to seek help for hot flashes, they will be told they are imagining them. For generations, before the function of female hormones was understood, some doctors told women that menopausal symptoms were imagined or strictly psychological. Now, however, hormonal replacement therapies are available to help relieve severe cases of hot flashes.

Understanding what happens in their bodies during and after menopause can reduce the fear of hot flashes for many women.

Women who fear hot flashes can reduce their anxieties by making themselves as comfortable as possible at times when they think hot flashes might occur. For example, they can layer their clothing so that they can remove a jacket or sweater if they become warm. They can learn to use relaxation techniques so that they will feel in control if a hot flash does occur while they are in public. Keeping windows open or a fan on may alleviate some of their feelings of excessive warmth. Above all, having support and understanding from family and friends can be helpful. Many menopausal women seek help from psychotherapists because hot flashes are one of many situations that cause them stress during this period of their lives. When they learn to cope better with other stressors in the lives, they also may become less anxious about hot flashes.

Many women fear menopause, with the accompanying symptoms, such as hot flashes, because they fear growing old and less attractive. While for generations many women based their self-worth on an ability to bear children, this is becoming increasingly less the case as women carry on important jobs in business and industry well past their childbearing years.

See also AGING, FEAR OF; GROWING OLD, FEAR OF; MENOPAUSE, FEAR OF.

hot lines   Hot lines are telephone lines maintained by trained personnel to provide crisis-intervention service, or information on a given topic. Throughout the United States, hot lines cover many concerns related to anxieties and mental health. In many cases, the numbers for information and help are toll-free and usually operate on a 24-hour basis.

Most city telephone directories list some of the available hot lines.

See also SELF-HELP GROUPS; SUPPORT GROUPS.

house, fear of being in a   Fear of being in a house, or fear of a specific house, is known as domatophobia. This term relates to the fear of the house itself; the term "ECOPHOBIA" pertains to the things inside the house.

See also HOME, FEAR OF RETURNING; HOME SURROUNDINGS, FEAR OF.

human beings and human society, fear of   Fear of human beings and human society is known as anthropophobia.

See also PEOPLE, FEAR OF.

human immunodeficiency virus (HIV)   See ACQUIRED IMMUNE DEFICIENCY SYNDROME/HUMAN IMMUNODEFICIENCY VIRUS.

humanistic psychology   An approach to psychology that centers on the individual and his personal experience. Humanistic psychology opposes Freudian psychology, which holds that sexual drive is the sole motivating force, and behavioral psychology, which explains human behavior as the product of a multiplicity of organismic and environmental relationships, each of which in turn dominates the others at certain times. In humanistic psychology, emphasis is on human qualities such as choice, creativity, valuation, and self-realization; meaningfulness is the key to selection of problems for study, and therapists oppose primary emphasis on objectivity at the expense of significance. The ultimate concern of humanistic psychology is the development of each person's inherent potential. According to humanistic psychologists, man has a hierarchy of many needs, beginning with physiological needs; safety; love and "belongingness"; esteem needs; esthetic needs; the need to know and understand; and ending in the essential need for self-actualization. The American Association for Humanistic Psychology was founded in 1962 by Abraham Maslow, Kurt Goldstein, Rollo May, Carl Rogers, and others.

See also HIERARCHY OF NEEDS.

humor, fear of   Humor has been studied by psychologists as a form of human behavior and does have some relationship to fears and anxieties. Humor is feared by some individuals who view laughing at rather than with someone as a form of attack. Belittling, sarcastic, or derisive remarks are high on the list of fear producers for individuals who are socially insecure or socially phobic. Laughter can be disturbing if it is an indication that sincere remarks are not being taken sincerely. Laughter and a light joking attitude also may be objectionable and manipulative when used to convince someone that he is not being a good sport about a truly negative, distressing situation. Insincere laughter used to flatter and gain social or professional favor often causes tensions. Laughter may also promote rifts and misunderstandings between social and ethnic groups because what may be funny in one culture and language may not even be amusing in another.

See also HUMOR, USE IN THERAPY.

humor, use in therapy   Humor can be a useful way of releasing tension, dispelling anxieties, and momentarily relieving depression during therapy sessions. Humor promotes an individual's hopeful feelings about himself. If an individual can laugh during a therapy session, he will probably be more inclined to open up and reveal more about himself. Humor has known properties of healing. A therapist can employ humor as exaggeration or as a way of adding emphasis. Using a technique called paradoxical therapy, a therapist gives the individual perspective on his or her problems by exaggerating them until they become funny. With a similar exaggeration technique, a therapist assigns the individual a certain time of day to be anxious, depressed, or jealous. Often the silliness of the situation helps to alleviate the individual's distressed feelings. Humor can be used with individuals who are depressed or angry but who will not admit to their true feelings. Thus humor allows the therapist to explore without generating resistance. Since humorous remarks and stories have layers of meaning, such stories can at times be used to reach into the individual's unconscious.

See also HUMOR AS ANXIETY RELIEF.

humor as anxiety relief   Humor serves to relieve the pressures of anxiety and stress in many ways. Comedians have indicated that they entered the profession because it affords an emotional release and a way of attracting positive attention. The simple absurdity and irrationality of humor is a welcome relief in the usual orderly, serious process of living. If some humor can be found in a negative situation, such as a setback at work or a minor accident, the victim can laugh about it, relax momentarily, and then pick up the pieces instead of uninterruptedly sustaining the stress of the situation. Because of the element of detachment inherent in humor, humor can reduce the stress of an ambitious person trying to reach a goal. Thus having a sense of humor allows the highly motivated person to be objective about the amount of effort and sacrifice necessary to reach the top.

Humor also provides a sense of freedom from political and social constraints. If a powerful figure or government program can be viewed as amusing, the stressful sense of autocratic control is reduced. Studies have shown that BRAINWASHING is impossible as long as the victim retains his ability to laugh. Humor also affords relief from anxieties related to social situations. A witticism can cover complaints and awkward situations that would cause hostility or tension if approached directly.

Shared humor is also a great reliever of anxiety in stressful group situations such as delayed trains. Humor relieves the stress that can result from boredom. When there seems nothing left to talk about, familiar topics can be made new by the use of humor.

Late-20th-century studies indicate the actual physical and psychological effects of laughter. The simple act of laughing may actually promote well-being. Norman Cousin's book, *Anatomy of an Illness* (1977), although concerned with physical disease, stimulated interest in the use of humor in recovery from both mental and physical illness.

See also HUMOR, FEAR OF; HUMOR, USE IN THERAPY.

Morreall, John, *Taking Laughter Seriously* (Albany: State University of New York, 1983).

Ziv, Avner, *Personality and Sense of Humor* (New York: Springer, 1984).

hurricanes, fear of   Fear of hurricanes is known as lilapsophobia. Those who fear hurricanes will stay indoors with windows, shades, and shutters closed during any period of time in which hurricanes are possible. Some will leave the area and remain in another geographic location for fear of being in the path of a hurricane. Some who fear hurricanes fear not only the destruction of property that occurs, but also a threat to their physical safety. Some fear that they might die as a result of the hurricane.

See also CLIMATE, FEAR OF; LANDSCAPE, FEAR OF.

hyalophobia or hyelophobia   Fear of glass.

See also GLASS, FEAR OF.

hydrargyrophobia   Fear of mercurial medicines.

See also MERCURIAL MEDICINES, FEAR OF.

hydrophobia   Fear of water. Hydrophobia is also the technical name for rabies. An individual in the early stages of the disease experiences throat spasms, pain, and fear at the sight of water.

See also RABIES, FEAR OF; WATER, FEAR OF.

hydrophobophobia   Fear of rabies.

See also RABIES, FEAR OF.

hygrophobia   Fear of dampness, humidity, or moisture.

See also DAMPNESS, FEAR OF.

hylephobia   Fear of epilepsy. Also, fear of matter (materialism) and wood (forests).

See also EPILEPSY, FEAR OF; FORESTS, FEAR OF.

hylophobia   Fear of a forest, or fear of materialism. Also known as ylophobia. In metaphysical thinking, matter is regarded as the principle of evil.

See also FORESTS, FEAR OF; WOODS, FEAR OF.

hypengyophobia (hypegiaphobia)   Fear of responsibility.

See also RESPONSIBILITY, FEAR OF.

hyperarousal   A state of increasing excitement and sensitivity to stimuli that can be a precursor to ANXIETY.

hyperinsulinism   A condition in which too much insulin is produced and secreted by the body. Hyperinsulinism is often due to an overgrowth of the islets of Langerhans, from which insulin is secreted. As insulin promotes the removal and utilization of blood glucose, individuals who have hyperinsulinism become hypoglycemic and must be given massive amounts of glucose. The hypoglycemic condition can produce anxiety symptoms characteristic of anxiety states. Without this therapy individuals will experience "insulin shock," just as a diabetic does if given too much insulin. In such shock, the individual experiences hallucinations, extreme nervousness, trembling and may have convulsions, lose consciousness and pass into a coma. If treatment by injection of glucose is not rapid, there may be permanent damage to nerve cells, which need constant nutrients. Hyperinsulinism can be measured with a glucose tolerance test and a plasma insulin test.

See also DIABETES, FEAR OF.

hypertension   See HIGH BLOOD PRESSURE.

hyperthyroidism   A metabolic condition of too much thyroid hormone in the body's system. Based on an exhaustive study of more than 17,000 people, reported in 2002 in the *Journal of Clinical Endocrinology & Metabolism,* an estimated 1.3 percent of the population in the United States, or about 4 million people, have hyperthyroidism.

The individual with hyperthyroidism often appears extremely nervous and agitated to others and may be misdiagnosed with an ANXIETY DISORDER or with ATTENTION-DEFICIT/HYPERACTIVITY DISORDER.

Graves' disease, an autoimmune disorder, is the most common type of hyperthyroidism. Individuals with Graves' disease often have a characteristic bulging neck that signifies a goiter and they may also have bulging eyes. The late actor and comedian Marty Feldman had severe hyperthyroidism, with bulging eyes.

Other causes of hyperthyroidism include a multinodular goiter, thyroiditis (inflammation of the thyroid gland), and some medications such as lithium, a drug that is given to treat BIPOLAR DISORDER. (Lithium can also cause HYPOTHYROIDISM.)

Symptoms and Diagnostic Path

Hyperthyroidism is a common problem and some of its symptoms resemble those of anxiety disorders, such as an excess of energy, restlessness, nervousness, headaches, excessive sweating, and shaky uncoordinated movements.

A hyperthyroid individual may have difficulty sleeping at night and may experience wide changes in mood, varying from very happy to very depressed. An individual who has hyperthyroidism burns up food rapidly so that the appetite may become ravenous at the same time that weight loss occurs. There may be muscle weakness, loss of calcium, and diarrhea or loose bowels.

A hyperthyroid individual has a rapid heartbeat and, in severe cases, congestive heart failure can occur because blood cannot be pumped out of a heart chamber fast enough and collects there.

Other symptoms that may occur include

- heat intolerance
- menstrual disturbances, such as infrequent periods or no periods
- weight change (usually a loss but some patients gain weight)
- warm and moist skin with a velvety texture
- the presence of a goiter

The physician who suspects hyperthyroidism will order a test of thyroid-stimulating hormone (TSH). The normal range for the TSH test is between 0.3 and 3.0 mIU/L. The individual with hyperthyroidism will test at a rate *less than* 0.3.

The doctor may also order a radioactive iodine uptake text, and a finding of a high level indicates hyperthyroidism.

Hyperthyroidism is a serious condition that requires medical attention and, once diagnosed, continued close monitoring of treatment.

Treatment Options and Outlook

Treatment is aimed at bringing down the excessively high thyroid levels. If the patient is diagnosed with Graves' disease, he or she may be prescribed antithyroid medications, such as methimazole (Tapazole) or propylthiouracil (PTU). The condition is also treated with radiation or surgical removal of part of the thyroid gland (thyroidectomy). Often tumors on the thyroid cause dysregulation of the gland. After treatment, the individual is at risk for the development of hypothyroidism and, if it develops, must take supplemental thyroid medication.

Risk Factors and Preventive Measures

Individuals with a family history of any form of thyroid disease may be at risk for inheriting hyperthyroidism. There is no known method to prevent the development of hyperthyroidism in susceptible individuals.

Hallowell, Joseph G., et al., "Serum TSH, T$_4$, and Thyroid Antibodies in the United States Population (1988 to 1994): National Health and Nutrition Examination

Survey (NHANES III," *Journal of Clinical Endocrinology & Metabolism* 87, no. 2 (2002): pp. 489–499.

Petit, William A., M.D., and Christine Adamec, *The Encyclopedia of Endocrine Diseases and Disorders* (New York: Facts On File, Inc., 2005).

hyperventilation   Very rapid and deep breathing and a feeling of shortness of breath that can bring on high levels of ANXIETY. Hyperventilation causes a reduction in the level of carbon dioxide in the blood, which in turn can lead to feelings of numbness, tingling of the hands, dizziness, muscle spasms, and fainting. Individuals who are anxious or aroused begin to breathe in a rapid, deep manner with shallow exhalations. Gasping may occur. Although they have the sensation of shortness of breath, they are actually overbreathing. Sometimes this experience is accompanied by a feeling of constriction or pain in the chest.

The symptoms of hyperventilation and hyperventilation syndrome are frightening, and sufferers may fear that they are having a heart attack or that they will die. Some agoraphobics experience hyperventilation when they attempt to leave home or even think of going out, particularly unaccompanied by a companion upon whom they depend for security. Hyperventilation, or overbreathing, is also a common symptom among phobics when they face (or even think about) their phobic stimuli. For example, height phobics may hyperventilate when they think about looking out from the top of a tall building.

Hyperventilation is more common in women than in men. Usually, hyperventilation occurs in individuals who are nervous, tense, or having an anxiety or panic attack. Repeated attacks of hyperventilation may occur. Once the individual recognizes that the hyperventilation syndrome is a reaction to anxiety and not a disease itself, the attacks may become fewer or stop because the panic component will be somewhat reduced.

An individual who hyperventilates can help himself by understanding what happens during an attack. By voluntarily hyperventilating (about 50 deep breaths while lying down) and reproducing the symptoms felt during an anxiety attack, the sufferer will see that the symptoms do not indicate a heart attack or a "nervous breakdown." When the fear is reduced, hyperventilation during an anxious time may decrease.

Hyperventilation may also be a response to severe pain, particularly abdominal pain. When there is doubt about the cause of hyperventilation, the sufferer should be examined by a physician.

An Australian investigation of hyperventilation symptoms reported during 1986 compared responses to voluntary hyperventilation by individuals who had panic disorder and generalized anxiety disorder. Those who had panic disorder reported greater distress, a greater number of symptoms, and a lower level of carbon dioxide. Hyperventilation symptoms reported by the panic disorder patients and the generalized anxiety patients are compared in the chart on page 291.

See also HEART ATTACK, FEAR OF.

hypnophobia   Fear of being hypnotized, or fear of hypnosis in general. The fear may relate to watching another person become hypnotized, or just thinking about HYPNOSIS.

hypnosis (hypnotherapy)   Hypnosis is a form of focused attention in which the individual becomes relatively open to receiving new information and exploring the mind-body relationship. It is not a "therapy" but can be a useful supplement to an appropriate anxiety-reduction therapy. Under hypnosis, the individual is in a trancelike state resembling sleep, during which he or she will be more susceptible to suggestion than during the "normal waking" state. While there are theories, no one knows exactly what the trance state represents physiologically or psychologically. Any hypnotizable individual may experience one or more of many hypnotic phenomena. These include sensory, motor, and psychological changes, such as an ability to alter perceptions, capacity to dissociate, amnesia for part or all of the hypnotic experience, a tendency to compulsively comply with suggestions given during the hypnotic state, and a willingness to accept logical incongruities.

There are two types of hypnosis. One is directive or authoritative hypnosis, in which the individual

HYPERVENTILATION-RELATED SYMPTOMS

This table indicates symptoms of hyperventilation and differentiates panic and generalized anxiety disorder. Following are symptoms listed in the Hyperventilation Questionnaire, showing the percentage of subjects in each group reporting each symptom and the mean distress experienced during the voluntary hyperventilation. (M = level of distress, a degree of concern or anxiety about the symptom.)

Symptom	Panic Group		Generalized Anxiety Group	
	% Reporting	M Distress	% Reporting	M Distress
Dizziness	100.0	4.8	69.2	3.2
Breathless	89.5	2.9	53.8	3.3
Tingling hands/feet	73.7	3.6	0.0	—
Dry mouth	100.0	4.3	61.5	3.6
Unsteady on feet	84.2	4.9	3.1	3.3
Nausea	31.6	2.2	7.7	4.0
Little stamina	78.9	3.9	46.2	3.3
Trouble thinking clearly	73.7	3.4	30.8	2.5
Trembling hands/legs	78.9	4.0	7.7	2.0
Tight/pain in chest	31.6	3.3	15.4	2.0
Seeing double	26.3	1.6	15.4	1.5
Fear heart attack	15.8	4.3	0.0	—
Depersonalization/derealization	68.4	2.4	15.4	2.5
Headache	10.5	2.5	7.7	2.0
Tetany (ringing in ear)	26.3	1.8	15.4	1.5
Tingling face	47.4	2.6	7.7	1.0
Breathing too much	68.4	4.2	53.8	3.7
Cold hands	26.3	3.8	7.7	4.0
Difficulty talking	42.1	3.3	15.4	2.0
Feeling far away	57.9	3.0	30.8	2.3
Crying	21.0	3.0	0.0	—
Lump in throat	36.8	3.6	30.8	2.8
Passing out, collapsing	78.9	5.1	38.5	2.8
Blurred vision	42.1	3.0	23.1	1.7
Panic	94.7	3.8	15.4	3.0
Pounding, racing heart	78.9	3.7	38.5	1.8
Nervous stomach	52.6	2.7	23.1	3.3
Burning, tingling, crawling	57.9	2.9	7.7	5.0
Rising agitation	73.7	4.4	30.8	2.5
Feeling want to run	52.6	3.5	0.0	—
Muscular tension	52.6	3.3	38.5	3.4
Feeling of wetting pants	5.3	1.0	0.0	—
Diarrhea	10.5	1.0	0.0	—
Feeling hot or flushed	73.7	2.9	30.8	3.0
Fear may die	21.0	2.8	0.0	—
Feeling trapped/helpless	47.4	3.4	38.5	1.8
Feeling ground moving	21.0	2.5	15.4	2.5
Exhaustion	63.2	3.5	23.1	2.0
Feeling going mad	15.8	2.3	0.0	—
Feeling losing control	31.6	4.2	7.7	2.0
Causing a scene	26.3	4.2	0.0	—

Ron Rapee, "Differential Response to Hyperventilation in Panic Disorder and Generalized Anxiety Disorder," *Journal of Abnormal Psychology*, 95:1 (1986), p. 27.

is ordered to give up a symptom, such as a phobic behavior. The second is cathartic hypnosis, in which the individual searches for hidden memories.

Hypnosis is a relatively safe procedure when used by a competent therapist who is specially trained in hypnosis. Practitioners do not have to be medical doctors.

While some people fear that under hypnosis they will do something that they would not do under conscious circumstances, it is generally thought that hypnotized individuals cannot be coerced into actions that go against their values and beliefs.

Most hypnosis is used to help relieve symptoms. Some therapists teach individuals to self-hypnotize themselves, while other therapists prefer to have repeated sessions during which suggestions are given, behavior is supported, and therapeutic gains are rewarded.

Many individuals who have forms of anxiety and phobias are hypnotizable. Individuals can learn to put themselves into the trance state to relax and dissociate psychological and body tension. This can be particularly helpful for those who have specific or simple phobias or performance anxiety. The trance experience can be used to induce physical relaxation in the face of the anxiety-provoking stimulus and to help an individual prepare for an anxiety-producing encounter by focusing on aspects of the experience that are less anxiety-provoking. For example, individuals who fear flying in an airplane can prepare themselves for flight by going into the trance state, thinking about the flight and themselves in the plane, and viewing the plane as an extension of their body, just as a bicycle or car is an extension of their body that enables them to get from one place to another more quickly. Individuals learn to restructure flying from an experience of being trapped in the plane into one of using the plane for their own benefit. Individuals can choose to enter the self-hypnotic trance state repeatedly during the trip, especially at stressful times, such as takeoffs and landings. Hypnosis may also be useful in conjunction with exposure therapy for simple phobias.

Hypnosis is useful in a variety of pain conditions, such as headache and dentistry. Individuals can be hypnotized to begin their relaxation techniques when they feel a headache coming on. Hypnosis

has been used in dentistry with fearful patients. The technique enables such individuals to have necessary care performed without use of drugs and the side effects from them.

It is sometimes helpful to induce hypnosis as an adjunct in psychotherapy to help an individual intensify memories or to relive aspects of the past. However, only individuals who are highly hypnotizable are capable of such regression. Age regression and/or recall can be accomplished with hypnosis when the therapist, usually a psychiatrist, wishes a subject to return to any age in his or her childhood and react as he did then. Regressed to the state of an infant, the individual will go through sucking motions; regressed to age two, he will draw a crude picture as he did at that age and will react to frustrations as he did then. With this method, childhood traumas that might have led to phobic behavior in adulthood but have been consciously forgotten can be uncovered.

See also DENTAL FEARS; HEADACHES.

hypnotic drugs Drugs used to induce sleep by depressing the central nervous system to a greater degree than a sedative. The effect of hypnotic DRUGS is of short duration. They are used for some hospitalized patients and for cardiac patients who cannot sleep through the night because of ANXIETY. An example of a hypnotic drug is sodium secobarbital (Seconal). Because of drug abuse, barbiturates are not prescribed as frequently as in the past. Instead, BENZODIAZEPINES are used more routinely as hypnotics.

hypochondriasis Preoccupation with the fear of having, or the belief that one has, a serious disease, based on the individual's interpretation of physical signs or sensations. This is sometimes referred to as hypochondriacal phobia. A thorough physical examination does not support the diagnosis of any physical disorder that can account for the physical signs or sensations or for the individual's unwarranted interpretation of them, although a coexisting physical disorder may be present. The unwarranted fear or belief of having a disease persists despite medical reassurance, but is not of delusional intensity, in that the person can acknowledge the possibility that he or she may be exaggerating the extent of the feared disease or that there may be no disease at all.

The preoccupation may be with bodily functions, such as heartbeat, sweating, or digestion, or with minor physical abnormalities, such as a small sore or an occasional cough. The individual interprets these sensations or signs as evidence of a serious disease. The feared disease, or diseases, may involve several body systems, at different times or simultaneously. Alternatively, there may be preoccupation with a specific organ or a single disease, as in "cardiac neurosis," in which the individual fears or believes that he or she has heart disease.

Individuals with hypochondriasis frequently show signs of anxiety, depressed mood, and obsessive-compulsive personality traits. The most common age of onset is between 20 and 30 years, and it seems equally common in males and females.

See DISEASE, FEAR OF.

hypoglycemia   A reduced level of glucose in the blood. Hypoglycemia can produce extreme nervousness, trembling, and hallucinations and many characteristic symptoms of anxiety states. Hypoglycemia was thought to be the medical basis for many anxiety disorders, but research has indicated that true hypoglycemia seldom occurs in anxiety disorders. Some individuals with known blood-sugar-level abnormalities fear reactions to their body's own chemistry. In normal individuals, lowering of blood sugars is performed by the body's insulin, which is produced by the islets of Langerhans in the pancreas. In an individual who has diabetes, the insulin is lacking or is incapable of transporting glucose across cell walls for utilization. In other cases, excessive amounts of insulin may be produced so that blood sugar is almost depleted. If glucose levels fall below certain limits, insufficient amounts are available in the blood for transport to the brain. Unconsciousness can result from too little insulin or too much insulin. It is difficult to tell the difference between the two cases, but the acetone smell on the breath and deep, heavy, rapid breathing are present only in diabetic coma.

See also DIABETES, FEAR OF; HYPERINSULINISM.

hypothalamus   A part of the brain responsible for emotional control, thirst, temperature, and certain endocrine functions. It is the lower part of the thalamus and relays stimuli for most sense organs (except olfactory). The hypothalamus is an endocrine gland.

hypothyroidism   A common metabolic condition in which the production of thyroid hormone by the thyroid gland, a butterfly-shaped gland in the neck which is located below the Adam's apple, is below normal. Based on an exhaustive study of more than 17,000 people, reported in 2002 in the *Journal of Clinical Endocrinology & Metabolism,* an estimated 4.6 percent of the population, in the United States (about 14 million people), have hypothyroidism. However, many individuals with hypothyroidism have not been diagnosed. Hypothyroidism may be mild, moderate, or severe.

Patients with hypothyroidism may be misdiagnosed with DEPRESSION, because they may be apathetic and listless. However, in some cases, the patient with hypothyroidism actually is clinically depressed. Other individuals who care about the hypothyroid patient may become anxious about the condition, as may the patient himself. In contrast to patients with hypothyroidism, however, patients with HYPERTHYROIDISM, a condition that causes an excess of thyroid gland, may appear extremely anxious and distressed, and may be misdiagnosed with an ANXIETY DISORDER.

The most common cause of hypothyroidism is Hashimoto's thyroiditis, an autoimmune disorder that may be inherited and that harms the thyroid gland over years, impeding its ability to produce sufficient thyroid hormone. After several years, most people with Hashimoto's thyroiditis develop a goiter, or an abnormally enlarged thyroid gland. Later, the thyroid gland may shrink and even atrophy.

There are other causes of hypothyroidism in addition to Hashimoto's thyroiditis; for example, external radiation to the neck may cause hypothyroidism. The removal of the thyroid gland for any reason will lead to hypothyroidism. Some medications may cause hypothyroidism, particularly lithium, which is used to treat BIPOLAR DISORDER. Interferon, a drug used to boost the immune system, may also cause hypothyroidism. Some infants are born with congenital hypothyroidism, a serious condition that requires immediate treatment.

Symptoms and Diagnostic Path

According to Dr. Petit in *The Encyclopedia of Endocrine Diseases and Disorders,* the primary symptoms of hypothyroidism include the following

- fatigue
- cold intolerance
- chronic constipation
- decreased appetite
- anemia
- muscle cramping and weakness
- reduced sexual libido
- decreased perspiration
- weight increase
- decreased memory/concentration
- slowed movements
- thinning of the outer third of the eyebrows
- puffy face
- excessively heavy menstrual cycles (menorrhagia)
- enlarged tongue (macroglossia)

In addition, if the hypothyroidism is severe and not treated, the following signs and symptoms may occur

- hypoglycemia (low blood sugar)
- hypothermia (below-normal body temperature)
- hyponatremia (below-normal levels of sodium in the blood)
- water retention
- slow heartbeat
- coma

Physicians diagnose hypothyroidism on the basis of the patient's complaints and appearance as well as on the results of thyroid blood tests and other tests. The most commonly used laboratory test to measure thyroid levels is the thyroid-stimulating hormone (TSH) test. With this test, if levels are elevated,

the individual is hypothyroid, whereas if they are below-normal, the individual has hyperthyroidism. The blood level at which hypothyroidism is diagnosed varies from laboratory to laboratory but the recommended TSH from the American Academy of Clinical Endocrinologists (AACE) is between 0.3 and 3.0 mIU/L. Thus, levels exceeding 3.0 indicate hypothyroidism and the higher the level, the more likely it is that the patient has hypothyroidism.

The doctor may also order a radioactive iodine uptake test. The patient swallows a small dose of radioactive iodine and special equipment measures the amount of radioactivity that the thyroid gland takes up, or the radioactive iodine uptake (RAIU) level. A low RAIU indicates hypothyroidism while a very high RAIU indicates hyperthyroidism.

The physician may also order an ultrasound of the neck and thyroid as well as imaging tests, such as a computed tomography (CT) scan or a magnetic resonance imaging (MRI) scan of the neck.

Treatment Options and Outlook

Most patients with hypothyroidism can be readily treated with levothyroxine, an oral synthetic thyroid hormone that is used to supplement the thyroid hormone that their body makes or to totally replace it, if necessary. Synthroid is the most commonly used brand name of levothyroxine, but there are other brand names, including Levolet, Levo-T, Levoxyl, Levothroid, Novothyrox, and Unithroid. Some patients take Armour thyroid, which is a natural form of thyroid that is derived from pigs.

If the cause of hypothyroidism is a medication, such as lithium, then the medication is changed to a drug that does not affect the thyroid gland.

The TSH blood test should be administered periodically to hypothyroid patients, because they may need their dosages of supplemental thyroid hormone adjusted up or down.

Risk Factors and Preventive Measures

Hypothyroidism is often an inherited medical problem, and individuals with parents or siblings with thyroid disease should have periodic checks of their TSH levels.

Women have a greater risk of developing hypothyroidism than men, particularly women who are older than 40 years old. According to the AACE, women are five to eight times more likely than men to be hypothyroid, and more than 80 percent of all patients with any thyroid disease are female.

According to the AACE, the risk for hypothyroidism increases with age and, by the age of 60, up to 17 percent of all females and 9 percent of males have hypothyroidism. As a result, it is a good idea for physicians of older individuals to order a TSH test if the patient is not feeling well.

Based on the data from the NHANES III study, reported in the *Journal of Clinical Endocrinology & Metabolism,* whites and Mexican Americans have a greater risk for thyroid disease than individuals of other races and ethnicities.

Hallowell, Joseph G., et al., "Serum TSH, T$_4$, and Thyroid Antibodies in the United States Population (1988 to 1994): National Health and Nutrition Examination Survey (NHANES III)," *Journal of Clinical Endocrinology & Metabolism* 87, no. 2 (2002): pp. 489–499.

Petit, William A., M.D., and Christine Adamec, *The Encyclopedia of Endocrine Diseases and Disorders* (New York: Facts On File, Inc., 2005).

hyprophobia   Fear of sleep.
See also SLEEP.

hypsiphobia   Fear of heights.
See also HEIGHTS, FEAR OF; HIGH OBJECTS, FEAR OF; HIGH PLACES, FEAR OF LOOKING UP AT.

hysterectomy, fear of   Many women fear hysterectomy, or surgical removal of the uterus. Although it is one of the most common operations in the United States, it is also sometimes a controversial one, because there are often differences of opinion concerning appropriate indications for hysterectomy and the surgical technique used. Some women fear being advised to have a hysterectomy when they do not really need one. Others fear having a premature menopause induced by the removal of the uterus. Actually, if the ovaries are left in place, the hormonal changes women fear with menopause do not occur. Some fear hysterectomy because of lack of information or misinformation. For example, many women fear that they will gain weight after the operation

or that their sex lives will change; however, studies have indicated that, in general, hysterectomy has little adverse effect on sexual function and no relation to weight gain. Some women fear pain during sexual intercourse, particularly upon resuming sexual intercourse after surgery. There may be some discomfort at first if there has been some vaginal repair, but this should disappear within a few weeks. Painful intercourse is unusual. Some women may fear depression when they realize that they can no longer bear children. Some fear being less desirable to men when they are no longer able to bear children.

Women who fear hysterectomy can help themselves overcome their fears by getting a second opinion if surgery is recommended and becoming informed about the diagnosis, the reason for the operation, the treatment options, the risks and the benefits of the operation, and the desired improvements in health that will result.

See also MENOPAUSE, FEAR OF; SURGICAL OPERATIONS, FEAR OF.

hysteria   Hysteria is a medical diagnostic term for illnesses characterized by the presence of physical SYMPTOMS, absence of physical SIGNS or any evidence of physical pathology, and behavior suggesting that the symptoms fulfill some psychological function. Hysteria, considered a neurotic disorder, may be characterized by emotional outbursts, repressed anxiety, and transformation of unconscious conflicts into physical symptoms such as blindness, paralysis, and loss of sensation. These symptoms help the individual blot out primary anxieties and elicit attention and sympathy.

The term hysteria comes from the ancient Greek word *hysteron,* meaning uterus. The Greeks used the term to refer only to diseases of women that they explained as arising from malfunctions of the uterus. Up until the late 1800s, hysteria was thought to be solely a female problem. Sigmund Freud presented a case in the late 1800s of male hysteria that his colleagues did not believe. Now male cases of hysteria often relate to job problems.

From the psychoanalytic point of view, there are two forms of hysteria: conversion hysteria, which corresponds to the traditional medical concept, and anxiety hysteria, the term used at times to denote phobias. Hysteria was first described in medical literature in Freud and Breuer's *Studies on Hysteria* (1895), in which hysterical symptoms were explained as the result of repressed memories and the conversion of ideas into physical symptoms. Freud suggested that symptoms were defenses against guilty sexual impulses, but contemporary therapists recognize many conflicts.

See also CONVERSION; PRIMARY GAIN; REPRESSION; SECONDARY GAIN.

hysterical disorder   A disorder characterized by involuntary impairment of certain physical functions, such as an inability to speak normally after a highly charged emotional experience. Other hysterical disorders might be a sudden loss of vision, hearing, sense of smell, or sensation in parts of the body. Individuals who have anxiety disorders, phobias, and obsessive-compulsive disorder usually do not have hysterical disorders.

See also HYSTERIA.

iatrogenic illness An illness induced by the examination or comments of a physician, medical practitioner, or therapist. Iatrogenic illness can be real or imagined. Fear of doctors is known as iatrophobia.

See also DOCTORS, FEAR OF; ILLNESS PHOBIA.

ice, fear of Fear of ice is known as cryophobia or papophobia.

See also COLD, FEAR OF; FROST, FEAR OF.

icthyophobia See FISH, FEAR OF.

id, and id anxiety The psychoanalytic term for the instinctual, biological drives that give the individual his basic psychic energy. Freud suggested that the id is the most primitive component of PERSONALITY and operates in the deepest level of the UNCONSCIOUS. Freud believed that the id's psychic energy (a hypothetical energy that runs psychic processes) was derived from biological processes, but he did not understand or speculate on how they worked. According to Freud, the id operates irrationally in accordance with the pleasure principle—i.e., immediate discharge. Thus the infant's life centers around the desire for immediate gratification of instincts, such as hunger, thirst, elimination, rage, and sex, until the conscious ego develops and operates in accordance with reality and the SUPEREGO.

Goldensen, Robert M., ed., *Longman Dictionary of Psychology and Psychiatry* (New York: Longman, 1984).

ideaphobia Fear of ideas.

ideas, fear of Fear of ideas is known as ideaphobia.

ideas of influence A type of DELUSION. Ideas of influence involve ideas that something—usually television messages, voices from audio speakers, animals, or other potential sources—is telling the individual what to do or is having an influence over his or her behavior. The New York murderer known as "Son of Sam" said he heard a dog that told him to kill people.

See also IDEAS OF REFERENCE; PARANOID.

ideas of reference Ideas of reference, also referred to as DELUSIONS of reference or delusions of observation, are misinterpretations in which one believes that others are smiling, talking, or whispering about one, or that one is being referred to in the newspaper, on television or radio news, or in movies. Ideas of reference are projections of feared situations onto the outside world; phobic individuals thus attribute their fears to an outside source rather than to their own experience. Ideas (or delusions) of reference commonly occur in paranoid SCHIZOPHRENIA.

idée fixe A rigidly held idea, such as an irrational fear. An idée fixe may become an OBSESSION and dominate the individual's mental life. For example, COMPULSIVE handwashing may stem from an idée fixe that the water is CONTAMINATED. The term was used by Pierre Janet in 1882.

See also CONTAMINATION, FEAR OF; OBSESSION; OBSESSIVE-COMPULSIVE DISORDER.

illiteracy Illiteracy is the inability to read or write. It is a personal source of anxiety for many people, contributing to their poor self-image and affecting their ability to obtain employment. People who are unable to read or write or who do one or both poorly may develop techniques to hide or compensate for their lack. Embarrassment may keep them from seeking help. For children, the illiteracy of a parent also can be a source of embarrassment and cause them a great deal of stress and anxiety.

Illiteracy is a fairly common problem in the United States. Estimates are that 75 percent of unemployed Americans are illiterate. In the early 1990s, the New York Telephone Company had to give 60,000 people an entry level exam in order to hire 3,000 employees. Some major corporations have had to use graphics on assembly lines to compensate for workers' inability to read simple phrases. As jobs have become increasingly complex and the economy has shifted from an industrial to service base, more jobs will require reading and writing ability.

Illiteracy is strongly related to poverty, drug use, and crime. It has been reported that about 75 percent of adult prison inmates are functionally illiterate. According to a survey by the National Advisory Council on Adult Education, in the late 1980s, 40 percent of all armed services enlistees read below a 9th grade level.

A study of emergency room and clinic patients at two public hospitals reported that a high proportion of them are unable to read and understand basic written medical instructions, according to an article in *The Journal of the American Medical Association* (December 5, 1995). The study raises the question of whether the estimated 40 to 44 million adults in the United States who are functionally illiterate and another 50 million adults who are only marginally literate are leaving doctors' offices and hospitals without understanding the steps to take to ensure their good health.

The authors commented that patients with limited literacy skills who have difficulty reading informed consent forms present a troubling ethical issue. "The ethical obligation of physicians to explain the risks and benefits of any procedure or treatment is fundamental to the physician-patient relationship. Patients unable to understand informed consent forms cannot intelligently participate in their own care."

LEARNING DISABILITIES account for illiteracy in some; however, there is not always agreement among educators as to the extent they affect literacy. There is a growing movement in American education to reduce illiteracy by treating reading and writing as learning disabilities at an early stage in schooling.

At the end of the 20th century, many community organizations have taken on illiteracy as a project. Volunteers work with people who need help reading and writing with good results.

See also SELF-ESTEEM; VOLUNTEERISM.

illness phobia   Fear of illness is known as nosemaphobia and nosophobia. Individuals who have illness phobia are frequently anxious and worry about having a disease. They fear dying and illnesses such as cancer, heart disease, and venereal disease. They may avoid anything that reminds them of diseases, such as programs on television or articles in newspapers. These individuals may frequently search their bodies for outward signs and misinterpret unusual sensations. They may seek frequent medical examinations because of their fears. Some illness phobics fear a disease that is most popular at a given time. For example, in earlier generations, many people feared tuberculosis or poliomyelitis. During the latter half of the 20th century, the most frequently feared diseases seem to be cancer and AIDS (acquired immunodeficiency syndrome).

Fear of illness is most prevalent among middle-aged and older persons. Women seem to fear illness more than men. Illness phobia may be considered as intermediate between simple phobia and obsessive-compulsive disorder, and it may also be regarded as a form of focused hypochondriasis.

See also CANCER, FEAR OF; HYPOCHONDRIASIS; INJECTIONS, FEAR OF.

illyngophobia   Fear of vertigo, or fear of feeling dizzy when looking down from a high place.

See also ACROPHOBIA; VERTIGO.

imagery   See GUIDED IMAGERY.

immigration   See ACCULTURATION; MIGRATION.

immobility of a joint, fear of   Fear of immobility of a joint is known as ankylophobia.

immune system   A collection of cells and proteins that protect the individual against possibly harmful microorganisms such as viruses, bacteria, and fungi. It is involved in problems related to ALLERGIES and hypersensitivity, rejection of tissues after grafts and transplants, and probably cancer. Suppression of the immune system can occur as an inherited disorder or after infection with certain viruses, including HIV (the virus that causes AIDS), resulting in lowered resistance to infections and to the development of malignancies. There is evidence that severe ANXIETY, STRESS, and DEPRESSION may inhibit normal immune function, although this has not been proven.

Relationship of Anxiety and Stress and the Immune System

There are possible physiological and behavioral explanations for changes in the immune system due to stress and negative emotional states. Stress is associated with activation of several systems, including the hypothalamic-pituitary-adrenal axis and the SYMPATHETIC NERVOUS SYSTEM.

Certain lifestyle factors influence the immune response. For example, lack of SLEEP or EXERCISE and use of alcohol and drugs affect the immune system in adverse ways. The best ways for a person to maintain immune system health is to have a balance of exercise, rest, RELAXATION, recreation, fun and LAUGHTER, a nutritionally healthful diet, and positive connections with family and/or friends.

Writing in *World Health* (March–April 1994), Dr. Tracy B. Herbert, Carnegie Mellon University, reported on studies relating stress and the immune system. Factors such as bereavement, DIVORCE, UNEMPLOYMENT, and caring for a relative with ALZHEIMER'S DISEASE were investigated. Generally, studies found that there is a large decrease in both lymphocyte proliferation and natural killer cell activities in individuals who have experienced anxieties and stress.

The duration of stress also affects the amount of immune change; the longer the stress, the greater the decrease in the number of specific types of white blood cells. Dr. Herbert also reported that interpersonal stress seems to produce different immune outcomes when compared with the stress due to unemployment or exams.

Researchers have also looked at relationships between anxiety and depression and the immune system. Results suggest that depression and anxiety are associated with decreases in lymphocyte proliferation and natural killer cell activity, changes in the numbers of white blood cells, and the quantity of antibody circulating in the blood. It seems that the ability of the body to produce antibody to a specific substance is related to the level of anxiety. More anxiety results in less antibody production after exposure to a potentially harmful substance.

See also AUTOIMMUNE DISEASES; COMPLEMENTARY THERAPIES; GUIDED IMAGERY; HUMAN IMMUNODEFICIENCY VIRUS; MEDITATION; MIND-BODY CONNECTIONS; PSYCHONEUROIMMUNOLOGY.

Herbert, Tracy B., "Stress and the immune system," *World Health,* March–April, 1994.
Locke, Steven, and Douglas Colligan, *The Healer Within* (New York: New American Library, 1986).
Sapolsky, Robert M., *Why Zebras Don't Get Ulcers. A Guide to Stress, Stress-Related Diseases, and Coping* (New York: W. H. Freeman, 1994).

imperfection, fear of   Fear of imperfection is known as atelophobia. Some individuals who have OBSESSIVE-COMPULSIVE DISORDER fear that they are not doing everything "right," or that they will make some ERROR in their daily routines unless they check and recheck. Many phobias stem from a fear of being imperfect. Many individuals are unduly concerned with what others think of them and hence develop a phobia of imperfection. Examples of fears of imperfection are talking on the telephone, going for a job interview, writing in front of others, eating in front of others, or speaking in public.

See also SOCIAL PHOBIAS.

implosion/implosive therapy   A behavior-therapy technique in which the individual is exposed to anxiety-producing stimuli by thoughts and imagery rather than the real situation. Implosion is also called FLOODING. The technique is based on CLASSICAL CONDITIONING principles, with ANXIETY as the CONDITIONED RESPONSE to images and thoughts about fearful situations or objects as the CONDITIONED STIMULI. The real situation is the unconditioned stimulus. The purpose of implosion is to prevent the individual from avoiding the conditioned stimuli. Implosion is based on principles of learning theory and psychoanalytic theory. The latter is used as a theoretical guide to develop fantasies or fantasy images about the phobic event that relate to conscious fears (such as castration, separation, etc.). This method was developed by Thomas Stampfl and Donald Levis, two American psychologists.

See also ABREACTION; BEHAVIOR THERAPY; CATHARSIS; SYSTEMATIC DESENSITIZATION.

impotence, fear of   Fear of impotence is a relatively common SEXUAL FEAR. Primary impotence is the physical or psychological condition of a man who has never had an erection sufficient for penetration or sexual intercourse. Secondary impotence is an inability of the male to have an erection sufficient for intercourse, although he has a history of at least one successful intromission.

incest, fear of   Some individuals fear incest, or sexual relations between blood relatives. Each society determines the prohibited degree of relationship. Many victims of child abuse realistically fear sexual assault by a blood relative. In many cases, fear of incest and retribution keeps children from reporting attempted molestation by relatives.

See also CHILD ABUSE, FEAR OF; RELATIVES, FEAR OF.

incontinence, fear of   Incontinence is an inability to control the evacuation of liquids or solids from the body. Incontinence may occur for many reasons, such as problems related to muscles, the nervous system, or infection, as well as an injury or complications of surgery. Many individuals at an advanced age fear incontinence and may become fearful of going out socially because they will be embarrassed if they wet themselves in pub-

lic. Incontinence is one of many fears associated with aging. Women around the age of menopause also fear incontinence; many notice loss of slight amounts of urine during physical stress, such as running, laughing, or coughing. Incontinence in men and women, in many cases, can be improved by surgical means.

See also AGING, FEARS OF.

incubation of fears   The period between the time an individual experiences events that cause ANXIETY or GUILT and the subsequent PHOBIAS or RITUALS that arise from the experience. In many cases, the problem begins even years after the first event. Some individuals relive the event in their mind and begin avoiding the painful situation. They go through an addictive cycle of avoidance to lessen tension and thus strengthen the tendency to further avoidance. An example is a fearful woman who, when given improper change in a store, was too uneasy to complain. After a few weeks she felt uncomfortable when returning to the store and later avoided going into the store or even passing the store for fear that she might see the man who had shortchanged her.

incubus   Historically, a male demon feared because he seduces sleeping women. In reality, incubus is a sleep disorder recognized since the time of Aristotle in which the victim has feelings of suffocation and impending death, exhaustion and fear upon awakening.

The term "incubus syndrome" has been used to describe patients suffering from the DELUSION that they have been sexually approached at night by an unseen lover.

See also SUCCUBUS; WITCHES AND WITCHCRAFT, FEAR OF.

indecision   See DECISION MAKING.

indigestion   A variety of symptoms brought on by eating, including FLATULENCE, HEARTBURN, abdominal pain, and NAUSEA. It causes a burning discomfort in the stomach because the individual has eaten too much, too fast, or too rich, spicy, or fatty foods. Nervous indigestion is a common cause of anxiety. This anxiety generally results from anything that causes ANGER, PAIN, and FEAR. STAGE FRIGHT, going on a job interview, or going on a first date are sometimes stressful situations that can cause indigestion.

To keep anxiety levels in line, eat a balanced diet, and do not overeat. Allow plenty of time for eating. Limit foods that cause indigestion; eat small meals four times a day. Get adequate sleep and practice deep breathing, visualization, and other anxiety-reducing techniques.

Belching

Belching, or common burping, comes from the swallowing of air or from gas in the stomach caused by the chemical reactions of food and digestive juices. Many individuals feel stressed by the embarrassment that results from belching in a social situation or public place. To overcome the embarrassment, as well as the source of the problem, careful attention to diet may make a difference. Also, taking more time to select foods carefully and eat slowly may reduce the incidence of this annoying reaction.

Belching may occur more frequently when an individual feels stressed because he or she either eats too fast or selects foods that contribute to heartburn, bloating, and belching. In addition to diet, relaxation techniques may be useful.

Bloating

The term *bloating* applies to the full, distended feeling in the abdomen that occurs after overeating.

TIPS TO RELIEVE ANXIETY DUE TO BLOATING

- Relax before eating; eat and drink slowly.
- Limit foods/beverages that contain air, such as carbonated drinks, baked goods, whipped cream, and souffles. Don't smoke, chew gum, suck on hard candy, or drink through straws or narrow-mouthed bottles.
- Correct loose dentures.
- Eat fewer rich foods, such as fatty meats, fried food, cream sauces, gravies and pastries.
- Don't lie down immediately after eating.
- Don't try to force yourself to belch.

Many people react to anxiety by overeating, eating too fast, or eating spicy, greasy foods, all of which contribute to bloating. The discomfort causes further anxieties, as bloating leads to belching or burping, which can be socially embarrassing.

See also IRRITABLE BOWEL SYNDROME; NUTRITION; RELAXATION.

Individualized Behavior Avoidance Tests (IBATs)
Tests used by researchers in AGORAPHOBIA. Some researchers prefer IBATs over STANDARDIZED BEHAVIORAL AVOIDANCE TESTS (SBATs) because agoraphobics have so many different phobic difficulties that may be measured. Another advantage of the IBAT is that it assesses personally relevant behaviors in naturalistic situations in phobic individuals' homes and clinics. An example of an individualized test is one that is initially developed from a 10-item hierarchy of phobic situations. Five items representing a range of severity are selected from this hierarchy, and assessment is conducted from the phobic individual's home. The individual is instructed to attempt all five items in the order of increasing difficulty. Each item is scored on a three-point scale, with the interpretation of each score as follows: (0) individual avoided the item; (1) partial completion of the item (escape); (2) successful completion of the item. The total score, therefore, has a range from one to 10. Additionally, Subjective Units of Disturbance (SUDS) ratings on a scale of zero to eight points may be obtained for each item. The IBAT allows assessment in many personally relevant situations and should, if the phobia hierarchy is properly constructed, possess a high enough ceiling to deal with distraction levels, sensitivity to treatment changes, and generalizability to other situations.

Himadi, William G., et al., "Assessment of Agoraphobia— II, Measurement of Clinical Change," *Behavior Research and Therapy* 24 no. 3 (1986), pp. 321–332.

individual psychology An approach to PSYCHOTHERAPY and PERSONALITY. Individual psychology is based on the theory that each individual is governed by a conscious drive to develop goals and create his or her own style of life, as opposed to the view that individuals are dominated by UNCONSCIOUS instincts. The term was introduced by ALFRED ADLER. The goal of individual psychology is to help the individual adopt a more socially useful lifestyle and thus improve interpersonal relationships. ANXIETIES and PHOBIAS can be overcome with changes in lifestyle brought about by therapy.

See also COMPENSATION.

infants, fear of   Fear of infants is known as pedophobia.

See also CHILDREN, FEAR OF.

infection, fear of   Fear of infection is known as molysmophobia or mysophobia. Some individuals who fear CONTAMINATION or GERMS or have ILLNESS PHOBIA fear infection. Also, those who fear BACTERIA or BACILLI usually fear infection. Those who have a phobia about contracting autoimmune deficiency syndrome (AIDS) fear infection, as do some individuals who have OBSESSIVE-COMPULSIVE DISORDER.

inferiority complex   Originally this was a term used by Alfred Adler to describe the cluster of ideas and feelings that arise in reaction to the sense of "organ" inferiority. Now it is a popular term for a general sense of inadequacy. A sense of inadequacy accompanies DEPRESSION or a mood disorder in which the individual feels a low sense of self-esteem and low self-worth. The opposite of the inferiority complex is a superiority complex; individuals who have BIPOLAR DISORDER or MANIC–DEPRESSIVE DISORDER often exhibit a superiority complex while they are in the manic phase of their illness.

See also COMPLEX.

infertility   The inability to produce an offspring. Usually the diagnosis of infertility is made in a couple after at least one year of sexual intercourse without contraception. Infertility is often a cause of STRESS and ANXIETY for many couples, particularly those who have delayed childbearing until their late 30s or early 40s. This frustrating and often anguishing problem affects about 15 percent of all couples of childbearing age. Only about one-half of the couples professionally treated for infertility achieve pregnancy.

Other anxieties produced by infertility can result in sexual problems, such as low or nonexistent sexual desire. Fortunately, for most couples, this is usually a situational problem, and when the infertility is resolved, it goes away.

According to William W. Hurd, assistant professor of obstetrics and gynecology, University of Michigan Medical Center, about one in 10 couples are considered "subfertile," which means that their chances of having a baby without professional intervention are slim. The infertility rate increases dramatically with age; couples between ages 30 and 35 have a 33 percent chance of being subfertile, and the odds jump to 50 percent by the time they reach 40. The probability of becoming pregnant the "old-fashioned way" is less than 10 percent among couples age 40 and older.

In approximately 40 percent of infertility cases, the problem is attributed to the female; in another 40 percent it is attributed to the male, and in the remaining cases, it stems from both partners. In about 3.5 percent of cases, infertility cannot be explained.

Female Infertility

Failure to ovulate is a common cause of female infertility. It may be due to a hormonal imbalance, anxieties and stress, or a disorder of the ovary, such as a tumor or a cyst. Disorders of the uterus and blocked Fallopian tubes are other causes of infertility. Chromosomal abnormality or allergy to a partner's sperm are rare factors also contributing to infertility.

Reasons why subfertility increases with time are largely based on changes that take place in a woman's body as she ages. For example, older ovaries in middle-aged women produce less fertility-enhancing hormones. Additionally, ova thus affected are not as receptive to sperm penetration and they tend to be spontaneously aborted once fertilized.

Male Infertility

Formerly, infertility problems were attributed exclusively to women. Now, however, sperm production and motility, hormonal imbalances, anatomical factors, infections, and inflammatory diseases are known to affect a man's ability to father a child.

According to Dana Ohl, M.D., assistant professor of surgery, University of Michigan Medical Center, anabolic steroids, which can lower sperm count drastically and sometimes irreversibly, will also leave an indelible mark on infertility statistics in the years to come; young men in high school who use steroids will have difficulty impregnating their partners five to 10 years later.

Some men perceive their infertility as a stressful threat to their masculine identity, which they may associate with their sexual prowess. One of the best ways to get men to accept infertility is to encourage them to talk about their condition, both with their partners and in support groups.

Diagnosing Infertility

Infertility does not always mean that conception is impossible. Today there are advances in treating many of the problems that might affect fertility. In diagnosing infertility, physicians look at medical factors that alone or in tandem could prevent pregnancy. They want to know, for example, if the ovaries release an egg each month, and along with it, a proper amount of hormones to allow for implantation. They also want to know if the male partner's sperm is of sufficient volume, motility, and quality to fertilize an egg.

Assisted Reproduction Techniques

Assisted reproduction techniques, which were developed during the 1980s and 1990s, offer hope to conceive a child, even for couples stressed by complex forms of infertility. These techniques originated in England with the birth of the first IVF (in vitro fertilization) baby, Louise Brown, in 1978. Since then, assisted reproduction procedures have been successfully performed worldwide, enabling thousands of couples with otherwise untreatable infertility to produce their own healthy babies.

Couples most suited for IVF are those in which the wife has a normal uterus and ovaries, but whose Fallopian tubes are damaged, blocked, or absent. Many patients in IVF programs have previously been treated for tubal disease that required surgery that proved unsuccessful or that required complete removal of the Fallopian tubes. Women suffering from endometriosis, or adhesions affecting reproductive organs, may be candidates for IVF or GIFT (gamete intra-Fallopian transfer). Couples in whom the husband has an infertility problem may also be suitable for IVF, TET (tubal embryo transfer), or ICSI (direct sperm injection into an egg cell).

Options with Technology

Understanding the options with assisted reproduction techniques helps relieve the anxieties of infertility for many couples. IVF is essentially a tubal bypass procedure. Mature eggs are retrieved from the ovary with ultrasound guidance. The eggs are fertilized in the laboratory. In special circumstances, IVF procedures may be performed using donated egg cells, sperm, or embryos. The resulting embryos are transferred into the woman's uterus or into her tubes via laparoscopy.

TET is performed through laparoscopy in an operating room. GIFT is similar to IVF, but the eggs and sperm, instead of being incubated in vitro, are placed together in the Fallopian tubes of the wife. GIFT can be performed if at least one of the tubes is healthy but an egg is unable to reach it.

Couples interested in exploring how medical technology can help them conceive should contact local medical centers and thoroughly check the credentials of the physicians who specialize in infertility or reproductive endocrinology, as well as the laboratories and facilities they are considering. Knowing that they are in the hands of experts will help relieve some of the stresses of undergoing the assisted reproduction procedures that may be emotionally and financially costly.

A support group started by infertile couples is RESOLVE.

See also BIOLOGICAL CLOCK; IMPOTENCE.

Berger, Gary S., Mark Goldstein, and Mark Fuerst, *The Couple's Guide to Fertility.* Rev. ed. (New York: Doubleday, 1994).

Corson, Stephen L., *Conquering Infertility: a Guide for Couples* (New York: Prentice Hall, 1990).

infinity, fear of Fear of infinity is known as apeirophobia. Individuals who fear infinity like to have terms defined and distances measured, and appreciate predictability in their lives. They may fear looking far into the distance where they cannot anticipate what lies ahead or looking ahead into time with UNKNOWN, unpredictable circumstances. This fear may relate to a fear of change or newness. Some agoraphobics may have fears related to infinity.

See also AGORAPHOBIA; CHANGE, FEAR OF; UNKNOWN, FEAR OF.

informed consent   Voluntary agreement to a therapy plan. Individuals who seek therapy for ANXIETIES or PHOBIAS should be informed about the types of therapy or treatment to be used, possible side effects, and desired outcome before going ahead with the therapy plan. Also, informed consent refers to the right of the therapist to give out information learned in therapy sessions only with the consent of the individual patient.

inhibition   Inhibition is an inner restraint that keeps an individual from following through on feelings or thoughts, such as anger or lust. Inhibition may be caused by real or imagined fear of the consequences of expression. Individuals who have inhibitions in specific areas may experience increased ANXIETY when confronted with the feared object or situation. Inhibitions often lead to SHYNESS; some social phobics have many inhibitions and consequently avoid many situations in which they feel uncomfortable.

See also SOCIAL PHOBIA.

injection phobias   Fear of injections is known as trypanophobia. A fear of injection may be one reason many individuals fear doctors and dentists. Many individuals say their fear of dentists arises from fear of injection of local anesthetic. Usually fear of injections begins before age ten or eleven and diminishes with age. Some who fear acupuncture do so because they fear needles. Some who fear donating blood or having blood transfusions also fear injection. Injection phobias include fear of vaccination and fear of inoculation and immunizations.

See also ACUPUNCTURE, FEAR OF; DENTAL ANXIETY; NEEDLES, FEAR OF.

Kleinknecht, Ronald A., *The Anxious Self* (New York: Human Sciences Press, 1986).
———, and D. A. Bernstein, "Assessment of Dental Fear," *Behavior Therapy,* 9 (1978), pp. 626–634.

injury, fear of   Fear of injury is known as traumatophobia.

See also BLOOD AND BLOOD-INJURY, FEAR OF.

inkblot test   See RORSCHACH TEST.

innovation, fear of   Fear of innovation, or of something new, is known as neophobia. Many anxious individuals like to keep to the same routine and avoid doing, seeing, or using anything new.

See also NEWNESS, FEAR OF.

inoculation, fear of   Fear of inoculation is known as trypanophobia. Those who fear inoculations fear needles. They fear being vaccinated or having any kind of immunization via a needle.

See also INJECTION, FEAR OF.

insanity, fear of   Fear of insanity is known as dementophobia, lyssophobia, and maniaphobia.

See also GOING CRAZY, FEAR OF; SCHIZOPHRENIA.

insects, fear of   Fear of insects is known as acarophobia and entomophobia. Some individuals are so afraid of insects that they seal off their windows, vacuum and sweep twice a day, and feel uncomfortable outside their "cleansed" environment. There is no instinctual basis or symbolism for fear of insects.

See also BEES, FEAR OF; STINGS, FEAR OF.

insight   A special kind of understanding of a situation. In therapy, the term implies depth and suddenness of understanding of, for example, the origins of one's PHOBIA or ANXIETY. Insight means seeing beneath the surface of one's behavior or ideas. In cognitive insight, an individual understands a relationship between cause and effect and achieves new ways to solve behavioral problems. In emotional insight, one gains new awareness about feelings, motives, and relationships. In PSYCHOANALYSIS, insight is an awareness of the relationship between past experience and current behavior, particularly with regard to UNCONSCIOUS conflicts brought into the CONSCIOUS. In all therapies, insight involves accepting the conceptual system of the therapist to a large extent. Insight therapies are not effective for anxiety disorders and are not the treatment of choice.

See also ATTRIBUTION THEORY; BEHAVIOR MODIFICATION; BEHAVIOR THERAPY.

insomnia, fear of Insomnia is an inability to sleep or stay asleep. Some individuals fear insomnia, and for others insomnia is a symptom of other disorders. Insomnia is a frequent symptom of individuals who have ANXIETIES. Many moderately or severely depressed individuals complain of fitful sleep with early-morning wakening. However, some depressed individuals sleep more than normal. Many people suffer from temporary insomnia when faced with a particular situation that causes them anxiety or great excitement, but there are also chronic insomniacs.

There are four main categories of insomnia: (1) light-sleep insomnia, characterized by an overabundance of light sleep and less or an inadequate amount of deep sleep; (2) sleep-awakening insomnia, in which the individual wakes up repeatedly during the night and spends at least thirty minutes trying to go back to sleep; (3) sleep-onset insomnia, in which the individual has trouble initially falling asleep; and (4) early-termination insomnia, in which the individual awakens after less than six hours and cannot go back to sleep at all.

Treatment Options and Outlook

Treatment of insomnia is usually focused on the main condition causing the sleeplessness, whether a physical condition such as pain or itching, or a psychological concern. Some depressed individuals react well to a sedative ANTIDEPRESSANT such as AMITRIPTYLENE,

DOXEPIN, or MIANSERIN taken at night. Similarly, some BENZODIAZEPINES have prolonged effects; one dose at night acts both as an immediate HYPNOTIC and as an ANXIOLYTIC the next day. For occasional use—for example, with travel and time-zone changes—a short-acting benzodiazepine is often recommended. However, use and misuse of sleeping pills is one of the greatest dangers facing chronic insomniacs. Since the pills are addictive and the body builds up a tolerance to them, the insomniac must take more and more of them to put him- or herself to sleep. Another danger of constant use of sleeping pills is that these drugs disturb the normal pattern of dreaming, which is essential to good mental health. Disturbing the dream pattern for several nights may result in neurotic daytime behavior.

Routine administration of drugs known as hypnotics is also a common cause of insomnia. If a drug is taken intermittently or the dose is not kept constant, mild withdrawal symptoms, including insomnia or nightmares, may follow. Drugs known as anxiolytics may make some children's sleep worse and may increase their anxieties. In children who have situational anxiety such as school phobia, anxiolytics may impair their intellectual function, outweighing any emotional benefits they might derive from the drugs.

In elderly individuals who have insomnia, barbiturates and benzodiazepines are sometimes prescribed for sleep problems, but their use should be limited to short courses related to definite periods of stress. To avoid toxicity, short-acting benzodiazepines or a chloral derivative are preferred.

Behavior treatment for insomnia has been effective in eliminating sleep disturbance within a relatively brief therapy duration. Behavioral therapists try to build an association between bed and sleep, and the individual who cannot sleep is asked to get out of bed until sleep is possible. Modification of cognitions (e.g., excessive worries) is often necessary, as well as training in relaxation (which is used preceding attempts to sleep).

See also BARBITURATES; DEPRESSION; DREAMS; SEDATIVES; SLEEP; SLEEP-WALKING; SYMPTOMS.

integrity groups SELF-HELP mental health groups developed by O. Hobart Mowrer during the 1960s.

Integrity groups were one of the early forms of self-helps for individuals who have anxieties. Mowrer believed that relationships with significant people in an individual's life can be affected by social ANXIETIES and FEARS, particularly the operation of guilt. He believed that the inability to keep commitments to other people was at the root of many psychosocial disorders. His idea in developing integrity groups was to provide a support group in which individuals could deal with these problems. In integrity groups, approximately eight persons met weekly for three-hour sessions during which they participated in open transactions with one another. Mowrer believed that shared honesty and involvement in the group encouraged a sense of community and raised self-esteem; group members thus developed a secure base on which they could then make changes in thoughts, feelings, and behavior toward others. The integrity group motto was: "You alone can do it, but you can't do it alone," which emphasizes the values of self-responsibility along with mutual support.

intergenerational conflicts   Because people live longer, it is not unusual to have family members representing as many as three or four generations. Having members of more than two generations living under one roof is less likely to occur today than in earlier times, but it is generally agreed that generational conflicts are often due to living together in one residence. However, no matter how close or far apart the generations live, as long as they continue to meet and share holiday and other family celebrations, some areas of generational conflict, often labeled as a *generation gap,* will persist.

Generation gap refers to the inability to communicate, view the same phenomenon with similar conclusions, and sensitively consider the feelings of others and their beliefs. While there is evidence of generation gaps as far back as the time of Jesus Christ, the gap, which usually extended between parents and children, has broadened to include grandparents as well. In these three-generational families, issues that most often involve all three generations in areas of disagreement include behavior.

Some young people often carry a stereotype of older adults as "living in the past," overly conservative, and unable to understand them and how much things have changed since they were young. While many young people admire and love older people and in specific instances (parents, relatives, friends, teachers) even use them as role models, the stress-filled intergenerational conflicts persist.

A good deal of stress emanating from middle-aged and older adults toward the young is, in fact, due to the overpowering youth culture of the 1990s. In addition, older people's view of the younger generation may be colored by their own feelings of self-achievement and life satisfaction. When they feel good about themselves, they are more likely to have higher expectations of the younger generation.

See also AGE DISCRIMINATION; AGEISM; BABY BOOMERS; COMMUNICATION; GENERATION X; ELDERLY PARENTS; LISTENING; PARENTING; PUBERTY.

Triebel, Axel, and Irmgard Luecking, "Laius and/or Odysseus: Divergent patterns of intergenerational conflicts," *International Forum of Psychoanalysis* 7, no. 1 (April 1998): pp. 19–23.

interpersonal anxiety   An old term used to describe SOCIAL ANXIETY.

See also PHOBIA; SOCIAL PHOBIA.

intimacy and fear of intimacy   Intimacy is marked by very close association and friendship between individuals. Emotional intimacy can exist between lovers, friends, siblings, or children and parents. There is evidence that intimacy can be linked to good health, but when a relationship turns sour, it can be a source of anxiety for many people.

Close Relationships and Good Health

There is evidence that suggests when individuals have happy relationships, the likelihood of disease and complications from disease are far less, according to Len Sperry, M.D., Duke University. A five-year study found that unmarried heart patients who did not have a confidante were three times more likely to die from cardiac disease than those who were married or had a close friend. Similar findings were presented in a Canadian study of 224 women with breast cancer. Seven years after they had been diagnosed, 76 percent of the women with at least

TAKING ANXIETIES OUT OF INTIMATE RELATIONSHIPS

- Don't plunge in. Relationships should develop slowly.
- Autonomy is important, don't lose control of your own needs.
- Don't expect perfection in yourself or the other person.
- Set boundaries and recharge, using periods of distance to strengthen your sense of self.
- Accept criticism, rejection, and disappointment as a fact of life.
- Maintain a life away from the relationship.

one intimate relationship survived. The explanation for this, Sperry says, is that feeling cared about and important helps maintain a person's optimism in times of stress. These emotional boosts translate into a strong immunity that helps fight disease.

The Stress and Fear of Intimacy

Author of the book, *Too Close for Comfort: Exploring the Risks of Intimacy,* Geraldine Piorkowski, Ph.D., explored the theory that the fears and stress of intimacy can be healthy when they are realistic and protective of the self. To do this, Piorkowski suggests that individuals reflect and learn from past experiences, schedule enough time to develop these relationships, be willing to share feelings with others, work at relationships but allow for failures, and be on intimate terms with more than one person.

Dr. Piorkowski comments, "there is a level of imperfect intimacy that is good enough to live and grow on. In good-enough intimacy, painful encounters occasionally occur, but they are balanced by the strengths and pleasures of the relationship. There are enough positives to balance the negatives. People who do well in intimate relationships don't have the perfect relationship, but it is good enough."

Piorkowski, Geraldine K., *Too Close For Comfort: Exploring the Risks of Intimacy* (New York: Plenum Press, 1994).

Thelen, Mark H., Michelle D. Sherman, and Tiffany S. Borst, "Fear of intimacy and attachment among rape survivors," *Behavior Modification* 22, no. 1 (January 1998): pp. 108–116.

intoxication   See ALCOHOL, FEAR OF.

introversion   Introversion is a personality characteristic marked by self-reliance. Introverts tend to be rather contemplative people, sensitive, and may seem aloof to others. The introvert is generally more interested in working alone or engaging in recreational activities alone than with others. Introverts may be stressed because they may become too preoccupied with their own inner thoughts and feelings.

See also PERSONALITY; SELF-ESTEEM.

Koszycki, Diana, Robert M. Zacharko, and Jacques Bradwejn, "Influence of personality on behavioral response to cholecystokinin-tetrapeptide in patients with panic disorder," *Psychiatry Research* 62, no. 2 (May 1996): pp. 131–138.

in vivo desensitization   A technique for treating phobias in real-life situations, as opposed to work in a laboratory or in imagination. Phobic individuals are led through the actual situations that arouse their ANXIETIES. The goal is for the phobic individuals to learn to relax in the presence of anxiety-causing stimuli. Whenever it is possible to use it, this is the more effective form of DESENSITIZATION therapy. Also known as *in vivo* therapy.

See also BEHAVIOR THERAPY; SYSTEMATIC DESENSITIZATION.

in vivo therapy   *In vivo* literally means "in life." This is the preferred form of desensitization, as contrasted with imaginal psychotherapies using images. *In vivo* desensitization was used by Wolpe, who then developed imaginal sensations as a more convenient tool in some situations.

See also EXPOSURE THERAPY; *IN VIVO* DESENSITIZATION.

iophobia   Fear of poisons, or of rust.

See also POISON, FEAR OF; RUST, FEAR OF.

iprindole   An antidepressant drug.

See also ANTIDEPRESSANTS; ANTIDEPRESSANTS, NEW; DEPRESSION.

irrational beliefs, fear of   Some individuals who have anxiety disorders harbor more irrational beliefs than those who do not have such disorders. Such irrational beliefs include thinking that it is important to be loved or approved by virtually everyone in one's community; that one must be perfectly competent, adequate, and achieving to consider oneself worthwhile; that past influences cannot be eradicated; and that some people are bad or villainous and therefore should be blamed or punished.

See also SUPERNATURAL, FEARS OF.

Davison, G. C., and J. M. Neale, *Abnormal Psychology* (New York: John Wiley, 1986), p. 123.
Encyclopedia of Unbelief (Buffalo, NY: Prometheus, 1985).

irritable bowel syndrome   A chronic gastrointestinal condition in which the individual experiences abdominal discomfort or pain and a change in bowel habits, such as cramping, DIARRHEA, or CONSTIPATION, without weight loss or gastrointestinal disease. The syndrome may affect eight to seventeen percent of the American population. Some physicians say that the condition is of "nervous" origin and have described irritable bowel syndrome patients as "neurasthenics." Among individuals who have irritable bowel syndrome, many have ANXIETY and depression. Conversely, functional gastrointestinal complaints are so common in individuals who have anxiety disorders that gastrointestinal distress has been included as a symptom of panic disorder in the American Psychiatric Association's *Diagnostic and Statistical Manual of Mental Disorders*. In both conditions, onset most often occurs in young and middle-aged adults. Both affect predominantly women, are associated with a variety of complaints, appear to be familial, and are often chronic conditions. In research studies, many individuals found relief from both irritable bowel syndrome and panic symptoms with anti-panic therapy. Panic disorder and irritable bowel syndrome both improved with BENZODIAZEPINES and tricyclic ANTIDEPRESSANTS. Researchers hypothesize that gastrointestinal symptoms experienced by some individuals may be symptoms of panic disorder or may be irritable bowel syndrome worsened by a coexisting anxiety disorder. PANIC DISORDER patients often report one particular symptom, such as diarrhea or DIZZINESS, as particularly troublesome and seek a specialist to treat that particular symptom.

Lydiard, R. Bruce, et al., "Can Panic Disorder Present as Irritable Bowel Syndrome?" *Journal of Clinical Psychiatry* (September 1986), pp. 470–473.

isolophobia   Fear of solitude or of being alone.

See also SOLITUDE, FEAR OF.

isopterophobia   Fear of termites or of other insects that eat wood and are destructive.

See also TERMITES, FEAR OF.

itch, fear of   Fear of itching, having itchy skin, or having the "seven-year itch" is known as scabiophobia or acarophobia.

See also SCABIES.

ithyphallophobia   Fear of seeing, thinking about, or having an erect penis.

See also PENIS, ERECT; SEXUAL FEARS.

Japan, stress in   See KAROSHI.

Japanophobia   Fear of Japan and Japanese things.

jealousy, fear of   Fear of jealousy is known as zelophobia. Jealousy is an emotion that includes feelings of loss of self-esteem, envy, hostility, and self-blame. Jealousy frequently first appears at the age of two or three when a new child arrives in the family. There may be hostile feelings toward the newborn because he or she is getting more attention. In adulthood, many types of jealousy persist. In the more extreme types it may take the form of a paranoid DELUSION. Many people have observed jealousy in others and may develop a fear of becoming jealous.

jet lag   Disruption of one's body rhythms (CIRCADIAN RHYTHM) resulting from traveling through several time zones within a short span of time. It takes many individuals several days or longer to recover from the stress of this type of travel. The sleep schedule, appetite, and ability to concentrate well while recovering from jet lag varies from individual to individual. Anxieties often result during a period of jet lag.

See also AIRPLANE.

Wingler, Sharon, *Travel Alone & Love It: A Flight Attendant's Guide to Solo Travel* (Willowbrook, IL: Chicago Spectrum Press, 1996).

job security   Lack of job security is a major cause of instability and stress for workers throughout the world. This was not so in the 1950s and '60s. Then, many employers had implicit or explicit long-term employment contracts with their workers, contracts that emphasized management's commitment and pledge to minimize the need for LAYOFFS. Wages and job benefits increased over the years, and it was not unusual for a company to pay the total cost of employees' health care and charge minimally for family coverage. This job security led workers to expect to remain in their jobs for many years, and it was not unusual for workers to devote their entire working lives to one company, retiring with the traditional gold watch and company pension.

During the later 1990s, DOWNSIZING, layoffs, MERGERS and other organizational changes greatly altered the job security picture. Employers are no longer sharing their wealth; raises and employee benefits have been scaled back. Full-time jobs are harder to find.

To cope with job insecurity, in addition to the option of operating his or her own business, *Money* magazine suggested that workers consider themselves free agents or skilled artisans; set new professional goals; look for new jobs while still employed; build portable skills; set up a board of directors (network) made up of five to 10 trusted colleagues, clients, former bosses, and other professionals who know the worker's track record and opportunities available in his/her field; create an escape hatch (options, lateral moves, further education); and be ready to accept change.

Job Change

Making the transition into a new position, whether within the same company or at a new one, can cause anxiety. Both situations have pros and cons. Coming from the outside means the individual does not have to worry about managing coworkers or friends. However, when the individual does not have a mentor or friend in a new company, he has no one to rely on, to show him or her the ropes, and provide introductions to corporate policies and politics. Starting out fresh also means not knowing other employees' strengths or weaknesses.

Promotion, whether from within or without, can also significantly raise anxiety levels because it raises fear of incompetence and fear of failure. Usually these fears and anxieties will go away once the new position is mastered and evidence of SUCCESS becomes visible.

See also WORKPLACE.

Catalano, Ralph, Raymond Novaco, and William McConnell, "A model of the net effect of job loss on violence," *Journal of Personality and Social Psychology* 72, no. 6 (June 1997): pp. 1,440–1,447.

deRoiste, Aine, "Sources of worry and happiness in Ireland," *Irish Journal of Psychology* 17, no. 3 (1996): pp. 193–212.

Snyder, Don J., *The Cliff Walk: A Memoir of a Job Lost and a Life Found* (Boston: Little, Brown, 1997).

journaling   Writing down thoughts and experiences in a daily or weekly journal is a way for the individual to relieve anxieties, sort out confusion, and deal with problems. Writing and reading what has been written sometimes exposes suppressed subconscious feelings that can be dealt with more constructively when they are recognized. In this sense, a diarist may get closer to his/her feelings and better understand self-motivations.

The cathartic effect of writing involves a distancing from negative feelings and experiences. Once the feelings or experiences are described on paper, the writer frequently has a sense of being rid of them, of being able to go on to something else. Writing may also help to bring repressed thoughts and attitudes out into the open and eliminate some of the restrictions that sap energy and limit productivity. Simply, the act of writing may give a sense of CONTROL, a way of giving some order and manageability to problems.

Symptoms such as ANXIETY, DEPRESSION and apathy may be masks for envy, JEALOUSY, and rage turned inward at the self. Some diarists have found it useful to write a portrait of a person whom they envy or who has angered them. The portrait sometimes reveals qualities of their own that they wish to either develop or change.

Making lists in a diary can be a good way of setting goals and giving order to what may seem to be an enormous or chaotic task. Journaling also can be useful for the person who is attempting to control addictive or obsessive behavior.

Journaling is used by many SUPPORT GROUPS for overeaters, as well as those who wish to stop SMOKING or drinking. The diary not only improves self-understanding and serves as a way to record progress but also gives the individual something to do over which he/she has complete control when he/she wants a drink, cigarette, or is about to give in to a desire to overeat, for example. Journaling on a regular basis, even for brief periods, has been shown to actually strengthen the immune system.

See also EATING DISORDERS; SELF-ESTEEM; SUPPORT GROUPS.

Adams, Kathleen, *Journal to the Self* (New York: Warner Books, 1990).

judeophobia   Fear of Jews and Jewish things.

judicial proceedings   Stresses endured by individuals serving on juries range from being away from their families (in the event of a sequestered jury) to the agonizing decision-making processes in which they will have to engage.

First there is the stress of the selection process, during which an individual faces the feeling of being out of CONTROL of his/her destiny for the next day or, perhaps, weeks. Then there is the concern about being sequestered for a period of time with a group of strangers. Some stress surrounds how well the individual will get along with fellow jury members. There is also the stress of making the right decision, particularly in a life or death matter, and having one's own judgment swayed by others in making a decision.

Anxieties Lawyers Face

Lawyers are the first to attest to the extreme anxieties that arise during a jury trial. These anxieties are often exhibited by loss of tempers on both sides of the issue. That is why stress management is a popular topic of seminars offered to lawyers nationwide. These seminars encourage lawyers to recognize the stressors, such as physical separation from their families and disruption of normal routines that may occur, particularly when a trial goes on for a long period of time, and to strategize ways to handle the stress. The seminars emphasize needs for lawyers to maintain themselves physically and emotionally and to try to talk out feelings, something that can be alien to those involved in legal work.

When asked about effective ways to handle anxieties and stress, many lawyers highly rate building a wall of separation between their professional and private lives. Others value a healthy regimen that includes not smoking or drinking, staying in shape by exercising, and establishing healthy lifestyle habits.

Anxieties Trial Judges Face

A study reported in the *Bulletin of the American Academy of Psychiatry Law* (vol. 22, 1994) examined work-related stress among American trial judges. A representative sample of 88 judges completed questionnaires addressing type and magnitude of specific work-related stressors, psychological stress symptoms, and psychosocial moderators of stress.

Types of stressors noted included cases, litigating parties, purposes and consequences of decisions, conflicts between professional and personal values, and seriousness of a criminal offense. The most stressful aspect of work related to poorly prepared or disrespectful counsel, exercising judicial management and discretion, and highly emotional cases under public scrutiny.

See also DECISION MAKING; LAWYERS.

Eells, T. D., and C. R. Showalter, "Work-related stress in American trial judges." *Bulletin of the American Academy of Psychiatry and Law* 22 (1994): pp. 71–83.

jumping (from both high and low places), fear of   Fear of jumping from both high and low places is known as catapedaphobia. This fear may be related to a fear of heights, a fear of falling, or a fear of being injured.

See also CLIFFS, FEAR OF; HEIGHTS, FEAR OF.

justice, fear of   Fear of justice or fear of seeing justice applied is known as dikephobia. Justice involves concepts of moral rightness, honor, and fairness.

See also AUTHORITY, FEAR OF.

K

kainophobia (kainotophobia) Fear of novelty, change, or newness.

See also CHANGE, FEAR OF; NEWNESS, FEAR OF; NOVELTY, FEAR OF.

kakorrhaphiophobia Fear of failure.

See also FAILURE, FEAR OF.

karoshi *Karoshi*—"death from overwork"—has become synonymous with stress in Japan. In an article by C. Frank Lawlis in *Alternative Therapies* (July 1995), "People (in Japan) are literally dying at their workstations. It appears that their entire physiological system collapses or shuts down."

Lawlis draws from a 1989 study by Chiyoda Fire and Marine Insurance, Ltd., one of the top insurance carriers in Japan. Chiyoda, which covers more than 100,000 Japanese corporations, conducted a major study on health problems Japanese people are likely to encounter. One important conclusion of the study was that in 40 percent of the health problems, stress played a major role.

As a result, Chiyoda established N.C. Wellness, a company that developed programs integrating Oriental medicine into health promotion for employees. Buildings housing the programs were constructed to focus on tranquil space and function similar to that of a "cocoon." At the same time, they were designed as places for nonordinary pleasure where "interference from everyday affairs is barred" and where the environment to practice the mind-body and awareness elements of balance is enjoyable and protective.

The first prototype center was opened in Kichjoji, Musashino-shi, Tokyo, in June 1994. The core program offered at this site incorporated five "direc-tions": self-management; self-promotion; self-discovery/purpose of life, fun and pleasure; interpersonal skills; and community.

See also ACCULTURATION; COMPLEMENTARY THERAPIES; MIND/BODY CONNECTIONS.

katagelophobia Fear of ridicule. This fear is related to a fear of criticism; both may be social phobias.

See also RIDICULE, FEAR OF.

kathisophobia Fear of sitting down.

See also SITTING DOWN, FEAR OF.

Kempf's disease See HOMOSEXUALITY.

kenophobia Fear of empty spaces.

See also EMPTY SPACES, FEAR OF.

keraunophobia Fear of lightning and thunder.

See also LIGHTNING, FEAR OF; STORMS, FEAR OF; THUNDER, FEAR OF.

kidney disease, fear of Fear of kidney disease is known as albuminurophobia. The major functions of the kidneys are cleaning the blood of metabolic waste products and controlling the amount of water in the body. Both functions are done by formation and excretion of urine. Some individuals fear that they have kidney disease when their urinary habits change or if they have vague pains in their abdomen or back. Some individuals worry that they are urinating too much, and others worry that they are not urinating enough. Urinalysis usually is part of routine physical examinations, and many phobic individuals are reassured when they learn test results.

See also DISEASE, FEAR OF; HIGH BLOOD PRESSURE, FEAR OF.

kinesics   The study of COMMUNICATION as expressed through facial expression and other body movements. Theories and techniques of studying this type of nonverbal communication were developed by Ray L. Birdwhistell (b. 1918), who found that certain gestures and expressions were specifically male or female and also related to regional and national groups. BODY LANGUAGE changes with age, health, mood, and the degree of STRESS or RELAXATION experienced by the individual. Birdwhistell developed his theories with the use of photography and a notation system of symbols called kinegraphs to describe gestures and expressions.

Birdwhistell, Ray L., *Kinesics and Context* (Philadelphia: University of Pennsylvania Press, 1970).

kinesophobia (or kinetophobia)   Fear of motion.
See also MOTION, FEAR OF.

kissing, fear of   Fear and anxieties about kissing range from feelings of social awkwardness, to rejection, to concern about disease. The AIDS (acquired immunodeficiency syndrome) epidemic during the 1980s has made actresses and actors fearful of engaging in the intimate kissing required in many films. Kissing is endowed with an element of performance anxiety for young people who may be more strongly motivated by a desire to appear adept and sophisticated than by genuine romance or passion. Kissing in social rather than romantic situations also creates a certain type of anxiety and confusion, since there is such a variation in method and expectations in different ethnic and social groups. Kissing is also an unpleasant prospect for some people because of a strong, but seldom freely expressed, social fear: bad breath.

The term "kiss of death," meaning a betrayal or generally damaging action, has its origin in the kiss given by Judas Iscariot to identify Jesus as the man to be arrested and ultimately crucified.
See also SOCIAL PHOBIA.

kleptomania   An uncontrollable impulse to steal, followed by a possible reduction in anxiety or tension during or after the act.
See also SHOPLIFTING.

Wiedemann, G., "Kleptomania: Characteristics of 12 Cases," *European Psychiatry* 13, no. 2 (April 1998): pp. 67–77.

kleptophobia, cleptophobia   Fear of stealing.
See also STEALING, FEAR OF.

knees, fear of   Fear of knees is known as genuphobia. While this fear seems quite unnatural to most people, sufferers feel equally perturbed. However, fears related to parts of the body do develop, just as fear of other objects develops. These fears, while rare, are treated with a behavioral, desensitization approach, with a high degree of success.

knives, fear of   Fear of knives is known as aichmophobia. Individuals who are phobic about knives usually are also phobic about various objects with points, such as letter openers, spears, and daggers. This fear may interfere with eating, since sufferers will avoid using knives or placing knives on a table.

koinoniphobia   See ROOM, FEAR OF.

kolpophobia   Fear of genitals, particularly female genitals.
See also GENITALS, FEMALE, FEAR OF.

koniophobia   Fear of dust.
See also CONTAMINATION, FEAR OF; DUST, FEAR OF.

kosmikophobia   Fear of cosmic phenomenon.

Kundalini   See YOGA.

kymophobia   Fear of waves.
See also WAVES, FEAR OF.

kynophobia   Fear of rabies.
See also RABIES, FEAR OF.

kyphophobia   Fear of stooping.
See also STOOPING, FEAR OF.

L-5-Hydroxytryptophan A drug used to treat individuals who have phobic disorders, with and without panic attacks and generalized anxiety disorders. It is abbreviated as 5-HTP. Research has indicated that some individuals experience a significant reduction in anxiety on this therapy in conjunction with carbidopa (a brain chemical). Clinical trials with other drugs used in controlled populations have not been conducted, so general utility of this drug has not been determined.

See also ANTIDEPRESSANTS; BIOLOGICAL BASIS FOR ANXIETY, TRYPTOPHAN.

lachanophobia Fear of vegetables.

See also VEGETABLES, FEAR OF.

lactate-induced anxiety Sodium lactate is one of the substances researchers have identified that can produce PANIC ATTACKS in people who have already experienced them. Chemical induction of panic provides a means of evaluating new treatments as well as the opportunity to closely monitor patients, both by psychophysiological and biochemical techniques, during the panic attack itself. Individuals who are subject to panic attacks may be biologically somewhat different than other people. For example, they may differ in sensitivity to sodium lactate or CARBON DIOXIDE and have differences in CHEMOCEPTOR activity.

Sodium lactate is one of the most studied of the known anxiety-producing chemicals. During the 1940s, researchers observed that individuals with chronic anxiety produced excessive amounts of lactate with standard exercise. For such individuals, exercise can actually set off a panic attack.

The anxiety level of anxiety-prone individuals increases as the level of lactic acid rises in their blood, while people in the nonanxious group experience no such anxiety. Researchers have injected chronically anxious patients with sodium lactate, which produces panic similar to their usual attacks, while normal individuals do not respond to the lactate. When lactate is given to anxiety sufferers in the form of an infusion (a constant flow of sodium lactate), their panic can be stopped by turning off the flow.

Researchers at Washington University School of Medicine (St. Louis, Missouri) observed a difference in blood flow in the brains of people who suffer panic attacks and of those who do not. Using positive-emission tomography (PET scans), they measured blood flow in seven areas of the brain that are thought to control panic and anxiety reactions. In one of these areas, the parahippocampal gyrus, researchers observed that in very lactate-sensitive people, blood flow on the right side of the gyrus was much higher than on the left side. Changes in blood flow appeared to reflect differences in the activity of nerve cells on the two sides. These differences were not seen in nonlactate-sensitive individuals.

Other researchers have suggested that sodium lactate triggers panic attacks in 80 percent of patients with panic disorder but in less than 20 percent of normal people. Lactate infusions were thought to provide a means of identifying people biologically prone to panic attacks and thus likely to respond to drug treatments. However, recent evidence casts doubt on the causative role of lactate, since susceptibility varies less after a person has completed behavior exposure treatments for anxiety. This suggests that lactate susceptibility is a variable factor and that psychophysiology can be altered by behavioral treatment and anxiety-coping skills. In light of this research, the most fruitful approach seems to be to study the relationship between physiology and emotion rather than each separately.

See also CARBON DIOXIDE SENSITIVITY; PANIC.

lakes, fear of   Fear of lakes is known as limnophobia. This fear may extend to being on a lake, looking at a lake, either in actuality or in a film or picture, or imagining a lake. Fear of lakes may relate to fear of water or fear of landscape.

See also LANDSCAPE, FEAR OF; WATER, FEAR OF.

laliophobia, lalophobia   Fear of talking, of speaking, or of stuttering.

See also TALKING, FEAR OF; SPEAKING, FEAR OF; STUTTERING, FEAR OF.

landscapes, fear of   Some individuals fear a particular kind of land arrangement or a specific locale—for example, mountains, the seaside, an open prairie, or a desert. Such individuals avoid a particular type of landscape that they may associate (consciously or unconsciously) with something extremely unpleasant or unfortunate in their past. Agoraphobics tend to experience more intense fear in landscape that is high and wide, but their fear tends to diminish when the view is interrupted by trees, irregularities in land, or rain.

See also LAKES, FEAR OF; RIVERS, FEAR OF; TREES, FEAR OF.

languages, fear of   Fears of foreign places are often manifested in the form of fears of foreign languages. Following are some commonly used terms relating to fears of specific languages (as well as those specific cultures):

China	Sinophobia
England	Anglophobia
France	Gallophobia
Germany	Germanophobia
Japan	Japanophobia
Russia	Russophobia

See also STRANGERS, FEAR OF.

large objects, fear of   Fear of large objects is known as megalophobia.

latent content   A term used in psychoanalytic theory for the unconscious material of a dream that the individual expresses in a disguised way through the symbols noticed in the dream. In some cases, an understanding of the latent content of a dream helps an individual understand the causes of phobias and anxieties. Latent content is contrasted with manifest content, which relates to the meaning of contemporary events in DREAM content.

See also DREAM SYMBOLS; DREAMS, FEAR OF.

laughter, fear of   Fear of laughter is known as geliophobia. This fear may be related to other fears, such as fear of gaiety, or cheerfulness, or good news.

Laughter is an individual's response—a smile, chuckle, or explosive sound—to something that inspires joy or scorn. The ability to laugh, and its companion, a sense of HUMOR, can provide psychological relief from stress, tension, ANXIETY, HOSTILITY, and emotional pain. Laughter helps individuals deal with stressful situations whether at work, in social situations, or in health care settings.

Laughter may be a defense against personal feelings of self-consciousness or embarrassment. An ability to laugh at oneself can be an important COPING mechanism against these stresses. However, many people find it difficult to poke fun at themselves and to acknowledge that they have made a mistake. Individuals suffering from DEPRESSION often lose their ability to laugh and see no humor in their lives or the world around them.

The Curative Powers of Laughter

Maintaining a sense of humor can help most people stay healthy. It causes the body to have a physiological response and the IMMUNE SYSTEM gets the benefit. For example, when one laughs, various muscles tense, then relax, which can result in toning. BREATHING gets faster, allowing the body to take in more oxygen and to get rid of more carbon dioxide. Heart and pulse rate and blood pressure also increase to promote more vigorous circulation, and an increase in the brain's chemical transmitters aids mental alertness.

Research shows that laughter, like exercise, can stimulate the brain to produce secretions known as ENDORPHINS. Endorphins increase one's sense of physical and mental well-being and, to some extent, relieve pain.

The curative power of laughter is not a 20th-century discovery. In the Book of Proverbs, it says: "A merry heart doeth good like a medicine." Norman Cousins (1915–90), former editor of the *Saturday Review* and later a member of the faculty of the medical school at the University of California at Los Angeles, used the curative power of laughter to help himself recover from a degenerative disease of the body's connective tissue. Following are a few excerpts from Cousins' *Anatomy of an Illness,* in which he described the benefits of laughter:

'I made the joyous discovery that ten minutes of genuine belly laughter had an anesthetic effect and would give me at least two hours of pain-free sleep . . . Exactly what happens inside the human mind and body as the result of humor is difficult to say. But the evidence that it works has stimulated the speculations not just of physicians but of philosophers and scholars over the centuries.'

Cousins checked out of the hospital and spent weeks watching the Marx brothers' movies and other comedies. He attributed his recovery to the positive feelings that laughter aroused in him.

Research in Laughter

In an article titled "Laughter" in *American Scientist* (January–February 1996), University of Maryland psychologist Robert R. Provine attempted to shed some light on laughter as a stereotyped, species-specific form of COMMUNICATION. Among other things, Provine's research provides a novel approach to the mechanisms and evolution of vocal production, speech perception, and social behavior.

The laugh tracks of television situation comedies—attempts to stimulate contagious laughter in viewers—and the difficulty of extinguishing "laugh jags," fits of nearly uncontrollable laughter, are familiar phenomena. "Rather than dismissing contagious laughter as a behavioral curiosity," Provine suggests, "we should recognize it and other laugh-related phenomena as clues to broader and deeper issues. Clearly, laughter is a powerful and pervasive part of our lives.

Provine and his assistants observed human laughter in various natural habitats, such as shopping malls, classrooms, sidewalks, offices, and cocktail parties. Among other things, they found that, contrary to their expectations, most conversational laughter is not a response to structured attempts at humor, such as jokes or stories. Most of the laughter seemed to follow rather banal remarks, such as "Look, it's Andre," and "Are you sure?" They found that mutual playfulness, in-group feelings, positive emotional tone, and not comedy, mark the social settings of most naturally occurring laughter. They also found that the average speaker laughs about 46 percent more often than the audience, and that females, whether they are speakers or audiences, laugh more often than males. "In some respects laughter may be a signal of dominance/submission or acceptance/rejection," Provine concluded. "In some situations, laughter may modify the behavior of others by shaping the emotional tone of a conversation."

See also GAIETY, FEAR OF; GOOD NEWS, FEAR OF; IMMUNE SYSTEM; PSYCHONEUROIMMUNOLOGY.

Peter, Laurence J., *The Laughter Prescription: The Tools of Humor and How to Use Them* (New York: Ballantine Books, 1982).

lavatories, public, fear of   Fear of public lavatories is common. Many individuals fear urinating or moving their bowels in a place where another person might be aware of what they are doing. Some fear contracting a disease from a toilet seat or from a towel or sink in a public lavatory. Some fear producing odors themselves, and others fear encountering odors in public lavatories. Some individuals have an inability to pass urine or move their bowels in a place other than their bathroom at home. With the advent of AIDS (acquired immunodeficiency syndrome), fear of public lavatories has increased, although the disease is not transmitted through casual contact.

See also CONTAMINATION, FEAR OF; DEFECATION, FEAR OF; URINATION, FEAR OF.

lawyers There are extremely high levels of anxieties associated with practicing law. Lawyers are frequently in adversarial situations and face deadlines and pressures from many people, including clients, partners, and opposing lawyers.

Litigators, lawyers who represent clients in lawsuits, must have a tough exterior to prevail in the situations they frequently encounter. In private life, some find it difficult to switch to a more passive role with personal partners or family, resulting in still another level of anxiety and tension.

Lawyers as individuals tend to be high achievers. Usually they have high expectations of themselves and others; often these expectations are unreasonable, causing a disparity. "Most lawyers are by nature compulsive people," said Nancy Weisman, general counsel, Rush North Shore Medical Center, Skokie, Illinois, in an article in the Chicago Bar Association's journal, *Record* (May 1994). "Lawyers are often the bringers of news, both good and bad. We bear the burden of delivering answers from other lawyers or the courts. It's easy to explain a win. Explaining a lost motion or case is a stressor lawyers face at times," said Weisman.

Additionally, lawyers must be good listeners and watch for BODY LANGUAGE and unspoken signals to try to anticipate the opposition's responses. Body language plays an equally important role in anticipating feelings of the judge or jury. At the same time, lawyers usually make efforts to hide signs of their vulnerability, which in itself is a stressful posture to take.

Different Anxieties at Different Career Stages

Lawyers face different stresses to their mental and physical health at various stages of their careers: just out of law school, in midcareer, and when nearing RETIREMENT. Personal stressors compound the tensions they encounter throughout their lives.

Most young lawyers begin careers as associates and are single. Though they may try to maintain an active social life, many young lawyers find it difficult while working 80 hours a week or more. The added demands involved in balancing the demands of new social relationships and those of bosses and clients can be overwhelmingly stressful.

Married lawyers, particularly those who have children, are often torn between wanting to do

their jobs well and enjoying family life. They may have experienced feelings of resentment about being absent from family events because of clients' needs.

As careers proceed, there is COMPETITION to advance. Some law firms' new family leave policies have great appeal for young lawyers; still they worry that they will be on a slower track than their peers.

Lawyers who are solo practitioners or in very small firms face the constant challenge of bringing in enough business to stay afloat. Lawyers whose firms have reorganized or merged with another firm may find being downsized a serious stressor. Those who do stay find that they have a new boss to report to, a new internal structure to adjust to, and new or additional responsibilities beyond their full workload.

As they near retirement, some lawyers feel threatened by younger partners in their firms. Others may regret not having reached the top echelon of their firm. They become concerned about what they will do after they retire. They face the stressful situation of having had too little time to develop outside interests or HOBBIES, which are usually the key to making a smooth transition from career to retirement.

See also JOB SECURITY; JURY DUTY; STRESS.

Paddy, Marsh, "The law and lawyers: Through psychodynamic eyes," *Psychodynamic Counselling* 2, no. 4 (October 1996): pp. 517–532.

lead poisoning, fear of Fear of lead poisoning is a 21st-century fear that is prevalent in many older neighborhoods in the United States. Lead poisoning, as well as all heavy metal poisoning, such as that by mercury and arsenic, is a significant problem, especially for children, who tend to put things in their mouths or chew on many things, such as toys, furniture and chips of paint that fall from ceilings or walls, especially in old buildings. Some newsprint such as colored comic pages, is made from leadbased paint. In some areas, there is a heavy concentration of lead in the air. Children are at greater risk than adults of permanent brain damage from lead and other heavy metal poisoning because their brains and nervous systems are still developing. They may become permanently mentally retarded. When an individual ingests too much lead, he may hallucinate and become delirious; he may have convulsions and uncontrollable tremors. To alleviate parents' fears regarding lead poisoning, children who live in high-lead areas can be tested. If high levels are found, children can be detoxified; the procedure may help to slow down and prevent continued brain deterioration.

See also AIR POLLUTION, FEAR OF.

learned helplessness   Feeling of fear and indecision and a sense of not being able to influence the external world. An individual may find that his helpless responses elicit sympathy and assistance from others. Martin Seligman (1942–   ), who developed the concept of learned helplessness during the 1970s, noted that self-initiated behavior is learned. If initiation is thwarted, the individual begins to feel helpless (that is, that he or she has no influence over his or her environment), and anxiety becomes intensified.

See also HELPLESSNESS.

learned optimism   A term coined by Martin E. P. Seligman in his book *Learned Optimism* (1991) describing attitudes and behaviors people exhibit when they face the stress of failures and disappointments that inevitably are a part of life's experience. According to Seligman, in childhood, individuals learn to explain setbacks to themselves. Some are able to say and believe: "It was just a matter of circumstance; life is speeding ahead and there is much more to look forward to." Scientific evidence has shown that this optimism is vitally important in overcoming defeat, promoting achievement, and maintaining or improving health. He documents the effects of optimism on the quality of life.

In his book, Seligman shows how to stop automatically assuming GUILT; how to get out of the habit of seeing the direst possible implications in every setback; and how to be optimistic.

The opposite of learned optimism is *helplessness*, a term Seligman coined earlier, which relates to an attitude of pessimism about the future and future activities.

See also COPING; GENERAL ADAPTATION SYNDROME; LEARNED HELPLESSNESS.

Seligman, Martin E. P., *Learned Optimism* (New York: A. Knopf, 1991).

learning, fear of   Fear of learning is known as sophophobia.

learning disabilities   A group of physical and psychological disorders that interfere with learning or make learning impossible. Because they may be taunted by their peers, young people who have such disabilities may suffer anxieties from a loss of SELF-ESTEEM and motivation. Learning disabilities are also a source of anxiety to parents who have high expectations of their children. Even when the disabilities are diagnosed, they may wonder why their children are not doing well in school and urge them to do better.

Learning disabilities include problems in learning caused by defects in speech, hearing, and memory; they do not include disabilities due to emotional or environmental deprivation or to poor teaching.

Children with minimal or borderline MENTAL RETARDATION generally have difficulty learning. Other children suffer from *hyperactivity*, which lowers the attention span; *dyslexia*, which is difficulty in reading; *dyscalculia*, an inability to perform mathematical problems; and *dysgraphia*, referring to writing disorders. Specific learning difficulties in children of normal intelligence may be caused by forms of *minimal brain dysfunction*, which may be inherited and have been untreatable.

Generally difficult to diagnose, children with learning disabilities should be observed and taught by teachers who have a degree in special education.

See also ATTENTION DEFICIT DISORDER; DISABILITIES; PARENTING.

Grey House Publishing, *The Complete Learning Disabilities Directory* (Lakeville, CT: Grey House Publishing, 1994).
Hall, David, *Living With Learning Disabilities: A Guide for Students* (Minneapolis: Lerner Publications Company, 1993).

Hoy, Cheri, Noel Gregg, Joseph Wisenbaker, et al., "Depression and anxiety in two groups of adults with learning disabilities." *Learning Disability Quarterly* 20, no. 4 (fall 1997): pp. 280–291.

learning theory   Learning theory is the study of the circumstances under which habits are formed or eliminated; it is the framework of behavior therapy and behavior modification. Learning theory is a set of principles that seeks to explain how behavior is modified in response to changes in the individual's environment. BEHAVIOR THERAPIES used to treat individuals who have anxieties and phobias are derived from the learning principles developed by PAVLOV, Thorndike, Watson, Tolman, Hull, SKINNER, WOLPE, and others whose work contributed to the theory of conditioning, motivation, and habit formation.

See also BEHAVIOR MODIFICATION; CLASSICAL CONDITIONING; CONDITIONING; MODELING; MOTIVATION; OPERANT CONDITIONING.

left, things to the, fear of   Fear of things to the left is known as sinistrophobia or levophobia. Rituals related to the rising sun may have contributed to the feeling that the left is the inferior side because the sun rises in the east, or on the right as one faces north. Many religious ceremonies contain a movement to the right, or toward the sun. By contrast, evil spells of witchcraft and black magic frequently involve a left or counterclockwise motion.

left-handedness   In religious symbolism and folklore, the left side is associated with the devil, and this attitude has permeated outlooks held by many people for centuries. Left handers often deal with subtle attitudes reflected in such phrases as a "left-handed compliment" that imply that something is wrong with being left-handed. Left-handed people are a minority in the United States, making up about 13 percent of the population.

In earlier generations, children were encouraged to use their right hands instead of their left, creating stressful situations for both parents and children. Studies of left-handedness in the population by age group show proportionally more young left-handers, probably an indication that parents and teachers are no longer trying to force these children into using their right hands.

Probably the biggest stress factor facing individuals who are left-handed is that handwriting techniques, scissors, and other kitchen and household tools are not designed with them in mind. However, special products are being made specifically for left-handers.

Scientists are unsure of what neurological factors cause handedness. There is some evidence that before birth all humans are potentially right-handed. Changes occur as the fetus develops or in the birth process that create left-handedness. The male hormone testosterone, produced by both men and women, may have something to do with left-handedness. The hypothesis is that an unusually high amount of testosterone produced by the mother before birth may enable the right side of the brain, the area that controls the left side of the body, to dominate. Studies have linked left-handedness with pregnancy in older mothers, cesarean deliveries, and difficult labor.

Studies also show that while there is a predominance of left-handers in the schizophrenic and retarded populations, left handers are statistically higher than in the general population among high scorers on standardized tests. Research of college students showed that left-handers entered fields such as graphic arts, architecture, and the sciences, which tend to be nonverbal. This is probably a reflection of the fact that the right brain controls spatial reasoning ability and other nonverbal skills.

Many famous criminals were left-handed. Evidence from the crimes of Jack the Ripper point to the fact that he was left handed, as were Billy the Kid, John Dillinger, Albert Henry DeSalvo, known as the Boston Strangler, and his lawyer, F. Lee Bailey. However, not all left-handers are infamous. Other well known left-handers include Pablo Picasso, Leonardo da Vinci, Benjamin Franklin, Babe Ruth, Marilyn Monroe, and Presidents Harry Truman and George Bush.

leprophobia, lepraphobia   See LEPROSY, FEAR OF.

leprosy, fear of   Fear of leprosy is known as lepro-phobia or lepraphobia. Leprosy is a communicable bacterial disease that primarily affects the skin and nerves, often producing severe disfigurement. This type of physical deformity is the main reason why the disease has been so feared in the past. In ancient times leprosy was well known and feared through Asia, Africa, and Europe. Today a few cases are still found in Europe and a few in the United States, particularly around the Gulf of Mexico and in Hawaii. The bacterium that causes leprosy was discovered in 1873 by G. Armauer Hansen, a Norwegian. The disease is also known as Hansen's disease. The factors influencing contraction of leprosy are unknown. There is some speculation that genetic factors determine a person's susceptibility to leprosy. Several drugs are used to treat leprosy.

See also DEFORMITY, FEAR OF.

lesbianism   The term for female HOMOSEXUALITY derived from the Greek island of Lesbos, home of the poetess Sappho. Lesbians prefer women as sexual partners, although some lesbians have or had heterosexual partners. In the late 1990s, lesbians still face anxieties related to lack of acceptance by their families, friends, coworkers and bosses, and members of the community at large.

Many lesbian couples have become parents (co-mothers) through artificial insemination and ADOPTION. While facing all the concerns and anxieties of parenthood, they may encounter particular stressors because of their sexual preference.

The gay liberation movement for civil rights for homosexuals during the 1970s and 1980s encouraged discussion of important issues and provided a political organization to work toward legal change to end discrimination. The National Gay Task Force is a clearinghouse for these groups and provides information on local organizations.

leukophobia   Fear of the color white.

See also WHITE, FEAR OF THE COLOR.

leukotomy, leucotomy   A surgical operation on the brain in which the nerve pathways in the pre-frontal lobes of the brain—the areas associated with emotion—are severed from the rest of the brain in an effort to reduce ANXIETY or violent behavior. Leukotomy is also known as prefrontal lobotomy. In recent years, this treatment has been replaced with tranquilizing medications and psychotherapy. In any case, it is not recommended as a treatment for phobias.

See also TRANQUILIZERS.

levophobia   Fear of things at the left side of the body.

See also LEFT, THINGS TO THE, FEAR OF.

libido   Sigmund Freud's term for the drives of the sexual instinct, love-object seeking, and pleasure. In many phobic and anxiety disorders, as well as affective disorders, particularly depression, there is a reduction of libido. The word is derived from the Latin words for "desire, lust." Freud believed that the libido was one of two vital human instincts, the drive toward self-preservation and the drive toward sexual gratification. Freud suggested that when an individual represses libido because of social pressures, continued repression leads to changes in personality and to neuroses such as ANXIETIES and PHOBIAS. Later, Freud gradually broadened the concept to include all expressions of love and pleasure. Jung expanded Freud's original concept to apply the term to the general life force that provides energy for all types of activities, including sexual, social, cultural, and creative.

See also SEXUAL ANXIETY.

Goldenson, Robert M. (ed.), *Longman Dictionary of Psychology and Psychiatry* (New York: Longman, 1984).

Librium   A trade name for CHLORDIAZEPOXIDE hydrochloride, an ANTIANXIETY DRUG.

lice, fear of   Fear of lice is known as phthiropho-bia or pediculophobia. Lice include a number of tiny insects that live on warm-blooded creatures, among them man. Though lice are more common in people among crowded conditions without good facilities for bathing, they are also found in all walks of life, particularly where many children congregate, such as schools and movie theaters. Head lice are particularly feared because anyone can pick up the pests from the clothing of another or from the headrest of a public vehicle. One of the first signs of lice is itching. There may be some skin eruptions containing pus. Bacteria may invade these lesions, leading to other skin diseases. Pesticides in shampoo, powder, or ointment form are available for eliminating lice.

The pubic louse (also known as crab) is found in the hairy region around the sex organs and the anus; this is transmitted by bodily contact with a person who is infested, or from toilet seats.

Individuals who fear contamination, dirt, filth, or public toilets may also fear contracting lice.

See also CONTAMINATION, FEAR OF.

life change events   See GENERALIZED ADAPTATION SYNDROME; LIFE CHANGE SELF-RATING SCALE.

life change self-rating scale   The original life change rating scale was developed by authors Holmes and Rahe as a predictor of illness based on stressful life events and presented at the Royal Society of Medicine in 1968. In many variations, this type of rating scale has been used to help individuals determine their composite stress level within the last year.

To take this test, mark any of the changes listed below that have occurred in your life in the past 12 months. Your total score indicates the amount of stress to which you have been subjected in the one-year period. Your score may be useful in predicting your chances of suffering illness in the next two years due to physiological effects of serious stressors.

What Your Score Means

A total score less than 150 may mean you have only a 27 percent chance of becoming ill in the next year. If your score is between 150 and 300, you have a 51 percent chance of encountering poor health. If your score is more than 300, you are facing odds of 80 percent that you will become ill, and as the score increases, so do the chances that the problem will

LIFE CHANGE SELF-RATING SCALE

Event	Value
Death of spouse	100
Divorce	73
Marital separation	65
Death of close family member	63
Personal injury or illness	53
Marriage	50
Fired from work	47
Marital reconciliation	45
Retirement	45
Change in family member's health	44
Pregnancy	40
Sex difficulties	39
Addition to family	39
Business readjustment	39
Change in financial status	38
Death of close friend	37
Change to different line of work	36
Foreclosure of mortgage or loan	30
Change in work responsibilities	29
Son or daughter leaving home	29
Trouble with in-laws	29
Outstanding personal achievement	28
Spouse begins or stops work	26
Starting or finishing school	26
Change in living conditions	25
Trouble with boss	23
Change in residence or school	20
Change in recreational habits	19
Change in church or social activities	19
Change in sleeping habits	16
Change in eating habits	15
Vacation	13
Christmas season	12
Minor violation of the law	11
Your total score:	

be serious. To avoid these consequences, attention to RELAXATION and STRESS relief can help.

(Adapted from Holmes and Rahe, *Life Change Measurements as a Predictor of Illness*, proceedings, Royal Society of Medicine, 1968.)

light, fear of   Fear of light is known as photophobia or phengophobia. This fear may be related to fear of light and shadows, fear of dawn, or fear of landscape.

See also DAWN, FEAR OF; LANDSCAPE, FEAR OF; LIGHT AND SHADOWS, FEAR OF.

light and shadows, fear of   Just as some individuals fear certain landscapes, some fear light-and-shadow effects. This may relate to a fear of twilight and the onset of darkness. From a psychoanalytic point of view, there may be deeper meaning to such fears. FENICHEL, an Austrian psychoanalyst (1899–1946), said, "Probably many phobias of darkness or twilight contain memories of PRIMAL SCENES."

lightning, fear of   Fear of lightning is known as astraphobia, astropophobia, and keraunophobia. Many people fear lightning so much that they will not go outdoors on days when lightning is predicted. When rain is forecast, many even call the weather bureau to check for the possibility of lightning. During a storm that includes lightning, many take refuge in a closet or in bed, feeling safer in an enclosed place. Fear of lightning is related to fear of storms in general, and many who fear lightning also fear thunder and noise.

Some individuals acquire the fear of lightning from observing their parents or grandparents. Others have experienced traumatic incidents in connection with lightning or thunderstorms.

Fears of specific natural phenomena, such as lightning, have been treated successfully in many cases with exposure therapy.

See also CLIMATE, FEAR OF; STORMS, FEAR OF; THUNDER, FEAR OF.

Ost, Lars-Goran, "Behavioral Treatment of Thunder and Lightning Phobias," *Behavior Research and Therapy* 16 (1978): pp. 197–207.

light therapy   See SEASONAL AFFECTIVE DISORDER.

ligyrophobia   Fear of noise.
See NOISE, FEAR OF.

lilapsophobia   See HURRICANES, FEAR OF.

limbic system   Part of the midbrain that controls expression of emotional behavior and basic motivational urges. The limbic system, part of the autonomic nervous system, also controls speed of heartbeat and breathing, trembling, sweating, and alterations in facial expression, as well as drives including defense, attack (fight or flight), hunger, thirst, and sex.

limnophobia   Fear of lakes.
See also LAKES, FEAR OF.

linonophobia   See STRING, FEAR OF.

listening   Listening, hearing with thoughtful attention, is a skill necessary for good COMMUNICATION between individuals. It is an active process in which one gives complete attention to what the other is saying and how they are saying it. According to Deborah Tannen, author of *Talking from 9 to 5: How Women's and Men's Conversational Styles Affect Who Gets Heard, Who Gets Credit and What Gets Done at Work,* "Listening taps two important areas, gathering information and developing relationships." Active listening can reduce the anxieties of communication not only in business but personal life as well.

By using nonverbal gestures such as a nod of the head or a smile, active listeners can convey concern

---

REDUCE ANXIETIES WITH BETTER LISTENING SKILLS

- Focus on the speaker; use eye contact. Keep interruptions, such as phone calls and other conversations to a minimum.
- It helps to question the speaker. You can gently guide a conversation, show that you are interested in what he/she is saying, and what you might want to learn.
- Don't judge the person speaking; concentrate on the information he/she is presenting.

and reinforce or encourage the other's verbalizations. Listeners contribute by asking good questions, providing FEEDBACK on what they hear, and seeking consensus or pointing out differences of opinion within a group. On the other hand, a person feels listened to when more than just their ideas get heard; they feel valued, and they will contribute a lot more to the conversation.

See also BODY LANGUAGE.

Tannen, Deborah, *Talking from 9 to 5: How Women's and Men's Conversational Styles Affect Who Gets Heard, Who Gets Credit and What Gets Done at Work* (New York: William Morrow, 1994).

Nichols, Michael P., *The Lost Art of Listening* (New York: Doubleday, 1995).

lithium carbonate A drug used in treating BIPOLAR DISORDER. Lithium acts by altering the metabolism of NOREPINEPHRINE in the brain. Lithium preparations are used routinely to treat manic and hypomanic individuals and to prevent attacks in individuals who have recurrent affective disorders. These attacks include both manic and depressive episodes in bipolar individuals, episodes of mania in recurrently manic patients, and depressive attacks in unipolar (only depressed) patients. Other conditions in which lithium treatment has been claimed effective include aggressive behavior, schizophrenia, epilepsy, alcoholism, Huntington's chorea, and premenstrual tension. However, as these claims are based mainly on clinical impressions and uncontrolled trials, they remain controversial.

Historical Background

During the 19th century, lithium salts were known as important constituents of some spa waters to which many medicinal properties were ascribed. In the 1940s, lithium salts were used as a taste substitute for sodium chloride for cardiac patients on saltfree diets. When severe side effects and some deaths were reported, its use was stopped. Then, in the late 1940s, researchers in Australia discovered that lithium had certain tranquilizing properties. In later experiments, lithium safely quieted manic patients to whom it was administered. However, because of the known toxicity of lithium, there

was little interest in it for almost a decade. In the 1950s and 1960s, several studies in Europe led to the acceptance of lithium in European and English psychiatric practices as a highly effective and safe treatment for manic-depressive illness. Lithium was accepted into American practice during the 1970s after the need for careful monitoring of blood levels to overcome side effects was understood.

Lithium also has been used in the U.S. since the 1970s because of its prophylactic qualities, preventing not only manic attacks and depressive episodes, but perhaps schizoaffective attacks as well. There is ongoing evaluation of the effectiveness of lithium in treating episodes of depression. Some uncontrolled studies suggested that perhaps 50 percent of depressed individuals might respond. Individuals who have endogenous depression—mainly those who have bipolar illnesses—respond best, but still at a lesser rate than with standard tricyclic antidepressant therapy. The improvement with lithium is often only partial, suggesting the value of combining lithium and tricyclic therapy; however, this is still controversial and under research.

How Lithium Works

The major ways in which lithium works are uncertain. However, it is known that lithium alters many electrolyte and neurotransmitter functions. For example, synthesis and release of acetycholine are depressed. Also, because lithium interferes with calcium, release of many neurotransmitters, including monoamines, is diminished. In normal individuals, lithium produces mild subjective feelings of lethargy and inability to concentrate. Sometimes it causes a decrease in memory function. Slow waves in the electrocardiogram increase.

Lithium as a Prophylactic

On current evidence, lithium therapy is most suitable for individuals who have a long history of many typical affective episodes. Any individual who has had two or more distinct manic-depressive episodes during one year or one or more separate attacks each year during the preceding two years should be evaluated and considered a candidate for lithium treatment. Individuals who have bipolar illnesses are more likely to respond than are patients who have unipolar depression, and the more closely the individual fits the bipolar stereotype, the better the chance of a good response. Some psychiatrists try maintenance therapy with tricyclic antidepressant, especially in unipolar individuals, before initiating lithium therapy. If an individual does not show an adequate response to lithium within the first year of treatment, the drug should be discontinued because it may be unwise to expose the individual to the risks of lithium treatment without benefit. While there is complete prevention for some individuals, lithium provides maintenance therapy for others, in whom the attacks are only reduced to the point at which the individual can be managed as an outpatient instead of being admitted to a hospital.

Dosage

Dosage depends on both the severity of the illness and the particular preparation; dosage should be governed by serum concentrations. Before initiating lithium therapy, the individual should have a complete physical examination. Suggested contraindications include chronic kidney failure, high blood pressure, and a history of heart problems, although in some cases individuals who have these symptoms can take lithium successfully if carefully monitored by their physicians. Lithium is not appropriate therapy for children.

Side Effects

Mild neurological side effects, especially during initial treatment, include general and muscular fatigue, lethargy, and mild shaking. The shaking, or tremor, usually begins early in treatment and may or may not resolve or lessen. Lowering the dose or adding a small dose of a beta-adrenoceptor antagonist such as propranolol usually minimizes the tremor. Early signs of toxicity include incoordination, difficulty in concentration, mild disorientation, muscle twitching, dizziness, and visual disturbances. Lithium affects thyroid function at several sites. The main effect is inhibition of release of thyroid hormones; hypothyroidism follows in some cases. Also, lithium use may be associated with alterations in bone-mineral metabolism, leading to osteoporosis in women.

See also AFFECTIVE DISORDERS; ANTIDEPRESSANTS; BIPOLAR DISORDER; DRUGS; ELECTROCARDIOGRAM; ENDOGENOUS DEPRESSION; HUNTINGTON'S CHOREA; HYPOTHYROIDISM; PREMENSTRUAL SYNDROME (PMS); PROPHYLACTIC; TRICYCLIC ANTIDEPRESSANTS.

Lader, Malcolm, *Introduction to Psychopharmacology* (Kalamazoo, MI: Upjohn Company, 1980).

litigaphobia Excessive fear of litigation or lawsuits. Twentieth-century American society has shown a rise in litigation as a means of solving interpersonal and societal difficulties. Many professionals now extensively document all procedures because of this fear.

Little Hans In the case of Little Hans, titled "Analysis of a Phobia in a Five-Year Old Boy," Sigmund Freud interpreted a young boy's horse phobias as a repressed fear of his father. In his conversation with Freud, Hans revealed that "what horses wear around their eyes" and "the black around their mouths" were disturbing to him. Freud related these remarks to the appearance of Hans's father, who had a mustache and wore glasses. Since Hans had a clinging relationship with his mother, Freud believed that Hans resented his father and also feared punishment in the form of castration because of his love for his mother. This case is significant because of the psychiatric implication that the phobic is not really disturbed by the thing ostensibly feared but has displaced his actual feelings onto something that can be avoided. Freud, who never saw Little Hans and really did not conduct therapy with him, obtained information through correspondence (and an occasional meeting) with Hans's father. JOSEPH WOLPE, who has reinterpreted this case from a classical-conditioning theory standpoint, convincingly demonstrates why this approach has a more powerful explanation.

Kaplan, Harold I., *Comprehensive Textbook of Psychiatry* (Baltimore: Williams and Wilkins, 1985).
Stoodley, Bartlett, *The Concepts of Sigmund Freud* (Glencoe, IL: The Free Press, 1959).

live-in A live-in is a common term for members of the opposite sex who share a domicile without the benefit of marriage. In many cases, anxieties arise when one individual decides he/she wants to get married and the other does not. Additionally, anxieties arise if the couple decides to break up. Besides the hurt feelings and blows to the ego, there may be mutually owned property or equipment, and live-ins may face the same dilemmas as a couple going through a DIVORCE.

Live-in is a term that evolved during the 1980s, when this practice became fairly common in the United States among men and women of all ages. The demographic term for this situation, used by the U.S. Census, is *POSSLQ* (person of the opposite sex sharing living quarters).

See also FRIENDS; INTIMACY; RELATIONSHIPS.

lizards, fear of   Fear of lizards is known as herpetophobia. This fear is related to fear of snakes.

See also SNAKES, FEAR OF.

lobotomy   A surgical operation on the brain in which the nerve pathways from the frontal lobes of the brain and the thalamus (part of the forebrain that serves as a relay point for nerve impulses between the spinal cord, the brainstem, and the cerebral cortex) are cut in the hope of bringing about beneficial behavior changes. This operation is not recommended as a treatment for phobias; the operation was rarely performed toward the end of the 20th century. Instead, psychotherapy and tranquilizing drugs are used to control unwanted behaviors. In the absence of any treatments, lobotomies were occasionally used on patients with chronic anxiety problems.

See also LEUKOTOMY.

lockiophobia   Fear of childbirth.

lockjaw, fear of   Fear of lockjaw, or tetanus, is known as tetanophobia. The condition is particularly feared because one of the first signs of the disease is a spasm or cramping of the muscles that close the jaw, making it difficult for the individual to open his or her mouth. The condition can be prevented by immunization.

locus ceruleus (coeruleus)   The locus ceruleus (also known as the pons) is a tiny organ in the brain that is thought to play a role in the development of fearful behavior. The locus ceruleus, rich in norepinephrine, contains nearly half the noradrenergic neurons and produces over 70 percent of the total adrenaline in the brain. Overactivity of the locus ceruleus and the noradrenergic system may be linked to the cause of anxiety attacks in some individuals.

Eugene Redmone's research on the relationship between brain activity and anxiety attacks at Yale University in the 1980s, using monkeys, indicated that when the locus ceruleus was electrically stimulated, the monkeys showed anxious and fearful behavior. However, when the same area was surgically stimulated, the monkeys were unresponsive to threats and did not show normal fear when approached by humans or dominant monkeys. In other studies, destruction of the locus ceruleus also reduced naturally occurring fear reactions. Findings from this research were significant because they indicated that the locus ceruleus is vulnerable to the influence of substances in the blood, indicating a possible physiological basis for panic attacks. Researchers speculate that panic, anxiety, and fear may be controlled by changes in norepinephrine metabolism in the brain.

Marks, Isaac M., *Fears, Phobias and Rituals* (New York: Oxford University Press, 1987).

locus of control   A concept that attempts to explain why some people behave the way they do and why some have more anxieties than others. An individual with an "internal" locus of control believes that whatever happens in his life is the direct result of his own actions, and that he has some control over these events and his behavior. A person who believes that God, destiny, or outside forces determine his fate is said to have an "external" locus of control. People who have an external locus of control are more likely to develop anxieties. Most people are not entirely internalists or externalists but feel more or less in control of their lives. An individual's belief about his locus of control affects his behavior, emotional condition, and manner of dealing with anxieties. The concept was developed in the late 1960s by Julian Rotter (1916–87).

logophobia   Fear of words.

See also WORDS, FEAR OF.

logotherapy   A technique for dealing with the spiritual and existential aspect of psychopathology. The therapist confronts individuals with their own responsibility for their existence and their obligation to pursue the values inherent in life. The technique, useful in treating some phobics, was developed by Viktor Frankl, a German-born American psychiatrist (1905–97).

See also EXISTENTIAL THERAPY; PARADOXICAL INTENTION.

lonely, being, fear of   Fear of being lonely is known as monophobia. This fear seems to increase with age as an individual sees friends and loved ones dying and anticipates having few contemporaries around. Fear of loneliness is compounded by the fear of illness.

Loneliness is a state of mind relating to lack of companionship or separation from others. It is different from being alone, which is a question of choice. It is this lack of choice that makes loneliness so filled with anxiety.

When people feel lonely, they are most likely to react in one of two ways. The first is sadness, indicated by too much time spent eating, sleeping, and crying. The other response is "creative solitude," where a person finds ways to deal with loneliness such as reading or watching a movie, listening to or playing music, using artistic talents to paint, crochet, quilt, weave or do ceramics, spending time in the garden, or pursuing other interests and hobbies. When people deal with loneliness creatively, they are in fact fighting BOREDOM and, in the process, they become happier, calmer, and less stressed.

Some lonely people fit the shy, retiring stereotype; others compensate for their feelings by trying to become the center of attraction whether it be in the classroom or at a party. Individuals who have spouses and families can be lonely even though they are surrounded by people. Adolescents and teenagers may become lonely when they long to be part of their peer group and are not. Many widowed or divorced people in their later years become lonely as their friends die and they find it increasingly difficulty to make new friends.

Conditions such as mental and physical DISABILITIES or language or ethnic barriers sometimes produce isolation that results in loneliness.

Research on Loneliness

In some cases, loneliness results from a sense of loss, a feeling that the past was better than the present. A 1990 Gallup poll showed that loneliness is most common among the widowed, separated, and divorced. Over half of this group felt lonely "frequently" or "sometimes" compared with 29 percent of the married participants. Adults who had never married fell in between. According to the survey, women are more likely to be lonely than men, possibly not because they genuinely have less companionship, but because they place more importance on friendship and are more willing to confess to being lonely.

Loneliness is often a factor in DEPRESSION, drug ADDICTION, and ALCOHOLISM. In recent years, many studies have shown that the more connected to life individuals are, the healthier—mentally and physically—they will be.

According to *The Complete Guide to Your Emotions and to Your Health*, results of a survey conducted by social researchers Rubenstein and Shaver indicate that loneliness has little to do with the number of people in a given living situation, but was more apt to be defined by people's expectations of life and reactions to their environment. Rubenstein and Shaver's questionnaire drew 22,000 respondents over the age of 18. The survey confirms that "feeling lonely"—regardless of living arrangement—is associated with greater health risks, including some psychological symptoms such as anxiety, depression, crying spells, and feeling worthless. Nearly one-quarter of the people who lived alone fell into the "least lonely" category. They had more friends on the average than people who lived with other people and were less troubled by symptoms of stress such as HEADACHES, ANGER, and irritability.

By comparison, young people who continued to live with parents after college appeared to be the loneliest of all respondents. Rubenstein explains, "A young person in this situation has different expectations. If there's no girlfriend or boyfriend in the picture, they face a social-psychological conflict. For young adults, in particular being alone—especially on Saturday night—can be a stigma. This makes them feel rejected and lonely."

Key to combating loneliness is maintaining a feeling of self-worth and the ability to care not only for yourself but for other people and other things. Altruistic people lose themselves in others. The process can block out depression, make us less aware of our own inadequacies, and help us surmount our personal problems. When you maintain a pattern of caring, whether for a house, a garden, pets, or other people, you are protecting yourself against despair. And in the process, you'll live a more happy and healthy existence—whether alone or in the company of others.

See also COPING; DEPRESSION; GENERAL ADAPTATION SYNDROME; GROWING OLD, FEAR OF; HOBBIES; VOLUNTEERISM.

Olds, Jacqueline, Richard S. Schwartz, and Harriet Webster, *Overcoming Loneliness in Everyday Life* (Secaucus, N.J.: Carol Publishing Group, 1996).

longitudinal study   A study in which observations of the same group of individuals are made at two or more different points in time usually after an initial intervention. An example of a longitudinal study is one in which observations are made about a group of agoraphobics and then the same variable is observed after a particular pharmacological therapy has been initiated.

See also CASE CONTROL; COHORT.

long waits, fear of   Also known as macrophobia. Some agoraphobics fear long waits, such as for buses and trains. This fear may prevent them from going out. In some cases, agoraphobics develop such a feeling of panic while waiting for a bus or train that when it finally arrives, they cannot board. However, if there is no wait, they can get on without anxiety.

See also AGORAPHOBIA.

looking-glass self   The concept of the self as a reflection of how other people react to and what other people think of the individual. The looking-glass-self concept is significant in many phobias, including agoraphobia and social phobias.

looking ridiculous, fear of   Fear of looking ridiculous is a social phobia that includes many specific fears, such as fear of shaking, blushing, sweating, fainting, vomiting, performing in front of an audience, entering a room, and looking inappropriate or unattractive. Some may not swim because they think they look ridiculous in a swimsuit. Some fear that their hands will tremble while writing a check or handling money in front of someone else. Fear of shaking may prevent a secretary from typing, or a teacher from writing on the blackboard. In such cases, the phobics fear that their hands or heads might shake; in reality, these fears rarely materialize. However, individuals who have tremors such as that of Parkinson's disease, who shake vigorously and unconsciously, usually do not fear doing anything in public despite their regular shaking. Generally, individuals who fear looking ridiculous have fewer positive and more negative thoughts and consider themselves awkward and less skillful. This fear is treated in the same ways social phobias and shyness are treated, specifically with behavior modification, cognitive modification, and other therapies aimed at improving the individual's self-esteem.

See also BEHAVIOR MODIFICATION; SELF-ESTEEM; SHYNESS; SOCIAL PHOBIA.

losing control, fear of   Many phobic individuals avoid their feared situations because they fear "losing control." For example, during a panic attack, some people fear that they might become totally paralyzed and not be able to move, or that they will not know what they are doing and will embarrass themselves or others in some way. Some agoraphobics who experience panic attacks have this fear. This feeling occurs because during intense anxiety the entire body becomes prepared for action and escape. This "fight or flight" response often makes people feel confused and distracted; however, individuals in such situations are still able to think and function normally. In fact, others rarely notice another individual experiencing a panic attack.

See also AGORAPHOBIA; PANIC.

lost, fear of being Fear of being lost is common among children as well as adults. In childhood, the fear of being lost is reinforced by such fairy tales as "Hansel and Gretel," in which the children lose their way in the forest. Fear of being lost is a fear of being out of control of one's destiny and may be related to fears of the dark, of animals, of injury, and of being far from safety. Fear of being lost may prevent individuals from visiting certain areas in major cities or from visiting the cities themselves. Fear of being lost also prevents many people from driving their cars in certain areas or on unfamiliar roads. Those who do not speak the language of the country in which they consider traveling may fear being lost and not being able to communicate well enough to ask for directions.

love, fear of Fear of love is known as philophobia. Love is a complex emotion comprising trust, respect, acceptance, strong affection, feelings of tenderness, pleasurable sensations in the presence of the love object, and devotion to his or her well-being. Love as an emotion takes many forms, such as concern for one's fellow humans, responsibility for the welfare of a child, sexual attraction and excitement, and self-esteem and self-acceptance.

See also COMMITMENT PHOBIA.

love play, fear of Fear of love play, or foreplay before sexual intercourse, is known as sarmassophobia or malaxophobia.

See also SEXUAL FEARS.

luiphobia A fear of lues, a synonymn for SYPHILIS. Lues is derived from the Latin word for "infection" or "plague."

See also SEXUALLY TRANSMITTED DISEASES.

lump in the throat A feeling of a "lump in the throat" (medically known as globus hystericus) is one of the most common symptoms of ANXIETY. Most people, whether phobic or not, have experienced this sensation at one time or another. Some people experience it before a job interview or a public speech and fear that they will not have their usual strong voice. The "lump" may actually cause some difficulty in swallowing, although the sufferer usually can make enough effort to eat. However, when one concentrates on swallowing, the problem may worsen. Lump in the throat is more often noticed in young adults, particularly women. The symptom, while unpleasant and uncomfortable, can usually be relieved with relaxation techniques and completion of the stressful event.

Lump in the throat should not be confused with symptoms of several serious diseases that can cause difficulty in swallowing first solid foods and then liquids, resulting in weight loss. In these cases, a physician should be consulted. X rays of the esophagus may be recommended.

See also GAGGING, HYPERSENSITIVE; SWALLOWING, FEAR OF.

lunaphobia Fear of the Moon.

lung disease, fear of Fear of lung disease is related to health anxieties in general and fear of illness. Some people fear lung diseases because the lungs are particularly vulnerable to particles floating in the air. Those who fear contamination by bacteria or other germs may fear lung diseases for this reason. Those who fear AIR POLLUTION, ACID RAIN, and ACID DEW may also fear lung disease. Fear of tuberculosis is included in many people's fears of lung diseases, but because of improved public health measures, pasteurization of milk, and routine examination of cattle, tuberculosis is becoming rare in developed countries. However, some individuals, particularly older people, still fear tuberculosis because they remember when the disease was widespread and less curable than it is today. At its height tuberculosis affected one half of the world population.

See also ASTHMA; TUBERCULOSIS, FEAR OF.

lutraphobia Fear of otters.

lygophobia Fear of being in dark or gloomy places. Derived from the Greek word *lyge,* meaning twilight.

See also DARKNESS, FEAR OF.

lying, fear of Fear of lying is known as mythophobia. Lying—making false statements with conscious intent to deceive—may be considered nonpathological or pathological. An example of nonpathological lying is when adults or children seek to avoid punishment or to save others from distress; these are sometimes referred to as "white lies." Pathological lying is a major characteristic of an antisocial personality and may be a symptom of many psychophysiological disorders due to guilt and fear reactions. The lie detector (polygraph) is based on physiological reactions. Many individuals fear lying because they fear being caught in a lie and being punished.

lyssophobia Fear of becoming insane or of dealing with insanity. This fear is also known as maniaphobia and lissophobia.

See also GOING CRAZY, FEAR OF; SCHIZOPHRENIA.

machinery, fear of Fear of machinery is known as mechanophobia. This fear is somewhat related to fears of technical things, such as computers.

See also COMPUTER PHOBIA.

macrophobia See LONG WAITS, FEAR OF.

mageirocophobia Fear of cooking.

magic, fear of Fear of magic is primarily concerned with the fear of and desire for supraconscious power and striving for connection with a greater power. Magicians consider themselves capable not of working miracles, but of using the powers of their minds and their knowledge of the laws and secrets of nature as a way of exerting control over nature and human events. Some magicians believe that man is a miniature replica of God and capable of expanding his powers accordingly, not in the rational path of progress provided by science, but by ascending a hierarchy of mysterious secrets; this process is an individual matter and cannot be taught.

Prehistoric cave paintings indicate that early man believed in and feared magic. The Egyptians, Greeks, and Romans combined magical beliefs and practices with their religious observances. Early Christians successfully claimed the superior power of their magic to gain pagan converts. For a time Christianity rejected magic, but the medieval church revived it, claiming the power to exert a certain degree of control over God's will and the course of events. During the Reformation Protestants branded as superstitions the use of holy water and belief in the intercession of the saints.

The power of black magic, to a certain extent, may be a self-fulfilling prophecy. An individual cursed by a person he believes to be a witch or magician may become mentally or physically ill from sheer anxiety.

See also WITCHES AND WITCHCRAFT, FEAR OF.

magical thinking A primitive thought process based on the illusion that thinking can influence events, fulfill wishes, or ward off evil or feared objects or situations. There is a lack of realistic relationship between cause and effect in magical thinking. Magical thinking begins in childhood and shows up later as obsessive thoughts, ritual acts, dreams, fantasies, and superstitions.

See also CHILDHOOD FEARS, PHOBIAS, AND ANXIETIES.

maieusiophobia Fear of childbirth.
See also CHILDBIRTH, FEAR OF.

malaxophobia Fear of love play.
See also LOVE PLAY, FEAR OF; SEXUAL FEARS; SEXUAL INTERCOURSE, FEAR OF.

mania An affective or mood disorder in which the individual is excessively elated, agitated, and hyperactive and has accelerated thinking and speaking. The more up-to-date term is manic episode or manic syndrome.

See also AFFECTIVE DISORDERS; BIPOLAR DISORDER; MANIC-DEPRESSIVE DISORDER.

maniaphobia Fear of INSANITY. Also known as lyssophobia.

manic-depressive disorder See BIPOLAR DISORDER.

manic episode A reaction characterized by a recurring period of extreme elation, extreme euphoria without reason, and grandiose thoughts or feelings about personal abilities. The manic episode may be a phase of manic-depressive disorder.

mantra A special word or phrase that one repeats over and over again, or an object on which one concentrates, while meditating. Meditation is a very self-disciplined routine and a way to learn more about one's own thoughts and feelings. Simple procedures can be learned easily. The basics include sitting in a quiet room with eyes closed, breathing deeply and rhythmically with attention focused on the breath.

See also MEDITATION.

many things, fear of Fear of many things is known as polyphobia. Individuals who are very anxious often have many phobias. Such individuals may have related phobias, such as fear of precipices, fear of heights, and fear of looking up at tall buildings. Others have unrelated fears, such as fear of water and fear of dogs.

See also EVERYTHING, FEAR OF.

MAOIs See MONOAMINE OXIDASE INHIBITORS.

maprotiline An antidepressant drug. Also known by the tradename Ludiomil, maprotiline is similar in action to the TRICYCLIC ANTIDEPRESSANTS but generally has fewer side effects.

See also ANTIDEPRESSANTS, NEW; DEPRESSION.

LaPierre, Y. D., "New Antidepressant Drugs," *Journal of Clinical Psychiatry* (August 1983): pp. 41–44.

marijuana The most commonly abused illegal drug in the United States. It is sometimes referred to as *cannabis.* Delta-9-tetrahydrocannabinol (THC)

TRENDS IN THIRTY-DAY PREVALENCE OF DAILY USE OF MARIJUANA FOR EIGHTH, TENTH, AND TWELFTH GRADERS, COLLEGE STUDENTS, AND YOUNG ADULTS (AGES 19–28)

	2000	2001	2002	2003	2004
8th Grade	1.3	1.3	1.2	1.0	0.8
10th Grade	3.8	4.5	3.9	3.6	3.2
12th Grade	6.0	5.8	6.0	6.0	5.6
College Students	4.6	4.5	4.1	4.7	4.5
Young Adults	4.2	5.0	4.5	5.3	5.0

Adapted from Johnston, Lloyd D., et al., *Monitoring the Future: National Survey Results on Drug Use, 1975–2004.* Volume II: College Students & Adults Ages 19–45. Bethesda, MD: National Institute on Drug Abuse, National Institutes of Health, 2005, p. 53.

is the active ingredient in marijuana that causes the intoxication. The green leaves of the marijuana plant (*cannabis sativa*) are dried and ground up to create the drug. Extraction and the further drying of the plant's resin is used to make hashish, a more powerful drug than marijuana with a higher concentration of THC.

Many individuals use and abuse marijuana under the assumption that it will help relieve their anxieties and stresses; however, in some cases, marijuana *increases* anxiety, particularly among heavy and chronic users. Marijuana use has been implicated in the onset of PANIC ATTACKS in some individuals.

Marijuana is usually smoked in cigarettes and pipes. It is also chewed and can be included in baked products, such as cookies.

Most marijuana that is used in the United States is trafficked from other countries such as Mexico, but some marijuana is illegally produced within the borders of the United States.

After alcohol, marijuana is the most popular drug of abuse among adolescents and young adults. Researchers report that marijuana use was slightly down in 2004 among students in the 8th, 10th, and 12th grades, as well as among college students and young adults, compared to the marijuana use of these same groups in 2003. (See table above.)

There were 14.6 million users of marijuana of all ages in the United States in 2004, according to the National Survey on Drug Use and Health, and about 2 million people tried marijuana for the first time in 2004.

Effects of Marijuana

Marijuana has positive effects and potential side effects. Some users say that they achieve a feeling of relaxation, mild euphoria, and sharpness in perception. Physiologically, there is a slight increase in the heart rate and an increased appetite. Some marijuana users believe that marijuana and other drugs make them more creative and allow them to think more clearly. Such claims are probably unfounded.

Smoking marijuana may have some of the same harmful health effects as smoking tobacco, which is now recognized to cause cancer and other severe respiratory illnesses. Another danger of marijuana use as a way to control anxieties is that users may become so dependent on it that they lose interest in all other aspects of life and develop a dependence on the drug. It is also dangerous for individuals under the influence of marijuana to drive motor vehicles, because the drug slows down normal reaction times and thus increases the risk for car crashes.

Many marijuana users combine marijuana with alcohol and other drugs, such as cocaine or methamphetamine, increasing their health risks further.

Marijuana use, particularly by women smokers, has been associated with panic attacks.

Chronic Marijuana Use

Chronic or frequent marijuana use is much more risky than occasional use. The frequent abuser of marijuana is at risk for the development of psychiatric symptoms, such as acute panic reactions, paranoia, and psychosis. Demotivation is a definite long-term side effect of chronic use. In addition,

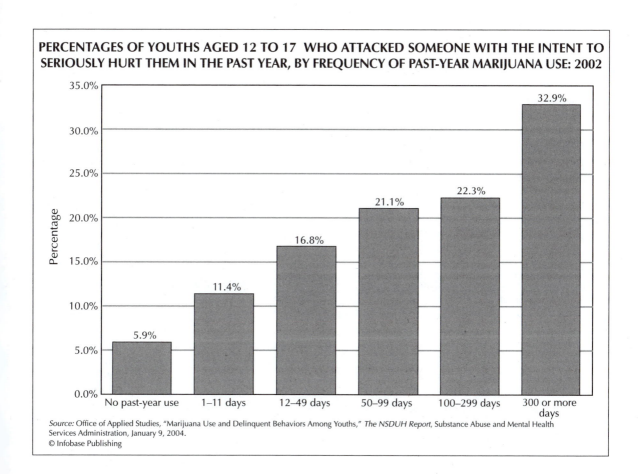

PERCENTAGES OF YOUTHS AGED 12 TO 17 WHO ATTACKED SOMEONE WITH THE INTENT TO SERIOUSLY HURT THEM IN THE PAST YEAR, BY FREQUENCY OF PAST-YEAR MARIJUANA USE: 2002

Source: Office of Applied Studies, "Marijuana Use and Delinquent Behaviors Among Youths," *The NSDUH Report,* Substance Abuse and Mental Health Services Administration, January 9, 2004.
© Infobase Publishing

contrary to its mythical image as a drug causing a person to become relaxed and/or euphoric, the chronic use of marijuana can lead to aggressive behaviors. Some studies have shown a clear link between an increased number of violent acts of adolescents and an increased frequency of marijuana use. (See the chart on page 333.) For example, in one study in 2002, 5.9 percent of adolescents who did *not* use marijuana attacked another person, with the intent to harm them. This percentage steadily climbed with increased use, up to 32.9 percent for individuals who used marijuana on 300 or more days per year.

Chronic marijuana use can impede memory, as demonstrated in studies with college students and other populations. It is unknown if the memory impairment is long term.

Medical Marijuana

Some states have passed laws whereby individuals with medical problems, such as cancer or chronic pain conditions, may use marijuana for medicinal purposes. This is a controversial issue and the Drug Enforcement Administration and other federal agencies have stated their public opposition to the use of marijuana for any purpose other than government-controlled and approved clinical studies. As of this writing, such a study is being conducted on the possible benefits of marijuana to control pain, but the results will not be available for at least several years.

See also DRUG ABUSE.

Gwinnell, Esther, M.D., and Christine Adamec, *The Encyclopedia of Drug Abuse* (New York: Facts On File, Inc., 2008).

Substance Abuse and Mental Health Services Administration, *Overview of Findings from the 2004 National Survey on Drug Use and Health.* Washington, DC, Department of Health and Human Services, September 2005.

marital therapy   Many individuals who have anxieties resulting from a difficult or troubled MARRIAGE choose to engage in marital therapy. This may involve couples or individual therapy, which may be directed toward overcoming specific problems, such as COPING with a spouse's DEPRESSION, help-ing one partner manage MONEY better, helping one partner overcome an unwanted compulsion—such as GAMBLING—or toward saving a marriage that might be headed for DIVORCE. Psychological counseling or SEX THERAPY, or a combination of both, may be involved in marital therapy.

In some cases, just the suggestion of marital therapy is a source of anxiety to one or the other partners. For the therapy to have a chance at succeeding, it is essential that both partners participate actively and honestly.

See also BEHAVIOR THERAPY; FAMILY THERAPY; INTIMACY; MARRIAGE; PSYCHOTHERAPY; RELATIONSHIPS; REMARRIAGE.

Trudel, Gilles, Lyne Landry, and Yvette Larose, "Low sexual desire: The role of anxiety, depression and marital adjustment." *Sexual and Marital Therapy* 121, no. 1 (February 1997): pp. 95–99.

marriage, fear of   Fear of marriage is known as gamophobia or gametophobia.

masked depression   Some people appear to be well but work hard at hiding DEPRESSION. For them, the hiding is a major source of anxiety. They outwardly do what they think is expected of them while inwardly they feel hopeless and even suicidal. They may have little facial animation, appear to have a fixed expression, and show little emotion. The terms *depressive equivalents, affective equivalents, hidden depression,* and *missed depression* are other terms used for this condition. Some mental health professionals use the term *borderline depression* to describe this situation.

See also AFFECTIVE DISORDERS; MANIC-DEPRESSIVE DISORDER; PHARMACOLOGICAL APPROACH.

massage therapy   A form of body therapy and complementary alternative medicine (CAM) in which the practitioner applies manual techniques such as kneading, stroking, and manipulation of the soft tissues of the body, including the skin, muscles, tendons, and ligaments, with the intention of positively affecting the health and well-being of the client. Massage therapy is also called *body work.*

Massage therapy helps many people relieve their anxieties, as well as the muscle and body aches that are often caused by tension and stress. The average massage therapy session lasts from 30–60 minutes.

A professional massage increases blood flow and also relaxes the muscles. Massage therapy can provide anything from soothing RELAXATION to therapy for specific physical problems. In addition, it can aid in recovery from pulled muscles or sprained ligaments. Massage therapy can also ease many of the uncomfortable stresses of child bearing and the discomforts of BACK PAIN and exhaustion, as well as the pains of certain REPETITIVE STRESS INJURIES related to on-the-job activities.

Once the massage is underway, many beneficial reactions are set in motion. Massage therapy can hasten the elimination of waste and toxic debris stored in muscles, increase the interchange of substances between the blood and tissue cells, and stimulate the relaxation response within the nervous system. Responses to massage therapy can help to strengthen the immune system, improve posture, increase joint flexibility and range of motion, and reduce blood pressure.

Some experts say that massage therapy may provide stimulation that blocks pain signals to the brain. Others say that it may shift the individual's nervous system from the sympathetic nervous system (which mobilizes the body for action) to the parasympathetic nervous system (in which the heart rate and breathing slow down). It may also increase the production of chemicals such as serotonin or endorphins, which can help to relax the body. Massage therapy may also promote sleep; the lack of sleep can contribute to muscle pain.

According to the National Center on Complementary and Alternative Medicine (NCCAM), a federal agency, a 2004 study revealed that of 31,000 participants, 5 percent had used massage therapy in the past year and 9.3 percent had ever used it. The survey also revealed that of those who used massage therapy, more than half or 60 percent thought that a combination of conventional medicine and massage therapy would improve their problem.

Precautions

Note that massage therapy is not recommended when patients have one or more of these conditions

- damaged blood vessels
- a bleeding disorder or the taking of medication that thins the blood, such as warfarin (Coumadin)
- deep vein thrombosis (a blood clot, most frequently in the legs)
- bones that are weakened by osteoporosis
- a fever
- any of these conditions in an area that would be massaged:
  - a tumor
  - damaged nerves
  - an open or healing wound
  - an infection or acute inflammation
  - inflammation caused by radiation treatment

In addition, individuals with the following conditions should consult their physician before receiving massage therapy

- cancer
- pregnancy
- heart problems
- fragile skin from diabetes, a healing scar, or another cause
- a history of physical abuse

Types of Massage

The most universally understood Western form of massage is Swedish massage. It consists of many types of strokes: gliding the hand across the skin, kneading, lifting, squeezing, and grasping the muscles, gentle pushing, friction, vibration, jostling, and rocking, and also percussion (hacking, chopping, and rapid pounding motions). A similar form of massage that uses long strokes is Esalen massage.

Eastern massage, sometimes referred to as *Shiatsu* or ACUPRESSURE, involves pressing at certain points along invisible energy meridians that run through the body; the practitioner looks for tight spots, knots, or anything that interferes with the flow of energy and concentrates on those areas.

Deep tissue massage uses slow strokes and deep finger pressure to combat aching muscles, such as a stiff neck or bad back. Sports massage is a combination of stretching and Swedish or deep-tissue massage, and it is performed before or after strenuous exercise.

Trigger point massage (also called pressure point massage) concentrates on muscular areas of the body that feel knotty and can cause pain everywhere. The therapist places pressure on these particular trigger points.

REFLEXOLOGY, the massage of the hands, feet and ears, is based on the belief that specific areas govern all parts of the body. For example, the tips of the toes are believed to correspond to the head, while the inside arch of the foot reflects the spine. The theory is that by stimulating the nerve endings of the different organs in the body changes can be affected.

Choosing a Massage Therapist

A qualified massage therapist should have a solid foundation in physiology and be knowledgeable about the inner workings of the body. Usually, therapists from an accredited school have completed 500 hours of training, including classes in anatomy, first aid, and cardiopulmonary resuscitation (CPR). Recommendations from others who have used a qualified massage therapist can also be useful in choosing the specific therapist.

An estimated 33 states and the District of Columbia have state laws regulating massage therapy, such as requiring therapists to pass a national certification examination in order to receive state licensing.

Experiencing a Massage

Most massage therapists work in small, semi-darkened rooms with soft music. Some therapists offer a choice of scented candles. During the massage, the entire body is draped in a sheet; only the portion that is currently being worked on is exposed. Oil or powder is used on the skin to reduce friction during the massage.

The massage therapist leaves the client alone to undress and lie down on a padded massage table. Quiet is an essential feature of the massage experience. While conversation with the therapist may be limited, a person should speak up if experiencing discomfort, feeling hot or cold, desiring more or less pressure, or wanting more attention paid to a certain area of the body such as an aching back.

Massage is productive "down time." During the massage, the body becomes very heavy and sinks into the table. As the therapist's hands locate the areas of tension, the individual consciously tries to let go and relax these areas. He or she lets go of a desire to control movement and instead allows the therapist to move the body and limbs into whatever position is required.

A good neck and shoulder massage may contribute toward better mental performance as well as relief of stress. One study reported that people who received 15-minute seated massages during their workday showed brain-wave patterns consistent with greater alertness. Those people were also able to complete arithmetic problems twice as fast and with half the errors as they did before the massage.

See also BODY THERAPIES; FIBROMYALGIA; MIND-BODY CONNECTIONS; ROLFING.

Field, Tiffany, Gail Ironson, Frank Scafidi, et al., "Massage therapy reduces anxiety and enhances EEG pattern of alertness and math computations." *International Journal of Neuroscience* 86, nos. 3–4 (1996): pp. 97–206.

National Center for Complementary and Alternative Medicine. "Backgrounder: Massage therapy as CAM." National Institutes of Health, 2006.

Shulman, Karen R., and Gwen F. Jones, "The effectiveness of massage therapy intervention on reducing anxiety in the workplace," *Journal of Applied Behavioral Science* 32, no. 2 (1996): pp. 160–173.

mass hysteria   Mass hysteria is also known as EPIDEMIC ANXIETY, a condition in which many people are simultaneously affected by extreme, often unfounded ANXIETY. Mass hysteria was recognized during the latter part of the Middle Ages, when whole groups of people were affected by similar anxieties—for example, dance manias involving raving, jumping, and convulsions. Some thought they had been bitten by a tarantula (spider) and would jump up and run out to dance in the street. This activity became known as *tarantism* in Italy and St. Vitus's Dance in the rest of Europe.

Another example of mass hysteria occurred during the 16th century when individuals imagined themselves being a wolf and then acted like a wolf. In the 1950s, there was also a mass hysteria incident in the state of Washington involving pitting of auto windshields. Groups of people feared that pitting (a normal phenomenon) developed from radioactive material in the air.

mastigophobia Fear of punishment.

masturbation Sexual self-gratification without a partner. Until recently, many people considered masturbation harmful. Many young people were told that masturbation would lead to bad consequences, ranging from acne to impotence. Because of the taboo against masturbation, many people became fearful and anxious about the practice. The more morally restrictive the culture or the environment in which people live, the more likely they are to develop fear and guilt about masturbation. Now it is recognized that masturbation is an almost universal practice before sexual maturity is reached, and a frequent practice in older age when a sexual partner is not available. In Kinsey's research in the 1960s, more than 90 percent of men reported masturbatory experiences in their adolescence. In the early 1980s, results of a research project by Shere Hite on female sexuality indicated that about 82 percent of American women masturbate. In most cases, men masturbate their penis and women the clitoris by hand.

See also SEXUAL FEARS.

Redlich, Fredrick C., and Daniel X. Freedman, *The Theory and Practice of Psychiatry* (New York: Basic Books, 1966).

material things Fear of materialism is known as hylophobia.

mathematics anxiety An individual's anxiety about mathematics can be broken down into three main components: numerical anxiety, mathematical test anxiety, and abstraction anxiety. Numerical anxiety involves the practical application of mathematics and numbers to one's everyday concerns (real-life "story problems")—items such as personal budgeting, timetables, counting change, and even odds for betting at a horse race.

Nearly everyone in an academic setting has experienced some degree of anxiety about mathematical tests—from multiplication flash cards to a pop quiz in a calculus class.

The third component, abstraction anxiety, is concerned with an individual's anxiety when confronted with methods of abstract mathematical reasoning involving mathematical schemas, theorems and proofs, or symbols and letters in place of numbers.

Questionnaires and anxiety scales can help to refine an approach to diminish or eradicate an individual's mathematics fears.

See also NUMBERS, FEAR OF.

Ferguson, Ronald D., "Abstraction Anxiety: A Factor of Mathematics Anxiety," *Journal for Research in Mathematics* (March 1986): pp. 145–150.

Maudsley Marital Questionnaire (MMQ) A questionnaire used in assessment of agoraphobic individuals. The MMQ is a series of questions grouped into five sections, including marital adjustment, sexual adjustment, orgasmic frequency, work and social adjustment, and warmth. The questionnaire is often given to the agoraphobic individual and his/her spouse before therapy and after therapy to measure changes and improvements. It was developed at Maudsley Hospital, London.

See also AGORAPHOBIA.

Monteiro, W., et al., "Marital Adjustment and Treatment Outcome in Agoraphobia," *British Journal of Psychiatry* 146 (1985), pp. 383–390.

Maudsley Personality Inventory (MPI) One of the most frequently used and widely standardized research instruments for personality assessment in Britain. The MPI is a 48-item self-rating questionnaire designed to measure two personality factors of neuroticism-normality and extraversion-introversion. The MPI is one of many tests therapists use in assessing an anxious or phobic individual's personality. The MPI was developed by Hans Jurgen Eysenck (1916–97).

See also PERSONALITY TYPES.

meat, fear of   Fear of meat is known as carnophobia. Some individuals fear the sight of raw meat or cooked meat; others fear eating meat in any form.

See also EATING, FEAR OF.

mechanophobia   See MACHINERY, FEAR OF.

medical model   Also known as "disease model." As applied in the treatment of ANXIETIES and PHOBIAS, the medical model is a set of assumptions in which abnormal behavior is viewed as similar to physical diseases. According to the medical model, symptoms of phobias (e.g., phobic object, anxiety, etc.) represent internally caused manifestations. The internal causes might be early childhood experience, psychodynamic interplay, and even biological predisposition. These internal (and usually unconscious) factors, given the right conditions, produce symptoms. In psychodynamic therapies, the symptoms symbolize something about the internal causes. In its simplest form, it presumes a single or limited number of causes (internal psychological or biological) for each "disease." In this sense it is a reductionist position that minimizes individual differences and multidetermined causation.

Psychodynamically, phobias are seen as displaced stimuli arising from unresolved Oedipal conflict. The classic case described by Freud was of Little Hans, a boy who developed a phobia about horses that Freud analyzed as a displaced fear of castration from his father.

The medical model, the dominant view of psychopathology, has influenced views of etiology, diagnosis, treatment, and research.

Contemporary psychology questions the medical model. Part of the dissatisfaction is that the diagnostic system and therapies based on this model have not proven reliable or effective in leading to behavior change methods.

Instead of the medical model, psychologists prefer a functional approach that relates behavior to environmental events including the internal cognitive environment of the individual either as trigger or consequence. The focus is individualized rather than categorized; treatment is based on principles of learning and behavior change developed through empirical study; the goals of therapy are defined and objectively evaluated. In the functional approach, diagnosis is an integral part of treatment (rather than a procedure in and of itself with little treatment relevance). The functional model is exemplified by the various behavior therapies that have revolutionized treatment and provided highly effective methods for treatment of all forms of anxiety.

See also FUNCTIONAL APPROACH.

medicine, fear of taking   See DRUGS, FEAR OF NEW; DRUGS, FEAR OF TAKING.

meditation   A learned technique to relieve anxieties involving deep RELAXATION brought on by focusing attention on a particular sound or image and breathing deeply. One directs thoughts away from work, family, relationships and the environment. During meditation, the heart rate, blood pressure, and oxygen-consumption rate decreases, temperature of the extremities rises, and muscles relax.

Meditation also has been shown to reduce a number of medical symptoms and improve health-related attitudes and behaviors. For example, people with chronic obstructive pulmonary disease (COPD) who practiced meditation reduced the frequency and severity of episodes of shortness of breath and numbers of visits to emergency rooms. People with heart disease, hypertension, CANCER, DIABETES, and chronic PAIN have reported feeling more self-confident, more in CONTROL in their lives, and better able to manage stress after mastering the meditation technique. Meditation has been used successfully by individuals who have PANIC ATTACKS AND PANIC DISORDER.

Meditation may bring out increased efficiency by eliminating unnecessary expenditures of energy. Individuals who practice meditation sometimes report a beneficial surge of energy marked by increased physical stamina, increased productivity on the job, the end of writer's or artist's "block," or the release of previously unsuspected creative potential.

Learning to Meditate

Meditation is a very self-disciplined routine and a way to learn more about one's own thoughts and feelings. Simple procedures can be learned easily. The basics include sitting in a quiet room with eyes closed, breathing deeply and rhythmically with attention focused on the breath. Also, there may be a focus on either a special word or MANTRA.

Meditation relies on the close links between mind and body. When one meditates, the alpha brainwaves indicate that the body is relaxed and free from physical tension and mental strain. BIO-FEEDBACK monitoring has indicated that meditation encourages the brain to produce an evenly balanced pattern of alpha and theta brain wave rhythms. This means that the body is relaxed and the mind calm yet alert. The "relaxation response" sets in, which is the opposite of the physical tension that results from stress.

Individuals who meditate frequently report that they are more aware of their own opinions after beginning meditation. They are not as easily influenced by others as they were previously and can arrive at decisions more quickly and easily. They may become more assertive and better able to stand up for themselves. Additionally, researchers have shown that the meditating person may become less irritable in his or her interpersonal relationships within a relatively short period of time after beginning meditation.

Types of Meditation

Modern meditation techniques are derived from spiritual practices in Eastern cultures dating back more than 2,000 years. Traditionally, the benefits of the techniques have been defined as spiritual in nature, and meditation has constituted a part of many religious practices. In the latter part of the 20th century, however, simple forms of meditation have been used for stress management with excellent results. Contributing to the rising interest is the fact that these meditation techniques are related to biofeedback (which also emphasizes a delicately attuned awareness of inner processes) and to muscle relaxation and visualization techniques used in BEHAVIOR THERAPY.

There are two basic types of meditation. One is *concentration* and the other, *insight*. Concentration

SITUATIONS IN WHICH MEDITATION MAY REDUCE ANXIETIES

- Chronic fatigue
- Insomnia and hypersomnia
- Abuse of alcohol or tobacco
- Excessive self-blame
- Chronic sub-acute depression
- Irritability, low tolerance for frustration
- Strong tendencies to submissiveness
- Prolonged bereavement reactions

types, such as TRANSCENDENTAL MEDITATION, often use a special sound or silently repeated phrase to focus attention and screen out extraneous thoughts or stimuli. *Insight-oriented meditations,* such as *mindfulness meditation,* accepts thoughts and feelings that arise from moment to moment as objects of attention and acceptance. The goal of mindfulness is an increased awareness of what is happening in one's mind and body right now. Recognition and acceptance of present reality provides the basis for changes of attitudes and conditions.

See also GUIDED IMAGERY; TRANSCENDENTAL MEDITATION.

Chopra, Deepak, *Creating Health: How to Wake Up the Body's Intelligence* (Boston: Houghton Mifflin, 1991).

———, *Creating Affluence: Wealth Consciousness in the Field of All Possibilities* (San Rafael, CA: New World Library, 1993).

Kabat-Zinn, Jon, *Full Catastrophe Living: Using the Wisdom of Your Body and Mind to Face Stress, Pain and Illness* (New York: Delacorte, 1991).

———, *Wherever You Go, There You Are: Mindfulness Meditation in Everyday Life* (New York: Hyperion, 1993).

Kerman, D. Ariel, *The H.A.R.T. Program: Lower Your Blood Pressure Without Drugs* (New York: HarperCollins Publishers, 1992).

Mahesh Yogi, Maharishi, *Science of Being and Art of Living: Transcendental Meditation* (New York: Meridian, 1995).

medomalacophobia   Fear of losing an erection.

See also ERECTION, FEAR OF LOSING; SEXUAL FEARS.

medorthophobia   Fear of an erect penis.
See also PENIS, ERECT, FEAR OF; SEXUAL FEARS.

megalophobia   Fear of large objects.
See also LARGE OBJECTS, FEAR OF.

melancholia   A term used throughout history to denote a severe form of DEPRESSION. The word derives from the Greek prefix *melas,* meaning black. In a state of melancholia, the individual feels loss of interest or pleasure in all, or almost all, activities, has low self-esteem, and is preoccupied with self-reproaches and regrets. *DIAGNOSTIC AND STATISTICAL MANUAL OF MENTAL DISORDERS* differentiates between the major melancholic type of major depressive episode and seasonal-pattern major depressive episodes. The long-standing lay definition of melancholia is close to the diagnostic criteria for the melancholic type of major depressive episode.
See also AFFECTIVE DISORDERS.

melissophobia   Fear of bees or insects.
See also BEES; INSECTS.

melophobia   Fear or hatred of music.

memory and memory loss, fear of   Fear of memories is known as *mnemophobia*. Many people feel stressed and anxious because of their inability to recall things at will. Some people fear they are developing ALZHEIMER'S DISEASE when their memory fails. During periods of extreme stress, many people experience difficulties with their memory.

The exact amount of retention depends on factors such as the thoroughness of the learning and repetition and the nature of the content. The more thoroughly the person learns, the greater the duration and amount of retention. Many people retain visual images of what they have learned, such as people, objects, pictures, or the printed page. Children have superior visual imagery, but this ability usually declines after about the age of fifteen.

There are various levels of recall. Immediate recall involves remembering within a few seconds to a few minutes; an example is remembering a phone number long enough to write it down. Short-term recall involves remembering within a few minutes to a few days. Long-term memory refers to recall from a period of a few days to a few years.

Verbalizing the memory involves finding the right words, which then calls into play the entire left side of the brain where words are stored. All parts of the brain are required for comprehension and storage of memory.

A poor memory may be due to poor learning, but sometimes there are psychological reasons for forgetting a fact, an event, or a person. This may be called *motivated forgetting,* as the person subconsciously tries to forget. Many people have a tendency to forget unpleasant things, but when forgetting becomes extreme it is called repression. When thoughts associated with GUILT, shame, or FEAR are pushed into the unconscious mind, tension and ANXIETY may result.

How Memory Works

There is ongoing research to determine just how the memory works. However, researchers agree that certain events occur in the central nervous system. It has been suggested that there are chemical and/or physical changes in brain cells and nerve pathways. Another theory is that memory is established in the cerebral cortex through a scanning process comparable to that of a computer. Memory is a cell-to-cell transmission of information across a synapse that has both electrical and chemical properties. This interaction and transmitting across cell walls takes place in a split second. Memories of smell, touch, and taste are placed in several places in the brain, awaiting a similar stimulus, such as the smell of a familiar food, to reactivate the memory.

Age-Related Memory Impairment

Older adults often fear memory loss as something that is inevitable. Health-care professionals use the term "age-associated memory impairment" to describe those minor glitches in memory that affect old adults' experience. Rather than remaining anxious and dwelling on this, many individuals find that written reminders, such as lists or repeating names or other information aloud, helps relieve these fears.

Many individuals are less able to remember certain types of information as they get older. Age-associated memory impairment (AAMI) is often most noticeable when an individual is under severe stress. When the person is relaxed, he or she will be able to remember the forgotten material with no difficulty.

See also AGING, FEAR OF; FORGETTING.

Kra, Siegfried J., *Aging Myths: Reversible Causes of Mind and Memory Loss* (New York: McGraw Hill, 1985).

Mark, Vernon H., *Reversing Memory Loss: Proven Methods for Regaining, Strengthening, and Preserving Your Memory* (Boston: Houghton Mifflin, 1992).

men, fear of Fear of men is known as androphobia or arrhenophobia. This fear may stem from a variety of factors, including unpleasant experiences with men or particular characteristics of men.

meningitophobia Fear of brain disease.

See also BRAIN DISEASE.

menopause, fear of Some women fear menopause, or the cessation of the menses. Some women fear that they will become unattractive to men at the time when they are no longer able to bear children. They fear having hot flashes and other symptoms of menopause, such as vaginal dryness, depression, and dry skin. Treatments involving estrogen replacement can alleviate many of the uncomfortable symptoms of menopause. Advances in estrogen products have made them safer to use with fewer side effects. Fewer women fear menopause than in earlier generations, because women now have longer life expectancies and anticipate satisfying lives after menopause. The average age for menopause in the United States is 50 to 51; in the United Kingdom it is 49 years and nine months.

See also AGEISM; AGING, FEAR OF; WRINKLES, FEAR OF.

menophobia Fear of menstruation.

See also MENSTRUATION, FEAR OF.

menstruation, fear of Fear of menstruation is known as menophobia. Some uninformed young women may fear menstruation because they have not learned about their bodies and sexuality. Since blood flow is usually a signal of physical injury, and a common fear of young children, adolescent girls may become alarmed at the first sight of monthly bleeding with the onset of menstruation at puberty. Some women who fear menstruation reflect anxiety felt by their mothers and generations of women before them: They feel shame if men around them know they are menstruating, they resent men for not having to endure menstruation, and they dread the repetition of what they regard as unpleasantness.

Historically, some men have had fears of menstruating women. Some men fear castration by having intercourse with a menstruating woman. They fear that menstrual blood should have formed the body of a child, and therefore it is charged with potent and dangerous energy. Some fear that menstruation is a punishment for sexual activity. Men who have blood phobia fear menstruating women. Others who fear menstruation are jealous of women's reproductive process. Some fear that women have cosmic power because of the connection of menstruation with the powerful rhythms of nature, such as the moon, sun, and tides.

In some cultures, largely as a result of men's fears of menstruating women, menstruating women were excluded from society during their periods and excluded from contact with religious people or ceremonies. Over centuries, women's fears regarding menstruation have included the notion that sexual intercourse during menstruation is harmful to both men and women's health, that deformed children result from intercourse at this time, that intercourse during menstruation is a sin against God; there has also been an assumption that women are not sexually aroused during menstruation.

Fears of menstruation can be overcome with appropriate information and reassurance that monthly periods are normal and part of female development. Notions that many people have that women are "unclean" during menstruation should be described and dismissed.

mental disorder, fear of Some individuals fear mental disorder or that they may be becoming mentally ill. This is a common—and commonly unfounded—reaction to PANIC ATTACKS. The American Psychiatric Association, in its *DIAGNOSTIC AND STATISTICAL MANUAL OF MENTAL DISORDERS,* conceptualizes each of the mental disorders as a clinically significant behavioral or psychological pattern that occurs in an individual and that is associated with present distress (a painful symptom) or disability (impairment in one or more important areas of functioning), or a significantly increased risk of suffering death, pain, disability, or an important loss of freedom. Additionally, to qualify as a mental disorder, this syndrome or pattern must not be merely the expected response to a particular event—for example, the death of a loved one. Whatever its original cause, it must currently be considered a manifestation of a behavioral, psychological, or biological dysfunction in the individual. Neither deviant behavior—political, religious, or sexual, for example—nor conflicts that are primarily between the individual and society are mental disorders unless the deviance or conflict is a symptom of a dysfunction in the individual.

Such fears often arise from lack of information regarding types of mental illness, the state of the mentally ill during episodes, forms of treatment, and rights of patients.

See also BEHAVIOR; DIAGNOSIS.

mental retardation   Mental retardation refers to impaired intellectual function that results in an inability to cope with the normal responsibilities of life. To be classified as mentally retarded, a person must have an IQ below 70 and impairment must be present before the age of 18. For families, anxiety results from COPING with the responsibilities of raising a retarded child. Early diagnosis is extremely important so that special education and training programs can be started and the child given every opportunity to learn.

It is crucial then that families seek professional help to define the retardation problem honestly and clearly. Next, they must gather information on community resources in order to make informed decisions about their child's future. While every state and most urban areas now have special governmental departments concerned with retarda-

tion where advice and consultation are available, accessing these agencies is not always easy and they are often bureaucratic.

Faced with the sadness and difficult problems of raising a retarded child, one of the first decisions families must make concerns institutionalization. Unless the child has debilitating physical problems as well as severe retardation, most families will opt to keep the child at home.

While the mentally retarded child remains a child all his or her life, he or she can experience feelings, concerns, emotions, fears, wonder, discovery, love, and laughter, as do all children. A retarded child does learn when given good training and support. If they are well cared for in a responsible and loving home, they will thrive; some may become reasonably independent and self-supporting.

Retarded adults, although often treated as children, experience normal adult feelings, including sexual desires. Unfortunately, caretakers often deny or try to suppress these feelings rather than teach appropriate behaviors, particularly those to prevent pregnancy and disease.

See also DISABILITIES.

Dolce, Laura, *Mental Retardation* (New York: Chelsea House, 1994).

Dunbar, Robert E., *Mental Retardation* (New York: Franklin Watts, 1991).

Grossman, Herbert J., et al. (eds.), *AMA Handbook on Mental Retardation* (Chicago: American Medical Association, 1987).

Stavrakaki, C., and G. Mintsiolis, "Implications of a clinical study of anxiety disorders in persons with mental retardation." *Psychiatric Annals* 27, no. 3 (March 1997): pp. 182–189.

mercurial medicines, fear of   Fear of mercurial medicines is known as hydrargyrophobia. This fear may be related to the fear of taking medicines. For example, mercury cyanide is a crystalline mercuric compound that is used as a medicine in small dosages but is quite poisonous in larger doses, hence inducing fear.

See also LEAD POISONING, FEAR OF.

merinthophobia   Fear of being bound or tied up.

mesmerism   An archaic name for HYPNOSIS. The term mesmerism was applied to work done by Franz Anton Mesmer (1734–1815), a German physician who used the power of suggestion, as well as magnetic rods, to treat anxious and mentally disordered individuals. Mesmer's work later led to the development of hypnotic techniques.

metals, fear of   This fear usually involves a reaction to particular metals or characteristics of some metals—for example, smooth or shiny surfaces, or such characteristics as color or the tendency to conduct cold. It is also known as metallophobia.
See also LEAD POISONING, FEAR OF.

metathesiophobia   Fear of changes; also known as neophobia.

meteorphobia   See METEORS, FEAR OF.

meteors, fear of   Superstitutions and traditional beliefs associate meteors, also known as falling stars, with death and bad luck. Meteors are chunks of matter from outer space, probably pieces of disintegrated comets that burn when they enter the earth's atmosphere. Meteorites are the remainders of meteors that are not completely destroyed by their blazing fall to earth. Asian tribes thought meteors were disembodied souls, some believing optimistically that they carried treasure, others that their purpose in coming to earth was to feed on the blood of the living. An American Indian belief links meteors with the moon; seeing a meteor was thought to cause one's face to become pockmarked like the surface of the moon.
Meteors are also feared because they can cause injury. A meteor may weigh over 2,000 pounds, and a shower may consist of 100,000 stones. There are unsubstantiated reports of human deaths caused by meteors from periods before the early 20th century. Meteorites have fallen through the roofs of houses, and animals have been killed by them.

Cavendish, Richard, ed., *Man, Myth, and Magic* (New York: Marshall Cavendish, 1983).

Heide, Fritz, *Meteorites* (Chicago: University of Chicago Press, 1964), pp. 60–61.

methyphobia   Fear of alcohol.
See also ALCOHOL, FEAR OF.

metrophobia   Fear of poetry.
See also POETRY, FEAR OF.

MHPG   3-methoxy 4-hydroxy phenylethylene glycol, a noradrenergic metabolite. It is increased during fear and panic attacks. After imipramine or clonidine is given, MHPG diminishes if phobic anxiety falls but not if it continues.

mice, fear of   Fear of mice is known as suriphobia or musophobia. Some people fear mice because they are considered to carry dirt and filth, because they can hide in small places, and because they destroy stored food and leave droppings around homes and stores. Some people who fear mice have fainted or run at the sight of one, or at least jumped away to avoid contact with them.

Feldman, S. S., "Fear of Mice." *Psychoanalytic Quarterly* 18 (1949): pp. 227–230.

microbes, fear of   Fear of microbes is known as bacillophobia. Those who fear microbes probably have a fear of contamination and a fear of germs.
See also MICROBIOPHOBIA.

microbiophobia, microphobia, mikrophobia   Fear of GERMS or SMALL OBJECTS. The word is derived from the Greek word *micros*, or small, and *bios*, meaning life.

migraine headaches   See HEADACHES.

migration   Leaving one's country or community to settle in another. Migration can set in motion a mourning process replete with anxieties similar to those that occur after losing a loved one.

At first, loss of country might appear to cause more anxieties for the involuntary emigrant; however, it is no less true for those who leave their country voluntarily. Relatives and friends feel abandoned and resent the person who is leaving. Although the emigrant may adjust to a new life in a new country, at the same time he or she may long for his or her former country.

Some may prolong their anxieties by holding to a fantasy of transience in the new country for as long as 30 years. For example, by not learning the language of the new country or, more subtly, by not becoming a citizen.

Culture Shock

Another aspect of migration that causes anxieties is culture shock, which is the result of a sudden change from a known environment to a strange, unknown one. The impact can be violent, and combined with the mourning process set in motion by the loss of that which is familiar, can cause a threat to the newcomer's identity. The sense of the continuity of the self and the sense of self-sameness, is threatened. At the same time, the consistency of one's own interpersonal interactions is disrupted. No longer is there the same confirmation of one's identity in interaction with the environment. As an example, an American living in a country hostile to the United States would be acutely aware of his nationality. Whether in a hostile country or not, environmental clues that normally confirm the emigrant's identity are absent and are replaced by unfamiliar phenomena, including language, architecture, housing, manner of dress, food, music, and smells.

One means of COPING with the anxieties of a new environment is to try to translate the unfamiliar into the familiar. For example, an individual from a forested country may look at tall buildings in a city and "translate" the tall buildings into a forest.

See also ACCULTURATION; CROSS-CULTURAL INFLUENCES; HOMESICKNESS; MOVING.

milieu therapy   Behavior change procedures that attempt to make the total environment conducive to psychological improvement. Milieu therapy is use-

ful in treating some agoraphobics and their families. While this form of therapy began as an approach to a large number of patients in a hospital ward, the term is now used in many different settings to describe generically environmental intervention.

See also BEHAVIOR THERAPY.

mind, fear of   Fear of the mind is known as psychophobia. This fear may be related to fear of thinking, fear of memory, or fear of memory loss.

mind/body connections   Links between the mind, brain, and other organ systems. Health philosophers in the late 20th century emphasize the mind/body relationships in health as well as disease. Research studies have demonstrated that psychological as well as physical stress has effects on health. Increasingly, physicians are recognizing that BEHAVIOR THERAPY and COMPLEMENTARY THERAPIES such as GUIDED IMAGERY, RELAXATION, BIOFEEDBACK and HYPNOSIS are useful adjuncts in the comprehensive care of patients, many of whom have anxiety-related disorders.

The term *mind/body medicine* relates to many treatments and approaches, ranging from meditation and relaxation training to social support groups planned to engage the mind in improving physical as well as emotional well-being.

ADVANTAGES OF MIND/BODY CONNECTIONS FOR ANXIETY RELIEF

- Can be used along with standard medical practices
- Financial cost of procedures is low
- Physical and emotional risk is minimal; potential benefit is great
- Many can be taught by paraprofessionals
- No high-tech interventions
- May improve quality of life by reducing pain and symptoms for people with chronic diseases
- May help control or reverse certain underlying disease processes
- May help prevent disease from developing
- May be useful when one is beginning psychotherapy

According to Herbert Benson, cardiologist and author of *The Relaxation Response,* "too often in the practice of modern medicine, the mind and body are considered to be separate and distinct, which is not in our best interest. Because of specialization, patients are no longer treated as whole persons. Instead, we are separated into groups of organs and specific symptoms are not considered in context."

In *The Mind/Body Effect,* Dr. Benson emphasized the need for practicing behavioral medicine, which incorporates the principles of medicine, physiology, psychiatry, and psychology. Patients are viewed in their entirety with the realization that what happens in their mind has direct bearing on the state of their physical health.

In *The Mind/Body Effect,* Dr. Benson makes it clear that psychological factors often induce physical ailments. He indicates that in extreme cases, fear and a sense of hopelessness can even induce death.

Many conditions have been found to respond to such techniques when they are used alone or in combination with standard medical and surgical treatments. These include HIGH BLOOD PRESSURE, coronary artery disease, CANCER, chronic PAIN, TMJ SYNDROME, HEADACHES, eczema, PSORIASIS, IRRITABLE BOWEL SYNDROME, ARTHRITIS, rheumatic diseases, ASTHMA, and DIABETES.

The Mind/Body Group at Boston's Beth Israel Hospital

The Mind/Body Group is part of a program of the Division of Behavioral Medicine at Beth Israel Hospital headed by Herbert Benson. It is one of many programs across the country to help individuals suffering from a variety of medical disorders, including cancer, arthritis, and diabetes.

The program uses a variation of the relaxation response, the meditation method pioneered by Dr. Benson. Since the early 1980s, the group has taught people to use the powers of their minds to help themselves bring about the relaxation response, learn how to change their own physiology, and finally have some sense of CONTROL over themselves and their lives.

See also MEDITATION; PRAYER; RELAXATION; RELIGION; SOCIAL SUPPORT SYSTEM; SUPPORT GROUPS; PSYCHONEUROIMMUNOLOGY (PNI).

Benson, Herbert, *The Relaxation Response* (New York: Avon Books, 1975).

———, *Beyond the Relaxation Response* (New York: Berkeley Press, 1985).

———, *The Mind/Body Effect: How Behavioral Medicine Can Show You the Way to Better Health* (New York: Simon & Schuster, 1979).

mindfulness meditation   See MEDITATION; MIND/BODY CONNECTIONS.

Minnesota Multiphasic Personality Inventory (MMPI)   A self-rating questionnaire to determine personality types. The MMPI may be of some use to therapists in helping anxious or phobic individuals. The MMPI was developed by Starke Rosecrans Hathaway (1903–84), an American psychologist, and John Charnley McKinley (1891–1950), an American psychiatrist, in 1942. Results of the questionnaire point toward nine personality scales: hypochondria, depression, hysteria, psychopathic deviate, masculine-feminine interest, paranoia, psychasthenia, schizophrenia, and hypomania. The subject of the test indicates agreement or disagreement with 550 statements; results are scored by an examiner or by computer to determine the individual's personality profile as well as any tendency to fake responses. The MMPI is widely used in clinical research.

See also PERSONALITY TYPES.

minor fears   Most people have minor fears that are not considered phobias; for example, they are nervous in a job interview or in some new social situations. They may be a little apprehensive as they drive along a road at the edge of a cliff. Such fears are common and even protective. Most people are clean and organized because they feel better, look better, and work better that way. Only when a habit becomes overwhelming—for example, avoiding going outdoors because one might see a bird, or endlessly washing hands—does the fear become abnormal and handicapping, and hence a phobia. Although it hasn't been studied extensively, clinically it is thought that minor fears can escalate.

mirroring   A BEHAVIOR MODIFICATION technique in which an individual sees himself portrayed by another person, usually the therapist, thereby acquiring a better idea of how he is viewed by others. Mirroring is used in helping some people overcome SOCIAL PHOBIAS. It is especially helpful in desensitizing a person to speech phobias.

See also BEHAVIOR THERAPY.

mirrors, fear of   Fear of mirrors is known as catoptrophobia, eisotrophobia, and spectrophobia. Many modern fears of mirrors are based on ancient fears and superstitions about reflections. The earliest known looking-glasses, or mirrors, were the still waters of lakes and pools. Primitive people believed that when a man saw his own image in a pool, or any other reflective surface, he saw not a mere reflection, but his soul looking back at him. The notion that the soul could be separated from the body without causing death, and that it was sometimes visible as a reflection or a shadow, was widespread in early times and appears in many well-known folktales. As long as the separated spirit was unharmed, the man whose body normally contained it was safe; but if it was injured in any way, misfortune, evil, and very often death would follow. The broken reflection of the human image has long been interpreted as a symbol of disaster. Many people fear seeing a broken or distorted image of themselves because they view distortion as a sign of disintegration, or of impending trouble and even death. Ancient Greeks considered it an omen of death to dream of seeing one's reflection in the water, because the water spirits might drag the soul into the dark depths below, leaving its owner to perish.

Basutos of southern Africa believe that crocodiles can kill a man by snapping at his reflection in water. Zulus of the Bantu nation of southeastern Africa consider it dangerous for anyone to look in a dark pool, because the spirit that dwells within it might seize the reflection and bear away the soul.

Some people fear breaking mirrors because they believe it brings seven years of bad luck, or a misfortune of a particular kind, such as the loss of a close friend, or a death in the house. Another superstition prohibits a child of less than a year from seeing its likeness in a mirror because to do so would cause it to languish, stunt its growth, or bring about an early death. The custom of veiling mirrors after a death is partly due to the fear that whoever sees his reflection then will die soon after, or if not he, then someone else in the house. Brides have been warned not to look at themselves in their wedding clothes, lest something happen to prevent the marriage. However, after the ceremony, it is considered lucky for the married couple to look at themselves together in the mirror. Actors fear looking into a mirror over another's shoulder. They fear seeing two reflections together, because doing so will bring bad luck to the one overlooked. Some individuals who have dysmorphophobia (a fear that part of their body is misshapen) fear looking in mirrors because seeing their reflection provokes anxiety.

Mythology and literature abound with references about fears of mirrors. For example, in a Greek myth, Narcissus's image reflected in a mirror was his own consciousness projected onto the world. In Lewis Carroll's *Alice in Wonderland—Through the Looking Glass*, a mirror symbolized the doorway through which the soul could pass to the other side. Merlin's mirror warned of treason, the mirror of Cambuscan in Chaucer's *Canterbury Tales* told of misfortunes to come, and the all-seeing mirror of Al-Asnam in the *Arabian Nights* indicated by the lightening or darkening of the mirror's surface whether or not the girl reflected was chaste.

In the 1600s and 1700s, catoptromancy, or mirror divination, was practiced, encouraging fears of mirrors and images. The seers dipped a metal mirror into water; depending upon whether the reflection of the sick person who looked into it was disfigured or clearly defined, the seer would decide if the person would live or die. During the Elizabethan era, mirror divination was used to detect witches.

The use of the mirror to deflect the rays of the Evil Eye was once a very common European practice. Among the Chinese, small mirrors were hung up in the house to scare away evil spirits because presumably the spirits would be shocked at the sight of their own reflections.

In dreams the mirror may be a symbol of sight, of the imagination, or of thought, as thought is a reflection of the universe. Also, mirrors may symbolize self-examination, truth, or vanity.

Mirrors have been thought of as doors through which the souls may find freedom. However, the Greek legend of Narcissus does not follow this pattern. Narcissus became enamored of his reflection in a fountain, leaned down to embrace it, and then was embraced by death. Narcissism remains the symbol of self-love. The fear of mirrors is often a symptomatic complaint of schizophrenics.

See also EVIL EYE, FEAR OF; SYMBOLS.

miscarriage The spontaneous end of a pregnancy before the fetus is capable of surviving outside the uterus. Many women who experience miscarriage also experience symptoms of extreme ANXIETY, GRIEF, and DEPRESSION for a period of time after the event. They feel the LOSS, even though the child was never born or seen.

Family and friends sometimes may seem less sympathetic toward women who have suffered miscarriages than toward those whose babies are stillborn or die in early infancy. Frequently, women who have miscarried are encouraged to try to become pregnant again soon. Those who do often overcome their depressions, but those for whom another pregnancy is difficult to achieve, mourn their lost child even more.

Understanding Miscarriage

Understanding the physiology involved in the process may help women who experience miscarriage to mentally adjust to the situation. Early miscarriages are usually the results of defects in the fetus. Later miscarriages, which occur in the middle trimester, are more likely to be caused by an incompetent cervix, uterine abnormalities, toxemias, or preexisting chronic disease.

Women who miscarry after some strenuous activity may experience guilt feelings, and some even believe that they induced the miscarriage. Usually this is not the case. Normal exercise does not usually induce miscarriage. Most women who play tennis, hike, or swim usually are advised by their obstetricians to continue exercising throughout their pregnancy (or until the last two months).

The first sign of a possible miscarriage is vaginal bleeding, with or without cramping; however, not all vaginal bleeding indicates miscarriage. Some bleeding may be associated with implantation, or it may come from the vagina, vulva, or cervix. If bleeding occurs from the uterus without any dilation of the cervix, and usually without pain, the situation is termed *threatened abortion*. With appropriate medical care, cases of threatened abortion can be salvaged, and many women have had healthy babies who were at the "threatened" stage during pregnancy. Treatment includes rest.

Late miscarriage may be the most anxiety-producing and difficult for a prospective parent to accept. If a woman has had good medical care and followed her obstetrician's advice, she should not feel responsible for the miscarriage. A later miscarriage, when the placenta and embryo are totally evacuated, is called a *complete abortion*. When placental tissue remains in the uterus, the term *incomplete abortion* is applied. The tissue must be removed by curettage.

Miscarriage is also known as *spontaneous abortion;* the term *miscarriage* is more commonly used because it is more socially acceptable. Both terms refer to the loss of an embryo or fetus before maturity.

See also POST-PARTUM DEPRESSION; PREGNANCY.

Lee, Dominic, T. S. Wong, C. K. Ungvari, G. S., et al., "Screening psychiatric morbidity after miscarriage," *Psychosomatic Medicine* 59, no. 2 (March–April 1997): pp. 207–210.

misophobia Fear of contamination with dirt or germs is known as misophobia.

See also CONTAMINATION, FEAR OF.

missiles, fear of Fear of missiles is known as ballistophobia. Those who fear missiles may fear nuclear war, or war in general. Many who have lived through wars fear missiles. Ballistophobia also refers to a fear of being shot.

See also POST-TRAUMATIC STRESS DISORDER; SHOT, FEAR OF BEING.

mist, fear of The fear of moisture is known as hygrophobia, and this fear may extend to mist and fog, forms of moisture. Both obscure one's view, which can create feelings of uncertainty, power-lessness, and loss of control, thus serving as sources of isolation, loneliness, and disorientation.

See also FOG, FEAR OF; WATER, FEAR OF.

mites, fear of Fear of mites is known as acarophobia.

mitral valve prolapse (MVP) A heart defect that has sometimes been linked with anxiety. In this condition, the mitral valve does not close sufficiently, and blood is forced back into the atrium as well as through the aortic valve. About 5 percent of normal adults have MVP. The condition can lead to a feeling of palpitations, anxiety, and difficult breathing. Research to study the relationship between anxiety disorders and mitral valve prolapse has unequivocally demonstrated that MVP is not a precursor, cause, or even related to panic and agoraphobia. While there is some symptom overlap, the overwhelming majority of MVP reactors do not develop panic or anxiety. However, individuals who have an anatomic vulnerability of their mitral valves may develop prolapse as a result of increased demands placed on their cardiovascular systems by anxiety.

See also LACTATE-INDUCED ANXIETY; PANIC ATTACK.

Reddy, Geetha, and Donald D. Tresch, "Mitral Valve Prolapse: A Different Disorder in the Elderly?" *Clinical Geriatrics* 6, no. 10 (September 1998): pp. 43–62.

mnemophobia Fear of memories.

See also MEMORY AND MEMORY LOSS, FEAR OF.

modeling The acquisition of behavior by observation of a real or symbolic model. Acquisition can occur in one observation if the individual identifies with or is attracted to the model. Modeling or observational learning may be produced by stories, television, or movies, or by direct observation (e.g., of a parent or friend). It is also possible to acquire emotional responses through observation. In this case, the model would be displaying emotional reactions in a particular stimulus situation, such as the ocean or showers. Many people, for example, developed fears of swimming in the ocean after seeing the movie *Jaws*. Likewise, people developed fears of taking showers alone after seeing the Hitchcock thriller *Psycho*. Behavior theorists make a distinction between acquisition (which occurs through observation) and performance (which requires repeated trials, reinforcement, etc., and is affected by the individual's learning history). In other words, a person might acquire a fear through observation, but whether they avoid the situation and consequently become phobic might depend on other factors, such as reinforcement.

See also BEHAVIOR THERAPY.

molysmophobia, molysomophobia Fear of contamination or infection.

See also CONTAMINATION, FEAR OF; INFECTION, FEAR OF.

money, fear of Fear of money is known as chrematophobia. Money can help an individual maintain esteem. Fear of loss of money represents a fear of losing the external validation of one's worth provided by money. After the Great Depression, many people committed suicide because they viewed lack of money as a loss of self-worth.

monoamine oxidase inhibitors (MAOIs) A class of ANTIDEPRESSANT drugs (used to treat depression). MAOIs reduce excessive emotional fluctuations and may stabilize brain chemistry by inhibiting the action of the enzyme monoamine oxidase, which in turn inactivates NOREPINEPHRINE. When more norepinephrine becomes available in the SYMPATHETIC NERVOUS SYSTEM, mood is elevated. MAOIs are rarely used because individuals taking them must avoid the foods listed in the chart of foods to be avoided by migraine sufferers.

See also HEADACHES.

monopathophobia Fear of definite disease.

See also DISEASE, FEAR OF DEFINITE.

monophobia Fear of being lonely; also fear of desolate places; fear of one thing.

See also BEING ALONE, FEAR OF; ONE THING, FEAR OF.

monotony, fear of Fear of monotony is a fear of sameness or unchanging situations and consequently has been called homophobia. (This term has also been applied to fear of homosexuality.) This may be related to a fear of boredom and a fear of time, known as chronophobia. Interestingly, monotony—or lack of stimulation—can trigger anxiety in agoraphobic individuals susceptible to react to lack of stimulation.

monstrosities, fear of Fear of monstrosities is known as teratophobia. Teratophobia also refers to fear of giving birth to a monster.

See also CHILDBIRTH, FEAR OF.

mood A sustained or pervasive emotion that markedly colors the individual's perception of the world. Examples of moods include depression, anxiety, anger, or elation. Moods may be significant in diagnosing anxieties and phobias, and therapists discuss moods with individuals who seek help for such problems. The American Psychiatric Association (in DIAGNOSTIC AND STATISTICAL MANUAL OF MENTAL DISORDERS) describes moods as:

Dysphoric: An unpleasant mood, such as depression, anxiety, or irritability.

Elevated: A mood that is more cheerful than normal. It does not imply pathology (as in manic-depressive illness).

Euphoric: An exaggerated feeling of well-being. Euphoria occurs in manic-depressive disorder. As a technical term, euphoria implies a pathological, or diseased, mood. Whereas an individual with a normally elevated mood may describe himself or herself as being in "good spirits," "very happy," or "cheerful," the euphoric person is likely to exclaim that he or she is "on top of the world," "up in the clouds," or "high."

Euthymic: A mood in the "normal" range, which implies the absence of depressed or elated mood.

Irritable: Internalized feeling of tension associated with being easily annoyed and provoked to anger.

See also AFFECTIVE DISORDERS; BIPOLAR DISORDER; MANIC-DEPRESSIVE DISORDER; MOOD DISORDERS.

American Psychiatric Association, Diagnostic and Statistical Manual of Mental Disorders, 4th ed. (Washington, DC: American Psychiatric Association 1994).

mood disorders In *Diagnostic and Statistical Manual of Mental Disorders* (American Psychiatric Association), AFFECTIVE DISORDERS are classified as mood disorders. Mood disorders include depression, manic-depressive disorder, bipolar illness, hypomanic episodes, cyclothymia, and others.

See also BIPOLAR DISORDER; MANIC-DEPRESSIVE DISORDER; MANIC EPISODE.

moon, fear of Fear of the moon is known as selenophobia. The effects of the moon on human behavior, especially as causing insanity, have been noted for centuries. The word "lunatic," coined by the physician Paracelsus in the Middle Ages, derives from the Latin word for moon. In some countries there is a fear that the man in the moon is the biblical Cain, accounting for the observation that as the moon becomes fuller and stronger, human behavior becomes more violent and erratic. People who are mentally unstable are thought to be particularly affected by the moon. Although scientific proof is lacking, professionals such as nurses, police, and firemen who deal with large numbers of people in emergency situations report an upsurge in activity and more extreme behavior at the time of the full moon.

Ancient Greeks and other cultures believed that the rays of the moon contained damaging power that could be collected by witches and magicians and used for their own evil purposes.

The observation that the moon's cycles parallel those of a woman's body led to the belief in some cultures that the moon was a lecherous man who ravished women and caused abortive or abnormal pregnancies each month. Other cultures identified the moon with a feminine emotional influence. In medieval Europe, the Roman moon goddess Diana became the patroness of witches.

Many fear-inducing superstitions are connected with the moon. For example, a full moon on Christmas prophesies a poor harvest; on Sunday, bad luck. A red moon foretells murder or war. Sleeping in the moonlight is thought to produce a twisted face.

Fear of the moon is often related to fear of the night or situations that might occur at a full moon. In any case, critical anxiety stimuli can be seeing darkness or emptiness, being out at night, looking at pictures of the moon, and sometimes, even seeing circles or circular objects that resemble the shape of the moon.

Morita therapy   A form of behavior therapy originated by Shoma Morita (1874–1938), a Japanese psychiatrist and contemporary of Freud. Morita therapy was developed as a treatment for many anxiety-related problems, which Morita referred to as "nervosity problems," characterized by hypochondriacal sensitivity and reactions to threats to health, introversion, self-preoccupation, perfectionistic self-expectations, intellectualized and dogmatic world views and expectations, and egocentric perceptions and reasoning. Morita therapy is centered on positive reinterpretation of anxiety in order to stimulate attentional, attitudinal, and behavioral change in self-preoccupied anxious individuals. This therapy promotes individuals' behavioral commitment to constructive and productive activities. It is currently practiced in Japan in various settings, such as supportive group guidance, directive outpatient therapy, correspondence guidance, guidance through diary commentaries, and also in structured residential treatment. Morita therapy is not widely integrated into Western therapy, largely because of the scarcity of literature on the outpatient application of the therapy.

Morita therapists have observed that Morita therapy often changes individuals' lifestyles. Instead of being mood-governed and feeling-oriented in thinking and action, such individuals become more purpose-oriented. They accept their emotional experiences as facts without suppressing or disputing them and start recognizing an abundance of tasks to be done in daily life that they have been neglecting because of their own self-preoccupation. Instead of allowing temporary moods and feelings to decide or interfere with action, individuals in Morita therapy learn to make pragmatic purposes their priorities. They learn to modify, by actual experiences outside therapy sessions, their acceptance of anxiety at cognitive, behavioral, and emotional levels.

See also BEHAVIOR MODIFICATION; BEHAVIOR THERAPY; COGNITIVE THERAPY.

Ishiyama, F. Ishu, "Morita Therapy: Its Basic Features and Cognitive Interventions for Anxiety Treatment," *Psychotherapy* (Fall 1986): p. 375.

Morita, S., *Nature and Treatment of Nervosity* (Tokyo: Hakuyosha, 1960). In Japanese.

mother-in-law, fear of   Fear of a mother-in-law is known as pentheraphobia. Fears of mothers-in-law frequently are expressed in jokes, which may perpetuate the mother-in-law mystique and fear. The most common themes are mothers-in-law as meddlesome troublemakers, ego deflators, unwanted guests, and often mean, unattractive women. Such jokes may have some historical basis, because some primitive societies actually prohibited contact between a man and his mother-in-law.

Hostile feelings toward the mother-in-law may arise from one spouse complaining to the other about mistreatment by his or her mother or a feeling that the irritating or unattractive qualities of the spouse are a direct result of his or her upbringing.

Though mothers-in-law are the butt of jokes, there seems to be some basis in fact for the belief that they present the most frequent in-law problems, with conflict most frequently arising between daughter-in-law and husband's mother. In some young couples, however, the conflict is between husband and the wife's mother because of the young bride's continuing dependence on her mother. In some cases, sources of these conflicts may be children's repressed resentments of their own parents being projected toward in-laws; ethnic, social and religious differences; and the mother-in-law's own difficulty in adjusting to the departure of her children and to the aging process.

See also FATHER-IN-LAW, FEAR OF; RELATIVES, FEAR OF.

mothers   Traditionally, mothers give their infants and children emotional warmth as well as sensory stimulation, both of which are necessary for developing a sense of self-worth and an ability to deal effectively with the stresses of the environment.

For many women, motherhood may serve purposes other than the simple desire for a child. For example, having children may seem to be a solution to an anxiety-filled or troubled MARRIAGE. Women may expect their children to succeed where they have failed and may live vicariously through their offspring. With their older children maturing and the threat of no longer being needed, some women will have another child rather than confront the next phase of life.

Images of Mother

The image of "mother" in the media has changed to reflect motherhood's changing role, or possibly the fact that the audience has grown more realistic and tolerant, even admiring, of different types of mothers. For example, in the 1950s and early 1960s, mothers depicted on television were always homemakers, dispensing wisdom and charm while impeccably dressed and groomed. At present unmarried mothers and working mothers are leading characters in television programs.

Many mothers undertake the double role of having a career and family, frequently out of economic necessity. However, even though women work, they still tend to be saddled with home, family, and social responsibilities, while men who may be willing to stay home with a sick child or leave work punctually because of a family obligation may not be met with the understanding they need from their employers.

Working mothers' responsibilities include getting themselves to work and quite often getting their child to a day care facility. Some mothers of school-age children may have to deal with the worries of leaving their children unattended. Careers that require travel or situations leaving mothers inaccessible may have to be passed over. HOBBIES, interests or just having time for oneself are almost nonexistent for many working mothers. Faced with these pressures more women are expressing an interest in limiting their family to one child or staying home with their children and/or trying to work from their home. Many women who completed their education in the late 1970s, began careers, married, and had children tried "HAVING IT ALL," meaning marriage, family, and career, and feel constantly stressed by all factors. Currently, women who work outside the house are opting for less aggressive career tracks so that they can spend more time with their families and have less anxiety in their lives.

See also ADOPTION; DAY CARE; MARRIAGE; MOTHERS-IN-LAW; REMARRIAGE; SINGLE PARENTS; STEPFAMILIES; UNWED MOTHERS; WORKING MOTHERS.

Jetter, Alexis, Annelise Orleck, and Diana Taylor, eds., *The Politics of Motherhood: Activist Voices From Left to Right* (Hanover, N.Y.: University Press of New England, 1997).

motion, fear of   Fear of motion is known as kinesophobia. Persons may fear motion for many reasons. They may fear the motion of race cars and roller coaster rides because of the danger involved. They may fear plane, train, car, or other vehicular motion because they fear motion sickness, and they may fear the physical discomfort they have previously experienced. Some fear having a lack of control over what may happen during the movement experience. Some individuals fear looking at or being in a whirlpool. Individuals who have balance problems or inner-ear disorders may have a greater fear of motion because of their reduced ability to accommodate to it physically. Some individuals who fear movement are startled by sudden changes, such as a loss of support, changes in altitude in an airplane, or being plunged into darkness. Infants and young children may react with fear when they see a live or toy animal rushing toward them. Movement also means increases in stimulation, and for anxiety-prone individuals, stimulation can be a trigger for anxiety.

See also AUTOMOBILES, FEAR OF; FLYING, FEAR OF; TRAINS, FEAR OF; WHIRLPOOL, FEAR OF.

Marks, I. M., *Fears, Phobias, and Rituals* (New York: Oxford University Press, 1987).

motivation   Motivation is the force or energy that causes individuals to behave in a particular manner. Motivation may include satisfaction of basic drives, such as hunger, thirst, or sex, or desire for praise, power, money, or success. Anxiety or fear may act as motivation for FIGHT OR FLIGHT, causing the anxious individual either to stand up to the feared stimulus or to flee from it. Anxiety may motivate very different behaviors in different individuals depending on their underlying personality structure.

Also, reduction of anxiety can serve as a powerful reinforcer or motivator for the behavior of avoidance. This built-in reinforcement for avoidance is what makes treatment of anxiety reactions difficult. Furthermore, only a small group of sufferers (less than 20 percent) ever seeks treatment.

See also STIMULUS.

motorphobia   Fear of automobiles. The fear may also extend to a fear of other vehicles, such as buses.

See also AUTOMOBILES, FEAR OF.

mottephobia   Fear of moths. Fear of insects in general is known as *entomophobia*.

movement, fear of   See MOTION, FEAR OF.

moving, fear of   Fear of moving or relocation is known as tropophobia. This fear may be related to a fear of newness or of new things. A move from one home to another brings with it the anxiety of facing the unknown. People anticipating a move fear the possibilities of hidden defects in a house or apartment and noisy or disagreeable neighbors. The sheer number of details and responsibilities in moving and the necessity of focusing energy on one project may be physically as well as mentally exhausting. Seeing their parents faced with unaccustomed anxieties and fears, children may sense the uneasiness and become anxious themselves.

A move that involves a complete change of location can cause many anxieties as the sense of the familiar vanishes. Differing customs, a change from rural to urban living or vice versa, or change of climate may create difficulties, including unexpected expenses. Activities that formerly were almost automatic, such as going to the grocery store, visiting the library, or getting a haircut, take more time and investigation in a new place. Children feel lonely and depressed after leaving friends and abandoning group activities such as sports and clubs in which they had created a place for themselves. Anxiety can arise from newness and from the emergence of these aversive feelings.

The reasons for moving may create anxieties. Some moves are made for negative reasons, such as death in the family, divorce, or a reduced economic situation. Even though the move may be an advantage to one member of the family, others may feel dragged along and become resentful and anxious.

See also LANDSCAPE, FEAR OF; NEWNESS, FEAR OF.

Nida, Patricia Cooney, and Wendy M. Heller, *The Teenager's Survival Guide to Moving* (New York: Atheneum, 1985).

moxabustion   See CROSS-CULTURAL INFLUENCE.

mugging, fear of   Mugging is a realistic contemporary fear. Many people fear mugging because victims are confronted unexpectedly and suffer physical harm as well as loss of possessions. Fear of being mugged leads many people to avoid wearing expensive, attention-getting clothing or jewelry on the street. In major cities, some individuals have been known to change their clothes before riding the subway, putting on clothes that "disguise" their mission as a business person or partygoer. They carry their "good clothes" in a plain paper bag so that they will not be the victim of a thief. Some individuals may carry this "avoidance" response to an extreme.

See also BAD MEN, FEAR OF; BURGLARS, FEAR OF.

Pasternack, Stefan A., *Violence and Victims* (New York: Spectrum, 1978).

multimodal behavior therapy A form of behavioral therapy developed by Arnold Lazarus (1932–) that views psychological disorders from seven modalities: behavior, affect, sensation, imagery, cognition, interpersonal relationships, and drug/biological aspects. The acronym BASIC ID was coined for these modalities. A comprehensive, individualized program is developed for each client to assess each of these modalities and to provide consecutive therapies in an eclectic array.

multiple personality disorder An old name for dissociative identity disorder in which the individual adopts two or more personalities. Multiple personalities may develop as a defense mechanism against extreme fears or anxieties and is always associated with a history of early sexual or physical abuse. According to *DIAGNOSTIC AND STATISTICAL MANUAL OF MENTAL DISORDERS*, diagnostic criteria for this disorder include the existence within the individual of two or more distinct personalities or personality states, each with its own relatively enduring pattern of perceiving, relating to, and thinking about the environment and the self. Further, at least two of these personalities or personality states recurrently take full control of the individual's behavior. Frequently, one or more of the personalities shows some symptoms of a coexisting disorder, such as a mood disorder, complaints of anxiety suggesting an anxiety disorder, or marked disturbance in personality functioning suggesting BORDERLINE PERSONALITY DISORDER. It is often unclear whether these in fact represent coexisting disorders or are associated features of dissociative identity disorder. Dissociative identity disorder occurs three to nine times more frequently in females than in males. Several studies have shown that the disorder is more common in first-degree biologic relatives of people with the disorder than in the general population.

See also DISSOCIATION.

Diagnostic and Statistical Manual of Mental Disorders, 4th ed. (Washington, DC: American Psychiatric Press, 1994).

Munchausen syndrome A condition in which an individual repeatedly fabricates clinically convincing symptoms and a false medical and social history. Some people do this in order to assume the SICK ROLE. The syndrome was named by R. Asher in 1951 after Baron Karl Friedrich Hieronymus von Münchhausen (1720–97) a German soldier-adventurer famous for his tall tales. A more up-to-date term for this condition is *factitious disorder.*

murophobia, musophobia See MICE, FEAR OF.

muscle relaxants Pharmacological agents that act on the central nervous system or its associated structures to reduce muscle tone and spontaneous activity. Many people experience tense, tight, or strained muscles as a result of anxieties or injury and some resort to these prescription medications instead of or in addition to using mind/body techniques for RELAXATION. Many skeletal muscle relaxants also function as minor tranquilizers.

See also PHARMACOLOGICAL APPROACH; MIND/BODY CONNECTIONS.

music, fear of Fear of music is known as musicophobia and melophobia. Music phobics usually fear only one type of music, such as organ music, which may have unpleasant associations for the individual. Historically, music has created a number of social fears and has been subjected to censorship. For example, operas hinting at revolution were censored in 19th-century Europe, as was music of Jewish composers in Nazi Germany and music expressing subjectivity or individuality in Soviet Russia. Social and religious leaders have objected to jazz because of its association with sensuous dancing and because of its development in lower-class dance halls that served as contact points for prostitutes. Jazz was particularly looked down upon by white southerners because of its origin in black culture, and some blacks attempting to rise in a white world have rejected it. Similarly, many have objected to and feared rock music for its associations with commercialization, violence, sex, unbridled primitive energies, and drugs. Folk music became associated with radical, left-wing political movements, frequently labeled subversive, in the United States in the 1930s and 1940s and again in the 1960s and 1970s.

In Hippocrates' (460–377 B.C.) writings, there is mention of a man frightened by the sound of a flute. Mozart is said to have feared the sounds of trumpets.

music as anxiety therapy   Since antiquity, benefits of music as a soother of anxieties have been known. Music probably has powers to relieve anxieties because it involves nonverbal communication and fills physiological and psychological needs for pattern, form, and sensory stimulation. Music is a way to make the external environment more appealing and acceptable to the individual. Music can provide a focus for therapeutic activity and motivate and reinforce participation in therapy.

In Greek mythology, Apollo was god of both medicine and music. Apollo's son, Aesculapius, god of medicine, was said to cure diseases of the mind by using music and song. The Greek philosopher Plato believed that music affected the emotions and could influence the individual's character. In the Bible, David played his harp to relieve King Saul's melancholy (depression). Music was used during the Middle Ages to exhaust crowds of people suffering from MASS HYSTERIA (probably because the music encouraged them to keep on dancing until exhaustion). Shakespeare made reference to the healing powers of music in his plays.

The first book in English on the subject was *Medicina Musica,* written by Richard Browne, an apothecary, in the early 1700s. In the book, music was said to "soothe the turbulent affections" and calm "maniacal patients who did not respond to other remedies."

During the 19th century, music therapy in the form of brass bands and concerts was used for patients with all the then-identified mental disorders, including anxiety. In the 20th century, particularly during World War II, many American psychiatric hospitals used active music therapy programs. The National Association for Music Therapy (NAMT) was organized in 1950, and in 1954 the NAMT recommended a curriculum for preparation of music therapists. Subsequently, organizations of music therapists were formed in England, Europe, South America, and Australia.

Contemporary music therapists use music and musical activities to bring about desirable changes in an individual's behavior and help the individual adjust to his environment.

See also POETRY AS THERAPY.

Hammer, Susan E., "The effects of guided imagery through music on state and trait anxiety," *Journal of Music Therapy* 33, no. 1 (Spring 1995): pp. 47–70.

McCraty, Rollin, Bob Barrios-Choplin, Mike Atkinson, et al., "The effects of different types of music on mood, tension and mental clarity," *Alternative Therapies* 4, no. 1 (January 1998): pp. 75–84.

musophobia or murophobia   Fear of mice.
   See also MICE, FEAR OF.

mycophobia   Fear of mushrooms.

mycrophobia   Fear of small things.

myctophobia   Fear of darkness.
   See also DARKNESS, FEAR OF.

myrmecophobia   Fear of ants.
   See also ANTS, FEAR OF.

mysophobia   Fear of dirt, germs, contamination, or filth.
   See also CONTAMINATION, FEAR OF; DIRT, FEAR OF.

mythophobia   Fear of FALSE STATEMENTS, lying, or myths.
   See also LYING, FEAR OF.

myxophobia   See SLIME, FEAR OF.

nail biting A difficult habit to break. In spite of the stereotype of the nervous nail-biter, nail biting does not correlate with specific personality qualities. However, many children as well as adults bite their nails when affected by anxieties. Situations that cause FEAR, BOREDOM, PAIN, or STRESS relate to nail biting.

With some people, nail biting continues because it is a routine and unconscious HABIT without a seemly underlying cause. Many people are embarrassed and only bite their nails when no one is around to see them. A somewhat universal habit, nail biting has no relationship to sex, race, or intelligence. It is estimated that more than 50 percent of the population has had the nail biting habit at some point in life. Nail biting usually starts in childhood after the age of three and frequently ends in adolescence when peer pressure and personal grooming become important. About 20–25 percent of adults remain nail biters. More women than men seek help to break the habit.

There seems to be a slight hereditary tendency to nail biting, but because family members are prone to mimic each others' habits, this is hard to establish. It seems, however, that a nail-biting parent is likely to have trouble correcting a nail-biting child.

See also ANXIETIES; HABITS; OBSESSIVE-COMPULSIVE DISORDER; NERVOUS HABITS.

naked body, fear of See NUDITY, FEAR OF.

names, fear of Fear of specific names is known as nomatophobia or onomatophobia. The fear may have developed from a primitive time when men guarded their first name as a precious secret and assumed another name to mislead those who might be able to gain power over them by knowing one's first name. Among gypsies, it is said, individuals were never told their first names, except at birth, when their mothers whispered it to them. Among ancient Hebrews, the name of God was never written down and never spoken.

In certain obsessive-compulsive individuals, hearing a name might stir up anxieties. Historically, names have been tied to numerology and astrology and the belief that names can determine the destiny of the individual. Fears develop about the effect of a name on a child and the outcome of the child's life, as well as the effect of the name on others.

See also WORDS, FEAR OF.

narcolepsy, fear of Some individuals fear sleep attacks, known as narcolepsy. An individual who has narcolepsy may fall asleep suddenly and involuntarily without warning. Sleep attacks appear to be triggered by strong emotions and may be accompanied by visual or auditory hallucinations at the onset. The attacks may occur up to several times per day and often include the type of muscle paralysis common in REM sleep. Individuals who have narcolepsy may experience increased anxiety throughout the day due to their inability to control their actions.

See also HALLUCINATIONS; SLEEP, FEAR OF; SLEEP, FUNCTION OF.

narcosynthesis See DEPTH PSYCHOLOGY.

narrowness, fear of Fear of narrowness is known as anginaphobia. This may relate to a fear of being in narrow places, of viewing scenery from a narrow vantage point, or of having any narrowing of the body, such as a narrowing of the arteries. The fear may also relate to fear of being in a tunnel and fear of crossing a bridge.

Fear of narrow places is known as stenophobia. This fear is related to the fear of narrowness and may be related to a fear of enclosed places, such as occurs in CLAUSTROPHOBIA. Some who fear narrow places also fear being in tunnels, riding on escalators, using moving walks at airports, and crossing bridges.

See also ANGINA PECTORIS, FEAR OF; BRIDGES, FEAR OF.

nature v. nurture controversy   An ongoing debate in psychology involving the relative importance of heredity, or nature, and learning, experience, or nurture, in determining human development and behavior. Currently, this is seen in the controversies between strictly biological and behavioral points of view in causes of agoraphobia, obsessive-compulsive disorder, other phobias, and many anxieties. No conclusions have been reached, but there seems to be mutual influence between biological and psychological factors.

nausea   Nausea is a common symptom of ANXIETY and anxiety disorders. Nausea is experienced as a feeling of sickness in the stomach and a feeling that one wants to vomit. Nausea may be accompanied by DIZZINESS or lightheadedness, SWEATING, and muscular weakness. Nausea may accompany anxiety attacks and can appear either as a precursor to or at the onset of an actual bout with anxiety. Nausea may occur on contact with a food that is associated with an anxiety-producing experience from childhood, or in response to certain odors. Nausea may be involved with many specific phobias, such as SOCIAL PHOBIAS, PERFORMANCE ANXIETY, SPORTS ANXIETY, and EXAMINATION ANXIETY. Many individuals experience nausea before an important appointment, before job interviews, before speaking in public, before playing an important game, and before taking tests, whether academic or a type of physical examination. Various forms of BEHAVIOR THERAPY are used to help individuals overcome nausea that does not have physical causes.

Some individuals whose religions proscribe meat (for Hindus) and pork (for Muslims and Jews) fear having reactions of nausea or actually do have nausea when they eat their forbidden food by mistake or coercion. Mahatma Gandhi, a vegetarian, described this reaction after eating meat.

See also FOOD AVERSION; ODORS, FEAR OF; SMELLS, FEAR OF.

nebulaphobia   Fear of fog.

See also FOG, FEAR OF.

necrophobia   Fear of corpses or dead bodies.

See also CORPSES, FEAR OF; DEAD BODIES, FEAR OF.

needles, fear of   Fear of needles is known as belonephobia. Some fear being pricked by a sewing needle, while others fear injections by hypodermic needles. Some fear dentists because they fear an injection of an analgesic substance with a needle. Some fear needles because needles have been strongly implicated in the transmission of acquired immunodeficiency syndrome (AIDS).

Because of fear of needles, some individuals are reluctant to donate blood. Some fear having or seeing a blood transfusion because of their needle fear.

Individuals who have a phobia of needles should, if possible, advise any health-care professionals who treat them. For example, if a dentist knows that a patient has a phobia of needles, he or she will ask the patient to relax first, or to look away, and will keep the needle out of the patient's view rather than provoke a panic attack or make the patient scream or faint. EXPOSURE THERAPY has been effective in successfully treating many individuals who fear needles.

See also ACUPUNCTURE; BLOOD AND BLOOD-INJURY PHOBIA; BLOOD DONATION, FEAR OF; BLOOD TRANSFUSION, FEAR OF; DENTAL ANXIETY; DOCTORS, FEAR OF; INJURY, FEAR OF; TOOTHACHE, FEAR OF.

negative ambition   A type of behavior in which the individual avoids competition, misses opportunities for success, and follows a line of maximum resistance. The term was coined by Theodor Reik (1888–1970), an Austrian-American psychoanalyst. This behavior leads to anxieties in some individuals.

negative practice A therapy procedure in which the individual is encouraged to intentionally repeat an error for the purpose of overcoming it. The technique was originally used to help individuals overcome stuttering. Deliberate repetition of a habit enables the individual to control it willingly at a later time. Researchers who have compared this practice to FLOODING suggest that negative practice is less effective.

See also BEHAVIOR THERAPY.

neglect of duty, fear of Fear of neglect of duty is known as paraliphobia. Those who have this fear may feel guilty if they do not do what is expected of them and what they expect of themselves. Such individuals may even be compulsive about fulfilling obligations.

nelophobia Fear of glass.
See also GLASS, FEAR OF.

neopharmaphobia Fear of new drugs.
See also DRUGS, FEAR OF NEW.

neophobia Fear of newness, novelty, innovation, or change.
See also CHANGE, FEAR OF; INNOVATION, FEAR OF; NEWNESS, FEAR OF; NOVELTY, FEAR OF.

nephophobia Fear of clouds.
See also CLOUDS, FEAR OF.

nervous An informal term indicating a state of tension, apprehension, and restlessness. Nervousness is a form of anxiety. The term comes from Freud's theory that neurological weaknesses (neur-

asthenias) developed as a result of unconscious conflicts.

nervous breakdown A popular term referring to any one or more of a variety of mental-health disorders in an acute phase. It is a type of collapse during which the individual has lost ability to function at his or her previous level of adjustment. Some phobic individuals fear a nervous breakdown when their fears increase or when they have a panic attack.

nervous habits Habits including involuntary twitches and facial tics and voluntary behaviors, such as nose picking, thumb sucking, and nail biting. These habits may be a reaction to anxiety or a means of relieving anxieties for some people. If the individual has a strong desire to overcome these nervous habits, in some cases, BEHAVIORAL THERAPY techniques will help.

See also ANXIETIES; HABITS; IRRITABLE BOWEL SYNDROME; NAIL BITING; STRESS; OBSESSIVE-COMPULSIVE DISORDER.

nervous stomach A common term for feelings of NAUSEA, diarrhea, and abdominal discomfort that an individual experiences when feeling anxious. Nervous stomach is also a common symptom of a panic attack.

See also IRRITABLE BOWEL SYNDROME.

nervous system An informal term for the AUTONOMIC NERVOUS SYSTEM. Neuro pharmacology is the study of the effects of drugs on the nervous system. Neuropathology is the study of diseases of the nervous system. Neuropathology may include examination of the brain, microscopic studies of tissue cells and laboratory analysis of the neurochemistry of tissues.

neurosis A now-obsolete term used interchangeably with neurotic disorder (also considered obsolete). A neurosis is a mental condition characterized by anxiety, fears, obsessive thoughts, compulsive acts, dissociation, and depression. Neuroses are considered exaggerated, unconscious ways of coping with internal conflicts. The symptoms are distressing and unacceptable to the individual. The more current term for neurosis is anxiety disorder.

See also ANXIETY DISORDERS.

neurotic disorders   An obsolete diagnostic term now replaced by several terms, including ANXIETY DISORDERS. The term "neurotic disorders" comes from psychoanalytic theory and was used in the first diagnostic systems.

See also FUNCTIONAL APPROACH; MEDICAL MODEL; NEUROSIS.

neurotic paradox   A term developed by O. Hobart Mowrer (1902–82) to account for the apparent paradox of why an individual would maintain a "self-defeating," limiting symptom. Mowrer suggested that the punishment or self-defeating nature of the behavior is less aversive than facing the anxiety situation. Facing the feared situation is more aversive than the avoidance, thus the paradox. The tendency is a paradox because in the long run, defenses prevent overall optimal function and development. An example is avoiding areas of life (such as shopping, driving, being alone, etc.) that are self-defeating. However, avoidance, although self-defeating, is more reinforcing than dread facing the fear situation and getting better.

neurotransmitters   Chemical substances that are important in transferring nerve impulses from one cell to another. Neurotransmitters are released at nerve-fiber endings to help nerve impulses across the gap between neurons. At least 30 different substances are known, produced in systems that link various parts of the brain. Several neurotransmitters are involved with fear and anxiety, particularly SEROTONIN, acetylcholine, and dopamine. (See chart on page 365.)

See also LOCUS CERULEUS; NOREPINEPHRINE.

newness, fear of   Fear of newness or of anything new is known as neophobia. Individuals who

NEUROTRANSMITTERS

For a chemical to be designated a neurotransmitter, several criteria must be met. It must be manufactured in the presynaptic terminal of a neuron and be released when a nerve impulse reaches the terminal. Its presence in the synaptic gap must generate a biological response in the next neuron, and if its release is blocked, there must be no subsequent response. Among the chemicals so far identified as neurotransmitters are the following:

Acetylcholine ("asséetil-cóleen")—found in many synapses of the central and peripheral nervous systems and the parasympathetic division. Excitatory at most central synapses and neuromuscular synapses; inhibitory at heart and some other autonomic nervous system synapses.

Serotonin—produced in the central nervous system, involved in circuits that influence sleep and emotional arousal. Can be either excitatory or inhibitory.

Catecholamines—chemicals found in synapses in the central nervous system and sympathetic division.
Dopamine—found in circuits involving voluntary movement, learning, memory, and emotional arousal. Inhibitory.
Norepinephrine or chemically similar noradrenaline—both a hormone and a transmitter. Found in circuits controlling arousal, wakefulness, eating, learning, and memory. Can be either excitatory or inhibitory.

Epinephrine or chemically similar adrenaline—both a hormone and a transmitter. Either excitatory or inhibitory; actions include increased pulse and blood pressure.

Amino acids—widely found in brain.
GABA—the main inhibitory transmitter in the brain.
Glutamic acid—possibly the chief excitatory transmitter in the brain.

Neuropeptides—chains of amino acids found in the brain.
Enkephalins—mostly inhibitory, as in pain relief, but excitatory in some locations.
Beta-endorphin—the most powerful pain reliever produced in the brain. Mostly inhibitory but excitatory in some locations; contained in the stress hormone, ACTH.

have this fear tend to have fairly routine lives and avoid doing new things, going to new places, or perhaps even wearing new clothes. This fear is related to fear of change, fear of traveling, and fear of moving.

See also INNOVATION, FEAR OF; NOVELTY, FEAR OF.

night, fear of   Fear of night is known as noctiphobia or nyctophobia. Fear of night is related to fear of the unknown, or fear of the dark. Night fear is common in young children. While children may fear the night because they fear separation from their parents, being alone, or imaginary monsters and DEMONS, adults may fear the night for more realistic reasons, such as BURGLARS, who operate under cover of darkness, fear of becoming lost in the dark, or fear of driving a car during the dark hours. Some who fear night fear SLEEPING and DREAMING or fear having NIGHT TERRORS. Some fear SLEEPWALKING or SLEEPTALKING. Some fear going to bed at night for fear that they will not wake up in the morning. People who fear the night usually begin to avoid their fear by going home as dark nears. Night to many primitive people symbolized death, the color black, and unknown forces.

See also DREAMS, FEAR OF; NIGHTMARES; WAKING UP, FEAR OF NOT.

nightmare   A frightening dream during the night. Nightmares resemble phobias in that they are unpleasant stimuli that individuals avoid thinking or talking about in detail. Those who have had a nightmare awaken with a vivid memory of the DREAM and a deep sense of ANXIETY. Nightmares affect about 6 percent of the population. A controlled study of students (as reported by Isaac Marks) found that desensitization decreased nightmare frequency and intensity more than did discussion of the nightmares or mere recording of their frequency. Those who suffer from nightmares often tend to have other forms of sleep disorders and high scores on the TAYLOR MANIFEST ANXIETY SCALE. Children as well as adults fear nightmares that leave them with acute feelings of extreme anxiety, terror, or helplessness. Normal children may have an occasional nightmare after an alarming experience, but constant nightmares may reflect more deep-rooted anxieties or emotional conflicts.

In some cases, nightmares may be the expressions of waking fears, such as BRIDGES or HEIGHTS, and can be reduced by gradual exposure to the frightening stimuli. EXPOSURE THERAPY, which helps phobias, also eases nightmares when applied as rehearsal relief.

Recurrent nightmares are a pronounced feature of acute and chronic POST-TRAUMATIC STRESS DISORDER, which often follows massive trauma and can persist for many years. Fantasy FLOODING, a form of behavioral therapy, has helped Vietnam veterans and victims of physical and sexual assault. Other sufferers of PTSD have improved with fantasy desensitization, and battle dreams have been reported to fade after the individual talks about them.

See also BEHAVIOR THERAPY; FEARS; NIGHT, FEAR OF; NIGHT TERRORS.

night terror   A nightmare, sometimes containing a phobic object or situation, from which the dreamer, usually a child, awakens screaming with fright. The terror may continue for up to 15 minutes while the child is in a state of semiconsciousness. He or she may scream or talk loudly and show intense fear. The child may appear to be asleep or in a trance, be difficult to awaken, be sitting up, walking around, or lying in bed thrashing about. If the child is wakened, he or she cannot recall what was frightening him or her. Night terrors can make parents anxious. Most children outgrow these episodes without treatment. The Latin name for night terrors is pavor nocturnus.

See also DREAM SYMBOLS; DREAMS, FEAR OF; NIGHT, FEAR OF; NIGHTMARE.

noctiphobia   See NIGHT, FEAR OF.

nocturnal panic   Panic attacks experienced during the night while asleep. According to researchers (Craske and Barlow, 1989), approximately 40 percent of people who have panic disorder have experienced nocturnal panic attacks. For many people, panic attacks occur more frequently between 1:30 A.M. and 3:30 A.M. than at any other time.

Nocturnal panic attacks have been studied in sleep laboratories where patients spend a few nights sleeping while attached to an ELECTROEN-CEPHALOGRAPH (ECG) machine that monitors brain waves. Various stages of sleep are indicated by different patterns on the ECG. Nocturnal panics occur during the delta wave, or slow wave, sleep stage, which typically occurs several hours after the onset of sleep. It is the deepest stage of sleep and people with panic disorder often begin to panic when they begin sinking into this deep stage of sleep, and then awaken in the midst of panic attack.

See also ANXIETY DISORDERS; NIGHTMARE; PANIC, PANIC ATTACKS; PANIC DISORDER; SLEEP.

noise, fear of   Fear of noise is known as acoustico-phobia or ligyrophobia. Noise PHOBIA goes beyond just being startled by loud noises. The individual reacts with FEAR because he feels that the environment is in control of him and he is powerless to stop it. Some individuals fear specific noises, such as sonic booms, whistling, or balloons popping. Some individuals with the last fear avoid going to birthday parties.

Some fears of noises may be related to POST-TRAUMATIC STRESS DISORDER. For example, soldiers who have been in battle may fear loud noises later on. Individuals who have been involved in serious automobile accidents may recall only the noise of the impact and fear loud noises later on. Behavior therapy can be helpful to such individuals.

See also CHILDHOOD ANXIETIES, FEARS, AND PHO-BIAS; NIGHTMARES.

nomatophobia   See NAMES, FEAR OF.

noradrenergic system   See LOCUS CERULEUS.

norepinephrine   A hormone and NEUROTRANSMIT-TER to the nervous system. It is also known as nor-adrenaline. It is found in circuits that control arousal, wakefulness, eating, learning, and memory. Norepi-nephrine can be either excitatory or inhibitory. Its actions include increased pulse and blood pressure.

Disturbances in the level of norepinephrine in the brain may be associated with DEPRESSION and MANIC states. One viewpoint suggests that depression is the result of too little norepinephrine (and too much leads to mania), while another viewpoint suggests that depression results from too little SEROTONIN, another neurotransmitter. There are receptors in the central and sympathetic nervous systems that are sensitive to norepinephrine or substances that mimic its actions. Some receptors accept agents that mimic or inhibit norepinephrine-like qualities. Norepineph-rine is a strong vasoconstrictor.

nosebleeds, fear of   Fear of nosebleeds is known as epistaxiophobia. Some blood phobics become fearful when they see anyone else having a nosebleed. For some of these individuals, the sight of blood lowers blood pressure, reduces breathing rate, and induces a feeling of weakness or even a fainting spell. Others fear having nosebleeds themselves, which may be related to a fear of more serious disease, or even fear of bleeding to death. Nosebleeds may have many causes. Among the most common causes of nosebleed are physical injuries to the nose, dryness of the nasal lining, picking at the nasal passage with the fingernails, or too-forceful blowing of the nose. However, persistent or recurring bleeding from the nose may be a symptom of a systemic disease, such as high blood pressure, or of an infection in the nasal passages.

See also BLOOD AND BLOOD-INJURY PHOBIA; INJURY, FEAR OF.

nosemaphobia   Fear of illness is known as nose-maphobia.

See also ILLNESS, FEAR OF.

nosocomephobia   Fear of hospitals is known as nosocomephobia. Some fear that they will go in healthy for an examination and later need treatment for an infection they contracted while in the hospital. This fear is related to a fear of ILLNESS, a fear of CONTAMINATION, and a fear of GERMS.

See also CONTAMINATION, FEAR OF; HOSPITALS, FEAR OF; ILLNESS, FEAR OF.

nosophobia Fear of disease is known as nosophobia.
See also DISEASE, FEAR OF; ILLNESS, FEAR OF.

nostophobia Fear of returning home is known as nostophobia.
See also HOME, FEAR OF RETURNING.

novelty, fear of Fear of novelty is known as cainophobia, cainotophobia, kainophobia, and kainotophobia; also as neophobia and centophobia. For some, novelty implies greater danger, and the strange and unfamiliar provoke fear in many individuals. Individuals who fear novelty tend to have repetitive patterns in their lives. They do not move often, usually live in the same place for a long time, keep the same job, and wear the same clothes. They tend to take vacations in the same places each year to avoid the novelty of something different. They tend to resist change of any sort.
See also CHANGE, FEAR OF; NEWNESS, FEAR OF.

novercaphobia Fear of a stepmother.
See also RELATIVES, FEAR OF; STEPMOTHER, FEAR OF.

nuclear war and nuclear weapons, fear of The fear of nuclear war has been found to be the greatest fear of children, after fear of death of their parents. Fear of nuclear weapons is known as nucleomitophobia. The same term applies to fear of atomic energy. This is a 20th-century fear related to the development of atomic and nuclear power. The fear is based on a feeling by individuals that they have no control over the fate of the world and that nuclear weapons can kill off all of human life and civilization. This fear is also related to a fear of DEATH and a fear of APOCALYPSE, or the end of the world.
See also APOCALYPSE, FEAR OF; DEATH, FEAR OF.

nucleomitophobia Fear of nuclear weapons.
See also NUCLEAR WEAPONS, FEAR OF.

nudity, fear of Fear of nudity is known as gymnophobia and nudophobia. Some individuals fear being nude themselves, fear seeing others nude, or fear having their bodies looked at by others. This fear may be related to a SEXUAL FEAR or may be a social fear of being without the superficial "cover-up" through which one obtains identity.

nudophobia See NUDITY, FEAR OF.

numbers, fear of Fear of numbers is known as numerophobia. Some individuals have fears of particular numbers, such as thirteen. Some individuals fear working with numbers, as in doing mathematics. Many people fear the modern tendency to give everything a number instead of a name. They fear namelessness and anonymity.
See also MATHEMATICS ANXIETY; THIRTEEN, FEAR OF THE NUMBER.

numerophobia See MATHEMATICS ANXIETY; NUMBERS, FEAR OF; THIRTEEN, FEAR OF THE NUMBER.

nutrition The study and science of the food people eat and drink and the way food and drink are digested and assimilated in the body. Anxieties play an important role in nutritional aspects of life. At times of certain mental or physical illnesses, an individual's nutrition may be less than optimal. For example, a severely depressed person may have little interest in eating, and lose weight, or a patient with a chronic illness, such as cancer, may have little appetite because of chemotherapy. ALCOHOLISM and substance abuse can suppress the appetite, leading to a decrease in food intake.

In Western societies today, many people become anxious about the relationship between diet and health. The focus is on the danger of too much fat in the diet, and the effects of food additives, coloring, and preservatives. Inadequate intake of protein and calories may occur in people who restrict their diet and try to lose weight. This can lead to EATING DISORDERS such as anorexia nervosa. It can also occur because of a mistaken belief about diet and health. Emphasis on thinness in our society has led many to poor nutritional habits in an effort to lose weight. Hence one's perception of BODY IMAGE may interfere with proper nutritional intake.

Psychotropic medications can contribute to inadequate nutrition for some individuals. For example, dry mouth, a side effect of some medications, may make eating less pleasurable than usual. Other side effects that interfere with one's ability to maintain good nutrition include glossitis, nausea, abdominal pain, vomiting, and diarrhea.

Mental impairment, caused by organic mental disorders and MENTAL RETARDATION or alcoholism and drug abuse can result in an inability to make decisions about eating. The lack of judgment may be reflected in inappropriate selection or preparation of meals. MEMORY impairment associated with some of these disorders may cause one to forget to eat, even after frequent reminders, or, forget that one has already eaten, and eat a second meal.

See also ALCOHOLISM; ANOREXIA; OBESITY; STRESS; WEIGHT GAIN AND LOSS.

nyctophobia   Fear of night or darkness.
See also DARKNESS, FEAR OF; NIGHT, FEAR OF.

obesophobia Fear of gaining weight is known as obesophobia.

See also BODY IMAGE, FEAR OF; WEIGHT GAIN, FEAR OF.

objective anxiety One form of ANXIETY, postulated by Sigmund Freud, that is due to a natural fear of a certain object or event. This is contrasted with neurotic anxiety (a signal that unconscious material is being stimulated toward consciousness) and moral anxiety (which is a feeling of deviating from superego standards).

obsessions The insistent, unwanted thoughts that recur despite active resistance against their intrusion. For example, a mother may be plagued by urges to strangle her baby while it sleeps. The word obsession is derived from the Latin word *obsidere,* meaning "to besiege." Individuals who have obsessions usually also have compulsive rituals that they feel compelled to repeat against their will—for example, checking and rechecking that the lights are turned off before leaving home.

See also OBSESSIVE-COMPULSIVE DISORDER; RUMINATIONS; SENSITIVE IDEAS OF REFERENCE.

obsessive-compulsive disorder (OCD) An anxiety disorder that usually comprises both chronic obsessions and compulsions that are detrimental to the individual's normal functioning. According to the National Institute on Mental Health (NIMH), an estimated 2.2 million adults age 18 and older have obsessive-compulsive disorder in the United States, or about 2.7 percent of the population in this age group. The first symptoms generally occur during childhood or adolescence, but the median age of onset is 19 years.

In contrast to those with other anxiety disorders, individuals with OCD are *less* at risk for substance abuse. In addition, a study in Sweden reported in *Comprehensive Psychiatry* indicated that individuals with OCD were less likely than others to smoke. Only 14 percent of the patients with OCD were current smokers, compared to 25 percent in the general population. Of the patients with OCD, 72 percent had never smoked.

OBSESSIONS are persistent, intense, senseless, worrisome, and often repugnant ideas, thoughts, images, or impulses that involuntarily invade consciousness. The automatic nature of these recurrent thoughts makes them difficult for the individual to ignore or restrain successfully. Furthermore, there is a strong emotional component that affects frequency and intensity. Obsessions increase or produce anxiety.

COMPULSIONS are repetitive and seemingly meaningless yet purposeful acts that reduce the anxiety brought on by the obsessions. The individual with obsessive-compulsive disorder performs certain acts according to certain self-made rules or in a stereotyped way in order to prevent or avoid adverse consequences. However, the compulsive act is not connected in a realistic way with what it is designed to produce or prevent, it is usually clearly excessive. While the individual may recognize the senselessness of the behavior and does not derive pleasure from carrying out the activity, doing so may provide a release of tension.

Obsessive PHOBIAS tend to have distinctive features. According to Isaac Marks, "They are usually part of a wide variety of fears of potential situations rather than objects or situations themselves. Because of the vagueness of these possibilities, ripples of avoidance and protective RITUALS spread far and wide to involve the patient's lifestyle and people around him. Clinical examination usually discloses obsessive rituals not directly connected with the professed fear; instead, the obsessive fear is part of a wider obsessive-compulsive disorder."

OCD was first described in a classic publication in 1903 by Pierre Janet, a French physician and psychologist. He used the term "psychasthenia" to describe the disorder. Later Sigmund Freud discussed obsessions and compulsions in his patients as complex psychological defenses that were used to deal with unconscious sexual and aggressive conflicts.

Symptoms and Diagnostic Path

Common obsessions are repetitive thoughts of violence, contamination, and doubt and when these obsessions interfere with normal functioning, a mental health professional may diagnose OCD. Two of the most common forms of obsessions are contamination of some sort and doubt (such as doubt as to whether the door was locked at home or the oven was turned off even though the individual checked these things before leaving home). Common compulsions involve handwashing, cleaning, counting, checking, touching, repeating, avoiding, slowing, striving for completeness, and extremely meticulous behavior. CHECKING and CLEANING are the two major forms of compulsive behaviors.

DEPRESSION and other forms of ANXIETY DISORDERS are often associated with obsessive-compulsive disorder. There may be a phobic avoidance of situations that involve the content of the obsessions, such as CONTAMINATION or DIRT.

Other common characteristics of individuals with OCD. Obsessive-compulsives usually fear LOSS OF CONTROL and experience a dissociation from the ongoing reality where they have no idea what they touched, what touched them, or whether they committed unwarranted acts. The obsessive-compulsive seems to need structure and rigidity more than others. He or she usually checks, filters, and censors all ingoing and outgoing stimuli. Obsessive-compulsives rarely drink ALCOHOL excessively because they fear becoming out of control while under the influence. Further, they endeavor to extend their sense of control to their immediate environment, and some try to force their family and close friends into ritualistic patterns.

In addition to fearing a loss of control, obsessive-compulsives fear uncertainty. They are constantly in doubt about how their behaviors will influence their environment and activities and they constantly ask for reassurance from others. Because of the fear of uncertainty and the need for reassurance, they are somewhat resistant to any form of medication. When medicated, sometimes they may resist the effects of a drug, which takes more effort in control, with the net result that they become more, not less, anxious.

Treatment Options and Outlook

Obsessive-compulsive disorder is treated in many ways. BEHAVIOR THERAPY gained favor as a treatment during the early 1960s, and many studies of advances in treatment modalities were carried out during the 1970s and 1980s.

In the course of research with obsessive-compulsives, scientists have found many differences between subgroups of obsessive-compulsive individuals. For example, researchers noted that those who have checking rituals differ significantly from those with washing rituals, and also that they respond differently to treatment. In addition, differences were found between those who display overt compulsive behaviors and those who do not show such ritualistic behavior. One subgroup was found to have slowness (a slow, methodical approach to the activities of daily living) as a primary characteristic, and they differed significantly from the checkers, washers, and ruminators. Several major studies have investigated these subgroups of obsessive-compulsives.

The anxiety caused by an obsession is partially the result of its unwantedness and intrusiveness. When the individual can gain mastery or control over it, such anxiety can be alleviated.

Antidepressants are often used to treat OCD, particularly clomipramine (Anafranil), a tricyclic antidepressant. In addition, selective serotonin reuptake inhibitors are also frequently used to treat the disorder, such as fluoxetine (Prozac), sertraline (Zoloft), escitalopram (Lexapro), citalopram (Celexa), and paroxetine (Paxil). BENZODIAZEPINES and beta blockers are sometimes used to treat OCD.

In general, pharmaceutical therapy must be administered cautiously to patients with OCD. Researchers have found that some obsessive thoughts may rapidly worsen after the individual takes a drug that stimulates a specific class of brain receptors. Behavioral treatments emphasize response prevention and exposure as intense but effective treatments. Response prevention involves not allowing the compulsive ritual to be acted upon so that anxiety is heightened until some resolution (change in thought) occurs. Exposure is the deliberate presentation of stimuli that trigger compulsive behavior, such as dirt, locks, etc. Obviously the client must be motivated to participate in this multiweek/multiday procedure.

Risk Factors and Preventive Measures

There are indications that there may be a genetically determined personality factor that influences obsessive-compulsive behavior. In a 2002 issue of the *American Journal of Medical Genetics*, researchers found suggestive evidence for a genetic linkage for OCD on chromosome 9p on a sample size of 56 people diagnosed with OCD.

Scientists have also suggested that there may be a biological explanation for some obsessive-compulsive disorders. There may be an imbalance in the frontal lobes of the brains of obsessive-compulsives that prevents the two brain regions from working together to channel and control incoming sensations and perceptions.

OBSESSIVE-COMPULSIVE SELF-TEST

Many individuals who have obsessive-compulsive symptoms have difficulty with some of the following activities. Answer each question by writing the appropriate number next to it. This is provided for education only and not for diagnosis. Only a mental health professional can make a diagnosis.

0   No problem with activity—takes me same time as average person, I do not need to repeat or avoid it.
1   Activity takes me twice as long as most people, or I have to repeat it twice, or I tend to avoid it.
2   Activity takes me three times as long as most people, or I have to repeat it three or more times, or I usually avoid it.

A high total score indicates the severity of the disorder.

Score	Activity	Score	Activity
——	Having a bath or shower	——	Visiting a hospital
——	Washing hands and face	——	Turning lights and tapes on or off
——	Care of hair (e.g., washing, combing, brushing)	——	Locking or closing doors or windows
——	Brushing teeth	——	Using electrical apparatus (e.g., heaters)
——	Dressing and undressing	——	Doing arithmetic or accounts
——	Using toilet to urinate	——	Getting to work
——	Using toilet to defecate	——	Doing own work
——	Touching people or being touched	——	Writing
——	Handling waste or waste bins	——	Form filling
——	Washing clothing	——	Posting letters
——	Washing dishes	——	Reading
——	Handling or cooking food	——	Walking down the street
——	Cleaning the house	——	Traveling by bus, train or car
——	Keeping things tidy	——	Looking after children
——	Bed making	——	Eating in restaurants
——	Cleaning shoes	——	Going to cinemas or theaters
——	Touching door handles	——	Going to public places
——	Touching own genitals, petting or sexual intercourse	——	Keeping appointments
——	Throwing things away	——	Looking at and talking to people
——		——	Buying things in shops
——	= —— Total	——	= —— Total

This speculation occurred after positron emission tomography (PET) scans were used on groups of obsessive-compulsives, depressives, and those with no diagnoses. PET scanning devices transform quantitative measures of metabolic activity through the brain into color-coded pictures. Metabolic rates in the forward portion of the frontal cortex were different in obsessive-compulsive individuals and individuals with serious forms of depression. Further studies on the range of environmental and physiological origins of obsessive-compulsive disorder are underway.

Obsessive-compulsive disorder also occurs at a high rate among victims of the brain disorder known as TOURETTE'S SYNDROME, which results in TICS and sometimes causes the involuntary shouting of obscenities.

Bejerot, S., and M. Humble, "Low Prevalence of Smoking among Patients with Obsessive-compulsive Disorder," *Comprehensive Psychiatry* 40, no. 4 (July–August 1999): pp. 268–272.

Hanna, Gregory L., et al., "Genome-Wide Linkage Analysis of Families with Obsessive-Compulsive Disorder Ascertained through Pediatric Probands," *American Journal of Medical Genetics* 114 (2002): pp. 541–552.

Marks, Isaac, *Fears and Phobias* (New York: Academic Press, 1969).

National Institute of Mental Health, "The Numbers Count: Mental Disorders in America." Available online. URL: http://www.nimh.nih.gov/publicat/numbers.cfm. Downloaded November 14, 2006.

ochlophobia   Fear of crowds or being in crowded places is known as ochlophobia.
See also AGORAPHOBIA; CROWDS, FEAR OF.

ochophobia   Fear of being in an automobile or other moving vehicle is known as ochophobia.
See also AUTOMOBILES, FEAR OF; MOTION; FEAR OF.

octophobia   Fear of the number eight.

odonophobia   Fear of teeth is known as odonophobia.
See also DENTAL ANXIETY; TEETH, FEAR OF.

odors, certain, fear of   Fear of particular odors is known as chromophobia, chromatophobia, olfactophobia, and osmophobia. Individuals may develop fears of certain odors because of traumatic experiences, associations with fearful situations or objects, or for many other reasons. Some fear odors of foods in general or those of particular foods. Usually the phobic individual reacts to particular smells, such as types of foods, perfumes, stale odors, etc., and becomes anxious in the presence of these odors. Some fear body odors from themselves or others. Some fear odors in nature, such as flowers, trees, grasses, or molds. Most develop this type of phobia through CLASSICAL CONDITIONING.

Benjamin Rush (1745–1813), American physician and author, commented on "the odor phobia": "The Odor phobia is a very frequent disease with all classes of people.

There are few men or women to whom smells of some kind are not disagreeable. Old cheese has oftenproduced paleness and tremor in a full-fed guest. There are odors from certain flowers that produce the same effects: hence it is not altogether a figure to say, that there are persons who 'die of a rose in aromatic pain.'"

See also SMELL, FEAR OF; TASTE, FEAR OF.

Runes, D. D., ed., *The Selected Writings of Benjamin Rush* (New York: The Philosophical Library, 1947).

odors, fear of body   Fear of body odors is known as osphreisiophobia or bromidrosiphobia.
See also BODY ODOR, FEAR OF.

odynesphobia   Fear of pain is known as odynesphobia, odynephobia, and odynophobia.
See also PAIN, FEAR OF.

Oedipus complex   Attachment of the child to the parent of the opposite sex, accompanied by envious and aggressive feelings toward the parent of the same sex. These feelings are largely repressed, or made UNCONSCIOUS because of the fear of displeasure or punishment by the parent of the same sex. Many individuals have PHOBIAS and ANXIETIES resulting from an unresolved Oedipus complex. The Oedipus complex, originally described by Sigmund Freud, is a crucial component of Freudian psychology. It derives from the Greek myth of Oedipus, who unwittingly killed his father and married his mother. In its original use, the term applied only to the boy or man in his relationship with his mother. The term Electra complex applied to girls and women and their relationships with their fathers.

oenophobia　Fear of wine is known as oenophobia or oinophobia.

See also ALCOHOL, FEAR OF; WINE, FEAR OF.

Ohashiatsu　A form of therapy based on the same system of Eastern medicine as ACUPUNCTURE. It is useful for relief of anxieties and tension for some people. Ohashiatsu addresses the body's energy meridians and points along those meridians called *tsubos.* Instead of using needles, however, the practitioner of Ohashiatsu uses hands, elbows, and sometimes even knees as tools. The goal is to achieve a feeling of deep RELAXATION, harmony, and peace.

Ohashiatsu adds psychological and spiritual dimensions to traditional SHIATSU, by incorporating Zen philosophy, movement, and MEDITATION to balance the energy of body, mind, and spirit.

See also ACUPUNCTURE; BODY THERAPIES; MEDITATION; MIND/BODY CONNECTIONS.

oikophobia　Fear of home surroundings is known as oikophobia.

See also HOME SURROUNDINGS, FEAR OF.

old, growing, fear of　Fear of growing old is known as gerascophobia.

See also AGING, FEAR OF; RETIREMENT, FEAR OF; WRINKLES, FEAR OF.

olfactophobia　Fear of odors is known as olfactophobia.

See also ODORS, FEAR OF; SMELL, FEAR OF.

ombrophobia　Fear of rain is known as ombrophobia.

See also RAIN, FEAR OF; STORMS, FEAR OF.

ommatophobia　Fear of eyes is known as ommatophobia and ommetaphobia.

See also BEING LOOKED AT, FEAR OF; EYES, FEAR OF.

oneirogmophobia　Fear of wet dreams is known as oneirogmophobia.

See also DREAMS, FEAR OF; SEXUAL FEARS; WET DREAMS, FEAR OF.

oneirophobia　Fear of dreams is known as oneirophobia.

See also DREAMS, FEAR OF; NIGHT TERRORS; NIGHTMARES.

oneself, fear of being　See BEING ONESELF, FEAR OF.

one's own voice　Fear of one's own voice is known as phonophobia. Some individuals fear hearing their own voice on a recording or in an ECHO. Some fear that their voice does not project a powerful image, and thus fear of one's own voice may be related to a fear of PUBLIC SPEAKING, speaking over the TELEPHONE, and in speaking out loud in social situations.

See also SOCIAL PHOBIA.

one thing, fear of　Fear of one thing is known as monophobia. Many individuals who have SIMPLE PHOBIAS, such as fear of DOGS, fear of THUNDERSTORMS, etc., have fear of only one thing. Some individuals who have SOCIAL PHOBIAS also fear only one thing, such as PUBLIC SPEAKING or entering a crowded room.

See also PHOBIA.

onomatophobia (ommatophobia)　Fear of names, or of hearing certain names.

See also NAMES, FEAR OF.

opening one's eyes, fear of   See EYES, FEAR OF.

open places and open spaces   See EMPTY ROOMS, FEAR OF.

open spaces   See AGORAPHOBIA.

operant conditioning   A method of learning. Operant conditioning involves the strengthening or weakening of some aspect of a response (for example, its form, frequency, intensity, etc.) based on the presentation of consequences. The two basic forms of operant learning are CONTINGENCY MANAGEMENT and operant shaping. Contingency management involves the manipulation of existing stimuli that precede or signal the behavior (such as taking cookies out of the cupboard to stop a child from climbing and opening the cupboard), or manipulation of stimuli that follow it as consequences (reinforcement or punishment). Shaping involves selective reinforcement for approximation to a particular behavior until the final behavior is emitted.

The term was coined by Burrhus Frederic Skinner, an American psychologist (1904–90), who applied understanding of operant conditioning to psychotherapy, language, learning, educational methods, and cultural analysis. In 1950, Ogden Lindsley, a student of Skinner's, made the first systematic attempts to apply the techniques of operant conditioning in a psychiatric ward to develop speech and cooperation. Teodoro Ayllon (1929–   ), a researcher at Anna State Hospital, Anna, Illinois, later developed a TOKEN ECONOMY that could be applied in a controlled setting such as a mental-hospital ward or a classroom setting. The principles of operant conditioning have been the basis for programs that successfully treat a wide range of human behavior problems, habit problems, and behavioral deficiencies, and that elicit and maintain new behavior development. Operant conditioning researchers have applied this methodology to study in the development and treatment of behavioral and cognitive manifestations of anxiety.

Shaping

A BEHAVIOR-MODIFICATION technique derived from operant conditioning. Shaping involves gradual and systematically reinforced responses toward a long-range desired new behavior. Shaping, also known as behavior-shaping, approximation conditioning, or reinforcement of successive approximations, was devised by B. F. Skinner, an American psychologist.

See also BEHAVIOR MODIFICATION; BEHAVIOR THERAPY; CONDITIONING.

ophidiophobia   Fear of snakes and/or reptiles. Fear of snakes is also known as ophiophobia, ophiciophobia, herpetophobia, and snake phobia.

See also SNAKE QUESTIONNAIRE; SNAKES, FEAR OF.

ophthalmophobia   Fear of being stared at.

See also STARED AT, FEAR OF BEING.

opinions, fear of others'   Fear of others' opinions is known as allodoxaphobia. Individuals who fear CRITICISM or RIDICULE fear opinions of others. Some social phobics have this fear.

See also CLASSIFICATION OF PHOBIAS; SOCIAL PHOBIA.

opposite sex, fear of   Fear of the opposite sex is known as sexophobia. Some individuals fear those of the opposite sex in business and/or social situations. For some this fear may be a fear of sexual activity, a fear of a mother, a fear of a father, or a repressed feeling of sexual desire toward the parent of the opposite sex. The fear seems unrelated to the development of homosexuality.

See also SEXUAL FEARS.

optophobia   Fear of opening one's eyes.

See also EYES, FEAR OF OPENING.

oral stage   In psychoanalytic theory, the first psychosexual stage of human development. The oral stage, as first described by Sigmund Freud in 1905, occurs during the first one to two years of life. During this period, the infant maintains a relationship with the outside world through its mouth. Also, the mouth acts as an erogenous zone from which the infant derives sexual pleasure from eating, sucking, and kissing. Successful transition through the oral stage is necessary for development into later stages. Without successful transition, later ANXIETIES, FEARS, and PHOBIAS may develop, according to psychoanalytic thinking.

See also ANAL STAGE; GENITAL STAGE; PHALLIC STAGE.

orderliness (as a ritual)   Some individuals, out of fear, feel compelled to organize and arrange objects in a particular way, such as items on a desk or on a kitchen counter. They become fearful and upset if anyone moves an item or attempts to interfere with their compulsion. The fear of disorder and disarray is known as ataxiophobia.

See also DISORDER, FEAR OF; OBSESSIVE-COMPULSIVE DISORDER; RITUAL.

organic approach   The theory that all disorders, mental and physical, have a physiological, biological, or biochemical basis. The organic approach is also known as organic viewpoint and organicism. In psychiatry, those who hold this view say that all psychotic disorders, including MANIC-DEPRESSIVE DISORDER and SCHIZOPHRENIA, as well as all anxiety disorders, result from structural brain changes or biochemical disturbances of the nervous or glandular system. The organic approach was suggested by Hippocrates (460 B.C.?) and Galen (Greek physician, A.D. 130?) and was systematically developed by Wilhelm Griesinger and Emil KRAEPELIN during the latter half of the 19th century. It has been the dominant but less obvious viewpoint in psychiatry within the last century.

See also BIOLOGICAL BASIS FOR ANXIETY.

orgasm   See SEXUAL RESPONSE CYCLE.

ornithophobia   Fear of birds is known as ornithophobia.

See also BIRDS, FEAR OF; FEATHERS, FEAR OF.

orthophobia   Fear of propriety is known as orthophobia.

See also PROPRIETY, FEAR OF.

osmophobia   Fear of odors is known as osmophobia.

See also ODORS, FEAR OF; SMELL, FEAR OF.

osphreisiophobia   Fear of body odor, either one's own or that of someone else, is known as osphreisiophobia.

See also BODY ODOR, FEAR OF; ODORS, FEAR OF.

ostraconophobia   Fear of shellfish is known as ostraconophobia.

See also FISH, FEAR OF; SHELLFISH, FEAR OF.

ouranophobia   Fear of heaven or thoughts related to heaven is known as ouranophobia.

See also GOD, FEAR OF; HEAVEN, FEAR OF; THEOLOGY, FEAR OF.

outer space, fear of   Fear of outer space is known as spacephobia. This fear is based on a fear of the UNKNOWN. Man has fearfully wondered for years if there is life in the alien, totally dark, soundless, and airless environment known as outer space. Discovery of the immensity and shape of the universe, the possibilities of other universes, theories about black holes, white holes, and "worm holes" that might connect one universe to another are disturbing because they are difficult concepts to comprehend. Scholarly theologians have interpreted these findings in light of their beliefs, but many people find these matters not only incomprehensible but somewhat frightening.

While some books and films portray extraterrestrials as highly advanced, nonthreatening beings, others have portrayed beings from outer space as violent invaders or exploiters of the earth. An example is Orson Welles's radio play of H. G. Wells's *War of the Worlds*, which caused a national panic in 1938 when listeners thought Martians had invaded Earth in spite of announcements preceding and during the program indicating that the broadcast was fictional.

Unidentified flying object (UFO) sightings started during World War II; these produced many theories of alien observation of Earth, including interest in the atomic bomb and in colonizing Earth. Kidnappings by extraterrestrials were reported. Fears were expressed that the United States government was covering up evidence regarding UFOs and even hiding the side of a crashed alien spaceship.

See SPACE TRAVEL, FEAR OF; UNKNOWN, FEAR OF.

overeating See EATING DISORDERS.

owls According to Jozefa Stuart in *The Magic of Owls,* in 18th-century Spain, the owl was a symbol of folly, stupidity, and irrational fears. It was linked to the bat as a threat to human tranquility. Bats were symbols of witchcraft. Owls had an ominous quality for early Native Americans.

pagophobia   Fear of ice or frost.

   See also FROST, FEAR OF; ICE, FEAR OF.

pain, anxiety and depression in   ANXIETY or DEPRESSION are rarely the only causes of pain. Both can make pain seem worse. Most people with pain have some emotional reaction to it. Some feel depressed, worried, or easily discouraged when they have pain. Some feel out of control, hopeless, or helpless. Others feel alone or embarrassed, inadequate, angry, or frightened.

   Anxiety or depression that accompany the pain of illness or injury may be caused by problems other than pain. For example, one may have concerns over family or friends, spiritual problems, or difficulties with insurance or money because of illness.

   Fatigue can intensify pain. If one is tired, one may not be able to cope with pain as well as when one is rested. Some individuals who have chronic pain fear fatigue or fear getting too tired to cope with their painful condition.

Relief of Pain and Accompanying Anxiety Drugs

In addition to prescription pain relievers and over-the-counter medications for pain, TRICYCLIC ANTIDEPRESSANTS such as Sinequan, Elavil, and Tofranil, taken daily, can help relieve depression associated with pain for some individuals. This antidepressant action is usually noticeable in about fourteen to twenty-one days. Antidepressants may also help stimulate appetite in a person whose pain or condition makes him or her uninterested in eating. Individuals with pain and depression who take antidepressant medications should be aware that the side effects of tricyclic antidepressants include dry mouth, bad dreams, dizziness, and nausea. The dizziness and nausea usually end within two weeks, but dry mouth may continue.

   Some individuals who have pain that makes them feel anxious and irritable take tranquilizers to calm them and make it easier for them to cope with pain. Tranquilizers can make nonmedical methods of pain relief more effective and might enable one to take lower doses of analgesics (pain relievers).

   Marijuana has been reported to reduce anxiety and control nausea so that a person in pain feels better. However, some individuals with cancer have reported that smoking marijuana actually increased their pain. In experimental studies, tetrahydrocannabinol (THC), the active substance in marijuana, has been found to have mild analgesic effects, but it cannot be recommended for pain relief because it causes HALLUCINATIONS and extreme drowsiness. THC is now available to physicians on an investigational basis for the treatment of nausea and vomiting in cancer patients who are receiving CHEMOTHERAPY.

   Non-medication techniques to relieve pain include relaxation, imagery, transcutaneous electric nerve stimulation (TENS), biofeedback, and acupuncture.

   Relaxation.   Relaxation relieves pain or keeps it from getting worse by reducing tension in the muscles. Relaxation can reduce ANXIETY and help one fall asleep, become more energetic or less tired, and make other pain-relief methods work better. For example, some people find that a pain medicine or a cold or hot pack works faster and better if they are able to relax at the same time.

   Imagery.   Imagery is a mental picture or situation an individual creates by using his or her imagination. How imagery relieves pain is not completely understood. Imagery can be thought of as a deliberate daydream that uses all of one's senses: sight, touch, hearing, smell, and taste. Some believe that imagery is a form of self-hypnosis. Certain images may reduce one's pain both during the time one imagines them and for hours afterward. When using imagery, one can decrease anxiety, relax, relieve boredom, and fall asleep more easily.

Transcutaneous electric nerve stimulation (TENS). TENS is a technique in which mild electric currents are applied to selected areas of the skin by a small power pack connected to two electrodes. The sensation is described as a pleasant buzzing, tingling, or tapping feeling; it does not feel like a shock. The small electric impulses seem to interfere with pain sensations. Pain relief usually lasts beyond the time that the current is applied.

Biofeedback.   Some individuals learn to control certain body functions such as heart rate, blood pressure, and muscle tension with the help of special machines that indicate how a part or function of the body is responding to stress. Biofeedback is sometimes used to help people learn to relax. Headache patients can use biofeedback techniques to reduce anxiety in order to help them cope with their pain. Usually biofeedback is used in combination with other pain-relief measures.

Acupuncture.   In acupuncture, special needles are inserted into the body at certain points and at various depths and angles. Particular groups of acupuncture points are believed to control specific areas of pain sensation. The procedure has been used in China for thousands of years, and elsewhere for a lesser time, to treat many types of pain and as an anesthetic.

Hypnosis.   Hypnosis is a trancelike state that can be induced by a person trained in the special technique. During hypnosis a person is very receptive to suggestions made by the hypnotist. To relieve pain, the hypnotist may suggest that when the person "wakes up" pain will be gone. Some cancer patients have learned methods of self-hypnosis that they use to control pain. However, the effectiveness of hypnosis for pain relief is unpredictable.

See also ACUPUNCTURE; BIOFEEDBACK; FATIGUE, FEAR OF; HYPNOSIS; PHANTOM LIMB PAIN; TRANQUILIZERS.

(Source: American Cancer Society)

pain, fear of   Fear of pain is known as algophobia, odynesphobia, and odynophobia. Pain is a sensa-tion that hurts enough to make one uncomfortable; it may be mild distress or severe discomfort, acute or chronic. Acute pain is usually severe and lasts a relatively short time. Chronic pain may be mild or severe and is present to some degree for long periods of time. Pain is often a signal that body tissue is being damaged in some way. Pain can only be defined by the person who is feeling it. It cannot be verified by someone else.

Mankind has suffered and feared pain since the beginning of time. Although a wide variety of drugs are now available to ease pain, pain is still a fearful subject, and the prospect of having pain makes people anxious. Fear of pain is evidenced by avoidance of potentially painful situations such as visits to doctors or dentists and dislike or avoidance of hospitals, rehabilitation centers, etc. The phobic individual's reaction is usually anticipatory and often not the result of any traumatic event in his or her life. This phobia is a good example of how reactions become sensitized and expanded by cognitive processes that operate during avoidance.

Some people find pain very difficult to explain. The fact that they cannot explain it to their doctor or others around them contributes to their anxiety and feelings of tension.

painful sexual intercourse, fear of   See DYSPAREUNIA, FEAR OF.

palpitations   Conscious sensations of the heart's beating harder and faster than normal or skipping beats. Whereas normally people are not aware of how their hearts beat, many of them experience palpitations when they participate in strenuous exercise or have anxiety-producing experiences.

Thumping or fluttering feelings in the chest do not normally indicate heart disease and may be a result of heavy use of caffeine, alcohol, or smoking. An arrhythmia (irregular beat) may cause a palpitation. Individuals may feel faint and breathless and their pulse may be as high as 200 beats per minute but remains regu-lar. Hyperthyroidism, overactive thyroid glands, may cause palpitation by speeding up the heartbeat.

Many individuals experience palpitations during PANIC ATTACKS or as a phobic reaction to a stimulus they fear. For example, a person who is phobic about dogs may experience palpitations just at the sight of a dog walking on the sidewalk. Although the dog is on a leash and does not pose any threat, the phobic individual may experience palpitations along with sweaty palms, weak knees, and DIZZINESS.

Those who experience palpitations may fear that they are having a heart attack or that they are going to die. For many people, just thinking these thoughts and becoming afraid of imagined consequences can cause palpitations to increase. Symptoms of ANXIETY, such as palpitations, are treated with BEHAVIOR THERAPY, and in some cases, drug therapy.

If an individual experiences palpitations for several hours or the feeling recurs over several days, or if they cause chest pain, breathlessness or dizziness, a family physician, general internist, or specialist in cardiology should be consulted as soon as possible. If palpitation episodes are brief, they are probably within the range of normal. Some medications may produce palpitations in individuals.

See also ANXIETY DISORDERS; PHARMACOLOGICAL APPROACH; PHOBIAS.

Eifert, Georg H., Stephanie E. Hodson, and Doreen R. Tracey, "Heart-focused anxiety, illness beliefs, and behavioral impairment: Comparing healthy heart-anxious patients with cardiac and surgical inpatients," *Journal of Behavioral Medicine* 19, no. 4 (August 1996): pp. 385–399.

Friedman, Bruce H., and Julian F. Thayer, "Autonomic balance revisited: Panic anxiety and heart rate variability," *Journal of Psychosomatic Research* 44, no. 1 (January 1998): pp. 133–151.

panic, panic attacks, and panic disorder Panic and panic attacks cover many discomforts, including an abrupt surge of anxiety with a feeling of impending doom that quickly peaks within about 10 minutes, although the time varies. Panic attacks strike some individuals with little warning and for no apparent reason. When panic attacks become chronic and debilitating, affecting the individual at work and at home, the person is said to have *panic disorder,* a form of ANXIETY DISORDER. An estimated 6 million adults ages 18 and older in the United States suffer from panic disorder or 2.7 percent of individuals in this age group. The median ages of onset is 24 years.

Spontaneous panic attacks also can be elicited by taking amphetamine or caffeine as well as during WITHDRAWAL from opiates, BARBITURATES, or other drugs. Marijuana use has also been associated with the onset of panic.

The word *panic* is derived from Pan, the god the Greeks worshiped as god of flocks, herds, pastures, and fields. The Greek word for "all" is also *pan.* Man was dependent on Pan to make the flocks fertile. Pan himself was a lustful creature known for his ability to reproduce. Pan's shape was that of a goat. A goat could traverse fields and dart through herds of cattle. Pan loved to scare people. He would dart out of the woods and frighten passersby in dark forests and at night. He would make eerie noises. The fright he created was known as "panic." Later, Pan fell out of favor because the Christian church portrayed the devil with the goat god's features—his two horns symbolized the philosophy of devil worship.

Symptoms and Diagnostic Path

Symptoms of a panic attack include lightheadedness, dizziness, rubbery legs, difficulty with breathing, a racing, palpitating heart, excessive perspiration, and choking and tingling sensations, as well as dissociation and feelings of helplessness and loneliness. Often the individual is convinced that he or she is having a heart attack or dying and seeks out medical attention, such as at an emergency room. The individual may feel a sense of unreality as well as one of impending doom.

Treatment Options and Outlook

Treatment for panic attacks and for panic disorder include psychotherapy and medications. Antianxiety drugs (BENZODIAZEPINES) are often helpful in treating panic disorder according to the National Institute of Mental Health (NIMH), particularly lorazepam (Ativan). ANTIDEPRESSANTS may also be used, including drugs in the serotonin reuptake inhibitor (SSRI) class, such as FLUOXETINE (Prozac), sertraline (Zoltof), Paroxetine (Paxil), escitalopram

(Lexapro), and citalopram (Celexa). When panic disorder occurs in combination with OBSESSIVE-COMPULSIVE DISORDER, depression, or social phobia, SSRIs are also often useful. Older drugs known as TRICYCLIC ANTIDEPRESSANTS are also used to treat panic disorder, particularly imipramine (Tofranil).

Individuals who have used excessive caffeine levels that have triggered panic attacks should taper off their usage. The outlook is good for most individuals, especially among those who are treated early in the disease. However, some individuals with panic disorder develop AGORAPHOBIA, and they become very reclusive and even homebound, as they seek to avoid those people or things that trigger a panic attack.

Risk Factors and Preventive Measures

Panic disorder is about twice as common among women as men.

Nearly all those with severe phobias (except some blood and food phobics) have phobic panic, making it difficult to classify phobias according to the presence of panic. During phobic panic, nearly all phobics feel changes in their heart rate, as well as experiencing tense muscles and sweaty palms. Spontaneous panic is most common among those with agoraphobia as well as in individuals with panic disorder without agoraphobia. However, between 33–70 percent of agoraphobics do not have panic disorder.

Nearly all phobics and individuals who have obsessive-compulsive disorder, panic disorder, generalized anxiety disorder, and severe depression experience panic at some time or other, although they do not necessarily develop a panic disorder. Many people will experience a panic attack in their lifetimes, but only a very few will develop panic disorder.

panphobia   Also known as panophobia, pantophobia, and pamphobia. A fear of anything and everything. Panphobia may be a form of ANXIETY rather than a true phobia.

panthophobia   Fear of suffering and disease.

papaphobia   Fear of the pope.
See also RELIGIOUS CEREMONIES, FEAR OF; RELIGIOUS OBJECTS, FEAR OF.

paper, fear of   Fear of paper is known as papyrophobia. This fear may include touching paper, seeing paper, being cut by the edge of paper, or even thinking about paper. Fear of paper may extend to wrapping paper, wallpaper, or drawing paper. It may be a fear of the paper itself or of writing or printing on paper. Fear of paper is classified as a SIMPLE PHOBIA, because it is a fear of one thing.
See also PHOBIA.

papyrophobia   See PAPER, FEAR OF.

paradoxical intention   A technique used to treat phobias. The phobic individual is instructed to think strongly and imagine himself in his phobic situation or facing the feared object. He is asked to magnify his fear reactions, such as rapid breathing in an actual phobic situation. Paradoxical intention is based on an understanding of the effects of anticipatory anxiety and the self-fulfilling prophecy. The goal of paradoxical intention is to teach individuals that they can control symptoms instead of allowing symptoms to control them; reverse the instinctive avoidance of the feared object, situation, or event; and break the cycle through which anticipatory anxiety produces symptoms.
See also ANTICIPATORY ANXIETY; EXISTENTIAL THERAPY; FLOODING.

paradoxical therapy   A method of therapy for phobias developed by Viktor Frankl (1905–97), a German-born American psychiatrist. In this method, the phobic individual magnifies his fear reactions, such as heavy breathing or sweating in an actual fearful situation, under the direction of a psychotherapist. Doing so enables the individual to see his symptoms objectively, particularly if he is able to see humor in the situation and laugh at himself. It also undoubtedly desensitizes the patient to the sensations of the body that occur with anxiety.

See also BEHAVIOR THERAPY; IMPLOSIVE THERAPY; PARADOXICAL INTENTION.

paraliphobia Also known as paralipophobia and hypengyophobia. Fear of neglecting duty, obligations, or responsibility.

See also RESPONSIBILITY, FEAR OF.

paranoid delusions See DELUSIONS; PARANOID THINKING.

paranoid thinking Relating to a mental disorder that is characterized primarily by DELUSIONS, a frequent symptom of SCHIZOPHRENIA. There are some aspects of paranoid thinking in AGORAPHOBIA and other phobic syndromes in which the individual wrongly believes that he or she is being watched or observed and may believe that others are plotting against him. The word *paranoia* comes from the Greek word meaning *derangement* or *madness.*

Paranoid delusions may include those of gradiosity or persecution. Individuals with grandiose delusions may believe that they have surgical powers or other abilities far beyond what they are capable of. Delusions of persecution involve suspicions based on the inaccurate belief that one is being harassed, persecuted, or in some way unfairly treated. In some instances the term *paranoid thinking* is used when the therapist is unsure of whether the disturbances are actually delusional. It is possible for relatively normally functioning people to have paranoid ideatiion regarding particular events and situations. Paranoid thinking is associated with often unrecognized feelings of fear and insecurity.

See also IDEAS OF REFERENCE; SENSITIVE IDEAS OF REFERENCE.

paraphobia See SEXUAL PERVERSIONS, FEAR OF.

parasites, fear of Fear of parasites is known as parasitophobia or phthiriophobia. This fear may extend to any tiny organism such as a virus, bacterium, or fungus that lives in or on another organism (the host) and at some time in its life takes all or part of its nourishment from the host. Some people fear that they may become infested with parasites but do not believe that they are currently infested. Some who believe that they are hosting parasites pick, scratch, and tear their skin until they develop sores out of fear of the damage the parasites will do. They may display bits of skin as examples of the parasites.

Fears of parasites are not totally unfounded, as some parasites are harmful to one's health and cause disease. Parasites may exist in the intestinal tract, where they have access to predigested food. Hookworms and tapeworms are examples. Parasites elsewhere in the body can damage cells, block organ ducts, cause toxic or allergic reactions, and stimulate the host's tissue to a point where abnormal growths are formed.

See also CONTAMINATION, FEAR OF; DISEASE, FEAR OF; GERMS, FEAR OF.

parasitophobia See PARASITES, FEAR OF.

paraskavedekatriaphobia Fear of Friday the 13th.
See also NUMBERS, FEAR OF.

parenting Caring for and nurturing children. The term may also apply to the function performed by grandparents who care for grandchildren because their parents can no longer assume the responsibilities of parenthood.

Of all the roles in life, parenting is one of the most important; it is one for which there is the least preparation and, therefore, brings with it a great deal of anxiety. For those with little instruction and no experience, the anxieties and fears of parenting begin with the basics of feeding, bathing, and caring for a baby. As role models, parents provide moral and ethical values; as disciplinarians, they reward good conduct and withhold reward when it is bad. They deal with family disputes, including sibling rivalry and, at the same time, try to avoid playing favorites, recognizing the needs of all their children. Keeping children safe throughout their lifetime is a constant concern.

Parenting involves responding to problems and concerns of children, both physical and mental. As children grow, parents must be vigilant yet recognize their children's capacities and respect their need to do things for themselves.

Parenting Adult Children

When children become adults, the parenting role often becomes one of friend and companion. Many adult children and their parents enjoy the same activities and hobbies.

Eventually the young people leave home and some parents are faced with the empty nest syndrome and no longer feel needed. While this may be a time of some degree of loneliness, it is a time when parents can explore their own interests and enjoy the intimacy they shared as newlyweds.

See also SIBLING RELATIONSHIPS; STEPFAMILIES; STRESS; WORKING MOTHERS.

parents-in-law, fear of   Fear of parents-in-law is known as soceraphobia.

See also RELATIVES, FEAR OF.

pareunophobia   Fear of sex.

parthenophobia   Fear of girls, or specifically of virgins.

See also GIRLS, FEAR OF; SEXUAL FEARS; VIRGINS, FEAR OF.

parties, fear of going to   Fear of going to parties is a SOCIAL PHOBIA. Some individuals fear making a bad impression, fear meeting new people, and fear being in a new situation. Some worry about criticism and ridicule of their appearance or speech. Although this is a fairly common fear in adolescence, for many individuals the fear continues into adulthood. Various forms of behavior therapy have been successful in treating many social phobics.

See also PHOBIA.

passive-aggressive personality disorder   A disorder characterized by being aggressive in a quietly passive way. For example, while outward aggression shows itself in a loud voice and possible physical force, passive-aggression is more calculated and expressed quietly. A passive-aggressive act may be one in which a person gives another directions to find a place but purposely leaves out an important detail. Another such act might be deliberately being late, causing others to wait and miss a train or other important opportunity. Characteristics of this personality disorder include putting off or forgetting to do a chore, or being purposefully inefficient. This procrastination or inefficiency gets in the way of job promotion and social acceptability.

See also AGGRESSION; PERSONALITY.

pathophobia   Fear of disease or illness.

See also DISEASE, FEAR OF.

patroiophobia   Fear of heredity.

See also HEREDITY, FEAR OF.

Pavlovian conditioning   A pattern of learning discovered near the end of the 19th century by Russian physiologist Ivan Petrovich Pavlov.

See also AVERSION THERAPY; CLASSICAL CONDITIONING.

pavor nocturnus   See NIGHTMARES; NIGHT TERRORS.

pavor scleris   See BAD MEN, FEAR OF.

peanut butter   Fear of peanut butter sticking to the roof of the mouth is known as arachibutyrophobia. This fear is related to fears of SWALLOWING and GAGGING. Spreading peanut butter on an apple slice prevents it from sticking.

peccatiphobia   Fear of sinning or wrongdoing. Also known as peccatophobia.

See also SIN, FEAR OF.

pediaphobia   Fear of dolls or small figures. This fear may also extend to a fear of small children or infants who look like dolls.

See also DOLLS, FEAR OF.

pediculophobia   Fear of lice.

See also LICE, FEAR OF; PHTHIRIOPHOBIA.

pediophobia   Fear of children, dolls, or infants.

See also CHILDREN, FEAR OF; DOLLS, FEAR OF; INFANTS, FEAR OF.

peer group   A group whose members are of equal standing. "Peer" refers to people who are of the same age, educational level, or have the same job or profession. A peer group can cause anxieties for an individual because it can arouse feelings of self-concept, low SELF-ESTEEM, and other negative attitudes, and behaviors.

Peer group relationships are important to children as well as adults. While children look to each other for acceptance and approval, so do adults.

Peers are crucial to psychological development of the individual throughout life. Children learn to cooperate, work together, handle aggressive impulses in nondestructive ways, and explore differences between themselves and their friends. Throughout the school years, children rely on their peers as important sources of information and may use peers as standards by which to measure themselves. Many look to their peers for role models and for social reinforcement as frequently as they look to their own families.

Some children who do not learn to combat LONELINESS by fitting into a peer group may develop emotional problems later in life. These children who feel "different" from their peers may endure particular stresses as they work toward "fitting in." Such children may be those who are in recently divorced families, recently "merged" families with two sets of parents, or adopted children of single parents. However, there are children who choose to shun their peers.

For adults, the increasing mobility that often cuts them off from family and longtime friends has made the development of peer relationships at work and other social and community activities extremely important.

Peer Pressure

Peer pressure is the influence of the peer group on the individual. It begins in adolescence, because teenagers want to belong to a group. Teenagers react to the physical changes they are going through, as well as their changing responsibilities and experiences, by close bonding with those in their own age group. Music, language, and clothing are important emblems of identity. The rallying cry of teenagers often is "everybody's doing it," or "everyone has it." Parents frequently become stressed by this peer pressure on their youngsters. They may also fear that the influence of friends may lead their children to genuinely damaging activities, such as experimenting with drugs, irresponsible sexual activity, criminal behavior, or dropping out of school.

Peer pressure doesn't end with teens but becomes more subtle in the way it affects adults. It may be caused by advertising that promotes a "keeping up with the Joneses" philosophy. It may also arise from COMPETITION.

See also PARENTING; PUBERTY.

peladophobia   Fear of bald people or of becoming bald oneself.

See also BALD PEOPLE, FEAR OF.

pellagra, fear of   Fear of pellagra is known as pellagraphobia. Pellagra is a chronic disease caused by niacin deficiency and characterized by skin eruptions, digestive and nervous disturbances, and eventual mental deterioration. Individuals with this fear may take large doses of niacin in an effort to combat their feared disease.

See also ILLNESS PHOBIA.

peniaphobia   Fear of poverty.

See also POVERTY, FEAR OF; RUIN, FEAR OF.

penis captivus, fear of   Fear of having one's penis held tightly by the female's vaginal muscles during sexual intercourse. This fear may be related to the male's fear of castration and to female castration impulses. It is possible for a female to deliberately produce strong spasmodic vaginal muscle tightening around the penis during intercourse, but this usually is not harmful to the penis.

See also CASTRATION ANXIETY; SEXUAL FEARS.

penis fear Fear of penises is known as phallophobia. These fears usually relate to anxiety regarding social judgment about the size of one's penis or social embarrassment about having an erection in public. Fear of an erect penis is known as ithyphallophobia or medorthophobia. Fear of the contour of a penis being visible through clothes is known as medectophobia.

See also PSYCHOSEXUAL FEARS.

pentheraphobia Fear of one's mother-in-law.

See also MOTHER-IN-LAW, FEAR OF.

people, fear of Fear of people, or of human beings or human society, is known as anthropophobia. Manifestations of this PHOBIA at its extreme would involve complete avoidance of people.

See also SOCIAL PHOBIA.

perfection The state of being expert, proficient, flawless, without fault or defect. It is an unrealistic goal, a drive toward the impossible and unattainable, and is a source of anxieties for many people. Perfectionists are very achievement-oriented. They are unable to determine what is important and operate under the false assumption that perfectionism equals quality.

The perfectionist faces anxieties and frustration with failure of any kind, imagined, real, large, or small. The obsession with perfection ultimately results in fragmentation of self; loss of efficiency; sleep deprivation, less time for exercise, rest, and quiet meals; increased use of alcohol and drugs, and, ultimately, exhaustion. The perfectionist ideal leaves out the important fact that people are only human and have limitations of body, mind, and spirit.

CONQUER PERFECTIONISM: AVOID ANXIETY

- Look for sources of satisfaction in simple pleasures.
- Pursue special interests such as painting, music, gardening, reading, handicrafts, etc.
- Take better care of the personal self with improved diet, rest, and exercise.
- Concentrate on the process of achieving a goal instead of the goal itself.
- Establish friendships outside work and family.
- Set personal priorities and stay with them.
- Find time to be alone and become better acquainted with yourself.

Many people believe the myth that overachieving will bring recognition and perhaps even love. Today's society measures individuals in terms of productivity and accomplishment. However, there is a delicate balance between the amount of work the human body and mind can do and the amount of time required for rest and regeneration. That balance differs for each person and is affected by feelings of stress, emotional overload, illness, and fatigue.

Overcoming Perfectionism

People who are plagued by the need to be perfect and its related stresses should realize their own limitations and reevaluate personal priorities. They must decide what is important and what is not and set realistic deadlines and short- and long-term goals, and adopt values that are not superficial.

See also OBSESSIVE-COMPULSIVE DISORDER; SELF-ESTEEM.

performance anxiety Performance anxiety, or stage fright, is a form of SOCIAL PHOBIA. Performance anxiety is a persistent, irrational fear of exposure to scrutiny in certain situations, particularly public speaking and musical, dramatic, or other types of performances. Some musicians are more prone to anxiety than performers in other disciplines because musicians have spent many years practicing by themselves, away from people. Actors, however, even though they train with other people, still may experience extreme performance anxiety when they appear before the public.

Some individuals experience performance anxiety in activities that are not scrutinized by the public, such as doing mechanical work or taking tests. Individuals who have this fear worry about doing something over which they might become embarrassed or humiliated. They tend to "catastrophize," or worry about what might happen in the worst possible cases. Catastrophizing thoughts might include: "I think I'm going to faint," "I don't think I will be able to get through to the end without cracking up," "I'm almost sure to make a dreadful mistake, and that will ruin everything," "I mustn't think about the possibility of making a mistake, or else I'll get into a state," "I don't feel in control of the situation; anything might happen," or "I think I'm going to be sick."

Symptoms may involve features of anxiety attacks, including dry mouth, lump in the throat, faintness, palpitations, rapid pulse, trembling, sweating, stomach upset, frequent urination, and inability to move. Some will avoid the situations, and some overcome these feelings and go through with their performance.

Treatment

Treatment includes positive thinking, with the individual—for example, a musician—repeatedly telling himself or herself, "I know I'm good and have prepared well for this; I'll go on and make them sit up and notice me," "I've prepared properly, so even if I do lose concentration for a bit my fingers can play the notes automatically," or "This concert is really going to be exciting."

Others use a mixed strategy—for example, thinking, "I will just concentrate on the music and ignore everything else," "I will just concentrate on staying relaxed," or "It's not the audience I worry about, it's my colleagues—if I mess it up, they are sure to notice."

To overcome audience sensitivity, some individuals use cognitive coping statements such as: "I will pretend the audience is not there and that it is a rehearsal," "The audience have paid their money; if I mess up I will be letting them down," or "I am in control; this tenseness I feel is an ally."

Learning to cope with performance anxiety includes cognitive therapy and repeated exposure

to an audience. Experience before an audience, for most performers, tends to reduce anxieties over time. However, it is difficult to determine whether the performances themselves enable people to be more comfortable or whether the most anxious performers, such as musicians, leave the field because of their anxieties.

Drug Treatment

Because many antianxiety drugs (such as benzodiazepines) cause drowsiness, other medications have been sought to combat performance anxiety. Beta-blockers have been tried with some degree of success. This class of drugs inhibits the activity of some NEUROTRANSMITTERS that are often associated with producing the physical symptoms of anxiety. The drug most often used in studies has been PROPRANOLOL. It has been helpful for musicians, public speakers, pilots, students taking examinations, and athletes. Preliminary studies have indicated that propranolol should be taken in a single dose just before exposure to the situation about which the individual feels anxious. However, some beta-blockers are not safe for individuals who have

---

BEHAVIOR OBSERVED IN PERFORMANCE ANXIETY

Paces
Sways
Shuffles feet
Knees tremble
Extraneous arm and hand movement (swings, scratches, toys, etc.)
Arms rigid
Hands restrained (in pockets, behind back, clasped)
Hand tremors
No eye contact
Face muscles tense (drawn, tics, grimaces)
Face "deadpan"
Face pale
Face flushed (blushes)
Moisten lips
Swallows
Clears throat
Breathes heavily
Perspires (face, hands, armpits)
Voice quivers
Speech blocks or stammers

ASTHMA or other lung disorders, cardiovascular disease, diabetes, or hypothyroidism.

personal filth, fear of   Fear of personal filth is similar to a fear of being dirty, which is known as automysophobia. This is a common fear of those who have obsessive-compulsive disorder.

See also CONTAMINATION, FEAR OF; DIRT, FEAR OF.

personality disorders   Patterns of relating to other people, perceiving, and thinking that are deeply ingrained, inflexible, and maladaptive. Such patterns are severe enough to cause the individual anxieties or distress or to interfere with normal functioning. Usually personality disorders are recognizable by adolescence or earlier, continue through adulthood, and become less obvious in middle or old age. The American Psychiatric Association's *DIAGNOSTIC AND STATISTICAL MANUAL OF MENTAL DISORDERS* categorizes personality disorders into three clusters:

Cluster A: Paranoid, schizoid, and schizotypal personality disorders. Individuals who have these disorders often appear odd or eccentric.

Cluster B: Antisocial, borderline, histrionic, and narcissistic personality disorders. Individuals who have these disorders often appear dramatic, emotional, or erratic.

Cluster C: Avoidant, dependent, obsessive-compulsive, and passive–aggressive personality disorders. Individuals who have these disorders often appear anxious or fearful.

The DSM-III-R also lists another category, "personality disorder not otherwise specified," that can be used for other specific personality disorders or for mixed conditions that do not qualify as any of the specific personality disorders. (See also charts that follow.)

See AVOIDANT PERSONALITY DISORDER; BORDERLINE PERSONALITY DISORDER; DEPENDENT PERSONALITY DISORDER; OBSESSIVE-COMPULSIVE DISORDER; PARANOID THINKING.

American Psychiatric Association, *Diagnostic and Statistical Manual of Mental Disorders* (Washington, DC: American Psychiatric Association, 1987).

personal odor, fear of   Fear of personal odor is known as bromidrophobia. This may relate to BODY ODOR, odor from soap, hair, perfume, clothing, or shoes, or anything else about the person. Some individuals fear personal odors from themselves; other individuals fear personal odors from others.

personal space   The invisible zone of privacy that individuals unconsciously put between themselves and other people. Although personal space is something rarely noticed, when it is invaded by someone approaching too closely, people may feel stressed and become anxious, irritated, and even hostile.

According to Lisa Davis, in *In Health* (September/October 1990), "we invite others in to our personal space by how closely we approach them, the angle at which we face them, and the speed with which we break a gaze. It's a subtle code but one we use and interpret easily and automatically, having absorbed the vocabulary since infancy."

Anthropologists have reported that people follow fairly established rules regarding how far apart they stand, depending largely on their relationship to each other. For example, friends, spouses, lovers, parents, and children tend to stand inside a "zone of intimacy," or within arm's reach, while a personal zone (about four feet) is comfortable for conversation with strangers and acquaintances.

The size needed for personal space depends on many variables, including the individual's cultural background, gender, and the nature of the occasion. Individuals from North European or British ancestry usually want about a square yard of space for conversation in uncrowded situations. However, people from more tropical climates choose a smaller personal area and are more likely to reach out and touch the occupant of another space. In Mediterranean and South American societies, social conversations include much eye contact, touching, and smiling, typically while standing at a distance of about a foot. In the United States, however, people usually stand about 18 inches apart for a social conversation; while they will shake hands, they tend to talk at arm's length.

Understanding cultural and gender differences in interpretations of personal space is becoming more important as intercultural trade and business

THEORIES ABOUT PERSONALITY DISORDERS

Theorist	Type	Emphasis	Viewpoint	Goal	Methods	Therapy
Freud	Traditional (Psychoanalytic)	Emotions, Biological Instincts, Unconscious Processes	(Biological) Intra-psychic	Explaining/Helping	Case Histories	Psychoanalysis
Erikson	Traditional (Psychoanalytic)	Emotions, Biological Instincts, Unconscious Processes (Conscious Processes)	(Biological) Intra-psychic Social	Explaining/Helping	Case Histories	Psychoanalysis
Jung	Traditional (Jungian Psychoanalytic)	Emotions, Biological Instincts, Unconscious Processes	(Biological) Intra-psychic Religious	Explaining/Helping	Case Histories	Jungian Psychoanalysis
Adler	Traditional (Psychoanalytic/ Humanistic)	Emotions, Biological Instincts, Conscious Processes	(Biological) Intra-psychic Social	Explaining/Helping	Case Histories (Experiments)	Adlerian Psychoanalysis/ Humanistic
Trait Theorists	Traditional	Underlying Traits or Dispositions	(Biological) Intra-psychic	Describing/ Predicting	Tests	Psychoanalysis/ Humanistic
Rogers	Personologist (Humanistic)	Cognitions, Conscious Processes, Self-Actualization	Intra-psychic	Explaining/ Helping	Case Histories	Humanistic
Maslow	Personologist (Humanistic)	Cognitions, Conscious Processes, Self-Actualization	Intra-psychic	Explaining/Helping	Case Histories	Humanistic
Murray	Personologist	Cognitions, Conscious Processes, Themas	Intra-psychic Social/ Behavioral	Helping/Predicting	Case Histories Personality Tests	Humanistic
Skinner	Personologist (Behaviorist)	Learned Responses (Denies Conscious & Unconscious Processes)	Social/Behavioral	Helping/Predicting	Experiments	Behavior Modification
Social Learning Theorists (Bandura)	Personologists	Perceptions, Cognitions, Conscious Processes	Intra-psychic Social/Behavioral	Helping/Predicting	Experiments	Cognitive Behavior Modification

James V. McConnell, *Understanding Human Behavior* (New York: Holt, Rinehart and Winston, 1986).

PERSONALITY DISORDERS

Disorder	Description
Histrionic (formerly hysterical personality)	Behaves in an exhibitionistic, immature manner, superficially charming and seductive, but after a relationship is established may become demanding and self-absorbed. Despite sexual flirtatiousness, is often naïve and sexually unresponsive.
Dependent	Does not want to have responsibility or to make decisions; non-assertive, lacking in self-confidence; difficulty being alone.
Passive-aggressive	Resists demands of others by noncompliance, inaction and procrastination; is forgetful, and makes weak excuses and apologies, never expressing true resentment and anger.
Compulsive	Has restricted ability to express warm and tender emotions. Preoccupied with rules, order, and detail.
Avoidant	Shows extreme sensitivity to rejection, ridicule, or disapproval. Avoids close personal attachments even though desires affection and acceptance.

transactions escalate. The interpretation of personal space leaves much room for misinterpretation. Consultants have developed businesses interpreting for people of all nationalities the meaning and use of personal space to prevent occurrences of stressful situations. It is possible that a culture's use of space is evidence of a reliance on one sense over another. For example, Middle Easterners get much of their information through their senses of smell and touch, which require a close approach, while Americans rely primarily on visual information, backing up in order to see an intelligible picture.

See also ACCULTURATION; CROWDING; MIGRATION.

Padus, Emrika, ed., *The Complete Guide to Your Emotions and Your Health.* Rev. ed. (Emmaus, PA: Rodale Press, 1994).

phagophobia Fear of eating or swallowing.
See also ANOREXIA NERVOSA; EATING, FEAR OF; FOOD, FEAR OF; SWALLOWING, FEAR OF.

phalacrophobia Fear of becoming bald.
See also BALD, FEAR OF BECOMING.

phallic stage In psychoanalysis, the third stage of psychosexual development, usually between ages three and six, when the child first focuses sexual feeling on the genital organs and masturbation becomes a source of pleasure. According to Sigmund Freud, the penis becomes the center of attention for both boys and girls. During the phallic phase or stage, the boy experiences sexual fantasies toward his mother and rivalry toward his father, both of which he eventually gives up due to castration fear. Similarly, the girl experiences sexual fantasies toward the father and hostility toward the mother, due to rivalry and blaming her for being deprived of a penis, but gives up these feelings when she becomes afraid of losing the love of both parents. According to the American psychoanalyst Erik Erikson (1902–94), if the child does not successfully advance out of the phallic stage into the genital stage, he or she experiences guilt and role fixation or inhibition, leading to later anxieties.

See also CASTRATION ANXIETY; DEVELOPMENTAL STAGES; ERIKSON, ERIK; GENITAL STAGE; OEDIPUS COMPLEX.

phallic symbol In psychoanalysis, any object that resembles or represents the penis. Structures that are longer than they are wide may be symbolic of the penis in dreams or in daily life. Examples include trees, skyscrapers, cigars, pencils, snakes, flutes and other musical instruments such as clarinets or trombones, motorcycles, airplanes, hammers, and many other similarly shaped objects.

See also CASTRATION ANXIETY; PHALLIC STAGE; SEXUAL FEARS; SYMBOLS, FEAR OF.

phallophobia Fear of the penis, especially an erect penis.

See also CASTRATION ANXIETY; GENITALS, FEAR OF MALE; PHALLIC STAGE; SEXUAL FEARS.

phantom limb pain Individuals who have had a limb (or a breast) removed by surgery may still experience pain as if it were coming from the absent limb. Doctors are not sure why this occurs, but phantom limb pain exists and is not imaginary. Individuals experiencing this kind of pain become anxious, irritable, and nervous because they often do not understand what is happening to them. There is no single method of relieving phantom pain in individuals who experience it, but the least invasive method seems to be relaxation techniques.

See also PAIN, ANXIETY AND DEPRESSION IN.

pharmacological approach See ANTIDEPRESSANTS; ANXIOLYTICS; BENZODIAZEPINES; LITHIUM.

pharmacophobia Fear of taking drugs or medicine.
See also DRUGS, FEAR OF TAKING.

phasmophobia Fear of GHOSTS.

phengophobia Fear of daylight or sunlight.
See also DAYLIGHT, FEAR OF; SUNLIGHT, FEAR OF.

philemaphobia, philematophobia Fear of kissing.
See also KISSING, FEAR OF.

philophobia Fear of love.
See also LOVE, FEAR OF.

philosophobia Fear of philosophy.

phobia A phobia is an irrational, intense fear of a person, object, situation, sensation, experience, thought, or stimulus event that is not shared by the consensual community and is thus out of proportion to any danger. The individual cannot easily explain or understand the phobia, has no voluntary control over the anxiety response, and seeks to avoid the dreaded situation or stimulus.

Not all phobias can be neatly classified because phobias of almost any situation can occur and may be associated with almost any other psychological symptom. However. when phobias occur as the dominant symptom, the condition is called a phobic state, phobic reaction, or phobic disorder. According to the American Psychiatric Association's *Diagnostic and Statistical Manual of Mental Disorders* (fourth edition, revised), phobias are classified as restricted or limited avoidance; AGORAPHOBIA, a form of panic disorder, is extensive avoidance.

Specific (Simple) Phobias

The essential feature of a simple phobia is a persistent, irrational fear of, and compelling desire to avoid, specific objects or situations. Simple phobia is characterized by a relatively specific fear of an object or a situation. The range of stimuli that may elicit a fearful response is narrower than in other phobic disorders. Simple phobias are therefore now also referred to as specific phobias.

The category of specific phobias contains an endless list of fears, as almost any object or situation can be phobic for a given individual. This is evident in this encyclopedia by the number of entries covering different phobias. Commonly recognized specific phobias are certain modes of transportation, such as driving, driving across bridges, or flying. Public speaking seems to be the most common phobic situation in the population. Heights and darkness seem to be the most common specific phobias. Other common phobic objects or situations include harmless animals such as dogs and cats, thunderstorms, darkness, and heights. All fears that do not fit into other phobic groups are categorized as simple phobias.

The individual with a specific phobia experiences physiological symptoms and behavior typical of many phobic disorders. However, because these fears are so specific, usually the individual can avoid contact with the phobic object, especially in instances in which the likelihood of a confrontation with the feared object or situation is low, as in snake phobias. On the other hand, individuals who fear common situations, such as elevators or heights, may not be able to avoid these stimuli easily.

Individuals with animal phobias usually only have symptoms in the presence of, or anticipated presence of, their phobic objects. Snakes, spiders, and birds have been the most reported animal phobias. Animal phobias are more prevalent among women.

Blood and injury phobias are special types of simple phobias. Unlike other phobias, which cause increased pulse and other physiological signs of arousal, blood and injury phobias produce lower pulse and blood pressure and bring on fainting spells.

The majority of specific phobias begin at any age. However, certain phobias are more common among certain age groups. For example, infants often fear loud noises and strangers. Children commonly fear darkness and injections. Fears of animals are common in preschool children around age five. Fear of aging occurs most commonly in people over age 50.

While the age of onset of different phobias varies widely, the average age at which patients seek treatment is age 24, according to Isaac Marks (1969).

How specific phobias start is not well understood. Researchers differ in their explanations; some report that direct conditioning—for example, a traumatic event—is an important factor, while others say that indirect learning experiences or exposure to negative instructions and vicarious experiences are also influential. Many individuals who have specific phobias do not recall the origin of their fear. Treatment of the phobic symptom, however, does not have to wait until the origin is uncovered.

Some specific phobias do not last long and improve as the individual gets older. Phobias in this category include doctors, injections, darkness, and strangers. However, fears of heights, storms, and enclosed places usually last longer. Fears of animals that are prevalent in children between the ages of nine and 11 remain with many girls after age 11 but disappear in most boys.

There are differences of opinions regarding effects of family influences on specific fears. While some experts say that the majority of specific phobics come from families in which no other member of the family shares the same fear, some studies have found relatively strong associations between the fears of mothers and children. Many specific phobics are dependent or anxious individuals, and their family backgrounds may have contributed to these characteristics.

Social Phobia

Individuals who have social phobias have excessive anxiety in social situations such as parties, meetings, interviews, restaurants, making complaints, writing in public, eating at restaurants, and interacting with the opposite sex, strangers, and aggressive individuals. They often fear situations in which they believe they are being observed and evaluated, such as eating, drinking, speaking in public, driving, etc.

Social phobia may be associated with fears of negative evaluation or embarrassing public behavior, such as making mistakes, being criticized, making a fool of oneself, sweating, fainting, blushing, speaking poorly, vomiting, or being rejected. Individuals with these phobias usually avoid the specific situations that they fear. Some individuals will participate in the activity only when they cannot be seen, for example, swimming in the dark.

Social phobias usually begin in late adolescence or early adulthood, although the range for onset is from 15 to 30. Usually social phobias are accompanied by heightened levels of generalized anxiety.

Some social phobias begin developing over many months or years, but sometimes a precipitating event can be determined. Some social phobics attribute their fears to direct conditioning, some to vicarious factors, and some to instructional and informational factors. Direct negative learning experience may play an important role.

Parental behavior may have some influence on social phobias. For example, parents who have few friends and are socially anxious in the presence of others may influence their children to react in similar ways. Also, the presence of anxiety in children is often associated with verbal punishment and criticism by parents.

Unlike specific or simple phobias, which tend to diminish as the individual grows into puberty and young adulthood, social phobias persist. Many such individuals have traits that interfere with social and marital adjustment. Some have ongoing problems with generalized anxiety, dependence, authority, and depression.

Social phobias often persist on a continuous basis, unlike agoraphobia, which tends to be episodic. Sometimes improving and sometimes worsening during periods of depression, social phobias also differ from the fears of crowds that agoraphobics suffer. Social phobics fear observation by individuals, while agoraphobics partly fear the masses of the crowds and feelings that might occur in crowds such as loneliness, separateness, or lack of identity.

Mixed and Other Classifications

Phobias of internal stimuli These are phobias within the individual with no external stimuli that can be avoided to reduce fear. Examples are fears of cancer, heart disease, venereal disease, and death. Fears of this type are often characteristic of depressive illnesses; in such cases, they improve when the depression improves. Illness phobias occur in both sexes. Some of these fears may be regarded as an extreme form of hypochondria.

Obsessive phobias These are fears that are disproportionate to the demands of the situation, cannot be explained by the individual, and are beyond voluntary control. Examples are fears of harming people or babies, fears of swearing, or fears of contamination that lead to obsessive hand-washing. Such phobias usually occur along with other obsessive-compulsive disorders.

See also AGORAPHOBIA ANXIETY; DIAGNOSTIC AND STATISTICAL MANUAL OF MENTAL DISORDERS; DIAGNOSTIC CRITERIA; FAMILY PATTERNS; HYPOCHONDRISM; OBSESSIVE-COMPULSIVE DISORDERS; PANIC; PHOBIC ANXIETY; PHOBIC CHARACTER; PHOBIC DISORDERS; PHOBIC REACTION; SOCIAL PHOBIA.

Adams, Henry E., and Patricia B. Sutker, *Comprehensive Handbook of Psychopathology* (New York: Plenum Press, 1984).

Barlow, David H., "Phobia," in *Encyclopedia Americana* (Danbury, CT: Grolier, 1984).

Marks, Isaac M., "The Classification of Phobic Disorders" *British Journal of Psychiatry* 116 (1970), pp. 377–386.

Turner, Samuel, *Behavioral Theories and Treatment of Anxiety* (New York: Plenum Press, 1984).

phobic anxiety A response of mind and body that the individual experiences only in the actual or imagined presence of the feared object, person, or situation. According to the American Psychiatric Association, there may be a sudden onset of intense apprehension and terror, feelings of unsteadiness, unreality, impending doom, dying, going crazy, or doing something uncontrolled. Also, there may be shortness of breath, sensations of choking and smothering, chest pain or discomfort, hot or cold flashes, faintness, and trembling. Freud applied the term to a type of anxiety that stems from unconscious sources but is displaced to objects or situations such as open areas, insects, or bridges that represent the real fear while posing little if any actual dangers in themselves. Behavioral theories emphasize the conditioned-associative learning that produces a bond between triggering stimuli and the response of anxiety.

See also ANXIETY; PANIC ATTACK; PHOBIA; PHOBIC DISORDERS.

Turner, Samuel, *Behavioral Theories and Treatment of Anxiety* (New York: Plenum Press, 1984).

phobic character Extremely inhibited, fearful persons. This term was coined by Otto Fenichel (1899–1946), an Austrian psychoanalyst, to apply to some individuals who resort to defense mechanisms of phobic reactions such as projection, displacement, and avoidance when facing internal conflicts. In a more generic use, the term would describe a shy, socially inhibited person who lacks assertive and expressive skills and reports excessive anxiety in his or her life, particularly in social contact situations.

See also PHOBIA; PHOBIC ANXIETY; PHOBIC DISORDERS; PHOBIC REACTION.

phobic disorders A group of disorders in which the significant features are persistent and irrational fears of specific objects, activities, or situations that result in a compelling desire to avoid the dreaded object, activity, or situation. The individual recognizes the fear as excessive or unreasonable in proportion to the actual dangerousness of the object, activity, or situation. Such feelings are so intense that they interfere with everyday functioning and are often a significant source of distress.

According to Stewart Agras (1969), about 77 out of 1,000 people suffer from some type of phobic disorder. Fears of illness or injury are the most common fears, while agoraphobia is the most frequent phobia for which individuals seek treatment.

The American Psychiatric Association, in *Diagnostic and Statistical Manual of Mental Disorder*, says: "Irrational avoidance of objects, activities, or situations that have an insignificant effect on life adjustment is commonplace. For example, many individuals experience some irrational fear when unable to avoid contact with harmless insects or spiders, but this has no major effect on their lives. However, when the avoidance behavior or fear is a significant source of distress to the individual or interferes with social or role functioning, a diagnosis of a phobic disorder is warranted."

Phobic disorders also used to be called phobic neuroses, but the "neuroses" classification was dropped in the DSM-III-R.

See also ANXIETY DISORDERS; DIAGNOSTIC AND STATISTICAL MANUAL OF MENTAL DISORDERS; SEPARATION ANXIETY; SEXUAL FEARS.

Agras, W. S., et al., "The Epidemiology of Common Fears and Phobias," *Comparative Psychiatry*, 10 (1969), pp. 151–156.

Adams, Henry E., and Patricia B. Sutker, *Comprehensive Handbook of Psychopathology* (New York: Plenum Press, 1984).

phobic neuroses   See PHOBIC DISORDERS.

phobic reaction   A group of persistent, intense, irrational, dominating fears that interfere with everyday life. Autonomic symptoms such as stomach upset and acutely distressing feelings may mount to panic proportions when the individual faces a phobic situation. Phobic situations that cause such reactions usually arise from traumatic or vicarious experiences.

See also PHOBIC DISORDERS.

phoboanthropy   Fear of human beings. Also known as anthropophobia.

phobophobia   Fear of fears
See also FEAR.

phonemophobia   Fear of thinking.

phonophobia   Fear of noise, talking, speaking aloud, or one's own voice. Also, fear of telephones.

See also NOISE, FEAR OF; ONE'S OWN VOICE, FEAR OF; SPEAKING ALOUD, FEAR OF; TALKING, FEAR OF.

photoalgia   Fear of pain in the eye.

photoaugiaphobia   Fear of glaring lights. Also known as photoaugiophobia.

See also GLARING LIGHTS, FEAR OF.

photographed, fear of being   The fear of being photographed, common in certain traditional ethnic groups such as American Indians and gypsies, is an extension of the belief that an individual's soul exists in his or her reflection. Being photographed puts the subject in the power of the photographer and may cause harm or even death.

Modern believers in magic and witchcraft have even more to fear from being photographed. Twentieth-century wizards and sorcerers have adapted and intensified the practice of using a doll to injure someone by attaching a photograph of the victim to the doll.

See also MIRRORS, FEAR OF.

photophobia   Fear of light. More commonly, however, the term for photophobia refers to an organically determined hypersensitivity to light that results in severe pain and tearing in the eyes when the individual is exposed to light. This may occur during many acute infectious diseases.

See also LIGHT, FEAR OF; LIGHT AND SHADOW, FEAR OF.

phronemophobia   Fear of thinking.

phthiriophobia   Fear of lice or parasites.

See also LICE, FEAR OF; PARASITES, FEAR OF; PEDICULOPHOBIA.

phthisiophobia   Fear of tuberculosis. This word is derived from the obsolete word (phthisis) for tuberculosis, which comes from the Greek word *phthisis* or *phthiein* meaning "to decay."

See also TUBERCULOSIS, FEAR OF.

pins and needles, fear of   Fear of pins and needles is known as belonephobia or enetophobia. The phrase "being on pins and needles" refers to feelings of anxiety, apprehension, and tension.

See also ACUPUNCTURE, FEAR OF; ANXIETY; NEEDLES, FEAR OF.

placebo   A preparation containing the form of treatment but not the substance; that is, a pretense of treatment without the actual ingredients being there. A placebo may be prescribed or administered to cause the phobic individual to believe he or she is receiving treatment. Placebo effects include the psychologic and physiologic benefits as well as undesirable reactions that reflect the individual's expectations. For example, if the individual believes that a medication will reduce anxiety, it probably will.

Placebos also influence the effects of psychotherapy. For example, research in psychotherapy includes placebo groups in the research design in order to determine the proportion of people who get better just because they think they are receiving a treatment. Surprisingly, depending on the research method and types of treatment presented, between 30 percent and 70 percent of people will significantly improve with just placebo treatment. Similar results have been obtained in drug research.

These results suggest that a powerful internal and personal energy is available to people who "suffer" from mental disorders that can produce positive change and growth.

See also DRUGS.

places, fear of   Fear of specific places is known as topophobia. This fear may be related to fears of landscapes, rivers, lakes, or specific geographic areas.

See also LAKES, FEAR OF; LANDSCAPE, FEAR OF; RIVERS, FEAR OF.

placophobia   Fear of tombstones.

See also CEMETERIES, FEAR OF; DEATH, FEAR OF; TOMBSTONES, FEAR OF.

plague, fear of the   Fear of the plague has been one of mankind's greatest fears of disease. There are several types of plague, including bubonic plague, which is characterized by the appearance of buboes, or swollen lymph glands of the armpits and groin, and pneumonic plague, which is the only type that is spread by means of airborne particles. In 14th-century Europe, the plague was referred to as the Great Dying or the Great Pestilence, the Black Death or Black Plague, and it killed about one out of every four persons, or 25,000,000 people. At other times in history, millions of others have died of plague throughout the world. The disease is still feared, although deaths from it are relatively rare.

Plague still occurs in parts of the world, particularly in Africa, South America, and the southwestern United States. In 1986, 10 cases were reported in the United States.

The bacteria that cause plague are usually transmitted to humans through the bites of fleas. The bacteria was identified in 1854 by Alexandre Yersin, a French bacteriologist. The carrier flea may be carried by a rat or other rodent; fleas carried by humans and dogs usually do not harbor the disease. The best way to reduce fear of the plague is through control of rodents and fleas. The risk increases when unsanitary conditions encourage the increase of the rodent population, such as during wartime or flood conditions. Military personnel and others who must live in areas where sanitary conditions are poor receive a vaccine to prevent infection.

Plague has always been highly feared because of the death rate among persons who contract the disease. Symptoms, which include infections in various glands, fever, chills, coughing, vomiting, and bleeding from the gastrointestinal tract, usually peak within a few days to a week. The term "black plague" came about because of dark purplish or black spots that appear on the skin.

At various times in the past the plague was thought to be caused by many sources, including unfavorable astrological combinations and contaminations by witches. Historically, different approaches have been taken to control the spread of the plague. One of these was quarantine, or keeping ill individuals confined at home. This led to contamination of others in the household. Passengers and goods arriving on ships were also quarantined at times.

Fears of the plague have been reduced during the last half of the 20th century because antibiotic drugs, including streptomycin and tetracyclines, and sulfa drugs help to control the disease. Epidemiologists now understand how the disease is spread and can take appropriate measures to prevent it.

In the 1980s, acquired immunodeficiency syndrome (AIDS) has been called the plague of the 20th century because of its rapid spread and the extensive physical devastation that results in the death of its victims. AIDS, which still has no cure, is now becoming just as feared as the plague was in earlier centuries.

plants, fear of   Fear of plants is known as botanophobia. Some fear plants because they believe that plants consume oxygen needed by man; some fear the allergies and skin rashes plants cause. Others fear plants because of personal associations. There is an old superstition about leaving flowers in the rooms of sick persons at night. Flowers and plants, according to this superstition, were the hiding places for evil spirits who at night, under cover of darkness, would take possession of the sick person and inflict harm.

pleasure, fear of   Fear of pleasure is known as hedonophobia. Some individuals who have guilt feelings about themselves fear enjoying themselves and hence fear pleasure. Some cannot enjoy an activity or event themselves because others less fortunate than they cannot do what they are doing.

See also GUILT, FEAR OF.

plutophobia   Fear of wealth.

See also MONEY.

pluviophobia   Fear of rain.

See also RAIN, FEAR OF.

pneumatophobia   Fear of spirits or noncorporeal beings.

pnigophobia, pnigerophobia   Fear of being smothered or of choking. The word is derived from the Greek word *pnigos,* meaning "choking."

See also CHOKING, FEAR OF; SMOTHERING, FEAR OF.

pocrescophobia   Fear of gaining weight.

See also WEIGHT GAIN, FEAR OF.

poetry, fear of   Fear of poetry is known as metrophobia. Some individuals have fearful and even aversive feelings about poetry because of its basic nature and because of the way it is taught and analyzed. In classical times, Spartans banned certain types of poetry because they thought it promoted effeminate and licentious behavior. The rhyme and figurative language of poetry is odd and distracting to some people. Frequently, poetry contains words, allusions, and obscurely stated thoughts and feelings that are confusing or incomprehensible to people who lack a scholarly, academic background.

poetry as therapy for anxiety Like MUSIC THERAPY, poetry therapy—the treatment of ANXIETY by the patient's reading or writing poetry—can help an anxious or fearful individual communicate feelings he or she might not otherwise be able to express. Poetry helps the individual uncover and release emotions that previously may have been repressed, consciously or unconsciously, and thus reduce anxiety and fears. In reading poetry, the individual realizes that someone else feels as he does; he feels less alone with his anxieties and fears. Making up poetry gives an individual a chance to express ideas in an indirect manner. Poetry therapy is used as an adjunct to other forms of therapy. It can be used in group or individual therapy.

Poetry therapy, like MUSIC THERAPY, has been used since antiquity. Chants of magicians and faith healers may be thought of as poetry because of their repetitions. It is said that ancient Egyptian chants were written on papyrus and then eaten by the patient in order that he or she might benefit from the power of the words.

The Association for Poetry Therapy was founded during the late 1960s.

pogonophobia Fear of beards or of men with beards.
See also BEARDS, FEAR OF.

poinephobia See PUNISHMENT, FEAR OF.

pointing the finger, fear of Some individuals fear pointing at their own body to show a place that is diseased or weak and fear pointing at their own body when talking about where another person is diseased; the fear is that the pointing individual will get the same complaint in the same place.

A second fear regarding pointing the finger relates to pointing the finger at someone else. Children are taught not to point their finger at anyone. This notion goes back to early times when man worshipped the phallus, which was the source of life. Man feared the outstretched finger as the image of the male organ, and thus the finger could prove equally productive in the creation of both good and evil. In primitive society, the phrase "to point the finger" became synonymous with killing a person.
See also POINTS, FEAR OF.

points, fear of Fear of points or pointed objects is known as aichmophobia or aichurophobia. This fear may relate to a fear of pins and needles or a fear of sticks. From a psychoanalytic point of view, pointed objects may be phallic symbols, and thus fear of pointed objects may be a sexual fear. Since pointed objects are also capable of inducing painful stimulation, with experience these can become aversive stimuli that trigger ANXIETY and AVOIDANCE.

poison, fear of Fear of poison is known as iophobia, toxiphobia, toxophobia, and toxicophobia. Fear of poison may be related to a fear of contamination, germs, or dirt.
See also CONTAMINATION; FEAR OF; OBSESSIVE-COMPULSIVE DISORDER.

police, fear of Individuals who have a fear of police and police personnel may fear authority, punishment, or entrapment. It is usual for those who break the law to fear police, because they probably fear being caught. Those who exceed the speed limit while driving fear being seen by police because they may have to pay a fine for their violation or go to court to defend themselves. However, when an individual becomes very anxious every time he sees a uniformed police officer, it may actually be a phobia that causes physiological effects such as rapid breathing, dizziness, and gastrointestinal symptoms. Some individuals who fear police fear that if they are apprehended, they will be subjected to extensive questioning and perhaps prison. Thus a fear of police may also be a fear of loss of control over one's own destiny.
See also AUTHORITY, FEAR OF.

poliosophobia Fear of contracting poliomyelitis.
See also DISEASE, FEAR OF.

politicians, fear of Fear of politicians is known as politicophobia. Those who fear politicians may fear authority or regimentation or fear hearing untruths and exaggerations.

See also AUTHORITY, FEAR OF.

pollution, fear of Fear of environmental pollution may come from the fear of bad health effects brought on by exposure to polluted air or water. Anxiety may be increased by an individual's personal lack of control over his exposure to pollution and his inability to avoid the many pollutants found in everyday life, such as exhaust from cars, wastes from industry, smoke from cigarettes, and toxins in drinking water. Some individuals deal with fears of pollution by using avoidance behavior, such as refusing to live in or travel to big cities, where pollution is more prevalent. Fear of air pollution may lead some individuals to develop agoraphobia.

See also ACID DEW, FEAR OF; ACID RAIN, FEAR OF; AGORAPHOBIA, FEAR OF; SMOKING, FEAR OF.

poltergeists, fear of Poltergeists are supernatural spirits that are heard but not seen. *Polter* is the German word for noise, *geist* for spirit. Poltergeists terrorize their victims by rapping, scratching, banging, speaking, whistling, and singing. Victims have reported seeing volleys of stones thrown by unseen hands and large pieces of furniture moved by an invisible force. Poltergeists pull off bedclothes and dump the occupants out of bed. The disappearance and reappearance of small household objects is thought to be the work of a poltergeist. Poltergeists are also blamed for breaking glass and china, and setting fires.

While poltergeists have been called ghosts and DEMONS, they seem to be resistant to the rite of EXORCISM and are considered by some to be a type of nature spirit, such as an elf.

Research has shown that poltergeists typically are associated with adolescent girls with high intelligence and usually excessive fantasy life and little self-awareness. Fraud or simply the tendency of teenagers to play pranks or the neurotic impulse to engage in irrational behavior are also factors, especially in view of the nature of poltergeist behavior. However, in some cases, responsible people have been reported to have eliminated these possibilities through careful observation. There is a theory that certain individuals, particularly the adolescent or the mentally unstable, may have uniquely intense powers of mind of which they themselves are unaware. These pressures, according to the theory, may build into a force that can perform what appear to be the supernatural acts typical of poltergeists. Because of these observations and theories, poltergeists have been called "the only demon left commanding even limited acceptance among the credulous."

polyphobia Fear of many things is known as polyphobia. Many phobic individuals have more than one phobia and hence are polyphobic.

ponophobia Fear of work or fatigue is known as ponophobia.

See also FATIGUE, FEAR OF; WORK, FEAR OF.

porphyrophobia Fear of the color purple. This may be related to a fear of colors in general.

See also COLORS, FEAR OF.

Positron Emission Tomography (PET) A BRAIN IMAGING TECHNIQUE. Using PET, researchers can measure blood flow in areas of the brain that are thought to control panic and anxiety reactions. Differences in blood flow between the two hemispheres of the brain are probably connected with differences in metabolic rates and reflect differences in the activity levels of nerve cells of the two sides. PET is useful in assessing the amount of psychoactive drug in various parts of the brain, as well as physiological abnormalities.

possession, fear of Psychological ailments were often ascribed to possession by DEMONS or evil spirits in many primitive cultures. Until the end of the 17th century, some ANXIETY disorders were considered demoniacal possessions, and treatments included beating and exorcism. Modern VOODOO beliefs include notions that possession by evil spirits can result in violent mental and physical symptoms.

See also EVIL EYE, FEAR OF THE; VOODOO, FEAR OF.

postcoronary bypass anxiety See CORONARY BYPASS ANXIETY, POSTOPERATIVE.

postpartum anxiety Many women experience postpartum anxiety, or depression after childbirth or delivery. Many women have "weepy" spells and feel somewhat "blue" at this time. Even though a woman may be elated with her new baby, some of the mild depression can be attributed to the letdown after months of eager anticipation. Also, a woman's anxiety may come about because she feels fearful of being a parent, fears being a failure as a parent, feels less loving toward her baby than she thinks she should, and feels less sexually attractive to her mate because her body has not regained its normal shape. The woman may also feel a loss of self-esteem if she has gone from a job outside the home into full-time motherhood. Because of the demands of the new baby she may feel exhausted, overwhelmed with chores, and deprived of sleep and may fear the chronic fatigue that seems to accompany her new status. Also, any tensions between the couple that existed before the birth of a baby may worsen after the baby's arrival in the household.

Hormonal changes after the birth of a baby may also affect a woman's mood. For example, rapidly plummeting estrogen and progesterone can lead to hot flashes and irritability, similar to the phenemona associated with menopause. Additionally, sleep deprivation caused by frequent waking during the night by the baby can lead to irritability and depression.

The degree to which a woman experiences postpartum depression also depends on her support system, including her husband, family, and additional caretaker for the baby. Also, the baby's temperament may affect her mood. For example, if the baby is colicky and cries frequently, she may become anxious and irritable. If the baby is calm, she will feel like a better mother and experience less anxiety.

See also CHILDBIRTH, FEAR OF; DEPRESSION; PREGNANCY, FEAR OF.

postpartum depression DEPRESSION immediately following the delivery of a baby. It is probably caused by hormonal changes after the birth as well as by anxieties. Postpartum depression ranges from extremely common and short-lived "maternity blues" or "baby blues" to a state of serious depression in which the mother may have to be hospitalized.

Some women become depressed after childbirth because they fear being a parent or being a failure as a parent. They feel less loving toward the baby than they think they should and feel less sexually attractive to their mates because their bodies have not regained their normal shape. Women may be overwhelmed with chores of a new baby and sleep deprivation, caused by the baby's frequent waking during the night, which can lead to additional stresses of irritability and chronic fatigue. If women go from careers outside the home into full-time motherhood, they may also suffer a loss of SELF-ESTEEM. With reassurance and support from family and friends, this type of "blues" lasts only two or three days. However, in about 10 to 15 percent of women, the depression is more marked and lasts for weeks. There is a constant feeling of tiredness, difficulty sleeping, restlessness, and loss of appetite. These symptoms are more likely to happen when there is a strained relationship with the father, financial or other concerns, no family support, or a personality disorder. First-time mothers, single mothers, or women who suffered from depression during pregnancy are likely candidates. The condition may end on its own or may be treated with antidepressant drugs. Persistent, severe depressions or bipolar symptoms (manic-depressive disorders) may require psychiatric treatment.

See also CHILDBIRTH; PREGNANCY.

Stuart, Scott, Greg Couser, Kelly Schilder, et al., "Postpartum anxiety and depression: Onset and comorbidity in a community sample," *Journal of Nervous and Mental Disease* 186, no. 7 (July 1998): pp. 420–424.

post-traumatic stress disorder (PTSD) A form of ANXIETY DISORDER that is a psychological response to an event perceived by individuals as severely threatening to them personally or physically or to those they love. With regard to combat veterans, one group suffering from post-traumatic stress disorder, the syndrome has variously been known as shell shock, battle fatigue, and war neurosis. Veterans of heavy combat are more likely to suffer from PTSD than military employed far away from combat zones.

PTSD also affects hundreds of thousands of individuals who have survived the trauma of natural disasters, such as EARTHQUAKES, or accidental disasters, such as airplane crashes. Furthermore, auto accidents and medical procedures contribute to civilian PTSD. PTSD is not confined to war and catastrophe victims. For example, adults who suffered severe abuse in childhood or adolescence may develop PTSD. Individuals who were raped or sexually assaulted or victims of domestic violence may also develop PTSD. The common denominator among all who suffer from PTSD is that the traumatized individual felt terrified and helpless.

According to the Substance Abuse and Mental Health Administration, of all those who experience the same traumatic event, about 7 percent will develop symptoms of PTSD. In considering the population of adults ages 18 and older in the United States, the National Institute for Mental Health (NIMH) estimates that about 7.7 million people suffer from PTSD in any given year. This is about 3.5 percent of the population of this age group. PTSD can develop at any age, but according to NIMH, the average age of onset is 23 years.

Symptoms and Diagnostic Path

Although its symptoms can occur soon after the event, PTSD symptoms often surface several months or even years after the traumatic event. Many sufferers experience the traumatic event in their minds repeatedly. This can happen in sudden, vivid memories that are accompanied by very painful emotions, such as anxiety, depression, fear, and guilt. The memory can be so strong that individuals feel that they are actually experiencing the traumatic event again. When a person has a severe flashback to the traumatic event, he or she is in a dissociative state, which sometimes can be mistaken for sleepwalking.

Sometimes the re-experiencing of the trauma occurs in NIGHTMARES that are powerful enough to awaken the person, who screams in terror. Individuals with PTSD often develop insomnia in an attempt to avoid these dreaded dreams. At times, the re-experience comes as a sudden, painful rush of extreme emotions that seems to have no apparent cause. These emotions often include grief, anger, or intense fear. Individuals say these emotional experiences occur repeatedly, much as the memories or dreams about the traumatic event.

PANIC and anxiety often result from PTSD experiences. These emotions may result from the great fear that the individual felt during the traumatic event, which fear has remained unresolved during later life events. During the PANIC ATTACK, the throat tightens, breathing and heart rate increase, and feelings of dizziness and nausea are present. The person with PTSD is at risk for developing other forms of ANXIETY DISORDERS and/or DEPRESSION.

Avoidance behavior is usually present among individuals with PTSD. This behavior affects the individual's relationships, because he or she often avoids close emotional ties with family, colleagues, and friends. Initially, the person feels numb, with diminished emotions, and can complete only routine, mechanical activities. Later, when re-experiences of the event begin, the individual often alternates between a flood of emotions and the opposite response of an emotional numbing and the inability to feel or express any emotions at all.

Some individuals who have PTSD report that they cannot feel emotions toward those to whom they are closest or, if they can feel emotions, cannot express how they feel to others. As the avoidance continues, the person may be misinterpreted by others as bored, cold, or preoccupied.

Some individuals with PTSD actively avoid any situations that might remind them of the traumatic event. For example, a survivor of an airplane crash might overreact in another plane as it seems to descend too rapidly. Others who have PTSD may have poor work records and poor relationships with their family and friends. Some have trouble concentrating or remembering current information.

Behaviors of War Veterans with PTSD. Some people—particularly war veterans—avoid accepting responsibility for others because they think that they failed to ensure the safety of those who were killed or injured during battle. War veterans may become suddenly irritable or explosive without provocation. This may result from leftover feelings of being exploited by superiors during the war or anger over their helplessness as they waited for orders or fulfilled illogical orders. Drug and alcohol abuse and dependence are common among war veterans and others with PTSD.

Hypervigilance is another indicator of PTSD. Some war veterans and others who have PTSD are always on guard for danger. As a result they have exaggerated startle reactions. War veterans may revert to their war behavior, plunging for cover when they hear noises such as backfiring cars or fireworks, which are similar to the sounds of battle. The person who survived a tsunami may panic upon seeing a lake or even a river.

Some individuals with PTSD feel guilty because they survived the disaster when others did not. In combat veterans, this guilt may be worse if they witnessed or participated in behavior that was necessary to survive but which is generally unacceptable in society (such as killing or harming others). Even when there was nothing that the individual could have done to help others, an irrational guilt may be present.

Such guilt can contribute to depression as the individual begins to look on him- or herself as unworthy, a failure, or a person who violated his own prewar values.

Treatment Options and Outlook

PTSD is treated with psychotherapy, EYE MOVEMENT DESENSITIZATION AND REPROCESSING (EMDR), and medication. Trained therapists can help individuals with PTSD work through the trauma and pain and resolve their unexpressed grief.

Individual psychotherapy often helps. PTSD results, in part, from the difference between the individual's personal values and the reality that he witnessed during the traumatic event. Psychotherapy helps the individual examine his or her values and how his or her behavior and experience during the traumatic event violated them. The goal is resolution of the consciousness and brain and body experiences that were created as a result of the trauma. Additionally, the individual works to build his or her self-esteem and self-control, develop a good and reasonable sense of personal accountability, and renew a sense of integrity and personal pride.

Therapists may recommend family therapy because spouse's and children's behavior may affect and be affected by the individual suffering PTSD. Spouses and children report that their loved one does not communicate, show affection, or share in family life. The therapist can help family members learn to recognize and cope with the range of emotions that each person feels. They do this by learning good communication and parenting skills and stress-management techniques.

EMDR and exposure are empirically tested effective therapies for PTSD. Another effective therapy involves support groups, in which survivors of similar traumatic events are encouraged to share their experiences and reactions. In doing so, group members help one another realize that many people have suffered the same or similar experiences and felt the same emotions. That realization, in turn, helps the individual realize that he or she is not uniquely unworthy or guilty. Over time, the individual reevaluates himself or herself and others and can build a new view of the world and redefine a positive sense of self.

Medications such as antidepressants and antianxiety drugs may be helpful over the short term, when the distress is new and extreme. According to the National Institute for Mental Health, selective serotonin reuptake inhibitors (SSRIs), a form of antidepressant, are commonly prescribed to treat PTSD, including fluoxetine (Prozac), sertraline (Zoloft), escitalopram (Lexapro), paroxetine (Paxil), and citalopram (Celexa).

Risk Factors and Preventive Measures

Combat veterans are at risk for PTSD. Among noncombatatants, women are more likely to develop PTSD than men. There are no known preventive measures to allay the development of PTSD, since it is difficult to impossible to predict ahead of time that a traumatic event will occur. When traumatic events can be predicted ahead of time, every eventuality to protect the individual should be taken. Research shows that preexisting psychiatric conditions and/or early abuse are high-risk predictors of subsequent PTSD.

See also ANXIETY DISORDERS; AVOIDANCE BEHAVIOR; DISSOCIATION; EYE MOVEMENT RESENSITIZATION AND REPROCESSING; FEAR.

Bower, Gordon H., and Heidi Sivers. "Cognitive Impact of Traumatic events." *Development and Psychopathology* 10, no. 4 (Fall 1998): pp. 625–653.

potamophobia   Fear of rivers or of sheets of water.

See also RIVERS, FEAR OF; SHEETS OF WATER, FEAR OF.

potophobia   Fear of alcohol.

poverty, fear of   Fear of poverty is known as peniaphobia.

See also RUIN, FEAR OF.

precipices, fear of   Fear of precipices is known as cremnophobia. This fear may be related to fears of heights, high places, and falling.

pregnancy, fear of   Some women fear becoming pregnant, not becoming pregnant, and pregnancy itself, for a wide range of reasons. Some unmarried women fear conceiving and bearing a child out of wedlock. Some women, although married, do not want to be burdened with a child; some fear the pain of childbirth, and some fear that they might die during pregnancy or childbirth. Thus fears of pregnancy stem from both psychological and physical sources. Some women fear being taken over by their pregnancy, as if they had no other purpose than to produce a child. They fear feeling victimized by motherhood, as though the child inside them is a parasite. While many women are delighted with the first fetal movement, some find it a frightening indication that they are harboring a separate life. Many women fear the interruption in their work and physical activity brought about by pregnancy. Some women fear that their physical appearance while pregnant will become comical and that they will not be attractive to their husbands and to men in general. A pregnant woman sometimes extends this fear to a feeling that she will never return to her original physical appearance. Some women fear a loss of interest in sexual activity during pregnancy, while others fear an increased interest in sexual activity.

Pregnant women often have intense dreams and fantasies about the child they are carrying. Some women fear that they are losing their minds. Mood swings during pregnancy, sometimes triggered by hormonal changes, disturb many women and their husbands. Well-meant advice and anecdotes from other women can also be a source of anxiety.

Many women become anxious and embarrassed by the physical symptoms associated with pregnancy. Morning sickness, food cravings, frequent urination, water retention, bloating, and swollen breasts are frequent complaints. First-time mothers fear that they may not be able to recognize the first movements of the fetus and as a result may fear that the baby is abnormal or dead. Although most mothers fear weight gain during pregnancy, others may feel that they are not gaining enough. Recent findings about the effects on the fetus of the mother's smoking and alcohol consumption have caused many pregnant women to abstain out of fear that they will have an unhealthy baby.

Clumsiness increases during the last months of pregnancy and, in addition to being unpleasant in itself, makes women fearful of accidents. Some men and women fear that intercourse during pregnancy will harm the fetus. Others may feel uneasy during intercourse in the belief that the fetus is watching and aware of what they are doing.

Some fears related to pregnancy have changed in recent years because of technology, changing social attitudes, and changes in society. The fear of unwanted pregnancy has been reduced by the variety of birth control techniques. Motherhood without marriage has become more socially acceptable in some circles. Couples who are fearful of an inability to conceive now have hope because of modern medical advances, including in vitro fertilization and artificial insemination. In spite of legal complications, surrogate motherhood is also gaining some degree of acceptance. Women who have delayed motherhood into their late 30s or early 40s because of their own or their husbands' careers or because of the attraction of the single life face diminished fertility and greater anxiety about the possibility of birth defects that come with increased maternal age. Amniocentesis (testing the amniotic fluid to detect abnormalities in the fetus) allays some fears of women who postpone motherhood. Fears of bearing a monster and fears of childbirth itself are related fears.

See also BIRTHING A MONSTER, FEAR OF; CHILD-BIRTH, FEAR OF.

premenstrual syndrome (PMS), fear of   Fear of the physical and mental symptoms of anxiety and tension that some women experience before getting their menstrual periods. Many women fear the discomfort associated with PMS, which may include water retention, tender breasts, headaches, body aches, food cravings, lethargy, and depression. Causes of premenstrual syndrome have not been determined and vary from woman to woman. The symptoms that occur several days before menstruation seem to be related to the interplay of hormones between ovulation and the beginning of menstruation.

Many fears about PMS are grounded in actual fact; some may be due to inhibitions and unpleasant associations. Sufferers of PMS sometimes fear that they are going crazy. Some women resent the regular loss of several days a month to PMS. Even nonsufferers dread the fact that a genuine emotional response or complaint may be chalked up to hormones. Since menstruation is not a subject that is discussed freely, many women feel isolated or misunderstood because they suffer in silence. Women are anxious and fearful about the possibility of hostile or even violent interaction with husbands, lovers, children, or employers because of PMS. Statistics on occupational and automobile accidents show that women are more likely to be clumsy, inattentive, and unable to judge distances just before their periods. Students fear that they may have to take an exam that will affect their scholastic records and ultimately their career at this time. Women fear that other occasions when they want to be at their best, such as employment interviews or athletic events, will fall just before menstruation. Since resistance to infection is lowered before the onset of menstruation, a woman has more reason to fear illness just before her period.

Until recently, the medical attitude that the discomfort of PMS was all in the mind has tended to increase rather than decrease anxiety. While attitudes are changing and PMS is a recognized physical condition, there is still some reluctance to take it seriously. Although there is no single successful treatment for PMS, many doctors now regard it as a challenging problem in need of solution. A variety of treatments such as hormones, vitamins, analgesics, and diuretics have been tried with varying degrees of success.

See also MENSTRUATION; FEAR OF.

prepared fears   A theory that individuals may be biologically prepared to develop certain fears and less prepared to develop others. Humans may be prepared for conditioned fear responses to certain stimuli that once evoked danger in our evolutionary cycle. An ability to readily develop fear to these stimuli helped our ancestors avoid such stimuli and therefore survive. This theory helps explain the disproportionately high number of certain phobias, such as snakes and small animals.

Researchers who have tested the preparedness theory of fears and phobias say that prepared fears are easily acquired with as little as a single conditioning trial. Once developed they will be quite resistent to extinction, and the prepared conditioned fear is not easily reduced by the information, for example, that spiders are not likely to be harmful. The theory was proposed by Martin Seligman, a research psychologist, in 1972.

See also CAUSALITY.

Seligman, M. E. P., "Phobias and Preparedness," in M. E. P. Seligman and J. L. Hager (eds.), *Biological Boundaries of Learning* (New York: Appleton-Century-Crofts, 1972), pp. 451–462.

primal scene   A term used by psychoanalysts to denote the real or fancied observation by the infant of parental or other heterosexual intercourse. Some therapists have suggested that such an experience, whether real or imagined, gives rise to later anxieties.

See also PRIMAL THERAPY; PSYCHOANALYSIS.

primal therapy   A technique developed by Arthur Janov (1924–   ), an American psychologist and author of *The Primal Scream*. Primal therapy, also known as primal scream therapy, treats neuroses, including anxieties and phobias, by encouraging the individual to relive basic or "primal" traumatic events and discharge painful emotions associated with them. Such events may have led to development of the anxieties and phobias and frequently involve feelings of abandonment or rejection experienced in infancy or early childhood. During therapy the individual may cry, scream, or writhe in agony and later experience a sense of release and freedom from "primal pain."

primal trauma   An early-life situation that the individual perceived as painful that is presumed to be the basis for anxieties later in life.
See also ANXIETY.

primary gain   The basic internal psychological benefit that the individual derives from having a phobic condition, anxiety, or emotional illness. If the individual develops mental symptoms defensively in largely unconscious ways to cope with or to resolve unconscious conflicts, then the symptoms provide a relief to the individual's system by reducing conflict between UNCONSCIOUS and defensive forces. The need for such gain may be the reason why a phobic condition or emotional problem develops. In contrast, secondary gain is that which is obtained from a symptom of an illness or phobia one already has. The term primary gain is derived from psychoanalytic and psychodynamic theories that emphasize the role of unconscious forces in ANXIETY.
See also AGORAPHOBIA; SECONDARY GAIN.

primeisodophobia   Fear of losing one's virginity.
See also VIRGINITY, FEAR OF LOSING ONE'S.

proctophobia   Fear of rectal diseases or anything having to do with the rectum.
See also RECTAL DISEASES, FEAR OF; RECTUM, FEAR OF.

progesterone   A HORMONE secreted by females during the luteal phase of the menstrual cycle (after ovulation). Progesterone may partially explain why more women than men have panic attacks and why some women suffer most from anxiety prior to menstruation. The same factors may help explain PREMENSTRUAL SYNDROME (PMS), which is characterized by many of the symptoms exhibited during PANIC ATTACKS: anxiety, irritability, nausea, headaches, and lightheadedness.
See also POSTPARTUM DEPRESSION.

progress, fear of   Fear of progress is known as prosophobia. This fear may be related to fears of novelty, newness, and innovation, and to technophobia and computer phobia.
See also NEWNESS, FEAR OF.

progressive muscle relaxation   An anxiety management procedure (also known as *progressive relaxation*) in which individuals learn to make heightened observations of what goes on under their skin. They learn to control all of the skeletal muscles so that any portion can be systematically relaxed or tensed by choice.

First, there is recognition of subtle states of tension. When a muscle contracts (tenses), waves of neural impulses are generated and carried to the brain along neural pathways. This muscle-neural phenomenon is an observable sign of tension.

Next, having learned to identify the tension sensation, the individual learns to relax it. Relaxation is the elongation (lengthening) of skeletal muscle fibers, which then eliminates the tension sensation. This general procedure of identifying a local state of tension, relaxing it away, and making the contrast between the tension and ensuing relaxation is then applied to all of the major muscle groups.

As an anxiety management technique, progressive relaxation is only effective when individuals have the ability to selectively elongate their muscle fibers on command. They can then exercise the self-control required for progressive relaxation and more rationally deal with the anxiety-producing thoughts or situations. Practice to competency usually takes three to four months.

Edmund Jacobson (1888–1983) was the developer of this technique and used it extensively with his medical patients.

See also BIOFEEDBACK; RELAXATION; RELAXATION RESPONSE.

Jacobson, Edmund, *Progressive Relaxation: A Physiological and Clinical Investigation of Muscular States and Their Significance in Psychology and Medical Practice.* 2d ed. (Chicago: University of Chicago Press, 1981).
———, "The origins and development of progressive relaxation," *Journal of Behavior Therapy and Experimental Psychiatry* 8 (1977): pp. 119–123.
Lehrer, Paul M., and Robert L. Woolfolk, eds., *Principles and Practice of Stress Management,* 2d ed. (New York: Guilford Press, 1993).

projection A DEFENSE MECHANISM the individual uses unconsciously to reject ideas or thoughts that are emotionally unacceptable to the self and attribute (project) them to others. Interpersonally, this is called blame as well as projection. This mechanism is a common form of protection with children. Unfortunately, it often remains in place into adulthood. The use of blame prevents the individual from making any significant personal changes. In phobias, an individual is projecting danger onto neutral objects or situations.

prophylactic maintenance Administration of drugs that may prevent or reduce the risk of recurrence of symptoms of a disorder. For example, lithium is taken by some individuals who have MANIC-DEPRESSIVE DISORDER to prevent recurrence of symptoms. Some beta-blocking drugs are taken by some headache sufferers to prevent occurrence of HEADACHES. Individuals who take drugs for these purposes should be carefully monitored by a physician to adjust dosage and watch for possible adverse effects.

See also BETA-BLOCKING AGENTS; LITHIUM.

propranolol A drug within the family of medications known as beta-adrenergic blocking agents, beta-blocking agents, or BETA BLOCKERS. It is commonly used to treat high blood pressure, migraine headaches, angina, and some heart conditions. Propranolol is also used in some cases to reduce symptoms of anxiety, such as rapid heartbeat (tachycardia), sweating, and general tension. It has been used successfully to help control symptoms of stage fright and fears of public speaking. Because it has few side effects, many tolerate it well. But there are some possible side effects, including dizziness, unusually slow pulse, insomnia, diarrhea, cold hands and feet, and numbness and/or tingling of fingers to toes. Propranolol should not be taken by individuals who have chronic lung disease, asthma, diabetes, or certain heart diseases, or by individuals who are severely depressed.

Propranolol and other beta blockers are sometimes prescribed for individuals who have MITRAL VALVE PROLAPSE (MVP), and for individuals who fear having rapid heartbeat.

propriety, fear of Fear of propriety is known as orthophobia.

prosophobia Fear of progress.
See also PROGRESS, FEAR OF.

prostate cancer A common malignant tumor that appears in the male prostate gland. The prostate is a walnut-sized gland that is involved in sexual erections and fertility. Prostate cancer is the second leading cause of cancer death in men, after lung cancer. (Among women, the second leading cause of cancer death is BREAST CANCER.)

The prostate gland lies in front of the rectum and just below the bladder. The urethra, the tube that carries urine from the bladder to the outside of the body, passes through the prostate gland in men. As men age, the prostate gland often enlarges, and as a result, it sometimes causes difficulty with urination. The prostate can also become infected, which is known as *prostatitis.* These disorders can be treated by a urologist.

When prostate cancer is diagnosed, the diagnosis causes considerable stress and anxiety among most males, as well as depression, not only because they fear dying from cancer, but also because they often fear the loss of their sexual potency, which is a real risk for some men, depending on the treatment that they need in order to combat the cancer. (See SEXUAL FEARS.) They may also fear the loss of love and affection from their significant other. However, if surgery is chosen as the best treatment, nerve-sparing surgery may enable some men to continue to have an active sex life subsequent to a radical prostatectomy (the removal of the entire prostate gland). However, this procedure is generally available only at major medical centers.

Many men are anxious subsequent to treatment because they fear that the cancer may still be present. In some cases, prostate cancer does recur, while in others, the treatment effectively and permanently eradicates the cancer.

About 200,000 men are diagnosed with prostate cancer each year in the United States. According to the National Center for Health Statistics, there were 29,554 deaths from prostate cancer in 2003 in the United States. The rate of deaths per 100,000 males was 20.7. In 2004, 161,000 men had radical prostatectomies (removal of the prostate gland).

Prostate cancer is usually found among men older than age 50, but this form of cancer can also occur in younger men, particularly if there is a history of prostate cancer in the family. More than 80 percent of all prostate cancers are diagnosed in men older than 65 years.

Symptoms and Diagnostic Path

Often there are no symptoms with prostate cancer, and the physician may become suspicious of cancer only upon an abnormal finding that is made in the course of a routine annual rectal examination. During the digital rectal examination (DRE), the doctor inserts a gloved and lubricated finger into the rectum to check the prostate gland for its size and any abnormalities. Many men actively seek to avoid the rectal examination, due to their embarrassment and very minor discomfort, but this examination can be a lifesaver when cancer is present in the prostate.

When there are symptoms of prostate cancer, they may include those listed below. Note that these symptoms may also be found with other diseases of the prostate or of the urinary tract and individuals should not assume that they have (or do not have) prostate cancer if these symptoms are present. Instead, they should check with their doctors for further information.

- a need for frequent urination
- pain or burning during urination
- a weak urinary flow
- difficulty with erections
- difficulty with urination
- blood in the urine or semen
- constant pain in the lower back, pelvis, or upper thighs

A simple blood test known as a prostate specific antigen (PSA) test can also help to detect whether a man is at risk for prostate cancer. Experts disagree considerably on the level of PSA beyond which cancer may be present and, consequently, when a biopsy should be done. In addition, some experts believe that when the PSA test has been performed at least several times a steadily rising PSA level is a more significant finding than the actual PSA number itself. However, PSA levels naturally increase with age. The "free PSA" is a new additional test that seems to have good diagnostic potential.

If the physician suspects that a man has prostate cancer, the doctor may conduct a transrectal ultrasound of the pelvic area by inserting a small probe through the rectum. This provides the doctor with a sonogram, or image of the prostate. The doctor may also order X-rays if he fears that the cancer cells may have already spread to the bones.

When the physician suspects that prostate cancer may be present, he or she will order a *biopsy*, or the removal of tiny tissue samples from the prostate gland. A pathologist will study these samples with a microscope to see if cancer is present. If this examination indicates that cancer is present, the cancer is *graded* and then it is *staged*.

The Gleason grading system, named after Dr. Gleason who created the system, is used to evaluate the aggressiveness of the cancer cells, and this scale ranges from a "1" (normal) to a "5" (the most abnormal).

Staging means that the cancer is evaluated based on the size of the tumor and how far cancer cells have spread in the body and, if cells have spread, the location of the spreading. The cancer may have remained within the prostate gland or it may have spread to the adjoining tissue or to distant tissue.

There are four stages of prostate cancer, ranging from Stage I to Stage IV. With Stage I, the cancer is limited to the prostate and is found only by accident. It cannot be felt during a rectal examination. With Stage II cancer, the cancer is more advanced, but it has not spread beyond the prostate. With Stage III the cancer *has* spread beyond the prostate, but has not yet spread to the lymph nodes. With Stage IV, the cancer may be located in organs and muscles near the prostate gland. It may also have spread to the lymph nodes and to other parts of the body.

The treatment for prostate cancer is based on whether the cancer has metastasized (spread) beyond the prostate or not, as well as how aggressive the cancer is.

For example, if the cancer has *not* spread beyond the prostate gland, then surgery or localized radiation treatment may be good choices for the patient. If cancer *has* spread beyond the prostate, such as to the bones, and is no longer curable, then radiation treatment can often improve the pain caused by the cancer.

The choice of treatment(s) depends on a variety of factors as well as on the patient's overall health status, age, and other factors. Patients diagnosed with prostate cancer should consult with their urologist and oncologist to discover the best choices for their own individual situations.

Treatment Options and Outlook

When cancer is identified, there are several basic options, including

- surgery (removal of the prostate gland, or prostatectomy)
- internal radiation (brachytherapy, the temporary insertion of radioactive material which is later removed) or external radiation therapy, a controlled bombardment of radiation waves to the exterior of the body
- hormone therapy

- cryotherapy (the use of a special probe that is used to freeze the cancer cells)

Each form of treatment has its own risk and benefits; for example, prostatectomy may rid the body of cancer, but it may also cause temporary or even long-term urinary incontinence as well as erectile dysfunction. External beam radiation may be effective in killing the cancer cells but it may also irritate the bladder significantly.

Sometimes a combination of treatments is used, such as hormone therapy and radiation therapy, in the case of a recurring prostate cancer. Hormone therapy is generally comprised of one or more long-acting injections, which are given to impede the production of testosterone by the testicles, since testosterone makes prostate cancer grow. Less testosterone translates into a lower risk for cancer cell growth and allows radiation treatment to be more effective against the cancer.

The choice of treatment depends on the severity and aggressiveness of the cancer as well as other factors. For example, if the man is younger than age 50 and the cancer appears to be contained within the prostate, then he may opt for radiation therapy or for a nerve-sparing prostatectomy which may enable him to continue having erections. The prostatectomy performed by most urologists does not spare the nerves needed for the man to continue to have the capacity to achieve erection. However, prostheses are available.

According to the National Cancer Institute, before treatment begins, men with prostate cancer should consider asking their doctor the following questions

- What is the stage of the disease? Do any lymph nodes show any indication of cancer? Has the cancer spread?
- What is the grade of the tumor?
- What is the goal of treatment? What are the treatment choices? Which treatment do you recommend and why?
- What are the expected benefits of each treatment?
- What are the risks and possible side effects of each treatment that I should consider? How can side effects be managed?

- What can I do to prepare for treatment?
- Will the treatment require me to stay in a hospital? If so, for how long?
- How will treatment affect my normal activities? Will it affect my sex life? Will I have urinary problems? Will I have bowel problems?
- What will the treatment cost? Will my insurance cover it?
- Would a clinical trial research study be the right choice for me?

Risk Factors and Preventive Measures

African-American men have a greater risk for the development of prostate cancer than men of any other racial group, although the reasons for this are unknown. In addition, men with a family history of prostate cancer, particularly men whose fathers and/or brothers were diagnosed with the disease, have an increased risk.

As mentioned, increasing age raises the risk of developing prostate cancer. (See table below.) For example, the risk of a prostate cancer diagnosis is one in 2,500 for men who are age 45, but the risk increases to one in 476 for men who are age 50. The risk is one in nine for a male who is age 75. If family members have prostate cancer or the man is African American, the risks are further increased.

It is unknown if or how men can prevent prostate cancer from occurring, although many studies are underway to determine if dietary or vitamin supplements may act as preventive measures. Some studies indicate that eating tomatoes may reduce the risk of developing prostate cancer. Ongoing studies seek to determine whether selenium or vitamin E may reduce the risk of prostate cancer.

Carroll, Peter R., MD, Carducci, Michael A., MD, Zietman, Anthony L., MD, and Rothaermel, Jason M., RN, *Report to the Nation on Prostate Cancer: A Guide for Men and Their Families* (Santa Monica, CA: Prostate Cancer Foundation, 2005).

Centers for Disease Control and Prevention. *Prostate Cancer Screening: A Decision Guide.* Available online. URL: http://www.cec./gov/cancer/prostate/prospdf/prosguide.pdf. Downloaded December 2, 2006.

Lange, Paul H., MD, and Christine Adamec, *Prostate Cancer for Dummies* (New York: Wiley, 2003).

National Cancer Institute, *What You Need to Know About Prostate Cancer* (Rockville, MD: National Institutes of Health, 2005). Available online. URL:http://www.cancer.gov/pdf/WYNTK/WYNTK-prostate.pdf. Downloaded December 2, 2006.

prostitutes, fear of   Fear of prostitutes is known as cyprianophobia. Fears of the practice of prostitution are a mixture of social, religious, and individual fears. Some men fear getting diseases from prostitutes, while others think that prostitutes are evil, without personal moral standards, and hence to be feared. Today, of course, this fear is also compounded by the possibility of acquiring acquired immunodeficiency syndrome (AIDS) from prostitutes. Businessmen and neighborhood residents fear prostitution because it damages the area where they live and conduct legitimate businesses. Prostitutes are a reminder of the negative influences in society, including unemployment, child abandonment, and broken families. Prostitution seems to increase in times of war and social disorder.

Women who contemplate prostitution as a form of employment have their own fears. For example, they may fear arrest or fear becoming victims of violence or venereal disease. Many prostitutes fear addiction to drugs or alcohol. Prostitutes may fear total control by a pimp and fear being in a situation they cannot control. On the other hand, in very repressive societies, women have become prostitutes out of fear of the life of the ordinary wife and mother who has no independence, freedom, or rights.

RISK OF BEING DIAGNOSED WITH PROSTATE CANCER BY	
Age 45	1 in 2,500
Age 50	1 in 476
Age 55	1 in 120
Age 60	1 in 43
Age 65	1 in 21
Age 70	1 in 13
Age 75	1 in 9

Source: Centers for Disease Control and Prevention. Prostate Cancer Screening: A Decision Guide. Available online. URL: http://www.cec./gov/cancer/prostate/prospdf/prosguide.pdf. Downloaded December 2, 2006, page 4.

As prostitution is often associated with other criminal activities, men may fear violence, theft, blackmail, and arrest. A woman may fear the involvement of her husband or lover with a prostitute because of the possibility of transmission of disease to her and the possibility that he may become emotionally involved with the prostitute.

Prostitution is as much a product of fear as a cause of fear. In the past, it was a form of contraception for couples who did not want more children. Men patronized prostitutes out of a fear that sex was a distasteful duty for a "good" woman. Men who are afraid to ask a wife or lover to act on unusual sexual preferences feel comfortable with prostitutes, as do some men who want assistance with sexual dysfunction. Men may also turn to prostitutes out of fear of intimacy and the usual romantic and domestic demands of a relationship with a woman.

See also SEXUAL FEARS.

Prozac The trade name for an antidepressant drug (fluoxetine) that has been available since the late 1980s. It is part of a class of selective serotonin reuptake inhibitors (SSRIs) with low toxicity and free of many side effects attributed to TRICYCLIC ANTIDEPRESSANTS. Fluoxetine is not sedative, has no anticholinergic side effects, and does not promote weight gain. Side effects may include possible nausea and weight loss—both usually time limited—insomnia, and anxious agitation that occurs rarely and is dose-related. Most people adjust to these side effects.

Martin, Andrew, "Psychopharmacology update: What's new in the treatment of depression," *Psychoanalysis and Psychotherapy* 15, no. 1 (1998): pp. 131–134.

psellismophobia See STUTTERING, FEAR OF.

pseudoscientific terms, fear of Fear of pseudoscientific terms is known as Hellenologophobia.

psychiatrist Physicians (medical doctors with an M.D. degree) specializing in mental/emotional treatment and research. Some psychiatrists tend to view mental "disorders" as chemical or biological in their source and hence medical in nature.

By virtue of their medical degree, psychiatrists can prescribe medications and conduct medically defined procedures (such as electroconvulsive shock therapy) and can admit patients to hospitals.

See also PSYCHIATRY, SCHOOLS OF.

psychiatry, schools of There are several theoretical frames of reference that have influenced and still influence psychiatrists' methods of treatment. The schools offer various explanations of how psychiatric symptoms or disorders develop, how they interfere with functioning, and how and why they can be changed by therapeutic interventions.

See also AVERSION THERAPY; BEHAVIORISM; CLASSICAL CONDITIONING; DESENSITIZATION; EXISTENTIAL ANALYSIS.

psychoactive drug A chemical compound that has a psychological effect and alters mood or thought processes. A tranquilizer is an example of a psychoactive drug. Some psychoactive drugs may be prescribed for individuals under treatment for phobias.

See also ANTIDEPRESSANTS; DRUGS; MAJOR TRANQUILIZER; MINOR TRANQUILIZER.

psychoanalysis A therapy developed by Sigmund Freud that stresses free association, dream analysis, transference, and the modification of defenses to allow the conscious expression of unconscious impulses, memories, emotions, experiences, etc. Psychoanalytic theory has had a powerful impact on our culture, art, movies, literature, advertising, child-rearing practices, views of mental and emotional disorders, and therapy. Anxiety was a key component of the therapy and the theory of human behavior. Psychoanalysis in theory was instrumental in developing anxiety as a diagnostic category.

psychodiagnostics Psychodiagnostics is concerned with the methods used to diagnose mental and emotional disorders, including anxiety and phobias.

Classification of mental disorders allows research-ers to conduct scientific experiments and helps therapists to choose the most appropriate course of treatment.

The process of labeling and discriminating between disorders is largely arbitrary and subjec-tive. The DIAGNOSTIC AND STATISTICAL MANUAL OF MENTAL DISORDERS, produced by the American Psy-chiatric Association, is periodically updated and revised to include reforms in the field. For exam-ple, the third edition included a multiaxial system of classification that forced a diagnostician to take a broader range of information into account when diagnosing a client.

The DSM includes many related disturbances in the "anxiety disorders" category. The first are the phobic disorders, followed by panic disorder, which includes generalized anxiety disorder, obsessive-compulsive disorder, and post-traumatic stress disorder. Demand for further reform of the DSM continues. Suggestions for changes include further study into the validity of the system, a modifica-tion of definitions, new organization, and a further increase in the number of conditions a person must fulfill before a diagnosis is reached.

See also DIAGNOSIS; DIAGNOSTIC CRITERIA.

psychodrama   A therapeutic technique in which individuals act out, or watch others act out, per-sonal problems, including phobias and anxiet-ies. Psychodrama is a type of group therapy that evolved in Vienna in the early part of the 20th century. Individuals create their own plays mirror-ing their personal problems and conflicts. Psycho-dramatic methods are applicable to many types of phobic individuals and may be used by therapists to help individuals overcome specific phobias or gen-eral anxieties.

See also ROLE PLAYING.

psycho-imagination therapy (PIT)   PIT is a tech-nique that uses waking imagery and imagination to effect personality changes and alter the ways an individual copes with anxieties. The basic proposi-tion of psycho-imagination therapy is recognizing people's needs to become aware of how they define

SCHOOLS OF PSYCHIATRY

I. Reconstructive
  A. Psychoanalysis—Sigmund Freud
  B. Neo-Freudian, modifications of psychoanalysis
    1. Active analytic techniques—Sandor Ferenczi, Wilhelm Stekel, the Chicago school (espe-cially Franz Alexander and Thomas French)
    2. Analytic play therapy—Anna Freud, Melanie Klein
    3. Analytical psychology—Carl Jung
    4. Character analysis, orgone therapy—Wilhelm Reich
    5. Cognitive—Jean Piaget
    6. Developmental—Erik Erikson
    7. Ego psychology—Paul Federn, Eduardo Weiss, Heinz Hartmann, Ernst Kris, Rudolph Loewenstein
    8. Existential analysis—Ludwig Binswanger
    9. Holistic analysis—Karen Horney
    10. Individual psychology—Alfred Adler
    11. Transactional analysis—Eric Berne
    12. Washington cultural school—Harry Stack Sullivan, Erich Fromm, Clara Thompson
    13. Will therapy—Otto Rank
  C. Group Approaches
    1. Orthodox psychoanalytic—S. R. Slavson
    2. Psychodrama—Jacob L. Moreno
    3. Psychoanalysis in groups—Alexander Wolf
    4. Valence systems—Walter Bion
II. Behavioral and humanistic—Joseph Wolpe
  1. Client-centered (non-directive)—Carl Rogers
  2. Conditioning, behavior therapy, behavior modification
    a. aversion therapy—N. V. Kantorovich, Joseph R. Cautela
    b. behaviorism—John B. Watson
    c. classical conditioning—Ivan Pavlov, Joseph Wolpe, Thomas Stampfl
    d. operant conditioning—Burrhus F. Skinner, Teodoro Ayllon, Ogden R. Lindsley
    e. sexual counseling—William Masters, Virginia Johnson
    f. systematic desensitization—Joseph Wolpe
  3. Cognitive behavior—Aaron Beck
  4. Family therapy—Nathan Ackerman
  5. Gestalt—Wolfgang Kohler, Kurt Lewin, Fritz Perls
  6. Logotherapy—Viktor Frankl
  7. Psychobiology (distributive analysis and synthesis)—Adolf Meyer
  8. Zen (satori)—Alan Watts

themselves in relation to others and how they think others define them.

See also COMPLEMENTARY THERAPIES; PSYCHO-THERAPIES.

psychologic tests Tests commonly used for diagnostic purposes. Some commonly used tests and their uses appear on the following pages.

psychologist In most states, a psychologist has a Ph.D. degree from a graduate program in PSYCHOLOGY. After World War II, psychologists began to perform psychotherapy for "mental illness" (up until the 1950s, psychotherapy was claimed to be a medical procedure) and now possess all the privileges of a mental-health professional in the form of licensing, insurance reimbursement, hospital privileges, and expert-witness designation.

Psychology, like medicine, has many areas of specialization. These include child, developmental, school, clinical, social, and industrial. The Ph.D. degree requires training in research skills. Clinical psychologists take further training in psychodiagnosis and psychotherapy and require supervision and an internship experience, as does psychiatry.

psychology The study of all behavior as part of the total life process. This includes the sequence of development, inherited and environmental factors, social interactions, conscious and unconscious mental processes, mental health and disorder, bodily systems associated with behavior, observation, testing and experimental study of behavior, and the application of psychological information to fields such as employment, education, and consumer behavior.

There are more than 20 subdivisions in the American Psychological Association's designated areas of specialization. Some of them are clinical, child, industrial, social, cognitive, animal-experimental, medical psychology, etc.

See also BEHAVIOR THERAPY.

psychoneuroimmunology (PNI) A relatively new branch of science that studies the interrelationships among the mind (pyscho), the nervous system (neuro), and the immune system (immunology). The aim of this field is to investigate and document interrelationships between psychological factors and the immune and neuroendocrine systems. Research efforts include looking at effects of anxieties on the immune system and health. In a general way, PNI seeks to understand the scientific basis of the MIND/BODY CONNECTION.

Authors Locke and Colligan, in *The Healer Within,* explain that a premise of PNI is that the immune system does not operate in a biological vacuum but is sensitive to outside influences. PNI researchers speculate that there is a line of communication between the mind and cells that are the immune system. Tendrils of the brain's nerve tissues run through important sectors of the immune system, including the thymus gland, bone marrow, lymph nodes, and spleen. Hormones and NEUROTRANSMITTERS secreted by the brain have an affinity for immune cells. Also, certain states of mind and feelings can have strong biochemical results.

The field began in 1981 with the publication of a book edited by Robert Ader (*Psychoneuroimmunology*). While most of the research presented was primarily based on animal models of stress and illness, the collection paved the way for clinical research with humans.

During the later 1980s and 1990s, researchers from various backgrounds were drawn to this new discipline. Social psychologists, experimental psychologists, psychiatrists, immunologists, neuroendocrinologists, neuroanatomists, biologists, oncologists, epidemiologists, among other specialists, have all made contributions to PNI research. Together, they seek to explain the way the brain and mind contribute to illness or keep people healthy.

See also COMPLEMENTARY THERAPIES; HUMOR; IMMUNE SYSTEM; LAUGHTER; PLACEBO; RELAXATION; STRESS; STRESS MANAGEMENT.

Kiecolt, Robert C., and Ronald Glaser, "Psychological influences on surgical recovery: Perspectives from psychoneuroimmunology," *American Psychologist* 53, no. 11 (November 1998): pp. 1209–1218.

Locke, Steven, and Douglas Colligan, *The Healer Within,* (New York: New American Library, 1984).

TABLE OF PSYCHOLOGIC TESTS

Test	Type	Assesses	Age of Patient	Output	Administration
Bayley Scales of Infant Development	Infant development	Cognitive functioning and motor development	1–30 months	Performance on subtests measuring cognitive and motor developmpment	Individual
Bender Visual-Motor Gestalt Test	Projective visual-motor development	Personality conflicts Ego function and structure Organic brain damage	5–Adults	Patient's reproduction of geometric figures	Individual
Benton Visual Retention Test	Objective performance	Organic brain damage	Adult	Patient's reproduction of geometric figures from memory	Individual
Cattell Infant Intelligence Scale	Infant development	General motor and cognitive development	1–18 months	Performance on developmental tasks	Individual
Children's Apperception Test (CAT)	Projective	Personality conflicts	Child	Patient makes up stories after viewing pictures	Individual
Draw-A-Person Draw-A-Family House-Tree-Person	Projective	Personality conflicts Self-image (DAP) Family perception (DAF) Ego functions Intellectual functioning (DAP) Visual-motor coordination	2–Adult	Patient's drawings on a blank sheet of paper	Individual
Frostig Develop-mental Test of Visual Perception	Visual perception	Eye-motor coordination Figure ground perception Constancy of shape Position in space Spatial relationships	4–8 years	Performance on paper-and-pencil test measuring five aspects of visual perception	Individual or group
Gesell Develop-mental Schedules	Preschool development	Cognitive, motor, language and social development	1–60 months	Performance on developmental tasks	Individual
Halstead-Reitan Neuropsycholo-gical Battery and Outer Measures	Brain functioning	Cerebral functioning and organic brain damage	6–Adult	Various subtests measure aspects of cerebral functioning	Individual
Illinois Test of Psycholinguistic Ability (ITPA)	Language ability	Auditory-vocal, visual-motor channels of language; receptive, organizational, and expressive components	2–10 years	Performance on 12 subtests measuring various dimensions of language functioning	Individual

Test	Type	Area measured	Age	Description	Administration
Michigan Picture Stories	Defensive structure	Personality conflicts	Adolescent	Patient makes up stories after viewing stimulus pictures	Individual
Minnesota Multiphasic Personality Inventory (MMPI)	Paper and pencil; personality inventory	Personality structure; Diagnostic classification	Adolescent-Adult	Personality profile reflecting some dimensions of personality; Diagnosis based upon actuarial prediction	Group
Otis Quick Scoring Mental Abilities Tests	Intelligence	Intellectual functioning	5-Adult	Performance on verbal and nonverbal dimensions of intellectual functioning	Group
Rorschach	Projective	Personality conflicts; Ego function and structure; Defensive structure; Thought processes; Affective integration	3-Adult	Patient's associations to inkblots	Individual
Senior Apperception Test (SAT)	Projective	Personality conflicts	Over 65	Patient makes up stories after viewing stimulus pictures	Individual
Stanford-Binet	Intelligence	Intellectual functioning	2-Adult	Performance on problem solving and developmental tasks	Individual
Tasks of Emotional Development (TED)	Projective	Personality conflicts	Child and Adolescent	Patient makes up stories after viewing stimulus pictures	Individual
Thematic Apperception Test (TAT)	Projective	Personality conflicts	Adult	Patient makes up stories after viewing stimulus pictures	Individual
Vineland Social Maturity Scale	Social maturity	Capacity for independent functioning	0-25+ years	Performance on developmental tasks measuring various dimensions of social functioning	Interview patient or guardian of patient, occasional self-report
Wechsler Adult Intelligence Scale (WAIS)	Intelligence	Intellectual functioning	16-Adult	Performance on 10 subtests measuring various dimensions of intellectual functioning	Individual
Wechsler Intelligence Scale for Children (WISC)	Intelligence	Intellectual functioning; Thought processes; Ego functioning	5-15	See above	Individual
Wechsler Preschool Primary Scale of Intelligence (WPPSI)	Intelligence	Intellectual functioning; Thought processes; Ego functioning	4-6½ years	See above	Individual

Reprinted with permission from *American Psychiatric Glossary* (Washington, DC: American Psychiatric Association, 1988).

psychophobia See MIND, FEAR OF THE.

psychosexual anxieties Psychosexual anxieties are disorders caused by mental attitudes about sexuality and physical conditions involving sexuality. Some anxieties are caused more by psychological attitudes while others come from physical aspects. Many psychosexual anxieties may have arisen because of new sexual freedoms that many individuals discovered in the latter decades of the 20th century. Sexual activity between men and women, unmarried as well as married, seemed to increase for a number of reasons. First, improved methods of contraception in the form of the birth-control pill became available. Secondly, previously known SEXUALLY TRANSMITTED (venereal) DISEASES, most notably SYPHILIS and gonorrhea, were curable with penicillin and other drugs.

During the last two decades of the 20th century, an increasing number of new sexually transmitted diseases (STDs) appeared, causing psychosexual anxieties that differed from previously recognized generalized SEXUAL FEARS. For example, when an individual discovers, feels, or suspects a genital lesion, he or she may lose interest in sexual intercourse or at least restrain himself/herself for fear of infecting the partner. Another situation is the concern faced by the innocently infected partner of an individual with a sexually transmitted disease who has had intercourse outside a stable relationship. The innocent partner may realize the implications of the STD but may not want to face the reality of the diagnosis.

Under the stress of having a sexually transmitted disease, a person may become angry, anxious, or depressed. Anger may be directed at the physician consulted as well as the person who transmitted the infection. Professionals in clinics specializing in sexually transmitted disease deal with this kind of anxiety by letting the individual voice his or her feelings and later by reassurance. In some individuals, anxiety is so severe that a short course of anti-anxiolytic medication is given.

GUILT and DEPRESSION over a sexually transmitted disease are not uncommon. In some cases, antidepressant medications are given. Many conditions, such as genital herpes, pelvic inflammatory disease, acute epididymitis, and hepatitis B, may cause anger, anxiety, guilt, and depression.

Physical symptoms of gonococcal and nongonococcal urethritis may be more easily and rapidly treated than the psychological symptoms. Resuming intercourse soon after tests indicate cure may help to heal the psychological wound that one or both partners in a stable relationship feel. Unfortunately, nongonococcal urethritis may be recurrent, and the patient may be told not to resume intercourse until the inflammation clears. This advice may put an extra strain on a relationship.

Pelvic pain and pain during sexual intercourse (dyspareunia) usually interfere with satisfactory sexual intercourse. Pelvic inflammatory disease also causes pain during intercourse and may lead to infertility. Along with dealing with a woman's feelings of loss of health and fertility, a physician may see the couple together to identify problems that have occurred because one or both partners has had sex with others, and to discuss the anger and resentment the woman feels if it is the man who has had casual sex (this is often the case).

Genital herpes may occur in one partner in a relationship when the other has never knowingly had the infection. Both may be confused about where the infection came from and may be angry, accusatory, or resentful of the other partner. Discussion guided by a trained therapist enables the couple to face the facts together. Such a couple should discuss whether herpes, once healed, might disturb further sexual relationships (usually not).

Women and homosexual men who have had anorectal herpes may develop maladaptive behavior after the primary attack. Vaginismus (tightening of the vaginal muscles) and anospasm (tightening of the anus muscles) may continue long after the ulcers have healed. SYSTEMATIC DESENSITIZATION (for example, using the partner's finger as a dilator) often is successful in overcoming this problem in a few sessions with an appropriately trained sex therapist.

Frequent recurrences of genital candidiasis (yeast infection) may leave both partners confused, frustrated, and angry about the supposed source of the problem. If the relationship is unstable, symptoms may assume dimensions out of proportion to the signs. Trichomonas vaginalis and Gardneralla vaginalis often involve offensive vaginal discharges, which may cause loss of interest by the male partner. After treatment the odor may disappear, but the woman may have lost confidence in herself, and the man may mistake the normal musky vaginal odor for the previous abnormal odor. The couple may need reassurance from a physician or sex therapist.

Syphilis, whether congenital or acquired, is feared by many people as "worse than cancer." Congenital syphilis that occurs in later life may devastate an individual when he or she realizes the implication of the disease with respect to his or her parents.

An individual who has a sexually transmitted disease or whose partner is unfaithful may lose interest in intercourse, particularly with the partner concerned. Loss of libido may be due to anxiety, depression, or just loss of interest in the partner. Individuals who are undergoing treatment for a sexually transmitted disease should discuss with their physician their attitudes about resuming sexual relations. Counseling with short-term psychotherapy may help the individual return to normal sexual function.

Some individuals may complain of symptoms of a sexually transmitted disease yet not have any illness. Some who have had an infection retain the symptoms after the infection has been cleared up with appropriate medication. Penile and urethral itching, penile and perineal pain, testicular pain, and pelvic pain may either be psychosomatic or represent symptoms of reactive sexually transmitted diseases.

Many individuals visit sexually transmitted disease clinics for checkups because they fear having acquired an STD. Some continue to believe or fear that they have contracted an infection in spite of extensive and frequent reassurance. Some of these individuals may have delusions of venereal disease, which are fixed ideas that the individual cannot be talked out of (found in schizophrenic disorders, psychotic depression, and monosymptomatic delusions), and phobias or obsessional fears. Individuals who have a fixed belief of venereal disease should be referred for psychotherapy.

See also SEX THERAPY.

Adapted with permission from: Goldmeier, David, "Psychosexual Problems," in *ABC of Sexually Transmitted Diseases* (London: British Medical Association, 1986), pp. 51–52.

psychosis A severe mental disorder that is characterized by gross impairment in the experience of reality. Individuals with SCHIZOPHRENIA exhibit psychotic symptoms, and sometimes those with BIPOLAR DISORDER are psychotic. These symptoms generally include HALLUCINATIONS, distorted thinking, and DELUSIONS.

Psychotic individuals mistakenly assume that their severely flawed perceptions and thoughts are accurate and, consequently, make incorrect inferences about external reality, even in the face of contrary evidence. The term *psychotic* does not apply, however, to minor distortions of reality that involve matters of relative judgment. For example, a depressed individual who lacks self-esteem and underestimates his or her achievements would not be described as psychotic. In contrast, a person who believes that he or she has caused a natural catastrophe such as an earthquake or a hurricane or who believes that interplanetary aliens have landed in the backyard would be described as psychotic.

Evidence suggests that psychosis is to a large extent (probably 50 percent or more) genetic but the skills one has developed and the quality of the environment have a significant impact on the extent, duration, and pervasiveness of psychosis. Coping skills and adaptation can counteract psychotic symptoms to a great extent. Medications such as antipsychotic drugs may also help.

See also NEUROSIS.

psychosurgery Sometimes called lobotomy, defined by the American Psychiatric Association Task Force on Psychosurgery as: "Surgical intervention to sever fibers connecting one part of the brain with another or to remove, destroy or stimulate brain tissue with the intent of modifying or altering disturbances in behavior, thought content, or mood for which no organic pathological cause can be demonstrated by established tests or techniques." The term "neurosurgery" is preferred when referring to the relief of pain due to organic diseases. The major type of psychosurgery is the prefrontal lobotomy or lesioning of the prefrontal area of the brain from the rest of the brain. Such surgeries, although rare, have been performed on anxiety patients to relieve these symptoms. However, there is no evidence that this surgery has any demonstrable effect on anxiety, panic, phobia, or agoraphobia.

Psychosurgery is still considered an experimental procedure that can be performed only after exhaustive attempts to modify thought, mood, or behavior. It is not at all appropriate with anxiety problems.

psychotherapy   A treatment of PHOBIA, ANXIETY, or mental disorder through a corrective experience resulting from the interaction between a trained therapist and the individual.

See also BEHAVIOR THERAPY; PSYCHIATRY; PSYCHOLOGY.

psychrophobia   Fear of being cold or of any cold thing. Also known as frigophobia.

See also COLD, FEAR OF.

pteromerhanophobia   Fear of flying.

pteronophobia   Fear of feathers or of anything bearing feathers or having a featherlike appearance. This fear is related to fear of birds, chickens, and other feathered things.

See ALSO BIRDS, FEAR OF; FEATHERS, FEAR OF; WINGED THINGS, FEAR OF.

puberty   The developmental stage between childhood and adulthood. It is the term used for the physical and emotional changes of adolescence: it generally occurs between the ages of 10 to 15 in boys and girls. This is a period filled with anxieties for many young people. Tensions exist between children's dependence on their parents and their increasing desire for independence from them.

Many young people feel anxious by the emotional ups and downs they experience. They may laugh, cry, or explode in anger without any apparent reason. Parents, teachers, and others need to be understanding, patient, tolerant, and sympathetic to help the adolescents weather this transition successfully.

Sexual and Physical Changes

Puberty, also defined as the period at which maturation of the sexual organs occurs, begins at about age 11 or 12 for girls and 13 or 14 for boys. However, there are wide variations; some girls begin to menstruate as early as age eight or nine and others as late as age 16. In Western cultures, the average age at which adolescents reach sexual maturity has been steadily decreasing over the last century, possibly as a result of better nutrition and medical care.

Many physical changes occur during puberty. In boys, this includes an increase in the secretion of male hormones and in testicular functions, and enlargement of the external sex organs. Nocturnal emissions or WET DREAMS, are a normal, automatic release at night for secretions that accumulate in the boy's sexual organs. Hair increases on the boys' legs, pubic area, chest, underarms, and face. Later their voices deepen. A spurt of growth in height and general filling-out usually occurs shortly before the start of this period.

Adolescents, particularly boys, often feel anxious by comparisons with their peers concerning physical development. Early-maturing boys seem to have advantages over later-maturing boys—they do better in athletics, are generally more popular, and have a positive sense of SELF-ESTEEM.

In pubescent girls, female hormone production and ovarian activity increase, the uterus matures and nearly doubles in size, the breasts develop, and mammary glands mature. The pelvis also widens and rounds, and hair begins to show on the legs, pubic area, and underarms. MENSTRUATION and ovulation begin, often irregularly at first.

Body weight may double during puberty, due to muscle growth in boys and increased fat in girls.

Communications between Generations

Adolescents need guidance and reinforcement. It is important that they and their parents keep the lines of communication open. They may have questions about the physical, sexual, and personality changes that they are experiencing as well as concerns about making appropriate choices and decisions. Today's teenagers face many external sources of anxiety, such as peer pressure, drugs and alcohol, HIV infection, and the possibility of teenage pregnancy. For some, internal sources of stress may lead to EATING DISORDERS and problems at school.

Recent surveys have found that anxiety and clinical depression are prevalent and possibly increasing in prevalence in the teen population. Research is beginning to examine this neglected area to establish effective interventions and to understand etiology.

See also COMMUNICATION; INTERGENERATIONAL CONFLICTS; LISTENING; PARENTING.

public speaking   Individuals can experience fears and anxieties relating to public speaking, or speaking to an audience, ranging from mild apprehension to true phobic reactions. The anticipation of giving a speech in public may arouse only a mild form of anxiety, which might be considered normal to feelings of rapid heartbeat, faintness, DIZZINESS, nausea, or other symptoms of a phobia.

An individual may suffer a mild degree of anxiety as a common reaction to being asked to give the speech, preparing it, and finally getting up in front of a group of people to give it. There may be apprehensions about how one looks or sounds and what people will think about the speech. All these apprehensions, however, could spur the individual to doing the best possible presentation.

A truly social phobic person who is reluctant to speak in public probably would not accept such an invitation, nor would an individual who has an extreme fear of FAILURE.

People who manage to give a speech in public but are extremely uneasy about it often exhibit behaviors such as shuffling the feet, pacing, no eye contact, facial tics or grimaces, moistening the lips and clearing the throat frequently, and noticeably perspiring.

Issues of self-confidence and SELF-ESTEEM are involved in the stress of public speaking. People who have given many speeches and feel confident

about the subject matter, as well as their appearance, will probably experience only a mild degree of stress.

See also PERFORMANCE ANXIETY; SOCIAL PHOBIA; STAGE FRIGHT.

punishment, fear of   Fear of punishment is known as poinephobia. This fear may relate to a fear of wrongdoing and getting caught, as well as telling untruths.

puppet therapy for anxieties and phobias   Use of puppets in therapy for ANXIETIES and phobias enables individuals, particularly CHILDREN, to express ideas and thoughts that they otherwise might think of as unacceptable to discuss with a therapist. The most popular kind of puppet in therapy is the one held on the hand because it is easy to manipulate and encourages spontaneity. Puppet therapy is also useful in FAMILY THERAPY: As each member of the family manipulates a puppet, a family's interactions can be enacted on an imaginary but representative level.

In puppet therapy, some puppets are realistic and some are fantasy figures. Based on the patient's choice of puppet, therapists can learn a great deal about such characteristics as aggression, caring, fearfulness, and the nature of conflicts.

See also CHILDHOOD ANXIETIES, FEARS, AND PHOBIAS.

purple, fear of   Fear of the color purple is known as porphyrophobia. This fear may be related to the fear of colors in general. The color purple is also associated with AIDS and homosexuality.

See also COLORS, FEAR OF.

pyrexiophobia   Fear of having a fever. Also known as pyrexeophobia and febriphobia.

See also FEVER, FEAR OF.

pyrophobia   Fear of fire, watching fires, or that one will start fires.

See also FIRES, FEAR OF.

rabies A virus-produced disease that destroys the brain nerve cells in both humans and animals. Rabies is also called hydrophobia (also the name for fear of water); fear of rabies is known as cynophobia, kynophobia, and lyssophobia. Although the dog is the most common transmitter of rabies, many domestic and wild animals such as cats, wolves, foxes, raccoons, bats, horses, and skunks may also carry it. People who fear rabies avoid outdoor activities such as hiking and camping. After a person has been bitten and infected by an animal carrying the virus, it usually takes twenty to ninety days for symptoms to develop. During the early part of the disease, the individual may be restless and anxious. The sight of water will produce throat spasms, pain, and fear of water. At this stage convulsions and delirium may occur, and the disease is almost always fatal in two to ten days. Immediate medical care after a dog or animal bite can be lifesaving. Cleansing of the bitten area removes much of the virus. Treatment consists of seven to fourteen daily injections, depending on the severity of the exposure.

See also HYDROPHOBIA.

radiation, fear of Fear of radiation is known as radiophobia. Some individuals fear harmful health effects from radiation. They fear that overexposure to rays may cause sterility, mutations, and damage to internal organs. These are legitimate fears but, if carried to extremes, or in the absence of radiation, are phobias. Some individuals fear radiation from emissions from color television sets, as well as from nuclear bombs.

Radiation has many beneficial characteristics that phobics overlook. Radioactivity in the form of X rays has been used for many years to diagnose and treat people for many injuries and diseases. Use of radiation has expanded to the use of radioisotopes to trace metabolic systems in the body, and to direct use of rays to treat cancer. Many elements, including radium and radioactive cobalt, are used to produce radiation for diagnostic and therapeutic purposes.

See also X RAYS, FEAR OF.

radiophobia Fear of radiation or of X rays.

See also RADIATION, FEAR OF; X RAY, FEAR OF.

radon, fear of An invisible radioactive gas emitted naturally by soil and rock containing uranium. Radon is colorless and odorless. Radon becomes diluted when emitted into outdoor air but seeps into homes, largely through cracks in the foundation, through some building materials and in sump pump and floor drain openings, where it may collect to dangerous levels. Radon is also present in groundwater used to supply drinking water. Fear of radon became prevalent during the 1980s when it was realized that inhaling the gas over a long period of time may cause lung cancer.

Individuals who are most fearful of radon are usually also fearful of air pollutants in general. They may fear disease and particularly fear developing cancer. Hypochondriacs, or those who believe they have symptoms or diseases, are another group of individuals who are likely to be fearful of radon.

According to the U.S. Environmental Protection Agency, 5,000 to 20,000 of the 135,000 U.S. lung-cancer deaths that occur each year can be attributed to radiation from indoor radon. Although radon in drinking water is a less serious risk than the radon seeping through the soil, this source of the pollutant is still estimated to contribute 30 to 600 excess lung-cancer deaths annually in the United States.

Those who want to allay their fears can detect the presence of this gas with appropriate detection kits; some communities perform home inspections for radon. Radon is measured in picocuries, a measurement of radioactivity. As of 1987, the EPA's federal standard was four picocuries of radioactive radon per liter of air.

Obviously, the fear of radon gases is not a phobia, since it is not an irrational fear. In this sense, it is in a group with many rational fears that people in a culture experience, such as fear of violence, crime, nuclear war, and radiation. If a significant amount of the individual's life is preoccupied with thoughts, anxieties, and ways to avoid such events, it comes closer to qualifying as a phobic reaction.

See also AIR POLLUTION, FEAR OF; CANCER, FEAR OF; DISEASE, FEAR OF; RADIATION, FEAR OF.

railroads, fear of Fear of railroads and trains is known as siderodromophobia. Some individuals may fear railroads because of the motion involved in riding on them. Others may fear them because they move fast and may not be able to stop for an object or person in their path.

See also MOTION, FEAR OF; TRAINS, FEAR OF.

rain Fear of rain is known as ombrophobia and pluviophobia.

random nuisances Annoying or unpleasant situations with which individuals cope. Such nuisances differ for each person, but if they produce anxieties, they take their toll.

Successful people regard random nuisances as "small stuff." There is a saying, "Don't sweat the small stuff; it's all small stuff." Random nuisances may seem small. However, the response to some of life's "small stressors" may escalate into physical responses, such as ANGER and rage, that are similar to responses to major stressors.

HANS SELYE explained the concept of STRESS with two basic ideas: the body has a similar set of responses to many of life's stressors; this he called the GENERAL ADAPTATION SYNDROME (G.A.S.). Also, stressors can make an individual ill. To prevent illness induced by stressors, keeping a positive perspective on life and everyday occurrences is essential. The individual should endeavor to cope with the small stressors and keep them from escalating into more serious consequences.

Many individuals find that MEDITATION helps them meet challenges. Others find that participating in regular EXERCISE helps them forget about the random nuisances of each day.

See also HARDINESS; RELAXATION; ROAD RAGE.

ranidaphobia Fear of frogs.

rape, fear of Fear of rape is known as virgivitiphobia.

See also GIRLS, FEAR OF; SEXUAL FEARS.

Rational Emotive Behavior Therapy (REBT) A therapy developed by Albert Ellis, an American psychologist (1913–2007). Also known as rational psychotherapy, rational emotive behavior therapy (REBT) is based on the premise that emotional problems are primarily caused by irrational attitudes and beliefs about oneself, others, and the world at large. This therapy helps the individual focus more clearly on specific irrational patterns of thought that produce unwanted disturbing behavior (ANXIETIES and PHOBIAS). REBT emphasizes that individuals are responsible for creating their own disturbing emotions, and that they are capable of rearranging their thoughts and beliefs in more rational ways that will reduce and eliminate anxieties and fears. Individuals are taught to "depropagandize" themselves in order to confront difficulties in a logical way. Action-oriented, REBT makes use of many techniques that work toward the practical aim of creating significant philosophical, emotional, and behavioral changes. The aim of REBT is to help individuals integrate their intellectual and experiential processes, to enhance their growth and creativity, and to rid themselves of unproductive and self-defeating habits.

Ellis wrote a book, *Growth Through Reason*, in which he details techniques used in rational emotive behavior therapy. He is noted for describing REBT as an ABCD process: A refers to an antecedent event that the individual usually thinks causes C, the emotional or behavioral consequent. Ellis points out that, in fact, it is our beliefs (B) that produce negative emotions and behavior. So individual beliefs may form an imperative (must, have to), catastrophic thought (wouldn't it be terrible) or exaggerated outcome event. It is these irrational beliefs that are the immediate cause of anxiety. Proper emotional or behavioral response requires depropagandizing (D) to bring thinking or internal beliefs into line with reality and the true nature of the situation.

See also BEHAVIOR MODIFICATION; BEHAVIOR THERAPY.

rationalization   A DEFENSE MECHANISM. The individual uses rationalization as an unconscious way to attempt to justify or make consciously tolerable by plausible means feelings, behavior, or motives that otherwise would be intolerable. Rationalization differs from conscious evasion.

See also PROJECTION.

rats, fear of   Fear of rats as well as mice is known as murophobia. This is a common fear. Rats are repugnant to many individuals for many reasons. Rats destroy food and carry disease. Rat bites may lead to rat-bite fever, a serious disease causing fever, chills, infection of the lymph glands, headache, swelling of the spleen, and other symptoms, including a rash. Prompt treatment with penicillin and other antibiotics reduces the danger of death. Bubonic plague, one of the oldest and most feared diseases in the world, begins with a bacillus carried by the rat flea, carried on the rat. The flea spreads the infection from rat to rat and from rat to man. Murine typus is another disease that fleas and rats transmit. Although there is reason to be careful about rats (due to the potential problems described above), phobias are exaggerated reactions often accompanied by preoccupations and associated excessive avoidance. In his book *1984*, George

Orwell gave his main character, Winston, this fear. Winston was forced to face his feared objects in an effort to make him change his political outlook.

See also ANIMALS, FEAR OF; MICE, FEAR OF; PLAGUE, FEAR OF THE.

Andelman, Samuel L., *The New Home Medical Encyclopedia* (New York: Quadrangle, 1973).

real anxiety   Anxiety caused by a true danger posed by the external environment. The term was used by Freud; also known as reality anxiety or objective anxiety.

reality therapy   A form of BEHAVIOR-MODIFICATION THERAPY. Reality therapy tries to help the individual get more closely in touch with the real world around him by providing assistance in learning new ways of fulfilling needs in real-life situations, such as managing anxieties and phobias. The method was developed by William Glasser, a Los Angeles psychiatrist, along with Dr. G. L. Harrington. In reality therapy, the individual is treated not as a patient with a disease stemming from some past crisis, but rather as someone needing guidance in facing the present conditions of his reality. Attention is directed to both present and future behavior with little emphasis on the past.

See also BEHAVIOR THERAPY.

rebirthing   A type of holistic therapy developed in the early 1970s by Leonard Orr. Rebirthing has been used to relieve anxiety disorders and many types of emotional and physical problems. Rebirthing is a breathing technique based on the belief in a connection between mind and matter. Persons who practice rebirthing with a trained rebirther as a teacher learn to inhale and exhale without pausing in between, emphasizing a longer inhale and a very brief exhale. Orr believed that after rebirthing has been carried out for about an hour, the person's thoughts will move from their focus on breathing to negative images and feelings from their past. As breathing continues these negative images are released, allowing the person to make decisions and take action in the present without the burden of unhealthy former belief systems. Powerful negative images may be connected with a person's birth, and the name "rebirthing" comes from the letting go of these.

reciprocal inhibition, law of   A principle based on the logical and physiological fact that two opposing emotions cannot be experienced at the same time, useful in combating many fears and emotions. For example, soldiers forget their fear when they are angry during combat. Many persons overcome the fear of flying by focusing on the pleasure they will derive during their good time at the end of the flight. Those who have elevator phobia manage to take the elevator up to their place of work because they enjoy thinking about what they will buy with their paycheck.

The term was introduced by Joseph Wolpe (1915–97), a pioneering psychiatrist in the use of behavior therapy. Wolpe's original book *Psychotherapy by Reciprocal Inhibition*, lead to the practical use of behavioral techniques with adults and children and accelerated the growth of behavior therapy. The principle of reciprocal inhibition is the basis of such widely diverse techniques as systematic desensitization (relaxation is the incompatible response to anxiety), assertive training (assertion is incompatible with fear and inhibition), and sexual responsiveness (treatment of impotence by introducing gradual sexual arousal to inhibit performance anxiety).

See also ANXIETY; ASSERTIVE TRAINING; BEHAVIOR THERAPY; COUNTERCONDITIONING; DESENSITIZATION; FEAR; PHOBIA; SOTERIA; SYSTEMATIC DESENSITIZATION.

rectal diseases, fear of   Fear of rectal diseases is known as protophobia, proctophobia, and rectophobia. The rectum is a short passage in the lower intestines between the colon and the anal canal through which solid digestive wastes are discharged. Infections and disorders of the rectum usually include those of the anal canal or the lower (sigmoid) colon. Some individuals fear infections in the rectum or damage to its tissues or muscles during a bowel movement or during childbirth.

Excessive strain during childbirth may result in a fistula (abnormal passage) from the rectum to the vagina, or other types of fistulas. Some individuals fear developing rectal hemorrhoids, and some who have them fear injuring themselves and seeing blood. Rectal disease fears may extend to fear of having bowel movements, of having pain during bowel movements, or of injuring oneself during a bowel movement. There are also obsessions about anal activity and appearance of buttocks.

rectophobia   See RECTAL DISEASES, FEAR OF.

red colors, fear of   Fear of red colors is known as erythrophobia and ereuthophobia. This may be related to a fear of blood or a fear of blushing in public. Some individuals become fearful when they see another individual wearing red clothing. Some who have this phobia may avoid wearing or being near anything red.

See also BLOOD AND BLOOD-INJURY, FEAR OF; BLUSHING, FEAR OF; COLORS, FEAR OF.

reflexology   A form of body therapy based on the theory that every part of the body has a direct line

---

USING REFLEXOLOGY TO REDUCE ANXIETY

- Choose a quiet place.
- Apply a few drops of a light, absorbent, greaseless lotion to your feet and massage them, continuing until the lotion is totally absorbed.
- Grasp the ankle, heel, or toes of one foot firmly in one hand, place the thumb of your other hand on the sole of your foot at the heel and apply steady, even pressure with the edge of your whole thumb.
- Keep your thumb slightly bent at the joint and use a forward, caterpillar-like motion. This is called *thumbwalking;* press one spot, move forward a little, press again, etc.
- When you reach the toes, start again at a new spot on the heel. Continue until the entire bottom of the foot has been worked. Then fingerwalk the top of the foot. Work your entire foot twice this way.

---

of communication to a reference point on the foot, hand, and ear. By massaging these reference points, professional reflexologists say they can help the corresponding body parts to heal. Through improved circulation, elimination of toxic by-products, and overall reduction of anxieties, the body responds and functions better because it is more relaxed.

See also BODY THERAPIES, COMPLEMENTARY THERAPIES.

Feltman, John, ed., *Reflexology: Hands on Healing* (Emmaus, PA: Rodale Press, 1989).

regression   Reversion to behavior appropriate during an earlier developmental stage. Regression is a defense mechanism the individual uses when threatened with anxiety-producing situations or internal conflicts. The regression may be general and long-standing, or it may be temporary and situation-specific. Individuals may react with earlier behaviors, such as fear, crying, thumbsucking, or temper tantrums, to gain attention or to force others to solve their problems. In working with phobic individuals, some therapists may encourage regression to determine the initial cause of the individual's phobic behavior. In psychoanalysis, regression is encouraged so that analyst and analysand can get in touch with the past. Individuals are also encouraged to regress in certain types of group therapy, such as primal therapy and rebirthing.

reinforcement   A procedure to change the likelihood or frequency of a phobic response or fearful behavior pattern. Reinforcement increases the strength of a conditioning or other learning process. In CLASSICAL CONDITIONING, reinforcement is the repeated association of the CONDITIONED STIMULUS with the UNCONDITIONED STIMULUS. In OPERANT CONDITIONING, reinforcement refers to the reward given after a correct response that strengthens the response or the punishment given after an incorrect response that weakens that response.

rejection, fear of   Fear of rejection is part of most SOCIAL PHOBIAS. It is a fear of being socially excluded or criticized, which would produce considerable emotional pain and self-degradation. For example, the avoidance of social situations may take obvious forms, such as extreme SHYNESS, avoidance of meeting new people, or fear of parties and crowds or it may take more subtle forms, such as avoidance of elevators and freeways. Individuals with extreme fear of rejection generally have a low sense of self-esteem.

See also SEXUAL FEARS.

relationships   Relationship are formed between individuals connected by affinity. These relationships include the individual's family, spouse, lovers, friends, and business or professional associates. Good relationships are healthy and nurturing and act as a buffer against outside sources of anxiety. However, even the most meaningful relationships can at times be unsupportive and sources of anxiety.

Relationships and Health

People who lack outlets for anxiety are susceptible to a list of anxiety-related illnesses. Having one or two close friends with whom one can feel free to discuss personal problems is invaluable. An objective view from a trusted friend can help relieve anxiety.

Romantic Relationships

Romantic relationships are far riskier and potentially more anxiety-producing to the individual's emotional and physical well-being than people realize. Not only are feelings likely to be hurt, SELF-ESTEEM damaged, and trust betrayed, but the there

---

HOW A HEALTHY RELATIONSHIP CAN AVERT ANXIETIES

- Realism: openness and honesty with each other
- Trust: allowing the individuals to share their feelings
- True friendship: having no hidden motives
- Forgiveness: accepting the individual as he or she is
- Security: knowing that individuals can count on one another
- Vulnerability: exposing weaknesses that allow the relationship to grow

---

can be physical and mental battery by an outraged spouse. America's high DIVORCE rate suggests that INTIMACY has painful consequences.

According to Geraldine K. Piorkowski, author of *Too Close for Comfort: Exploring the Risks of Intimacy,* romantic relationships can produce anxiety because they are related to the process of getting close to another person. As we become more intimate (both emotionally and sexually), we reveal our deepest secrets, hopes, inadequacies, and even fantasies. We become more vulnerable, and thus are easily wounded by a hostile comment, act of betrayal, or moment of rejection.

Further, Piorkowski says, anxiety arises in relationships when our emotional needs and expectations are unrealistic. Also, we may lose our AUTONOMY and wind up feeling suffocated by the other's demands; their neediness may drain energy needed to pursue our own desires and interests. We may be blamed for all the problems in the relationship and suffer GUILT and loss of self-confidence as a result.

Relationships and Support Groups

A lack of connections with other people can be detrimental to health, says Dr. Andrew Weil, author of *Spontaneous Healing.* "Surrounding yourself with supportive people is an important step for any healing you need to do. Whenever I take a family history from a patient, I always ask about people who are helping or hindering someone's illness. For example, sometimes a friend or family member who means well only makes matters worse, maybe by not wanting the patient to express sadness about being sick or show discomfort from pain."

In terms of building relationships through support groups, Dr. Weil urges patients to find and develop relationships with people who have overcome the same problems rather than simply join a SUPPORT GROUP. "I find that some support groups can be counterproductive and cause more stress for the individual," he says. "For example, some patients with cancer are horrified and extremely stressed when they see another person with a more advanced form of the disease. There is a similar phenomenon with chronic fatigue syndrome."

Some people are more fatalistic about their illness, while others tend to be positive thinkers. This should be factored into any relationships developed through a support group, and especially with family and friends, suggests Dr. Weil.

See also FAMILY; INTERGENERATIONAL CONFLICTS; LISTENING; LIVE-IN; MARRIAGE; PARENTING.

Dugas, Michel J., Mark H. Freeston, Robert Ladouceur, et al., "Worry themes in primary GAD, secondary GAD, and other anxiety disorders," *Journal of Anxiety Disorders* 12, no. 3 (May–June 1998): pp. 253–261.

Gilbert, Roberta M., *Extraordinary Relationships: A New Way of Thinking About Human Interactions* (Minneapolis: Chronimed Publishing, 1992).

Jaffe, Dennis T., *Healing From Within* (New York: Knopf, 1980).

Piorkowski, Geraldine K., *Too Close for Comfort: Exploring the Risks of Intimacy* (New York: Insight Books, 1994).

Weil, Andrew, *Spontaneous Healing: How to Discover and Enhance Your Body's Natural Ability to Maintain and Heal Itself* (New York: Knopf, 1995).

relatives, fear of   Fear of relatives is known as syngenesophobia. While extended families offer emotional and practical support, they are also promoters of fears and anxieties. Dependency and intrusiveness often are major issues in family anxieties. One's own family, as well as one's in-laws, often create anxieties and tensions for individuals at all ages and stages of life. Grandparents, while loving, may intrude in the upbringing of grandchildren by spoiling them, disciplining them in ways unacceptable to their parents, or siding with the child against his or her parents. Adult children may also burden their parents with unwanted babysitting responsibilities. Longer life spans are creating situations in which several generations of a family live with responsibilities of caring for elderly relatives. Some middle-aged individuals feel anxieties because they are the "sandwich" generation, with responsibilities to their own children as well as to their elderly parents.

Anxieties regarding relatives often arise because of nepotism in employment in both family-owned and nonfamily-owned organizations. Hiring and promotion of relatives may create anxieties and resentments from both other relatives and from other unrelated employees. Family-owned businesses often suffer because of the emotional stresses and strains inherent in the family relationship, and family members suffer because they feel locked into a certain way of life due to the nature of the business.

Issues related to inheritance also promote extended family anxieties and friction. One member may fear that another received more than he or she deserved from an estate. Positions of responsibility such as executor or trustee of a will also promote jealousy and conflicts. Occasions such as weddings, reunions, and holidays bring buried resentments and fears to the surface in some families, and situations that should be pleasant become filled with anxiety and tension.

Because of the high incidence of child abuse, some parents may fear leaving their children with relatives.

See also CHILD ABUSE, FEAR OF; "GENERATIONAL" ANXIETIES; FATHER-IN-LAW, FEAR OF; INCEST, FEAR OF; MOTHER-IN-LAW, FEAR OF.

relaxation   A feeling of freedom from anxiety and tension. Internal conflicts and disturbing feelings of STRESS are absent. Relaxation also refers to the return of a muscle to its normal state after a period of contraction.

People who are very tense and anxious can learn to relax using relaxation training, a form of BEHAVIOR THERAPY or alternative therapy. Relaxation techniques are methods used to unconsciously release muscular tension and achieve a sense of mental calm. Historically, relaxation techniques have included MEDITATION, T'AI CHI, MASSAGE THERAPY, YOGA, MUSIC, and AROMATHERAPY. More modern developments include AUTOGENIC TRAINING, PROGRESSIVE MUSCLE RELAXATION, HYPNOSIS, BIOFEEDBACK, and aerobic exercise.

Many of these techniques were developed to help people cope with anxieties brought on by the challenges of life. They are different approaches to relieving anxiety by bringing about generalized physical as well as mental relaxation. Relaxation techniques have in common the production of the relaxation response as one of their stress-relieving actions. Additionally, relaxation may counter some of the immunosuppressing effects of anxiety and stress and may actually enhance the activity of the immune system.

Relaxation training programs are commonly used in conjunction with more standard forms of therapy for many chronic diseases. The MIND/BODY CONNECTION between relaxation and ill health has been demonstrated in many conditions. Some of the physiological changes that occur during relaxation include decreased oxygen consumption, decreased heart and respiratory rates, diminished muscle tension, and a shift toward slower brain wave patterns.

The "Relaxation Response"

In the 1970s, Herbert Benson, M.D., a cardiologist at Harvard Medical School, studied the relationship between stress and hypertension. In stressful situations, the body undergoes several changes, including rise in blood pressure and pulse and faster breathing. Dr. Benson reasoned that if stress could bring about this reaction, another factor might be able to turn it off. He studied practitioners of TRANSCENDENTAL MEDITATION (TM) and found that once into their meditative states, some individuals could willfully reduce their pulse, blood pressure, and breathing rate. Dr. Benson named this "the relaxation response." This "relaxation response" relates to voluntary control of the parasympathetic system through extensive training. He explained this procedure in his book (written with Miriam Z. Klipper) *The Relaxation Response* (1976).

Applications for Relaxation

Relaxation training can be particularly useful for individuals who have "white coat hypertension," which means that their blood pressure is high only when facing a certain specifically anxiety-producing situation, such as having a medical examination or visiting a dentist. It can also help reduce hostility and anger, which in turn affect the body and the individual's physical responses to stress. Anxieties can lead to panic attacks, nausea, or gastrointestinal problems.

There are many applications of relaxation training to help individuals learn control over their mental state and body and in treating conditions as diverse as high blood pressure, cardiac arrhythmia, chronic pain, insomnia, premenstrual syndrome, and side effects of cancer treatments. Relaxation training is an important part of childbirth classes to help women cope with labor.

In a training program, individuals are instructed to move through the muscle groups of the body, making them tense and then completely relaxed. Through repetitions of this procedure, individuals learn how to be in voluntary control of their feelings of tension and relaxation. Some therapists provide individuals with instructional audio tapes for use during practice, while other therapists go through the procedure repeatedly with their clients.

To determine the effectiveness of relaxation training, some therapists use biofeedback as an indicator of an individual's degree of relaxation and absence of anxiety.

See also BIOFEEDBACK; EXERCISE; GUIDED IMAGERY; HOBBIES; IMMUNE SYSTEM; RECREATION.

Benson, Herbert, *The Relaxation Response* (New York: Avon Books, 1975).
———, *Beyond the Relaxation Response* (New York: Berkeley Press, 1985).
Goleman, Daniel, and Joel Gurin, eds., *Mind Body Medicine: How to Use Your Mind for Better Health* (Yonkers, NY: Consumer Reports Books, 1993).
Lehrer, Paul M., and Robert L. Woolfolk, eds. *Principles and Practice of Stress Management* (New York: The Guilford Press, 1993).
Locke, Steven, and Douglas Colligan, *The Healer Within* (New York: New American Library, 1984).

religious ceremonies, fear of   Fear of religious ceremonies is known as teletophobia. Such fears may be based on individual and/or historical concerns. Some people fear and dislike religious ritual because they were forced into meaningless, rigid observances as children. Others feel that an ethical, moral attitude toward religious practice, such as the observance of the Golden Rule, is more meaningful to them, and that ceremonies actually get in the way. Some fear religious ceremonies outside their own religious or ethnic group because they appear threatening, incomprehensible, or even ridiculous. Historically, Protestants have been fearful and distrustful of religious ceremony. One of the purposes of the Reformation movement was to cleanse the church of what were considered superstitious pagan elements represented in ceremonial behavior.

See also HOLY THINGS, FEAR OF; RELIGIOUS OBJECTS, FEAR OF; RITUAL.

Oyama, Oliver, and Harold G. Koenig, "Religious Beliefs and Practices in Family Medicine." *Archives of Family Medicine* 7 (September/October 1998): pp. 431–435.
Thomas, Keith, *Religion and the Decline of Magic* (New York: Scribner, 1971).
Thoules, Robert H., *An Introduction to the Psychology of Religion* (London: Cambridge University Press, 1971).

religious objects, fear of   Fear of religious objects or holy objects is known as hierophobia or hagiophobia. The awe- and fear-inspiring attributes of religious objects is evident in such customs as swearing on a Bible, which originated in the medieval church and is still in practice today. The individual tells the truth out of the fear that God will punish perjury in this life or the next. Some Protestants also fear and dislike religious objects, which they associate with what were considered pagan, superstitious practices of the Catholic church.

See also RELIGIOUS CEREMONIES, FEAR OF; SUPERNATURAL, FEAR OF.

remarriage   Marriage between partners when one or both of whom have been married previously. Bride and groom bring with them remembrances, some good and some bad, of former marriages. If there are children, establishing new family RELATIONSHIPS as well as maintaining old family ties are major concerns. Widows or widowers who experienced "good marriages" are less likely to have anxieties and apprehensions than those who are divorced.

Many people find their second marriage, particularly if it follows divorce, a source of anxiety. For example, some divorced men and women marry a person very similar to their first spouse and encounter similar difficulties. Others try very hard to find a quality that was lacking in their first spouse. As a consequence, they may marry a person who has that particular quality but be blinded to other ways in which he or she is actually incompatible.

Divorced or widowed persons may remarry out of emotional and financial need without understanding themselves first or resolving their feelings about their previous marriage. Ex-mates may interfere when one or the other remarries, and family members may make it obvious that they preferred the previous spouse. In some cases, men and women are stressed by feelings of GUILT about how the second marriage has affected their children or previous spouse.

In remarriages, the husband is frequently several years older than the wife and may not want more children, while she may be eager for a family. The financial strains on a man called upon to support two families is very often disruptive and is also source of stress.

Being accepted into the family, a stressor for many, may relate to the circumstances of the courtship. For example, if a woman was the "other woman" while the new husband was still married, his relatives may regard the wife as a "home wrecker." If a recently widowed woman marries too soon, her relatives may think the marriage was disrespectful to the deceased.

Statistics on Remarriage

According to a 1987 report, 46 percent of all marriages were remarriages for the bride or groom or both. More widows than widowers remarry, but divorced men are more likely to remarry than divorced women. Nineteen percent of divorced men remarry within a calendar year of their divorce; 8 percent of widowed men marry within a year of the death of their wives. Divorced men have good reason to remarry. Death rates for divorced men who remain single are far higher than for divorced women who do not remarry.

While divorced and widowed people remarry at a high rate, the divorce rate for these unions is higher than for first marriages. Responses to a survey concerning the failure rate of second marriages consistently listed two leading causes: children and money. Friction between stepparents and stepchildren is common.

In contemporary American society, some couples choose not to marry for a variety of reasons, ranging from not wanting to lose alimony payments to waiting for vesting in a pension plan to fear of making a mistake. Many older individuals who are past childbearing and child-rearing years opt for a LIVE-IN arrangement instead of remarriage.

See also MARRIAGE; DIVORCE; INTIMACY; STEP-FAMILIES.

Statistical Abstract of the United States, 1991 (Washington, DC: U.S. Department of Commerce, 1991).

Wilson, Barbara Foley, "The Marry-Go-Round," *American Demographics,* October 1991, pp. 52–54.

repeating (as a ritual)   Many individuals, out of fear of not doing an act correctly or sufficiently, become compulsive and ritualistic about repeating certain activities. For example, an individual may repeat stirring a cup of coffee a fixed number of times or washing a glass a number of times. About 40 percent of those who have OBSESSIVE-COMPULSIVE DISORDER experience repeating as a RITUAL.

repression   A defense mechanism by which one pushes impulses and thoughts into the unconscious.

See also PSYCHOANALYSIS.

reptiles, fear of   Fear of reptiles is known as ophidiophobia or batrachophobia. Ophidiophobia refers more to snakes; batrachophobia refers more to lizards and frogs.

See also FROGS, FEAR OF; SNAKES, FEAR OF; TOADS, FEAR OF.

resistance   An individual's efforts to obstruct the process of therapy. Resistance, a basic concept in PSYCHOANALYSIS, led Sigmund Freud to develop his fundamental rule of FREE ASSOCIATION, the need for neutrality on the part of the therapist, and recognition that the UNCONSCIOUS could be reached only by indirect methods. Freud viewed resistance primarily as the ego's efforts to prevent unconscious material from coming into the conscious; later, he considered resistance as a DEFENSE MECHANISM. Other therapeutic disciplines regard resistance in different ways. For example, behavior therapists view resistance from a social-learning point of view. Some behavior therapists explain both repression and resistance in terms of avoidance learning. When certain thoughts are repeatedly associated with painful experiences, such as situations that produce anxieties or fears, they become aversive. Strategic therapists and social influence theorists design strategies to overcome the individual's resistance to the therapist, to the process of treatment, and to the loss of symptoms.

See also BEHAVIOR THERAPY.

respiration relief therapy   A form of treatment that emphasizes respiration training and the use of respiratory relief (exhalation) as an antagonist to anxiety induced by specific phobias. There is some evidence that respiratory relief paired with presentation of a feared stimulus can produce extinction of the anxiety response.

respondent conditioning   Also known as CLASSICAL CONDITIONING or Pavlovian conditioning. Respondent conditioning is the eliciting of a response by a stimulus that usually does not elicit that response. The response (salivation or a change in heart rate) is one that is brought about by the autonomic nervous system. A previously neutral stimulus is repeatedly presented just before an unconditioned stimulus that normally elicits that response. When the response subsequently occurs in the presence of the previously neutral stimulus, it is called a conditioned response, and the previously neutral stimulus a CONDITIONED STIMULUS.

See also CONDITIONED RESPONSE; CONDITIONING.

responsibility, fear of   Fear of responsibility is known as hypengyophobia or hypeigiaphobia. Some individuals who have depressive disorders fear responsibility because they have a sense of self-worthlessness and inadequacy. Some individuals who have agoraphobia fear responsibility because they cannot make themselves go out to work or to social activities. Those who blame others for these reactions or situations are avoiding personal responsibilities.

retirement, fear of   Fear of retirement is a contemporary fear of many individuals as they grow older. The time of life when a person leaves his work or profession and devotes most of his time to leisure activities should be a time of enjoyment and reflec-tion. For many individuals, however, retirement becomes a time filled with anxieties and fears of the future, including fear of aging, fear of death, health anxieties, and fears of being alone without spouse, family, or friends. Some fear the loss of purpose, direction, and fulfillment they gained from working, as well as the loss of income. Many people who reach retirement age (usually considered in the upper sixties and beyond) suffer from diseases of older age, including heart disease, lung disorders, vision and hearing disabilities, diabetes, and neurological difficulties. Some individuals experience psychological and social problems connected with retirement that are medically related. The subsequent depression many people experience may require psychotherapy or drug therapy.

Some individuals fear feeling useless and fear boredom after they retire; men may experience this feeling more than women.

Individuals can relieve some of the stresses and anxieties of retirement by keeping in mind the following:

1. Don't wait until later to work on major fears such as traveling or being alone that would restrict retirement activity.
2. Prepare for retirement by planning financially. The further ahead you plan, the more realistic and prepared you will be.
3. Prepare psychologically by developing hobbies and interests that will support retirement.
4. Begin to detach from work, begin to see that your self-esteem does not have to be tied to a title or job activity. The better you feel about yourself the easier it will be to retire.
5. Develop meaningful retirement activities. See where you can contribute and give to others. Retirement tied to giving is much more rewarding.
6. Everything changes. This is a dynamic of life. You have to be able to let go of the past. Forgiveness is the key here.
7. Change emotions tied to illness. Seek help in resolving chronic emotional states (such as anxiety, depression, and fears).
8. Change your diet in both the type and quantities of food. As you age, your body will need fewer calories, less fat, less protein.

See also AGING, FEAR OF; BOREDOM, FEAR OF; DEATH, FEAR OF; HEART ATTACK, ANXIETY FOLLOWING; HEART ATTACK, FEAR OF.

"Any Cure for Retirement Phobia?" *Modern Maturity,* February–March 1988, p. 9.

Hayslip, Bert Jr., Michael Beyerlein, and Judith A. Nichols, "Assessing anxiety about retirement: The case of academicians," *International Journal of Aging and Human Development* 44, no. 1 (1997): pp. 15–36.

rhabdophobia   Fear of being beaten or punished with a rod, of fear of a rod.

See also BEATEN, FEAR OF BEING; RODS, FEAR OF; STICKS, FEAR OF.

rhypophobia   Fear of filth or dirt.

See also DIRT, FEAR OF; FILTH, FEAR OF.

rhytiphobia   Fear of getting wrinkles.

See also WRINKLES, FEAR OF.

ridicule, fear of   Fear of ridicule is known as catagelophobia or katagelophobia. Ridicule may take the form of unfavorable comments on one's appearance, behavior, or viewpoints. Some agoraphobics are afraid to venture out because they fear being ridiculed by people they meet in the street. Some telephone phobics are afraid to speak on the telephone because they fear that the caller will ridicule their speech mannerisms. Individuals who lack self-confidence fear ridicule. Those who have depressive disorder feel a lack of self-worth and thus believe that others will ridicule them.

risk taking, fear of   Fear of taking risks includes fears of gambling, of making decisions, of making errors, and of new things. People who fear taking risks prefer the security of known places and situations. Such individuals may fear losing control by taking risks. Those who fear losing money, for example, avoid risky investments such as the stock market.

See also CHANGE, FEAR OF; DECISIONS, FEAR OF; GAMBLING, FEAR OF; NEW THINGS, FEAR OF.

Ritalin   Trade name for a drug (methylphenidate hydrochloride) that has been used to treat hyperactivity in children and adults. It is a mild stimulant to the central nervous system and has helped some children increase their ability to concentrate in school or at work. However, use of the drug has been controversial.

See also ATTENTION-DEFICIT/HYPERACTIVITY DISORDER.

ritual   In psychopathology, a distorted or elaborate activity that an individual repeats as part of his or her daily routine. Individuals who have OBSESSIVE-COMPULSIVE DISORDERS commonly include some rituals in their routine—for example, frequent hand-washing or constant checking. Some individuals seek treatment to free themselves of the rituals, even though keeping up with the ritualistic behavior relieves their anxieties to some extent.

There are, of course, also rituals of daily life that are not indications of abnormalities and may actually have benefits in relieving anxieties. This type of ritual has been defined as "a symbol that is acted out" and "an agreed-upon pattern of movement"; such rituals are part of social, educational, religious, and athletic events. Rituals such as the use of good manners serve a positive social purpose as protection from aggressive, antisocial behavior. Religious rituals reduce feelings of guilt because of their cleansing, purifying quality. Rite-of-passage rituals, such as the engagement and marriage ceremony, provide a way to reduce the anxieties inherent in passing from one phase of life to another. Funeral rites provide companionship for the survivors and an organized way to behave at a time of grief and crisis. As rituals tend to be traditional, they also satisfy a need many people feel for a sense of continuity with the past and an avoidance of newness. Rituals make use of unique clothing and objects and exaggerated, repetitive, or unusual language to intensify communication, focus the attention of leader and participants, and exclude outside distractions.

Rituals may also promote fear and anxiety. Individuals may feel inhibited or anxious about conforming to certain types of rigid group-behavior patterns. Rituals that have become empty and meaningless or that are observed too rigidly may promote disaffection and disillusionment in individuals who perceive them as either time-wasting or tension-producing.

rivers, fear of Fear of rivers is known as potamophobia. Those who have this fear may fear being near or on a river (in a boat or swimming), seeing a picture or movie of a river, or even thinking about a river. This fear is related to fear of water and also to fear of landscape.

See also LANDSCAPE, FEAR OF; WATER, FEAR OF.

road rage Expressions of anger and hostility while driving a car. People are in a hurry and become frustrated because of traffic delays, being cut off by other drivers, or being given obscene signals by other drivers. Road rage is dangerous because drivers become excited and may accelerate their speed or make sudden and risky moves.

Road rage is a contemporary term, implying that impatience and competition have increased in our culture, perhaps due, in part, to increased population density.

robbers, fear of Fear of robbers is known as harpaxophobia. In modern urban centers this is a very real fear, as crime rates increase along with the population and social problems that come along with crowded conditions, a high cost of living, and lack of jobs for all who wish to work. Fear of robbers motivates many individuals to have elaborate burglar-alarm systems at their homes and places of businesses and several locks on their doors. Fear of robbers is a contemporary fear of many children. This takes the form of fearing being accosted on the street or that someone will enter their home.

rods, fear of being beaten with Fear of being beaten or punished with a rod or stick is known as rhabdophobia. The word rhabdophobia is derived from the Greek word *rhabdos,* or rod. Those who have this phobia fear injury as well as embarrassment and loss of control in the situation. Some

who fear police fear being beaten with the policeman's rod.

See also PUNISHMENT, FEAR OF; STICKS, FEAR OF.

role playing A technique used in PSYCHOTHERAPY in which the client acts according to a role that is not his or her own. Role playing is used in a variety of ways. For example, it can help a therapist determine how anxious or phobic individuals react to certain important social roles and how they see themselves in social situations. Role playing can help the individual gain insight into the conduct of others. It can also help the individual gain CATHARSIS, or release from phobic or other anxiety symptoms.

See also BEHAVIOR THERAPY.

Rolfing One of many contemporary BODY THERAPIES used to relieve anxieties and improve emotional and physical health. It is a form of deep tissue massage and is a combination of the disciplines of Eastern philosophical systems and practices and Western knowledge of muscular and skeletal structure.

The technique, which is often combined with other body therapy techniques, was developed by Ida P. Rolf (1896–1979), an American biochemist. As a young woman, she had an accident and was successfully treated by both an osteopathic physician and a yoga instructor. She combined these two techniques with the medical system of homeopathy, a practice which calls upon the patient's own healing powers rather than merely treating symptoms. The therapy gained recognition through Rolf's work at the Esalen Institute in California during the 1960s. From what had been considered fringe or one of many COMPLEMENTARY THERAPIES, Rolfing and other body therapies entered the mainstream of mental and physical treatments in the mid-1900s.

Rolfing focuses on the network of connective tissue—fascia, tendons, and ligaments—that contains the muscles and links them to the bones. Whenever connective tissue fails to work effectively, pain can result. For many, Rolfing helps to heal the body by bringing it into proper alignment and proper relationship to the forces of gravity. A Rolfing practitioner puts pressure on certain areas of the patient's connective tissue to improve the structure of the body. Certified Rolfers have had training in human anatomy, physiology, kinesiology, and various massage techniques.

Currently, Rolfing methods emphasize a gentler approach to client work.

Locating a Rolfing Therapist

The Rolf Institute, headquartered in Boulder, Colorado, has produced Rolfers since 1972. There are more than 600 practitioners across the United States and in 23 other countries. The institute provides a complete listing of its graduates, their addresses, and telephone numbers. The institute also has a free pamphlet that lists books, videotapes and audiovisual information currently available about Rolfing.

See also MASSAGE THERAPY.

Rolf, Ida P., *Rolfing: Reestablishing the Natural Alignment and Structural Integration of the Human Body for Vitality and Well Being* (Rochester, VT: Healing Arts Press, 1989).

room full of people, fear of   Fear of being in or entering a room full of people is known as koinoniphobia. Individuals who have this SOCIAL PHOBIA may also have agoraphobia, and vice versa. Some individuals may fear ridicule by others, fear being closed in without escape, or fear some type of social embarrassment, such as having to use the bathroom, fainting in front of others, vomiting, or being watched while they eat.

Rorschach test   A PSYCHOLOGICAL TEST developed by the Swiss psychiatrist Hermann Rorschach (1884–1922); also referred to as the inkblot test. An individual taking the test supposedly disclose conscious and unconscious personality traits and emotional conflicts by their associations of inkblots with objects, things, and situations. The Rorschach suffers from reliability and interpretation problems.

ruin, fear of   Fear of ruin or being ruined is known as atephobia. This fear may refer to financial or social ruin and may also apply to a fear of looking at historical ruins, or even ruins after a contemporary disaster, such as a fire or flood. This was a common fear during and following the Great Depression.

See also POVERTY, FEAR OF.

rumination   The act of persistently being excessively anxious about, worrying about, thinking about, and pondering one concern for an inordinate period of time. Ruminations produce anxiety and are repetitive, intrusive thoughts or OBSESSIONS about some aspect of one's life, such as fear of CONTAMINATION, fear of harming others, or fear of not doing certain tasks correctly. The thoughts may be evoked by external cues or come out of the blue. Ruminations impair concentration and are hard to drive out of one's mind. Rumination is a common symptom of OBSESSIVE-COMPULSIVE DISORDER.

See also CONTAMINATION, FEAR OF; THOUGHT STOPPING; WORRYING.

rum phobia   This phobia was mentioned by Benjamin Rush (1745–1813), an American physician and author known as the father of American psychiatry. "The Rum Phobia is a very rare distemper. I have known only five instances of it in the course of my life. The smell of rum, and of spirituous liquors of all kinds, produced upon these persons, sickness and distress. If it were possible to communicate this distemper as we do the smallpox, by inoculation, what an immense revenue would be derived from it by physicians, provided every person in our country who is addicted to the intemperate use of spirits were compelled to submit to that operation!"

Runes, D. D., ed., *The Selected Writings of Benjamin Rush* (New York: The Philosophical Library, 1947).

rupophobia   Fear of filth or dirt. Also known as rypophobia.

See also DIRT, FEAR OF; FILTH, FEAR OF.

Russia, fear of   Russophobia, a fear of Russia, the Russian language, and things relating to Russian culture.

rust, fear of   Fear of rust is known as iophobia.

sacred things, fear of Fear of sacred things is known as hierophobia. This fear includes holy or religious objects. The individual suffering from such a fear would avoid churches, shrines, museums, etc., where particular objects are displayed. Often this fear is quite specific, involving "holy" people or objects (such as crosses) that evoke anxiety.

See also HOLY OBJECTS, FEAR OF; RELIGIOUS OBJECTS, FEAR OF.

"safe sex" Refers to avoidance of behaviors that may lead to SEXUALLY TRANSMITTED DISEASES and AIDS and pregnancy. Safe sex involves avoiding exchange of bodily fluids, knowing one's partner, and using condoms and spermicidal agents properly. The concept of safe sex causes stress for many individuals, who either avoid sexual relationships or find preparations annoying. For some couples, use of a condom becomes an anxiety-producing issue.

See also AIDS; BIRTH CONTROL; CONDOMS.

samhainophobia Fear of Halloween.

"sandwich" generation The generation in midlife that has the responsibility of taking care of aging parents in addition to their almost adult or adult children. Anxieties abound due to the multiple roles it must assume. Stressors include living arrangements, financial constraints, and indefiniteness of roles.

See also INTERGENERATIONAL CONFLICTS; PARENTING.

sarmassophobia Fear of love play.

See also LOVE PLAY, FEAR OF; SEXUAL FEARS.

Satan, fear of Fear of Satan is known as Satanophobia. People fear manifestations of Satanic inter-ests, such as symbols, rituals, and possibly unknown destructive forces. The name Satan derives from the ancient Hebrew word for devil. Early men believed that the harmful forces of nature were demons and evil spirits, and they blamed such demons for all their troubles. In the Old Testament, Satan is not God's opponent; rather, he searches out the sins of men and accuses mankind before God. In the Apocrypha, Satan is the author of all evil and rules over a host of angels. In the New Testament, other names for Satan are devil, enemy, and Beelzebub. In the Middle Ages, Satan usually was represented with horns, a tail, and cloven hooves.

See also DEMONS, FEAR OF; DEVIL, FEAR OF; VOO-DOO, FEAR OF.

scabies, fear of Fear of scabies (also popularly known as the "seven-year itch") is known as scabiophobia. Tiny PARASITES, known as *Sarcoptes scabiei* and popularly known as the itch mite, are responsible for scabies, or "the itch." The mite looks like a white dot. The female burrows into the skin and creates a tunnel in which she lays eggs, resulting in a minute, narrow mark on the skin. Some individuals who are allergic to the mite and its secretions may also have tiny blisters, pus, or other blemishes. Eggs hatch in about a week; larvae appear and then develop into burrowing and egg-laying mites and spread over the body. The "seven-year itch" reached a peak of infestation during Word War II, but since then the incidence has dropped dramatically due to new pesticides and improved sanitation. Because it is less common now, this fear is more of historical than practical interest.

See also PARASITES, FEAR OF.

scabiophobia Fear of scabies or the "seven-year itch."

See also SCABIES, FEAR OF.

"scared stiff" During extreme fear, many people become "scared stiff," or "frozen with fear." These terms refer to a paralyzed conscious state with abrupt onset and end. This type of fear reaction has been reported by survivors of attacks by wild animals, shell-shocked soldiers, and rape victims. Characteristics of being "frozen with fear" include an inability to move (tonic immobility), body shaking, an inability to scream or call out, numbness or insensitivity to pain, and sensations of feeling cold. This term also refers to an involuntary erection that may occur under intense fear.

See also POST-TRAUMATIC STRESS DISORDER.

scatophobia Fear of fecal matter. The word is derived from the greek *skatos,* meaning "dung."

See also BOWEL MOVEMENTS, FEAR OF; FECAL MATTER, FEAR OF.

scelerophobia Fear of attack and harm by wicked persons, such as burglars and robbers. These "fears" have increased in prevalence and intensity such that fear of attack and harm by wicked persons are among the greatest fears of children today. Certainly, media programs with graphic depictions of violence have contributed to this increase.

See also BAD MEN, FEAR OF; BURGLARS, FEAR OF.

schizophrenia A mental illness with psychotic symptoms involving the withdrawal from reality, DELUSIONS, HALLUCINATIONS, and characteristic disturbances in both affect and form of thought. The person with schizophrenia may be fearful of and anxious with others. The word *schizophrenia* is derived from the Latin terms for "split mind" *(schizo + phrenia),* however, schizophrenia does *not* refer to a split personality, a term that is sometimes used to describe people with a dissociative identity disorder. On the other hand, it is a "splitting" off of affect (mood) from cognition.

According to the National Institute of Mental Health (NIMH), schizophrenia affects about 2.4 million people in the United States.

The symptoms of schizophrenia usually appear gradually over time, but the onset is usually not evident until about age 25. These symptoms create an inner turmoil and worsen to present as severe distortions in perception, speech, and thoughts. Individuals with schizophrenia may exhibit PARANOID THINKING, in which they suffer from delusions that others wish to harm them.

Most people with schizophrenia are not violent and if they had no criminal record before the onset of the illness, they rarely commit crimes afterward. Sometimes people who abuse drugs and/or alcohol exhibit symptoms that may be mistaken for schizophrenia, particularly those who abuse amphetamines or cocaine.

In most cases, the onset of schizophrenia occurs in late adolescence or early adulthood. Some sufferers experience only one psychotic episode (reactive), while others have repeated episodes throughout their lives. Individuals with schizophrenia have a high risk for suicide, and about 10 percent (mostly young adult males) succeed at ending their lives. It can be difficult, if not impossible, to know if talk about ending one's life is real, and, as a result, when a person with schizophrenia (or any other person) talks about a plan and a desire to commit suicide, professional help should be urgently sought for the person.

The cause of schizophrenia is unknown, but many experts believe that it may occur as a result of a combination of both predisposing genetic factors and an as yet unknown environmental trigger. Some experts believe that extreme stress can serve as an environmental trigger.

Many people with schizophrenia suffer from other psychiatric problems, such as DEPRESSION and ANXIETY DISORDERS. In addition, there is a high rate of substance abuse among individuals with schizophrenia. Some people with schizophrenia may abuse drugs and/or alcohol in an attempt to medicate their symptoms.

Symptoms and Diagnostic Path
Individuals with schizophrenia have both of what are called *positive* and *negative* symptoms. Positive symptoms do not refer to pleasant effects but rather they refer to HALLUCINATIONS, DELUSIONS, and disordered thinking. Some people with schizophrenia have disorders of movement, where they may have unusual mannerisms or grimaces. The most

extreme form of a disorder of movement is catatonia, in which the person does not move at all. This disorder is rare today as a result of medical treatments.

Negative symptoms refer to inactions, such as a lack of desire or an inability to express emotion, speak, or make plans. In addition, the person may have what is called a *flat affect,* or no expression of any emotion. Another negative symptom is an inability to take pleasure in everyday events. Sometimes the negative symptoms of schizophrenia are misdiagnosed as DEPRESSION.

Individuals with schizophrenia also have cognitive deficits and considerable difficulty with planning and organizing. Cognitive deficits can make it difficult to live a normal life, although with medication and therapy some individuals with schizophrenia can achieve a near-normal lifestyle.

Symptoms of schizophrenia may include some of the following

- paranoid delusions, which are unshakable personal thoughts that convince the individual that others are actively plotting against him or her
- delusions that one's thoughts are *broadcast* outside one's head so that others can hear them
- delusions that outside forces are controlling the person's thoughts, either inserting them into the individual's head or removing them from the individual's mind (delusions of influence)
- auditory hallucinations in which voices in the mind threaten, insult, or command the victim (less common are visual or tactile hallucinations)
- emotions that are blunted or inappropriate to the situation, such as laughing or smiling inappropriately

The symptoms of schizophrenia may come and go over periods of years, and sufferers may have some periods when they can function normally, particularly when they are receiving appropriate medical treatment.

Some phobics and their families worry about the possible development of schizophrenia. An examination by a psychiatrist is necessary to determine an appropriate diagnosis. Once diagnosed, treatment is essential.

Treatment Options and Outlook

Treatment is comprised of medication, and, when sufficient insight has been gained with medication, psychotherapy can be very helpful.

Antipsychotic medications may relieve the hallucinations and delusions, and newer antipsychotics, such as aripiprazole (Abilify), clozapine (Clozaril), or resperidone (Resperdal), are very effective in helping many people with schizophrenia attain normal or near-normal thinking.

Unfortunately, medication compliance is very poor for many patients with schizophrenia. They may take their medication for a period and then, believing that they are cured, stop taking the drug and suffer a relapse. Once the symptoms of the illness returns, the individual may refuse to believe that he or she is truly ill.

Another reason for medication noncompliance is that medications for schizophrenia sometimes cause side effects, such as weight gain, poor coordination, and other effects.

Individual therapy can help the person with schizophrenia who is improving with the use of medication and needs to learn to cope with the potential pain of past years of suffering as well as the feelings of grief and loss that may come from the stigmatization that they have experienced as a result of their mental illness. Therapy may help the individual create a life plan for the present and the future and learn to better understand others in their life and how to manage more effectively.

Family therapy may help spouses, parents, or siblings learn about schizophrenia and cope with the effects of dealing with a very ill person. Aside from the personal pain that the individual suffers, another real tragedy of schizophrenia is its effect on families. Often family members are burdened with a stubborn, confused, and marginally socialized young adult schizophrenic who, although not capable of independent life, is still able to attend school part-time, drive a car, and meet people. Family members may find themselves in the position of caretakers, often intervening at acute episodes when crises occur. There is little community or professional support for these families, although some groups such as the National Alliance for the Mentally Ill and its chapters provide support.

A tragic consequence of the reduced financing of professional support for schizophrenics is that many have been forced to live on their own, usually as *street people,* and as many as 30–50 percent of those who are homeless are also mentally ill, with a large proportion of this population suffering from schizophrenia.

See CLOZAPINE; GOING CRAZY, FEAR OF; PSYCHOSIS.

Risk Factors and Preventive Measures

Individuals with a family history of schizophrenia have an increased risk of developing schizophrenia, or about a 10 percent risk versus the risk of 1 percent when there is no family history.

There are no known preventive measures against schizophrenia, although a healthy family environment may play a positive role; for example, in studies of children adopted from families with schizophrenia, the adopted children had a significantly lower rate of developing schizophrenia than expected. In a study by Lowing et al. in 1983, the researchers found that when the child of a schizophrenic parent was adopted, the probability of the child developing schizophrenia fell to 3 percent, which was still higher than the rate for the general population, yet it was also significantly lower than the rate for a nonadopted child of a parent with schizophrenia.

Miller, Laurie M., MD, and Christine Adamec, *The Encyclopedia of Adoption,* 3rd ed. (New York: Facts On File, Inc., 2007).

Lowing, P., et al., "The Inheritance of Schizophrenia Disorder: A Reanalysis of the Danish Adoption Study Data," *American Journal of Psychiatry* 1400 (1983): pp. 1,167–1,171.

school phobia   School phobia is known as scolionophobia. School phobia is an exaggerated fear of going to school, or, more correctly, of leaving home or parents (separation fear). While many children show anxiety about school at one time or another, school phobics show frequent or long-standing fear and refusal to go to school.

In some individuals, school phobia develops from fears connected either with school or with the home. Some may have an irrational dread of some aspect of the school situation, such as fear of a teacher, principal, classmate, or examination. For most, however, the school phobia may be part of a SEPARATION ANXIETY syndrome.

School phobia is more common in elementary-school children than adolescents and is equally common in both sexes. According to the American Psychiatric Association, the extreme form of the disorder, involving school refusal, begins most often around ages eleven and twelve. The school-phobic child may be above average intelligence and average or above in achievement. Such children may otherwise be well-behaved and come from intact families with close-knit, concerned, caring parents. The disorder seems more common in some families on a transgenerational basis than in the general population. It occurs in children of every socioeconomic group and is not directly related to academic abilities.

In many children, this phobia develops after some life stress, such as a loss of a relative or pet through death, an illness of the child or a relative, or a change in the child's environment, such as a change of school or neighborhood.

In most cases, a school-phobic child should be treated as early as possible because fear of school interrupts the child's academic as well as social development. Also, the long-range outlook may depend on appropriate, early management. If school phobia becomes chronic, the phobic pattern of avoidance may continue into later life and be harder to control as the child gets older.

The child's phobia to school may or may not be overt. Young children may not verbalize reasons for refusing to go to school, while older children may attribute their fears to some specific aspect of school life. Often, school phobics are detected when they show physiologic symptoms on school days that are not present on weekends and holidays. Such symptoms may include headache, nausea, anorexia, vomiting, diarrhea, abdominal pain, feeling faint, sore throat, and others. There may be a lot of crying. The child may complain of being too ill to attend school, but when the mother says the child can stay home, symptoms often disappear. Often, when such children are sent to school despite complaints, the symptoms persist until the school nurse sends the child home.

There is a difference between truancy and school phobia. The truant stays away from both school and home; he avoids or leaves in order to pursue pleasures elsewhere. He keeps his truancy secret from his parents. On the other hand, the school phobic usually spends school hours at home, draws family attention to his problem, and may be ashamed to have others know about it. School-phobic children may refuse to see former friends or relatives to avoid explaining their difficulties in school or their absence from school, and the school phobic, unlike the truant, usually does not exhibit any other delinquent behavior. Researchers have found that the school-phobic child is likely to "fade into the woodwork," or even quietly disappear from school.

According to the American Psychiatric Association, school phobia is not included among its classification of phobic disorders because it has unique features and is characteristically associated with childhood.

Some authorities relate school phobia to separation anxiety, in which the child may have a combination of unconscious, unresolved hostility and feelings of dependency in his relationship with his mother, and at the same time, a fear of separation from her. This psychiatric viewpoint suggests that because the child unconsciously fears abandonment by the mother, he does not express his hostility toward her. He unconsciously fears that harm will come to the mother while he is in school and that if he stays home he can prevent his own destructive wishes from coming true. Behavioral viewpoints emphasize the parents' role in acquisition and maintenance of this behavior. Specifically, parents often reinforce school refusal subtly (or not so subtly) by complying with the child's wish to avoid (not wanting to "hurt" the child) or by wanting the child home (usually as a companion). Under stress, the child engages in refusal and thereby avoids school (and any stresses there) and receives a good deal of attention and sympathy. Some children become violent toward an individual who forces separation.

Experts differ on whether school phobia is a true phobia or should more properly be called *school refusal* and be considered a part of separation anxiety. Those who say it is a true phobia base their opinion on the fact that anxiety, originating from the child's fear of being separated from mother, is displaced to another object—the school and details of school life.

Not all school refusal is due to separation anxiety. When separation anxiety does account for school refusal, the child experiences difficulty being separated from home or family for a variety of purposes; school attendance is only one of them. In a true school phobia, the child fears the school situation, whether or not he is accompanied by the parent.

Some children have very specific, identifiable fears relating to school, and when these are determined and confronted, specific avenues may be taken to make the child more comfortable about attending school. For example, being bullied on the school bus, being teased about appearance or clothing, reciting in class, undressing in front of other children for gym, and going to the bathroom without privacy may be contributory factors to school phobia.

In a 1979 study, adolescent school phobics listed characteristics of the school that enabled them to function in it. First and foremost was the presence of an adult who was reliable and understanding. Next was flexibility in the school. They did not want to be hopelessly trapped in a particular classroom at a given time and did not want to have to experience anguish in returning after absence. They appreciated the involvement of their personal therapist with the school and its staff.

Treatment Options and Outlook

The type of help to seek depends on the child, the initial symptoms, the attitudes of parents, and school authorities. Efforts of parents and teachers with encouragement, indulgences, or even coercion may prove unsuccessful. If there has been a *real* event that frightened the child, such as a bully in the playground or an incident with an authority figure, parents and teachers can deal with this without involving a therapist.

In many cases, however, therapists can help the child, parents, and teachers. Treatment procedures vary, depending on the therapist, the age of the child, the duration of symptoms, the child's family situation, and other factors. Generally, school phobias are treated as interpersonal problems, rather than with the deconditioning techniques used with many other phobias, although management strategies are essential to achieve a positive outcome.

Therapists generally encourage returning to school as soon as possible so that the phobia does not become even stronger. However, others view early return to school as only a temporary solution that puts pressure on the child and makes him even more anxious.

Some therapists advocate use of pharmacological ANTIDEPRESSANT therapy for school phobics. This treatment originated when it was found that the antidepressant IMIPRAMINE relieves the panic attacks of AGORAPHOBIA, and many agoraphobics have a history of school phobia. The theory is that drug therapy, under careful supervision, enables the child to relearn behavior patterns and reorient attitudes, and when successful, the new behaviors will take over after the drug is no longer administered.

In some cases, lengthy psychotherapy is helpful for the child and the family. Some therapy programs involve support groups consisting of children, parents, and teachers who meet together to discuss their common problem and work out solutions. In one study, a group of adolescent school phobics reported that the existence of the group and the relaxation and comfort it provided was important to them. They appreciated sharing anxieties and garnering support from one another. Members of the group found that it was consoling to them to know that some of their fellow students were acutely sensitive to their problems and had parallel experiences that they customarily worked hard to hide. Some of the group members had fears related to being out of control and to having no power over their own school experience. Researchers found that it was important for students to exercise as much personal power as they could and learn to be masters of their own fate in school and outside it.

See also CHILDHOOD ANXIETIES, FEARS, AND PHOBIAS; DEPRESSION; DEPRESSION, ADOLESCENT.

American Handbook of Psychiatry (New York: Basic Books, 1977).

Coolidge, J. C., "School Phobia." In *Basic Handbook of Child Psychiatry.* Edited by J. D. Noshpitz (New York: Basic Books, 1979).

Diagnostic and Statistical Manual of Mental Disorders (Washington, DC: American Psychiatric Association, 1981), pp. 50–53.

Diamond, Stanley C., "School Phobic Adolescents and a Peer Support Group," *The Clearing House* (Nov. 1985), pp. 125–126.

DuPont, Robert L. (ed.), *Phobia* (New York: Brunner/Mazel, 1982), pp. 182–191.

Goodwin, Donald W., *Phobia, the Facts* (London: Oxford University Press, 1983).

International Encyclopedia of Psychiatry, Psychology, Psychoanalysis, and Neurology (New York: Van Nostrand Reinhold, 1977).

Marks, Isaac, *Fears and Phobias* (London: Heinemann Medical, 1969).

Sarafino, Edward P., *The Fears of Childhood* (New York: Human Sciences Press, 1986).

sciaphobia, sciophobia   Fear of shadows.
See also SHADOWS, FEAR OF.

scoleciphobia   Fear of worms.
See also WORMS, FEAR OF.

scolionophobia   See SCHOOL PHOBIA.

scopophobia, scoptophobia   Fear of being stared at.
See also BEING LOOKED AT, FEAR OF; STARED AT, FEAR OF BEING.

scotomaphobia   Fear of blind areas in the visual field.

scotophobia   Fear of darkness.
See also DARKNESS, FEAR OF.

scratched, fear of being   Fear of being scratched is known as amychophobia.

screen memory   A memory that the individual consciously tolerates to cover up a related remembrance that would be emotionally painful if recalled. Apparently, these memories are repressed or suppressed due to their painful or frightening nature and emerge only when the anxiety begins to lessen.

scriptophobia Fear of writing in public. This social phobia prevents many individuals from being able to write checks, use bank cards, or vote. When scriptophobics anticipate having to be seen writing, they experience physiological symptoms of heart palpitations, shortness of breath, trembling hands, sweating, and dizziness. Financial transactions have to be preplanned so that purchases can be made with cash (e.g., at grocery stores), or so that others do not see the individual writing (such as filling out deposit slips at home). Many rely on others to handle all financial matters involving writing. Some scriptophobics can cope better with writing in public when a trusted friend or relative is with them.

Many scriptophobic individuals also have other social anxieties, especially if they think they are being watched while doing some tasks and are afraid of doing something wrong, looking funny (by shaking or trembling), and becoming embarrassed. Scriptophobia represents a generalized fear of negative evaluation by others. Scriptophobia has been treated successfully with behavior therapy, graded exposure, and cognitive restructuring.

See also BEHAVIOR THERAPY; COGNITIVE RESTRUCTURING; PHOBIA; SOCIAL ANXIETY; SOCIAL PHOBIA.

sea, fear of Fear of the sea is known as thalassophobia. This fear may relate to a fear of water, fear of drowning, fear of waves, or fear of a particular type of landscape, such as the seashore, or just the sea's empty vastness and distance from land. It may also be related to a fear of salty water.

See also DROWNING, FEAR OF; LAKES, FEAR OF; WATER, FEAR OF; WAVES, FEAR OF.

seasonal affective disorder (SAD) A syndrome that is characterized by severe seasonal mood swings, with clinically depressed moods occurring for at least two weeks in the fall and winter, usually year after year, and with the individual's mood rebounding to normal or near-normal in the spring and summer. Periods within the year with less sunlight, later dawns, and early dusks appear to affect the circadian rhythms of individuals with SAD more severely than other individuals. It is believed that experiencing fewer hours of sunlight hours is a key factor in the development of SAD. The most difficult months for many individuals with SAD are January and February.

Researchers at the National Institute of Mental Health (NIMH) first began studying and defining the syndrome in the early 1980s. In 1987, SAD was first included in the *DIAGNOSTIC AND STATISTICAL MANUAL OF MENTAL DISORDERS*.

Symptoms and Diagnostic Path

Typically, SAD sufferers become clinically depressed with the approach of winter. In addition to gaining or losing weight, oversleeping, and feeling listless, they may also feel anxious and irritable and withdraw socially and lose interest in sex. As spring approaches, the depression subsides and behavior returns to normal. Other possible illnesses, such as major depressive disorder, bipolar disorder, hypothyroidism, hypoglycemia, and viral infections, should be ruled out before SAD is diagnosed. However, some individuals with SAD are misdiagnosed with depression or other disorders. There are no clinical laboratory markers for SAD, and the disorder is diagnosed based on the signs and symptoms in the individual.

Other symptoms of SAD include the following

- an intense craving for carbohydrates
- weight gain or loss
- fatigue
- loss of interest in normal activities

Treatment Options and Outlook

Light therapy (phototherapy) in which the individual is exposed to fluorescent light with five to 10 times the intensity of indoor lighting for 30 to 90 minutes per day has helped some SAD sufferers. Generally light therapy is given during the morning. Psychotherapy has also proven effective in patients with SAD. Antidepressants are helpful to many patients. In 2006, extended-release BUPROPION (Wellbutrin

XL) was approved by the Food and Drug Administration (FDA) for the treatment of patients with SAD.

Research studies have also shown that treating patients with SAD with a low dose of melatonin, a hormone naturally secreted by the pineal gland, may be sufficient to improve their condition. A study reported in *Proceedings of the National Academy of Sciences* indicated that melatonin could help to "reset" the circadian rhythm/biological clock of an individual.

The researchers found that among individuals without SAD, the time frame between the secretion of melatonin by their pineal gland and the middle of normal sleep was six hours. However, the researchers found that among their study subjects with SAD, in 71 percent of the cases, the subjects had interval secretion differences of melatonin in the fall and winter that were significantly greater than six hours. These individuals took melatonin capsules in the afternoon and they were able to bring their circadian levels back to normal, as well as improving their moods. The researchers also found that the closer those individuals were to secretion of melatonin at six-hour intervals, the less likely they were to suffer from SAD.

Risk Factors and Preventive Measures

SAD afflicts about four times as many women as men and usually appears in the early 20s. The age of onset for most individuals with SAD is between 18 and 30 years. However, the malady has been diagnosed in children as young as nine.

Latitude appears to be as important as season to individuals with SAD. The incidence and severity of SAD increase with distance from the equator, peaking at around 40 degrees north.

Researchers suspect there may be a genetic factor involved in SAD, because more than two-thirds of those with the syndrome have a close relative with a mood disorder. The role of the absence or presence of light in seasonal mood shifts is unclear. One theory attributes the disorder to a disturbance in the body's natural biological clock, resulting in an abnormal production of melatonin, a hormone manufactured in the brain, and serotonin, a chemical that helps transmit nerve impulses.

See also AFFECTIVE DISORDERS; CLIMATE, FEAR OF; DEPRESSION; MOOD.

Missagh, Ghadirian A., B. E. Murphy, and Marie-Josie Gendron, "Efficacy of light versus tryptophan therapy in seasonal affective disorder," *Journal of Affective Disorders* 50, no. 1 (July 1998): pp. 23–27.

Lewy, Alfred J., Bryan J. Lefler, Jonathan S. Emens, and Vance K. Bauer, "The Circadian Basis of Winter Depression," *Proceedings of the National Academy of Sciences* 103 (2006): pp. 7414–7419.

secondary depression   Depression occurring in an individual who has another illness, either mental or physical, that precedes the depression. Depression may accompany other disorders, such as obsessive-compulsive disorder, alcohol abuse or alcoholism (most common) and may occur after or in addition to a medical illness. Careful evaluation of secondary depression is essential to determine the cause and course of treatment to reduce the anxiety-producing effects of the disorder.

See also DEPRESSION; PHARMACOLOGICAL APPROACH.

secondary gain   An obvious advantage that an individual gains from his or her PHOBIA or anxiety disorder. Family and friends may be more protective and more attentive and may release the individual from responsibility. For example, agoraphobics experience secondary gains of having someone willing to accompany them outdoors and to do errands and other chores for them.

See also AGORAPHOBIA; PRIMARY GAIN; SICK ROLE.

secrets   Many people are hiding something they are afraid to tell and feeling anxious about keeping their secret. The word *secret* is derived from the Latin word *secretus*, meaning "separate," or "out of the way." The current definition, according to the *American Heritage Dictionary of the English Language*, comprises the following:

• Something kept hidden from others or known only to oneself or to a few

• Concealed from general knowledge or view

• Dependably close-mouthed; discreet

• Not visibly expressed; private; inward

Most of us guard something that fits the above categories that we don't reveal to others. But what the definition doesn't state is that many of us are uncomfortable and feel anxious about the secrets we keep. Many of us struggle lifelong with keeping of secrets. Some of us think that there is something wrong in having a secret, but we don't know what to do about it. Some of us even think there is something wrong with us.

As we continue to worry about hiding our secret, the anxiety produced by the hiding leads to body tension, thereby producing psychophysiological illnesses, such as headaches and stomachaches; behavioral symptoms such as irritability, short temper, and difficulty concentrating; and psychological reactions, such as depression and frustration.

Telling Secrets

People who hide secrets go around "what iffing" to themselves. They do what psychologists call "catastrophizing." That means they project the "worst case" scenario into the future and act on it as if it were true. It is predicting in your imagination the actuality of the negative event.

Secrets can be divided into those to keep, those to let go of, and those to share. Many couples share secrets—the intimacies of their relationship. Business associates share secrets. Mothers and daughters and fathers and sons share secrets. Many admit to shared secrets and for many their sharing has helped bond their loving and supportive relationship. Fortunately for them, their shared secrets are "constructive" secrets.

See also RELATIONSHIPS.

Kahn, Ada P., and Sheila Kimmel, *Empower Yourself: Every Woman's Guide to Self-Esteem* (New York: Avon Books, 1997).

security object   A special object, such as a favorite toy or blanket, that gives a child comfort and reassurance. If the object is taken away or lost, even temporarily, the child will experience great anxiety and probably cry inconsolably. Loss of a child's security object also causes anxiety for parents.

See also PARENTING.

sedative   An old term meaning a substance, such as a drug or herb, that relieves nervousness, anxiety, or irritability, sometimes to the point of inducing sleep. A sedative acts by depressing the CENTRAL NERVOUS SYSTEM. The degree of sedation depends on the agent, size of dose, method of administration (for example, oral or intravenous), and the physical and mental condition of the individual. A sedative used as a relaxant in small doses may be used to induce sleep with larger doses. BARBITURATES are common examples of sedative drugs used in this way.

selaphobia   Fear of flashing lights. This fear is often related to anxiety produced by excessive stimulation. For example, car headlights at night, crowds of people, and confusing buildings are all situations that involve stimulation and may provoke anxiety in an anxiety-prone individual.

See also FLASHING LIGHTS, FEAR OF.

selenophobia   Fear of the Moon.

See also MOON, FEAR OF; NIGHT, FEAR OF.

self, fear of   Fear of oneself is known as autophobia.

See also BEING ONESELF, FEAR OF.

self-efficacy (SE)   The concept that one can perform adequately; self-confidence. This concept as it relates to phobias and anxieties was researched during the 1970s by Albert Bandura, an American psychologist at Stanford University. SE measures how likely one believes one would be to succeed if one attempted a task. Such a rating can be used before, during, or after treatment for phobias. The SE rating correlates highly with performance in a behavioral test just after the rating. In phobics asked to rate SE concerning a phobic task, SE is low before treatment and rises after individuals improve with exposure treatment.

SE at the end of treatment may be the major mediator of fear reduction. However, a better way to increase SE is by exposure, the same procedure that reduces fear. In experiments, SE correlated highly not only with performance of a frightening task, but also with the fear expected during it. In one experiment with 50 snake-phobic students, most refused to try to hold the snake because they were frightened, not because they felt inept. They were certain that they could hold the snake if they really "had to." If a task is frightening, SE reflects an individual's willingness (rather than ability) to do it. When willingness rises, there is less anticipated fear.

SE can predict psychological changes achieved by different modes of treatment. Expectations of personal efficacy determine whether coping behavior will begin, how much effort will be expended, and how long it will be sustained in the face of aversive experiences. Persistence in activities that are subjectively threatening, but in fact relatively safe, produces, through experiences of mastery, further enhancement of self-efficacy and corresponding reductions in defensive behavior.

Individuals derive expectations of self-efficacy from four main sources: performance accomplishments, vicarious experience, verbal persuasion, and physiological states. The more dependable the experiential sources, the greater the changes in perceived self-efficacy.

Bandura, Albert, "Self-Efficacy: Toward a Unifying Theory of Behavioral Change," *Psychological Review* 84, no. 2 (1977): p. 215.

Marks, I. M., *Fears, Phobias and Rituals* (New York: Oxford University Press, 1987), pp. 500–501.

self-esteem   Self-esteem means accepting oneself, liking oneself, and appreciating one's self-worth. Self-esteem is built on personal feelings of accomplishment and skill. In the 1990s, self-esteem was targeted as a major characteristic of successful coping with anxieties. Low self-esteem can lead to mental and physical disorders, such as DEPRESSION, poor appetite, headaches, insomnia, and, in extreme cases, suicide.

Many people become anxious when they compare themselves with others, their own unrealistic standards, and standards set for them by others. Those who think they do not measure up develop low self-esteem. Such individuals may feel inferior, either intellectually or physically, while individuals with high self-esteem feel confident and capable. Some become workaholics and some become totally dependent on outside approval. People with low self-esteem often depend on approval from others.

Lack of self-esteem has been pointed to as a cause for many social ills, including juvenile delinquency, crime, and substance abuse. While it may not be the most important causative factor, it usually plays a role. Lack of self-esteem can be life-threatening. Particularly in young people, lack of self-esteem is a major factor in depression and suicide.

Causes of low self-esteem vary between individuals, but there are many common themes. For example, many people have low self-esteem because of physical appearance. Overweight is a common contributor to low self-esteem. This can be overcome by seeking counseling regarding a diet and exercise program. Some adults have lifelong low self-esteem because of a prominent facial feature, such as a misshapen nose or ear. With counseling and, possibly, cosmetic surgery, improvements can be made in both appearance and outlook.

A common cause of low self-esteem is having been abused as a child, either sexually or psychologically. Being an abused spouse or in a codependent relationship is also a cause. Being bullied or criticized in school can result in low self-esteem.

Some children lose their self-esteem on the athletic field because they do not compete well, or do not have the physical ability to keep up with others. Other children lose self-esteem in the classroom. Simple comments by teachers can produce anxieties for a child and ruin a child's self-esteem. In such cases, lack of self-esteem can lead to the anxiety disorders of social fears and phobias.

In a Gallup poll conducted in early 1992, 612 adults were interviewed by telephone. Respondents were asked about situations that would make them feel very bad about themselves. Situations included not being able to pay bills, being tempted into doing something immoral, having an abortion, getting a divorce, losing a job, feeling they had disobeyed God, being noticeably overweight, doing something embarrassing in public, and being criticized by someone they admired. Respondents above age 50 were more likely to feel bad about these situations than younger people. However, overall, 63 percent said that time and effort spent on self-esteem is worthwhile, while only 34 percent said that time and effort could be better spent on work.

See also BODY IMAGE; CODEPENDENCY; CRITICISM; DATING; INFERIORITY COMPLEX; RELATIONSHIPS; SOCIAL PHOBIAS; SUICIDE.

Kahn, Ada P., and Sheila Kimmel, *Empower Yourself: Every Woman's Guide to Self-Esteem* (New York: Avon Books, 1997).

Lee, Richard M., and Steven B. Robbins, "The relationship between social connectedness and anxiety, self-esteem, and social identity," *Journal of Counseling Psychology* 45, no. 3 (July 1998): pp. 338–345.

self-fulfilling prophecy   A belief that helps bring about its own fulfillment. For example, a feared event sometimes is brought about by predicting that it will happen.

self-help groups   Self-help groups and the self-help movement, with its growing strength and visibility, has helped many with concerns stemming from anxieties and has led to increased openness and understanding of many disorders, including anxiety disorders and chronic illnesses. Fighting anxiety or chronic illness can be a lonely and discouraging effort. Participating in a group offers regular connection with others who appreciate one's struggles in a very personal way.

The focus of a self-help group is the idea of sharing feelings, perceptions, and concerns with others who have had or still have the same experience. Members of the group can give each other practical advice, ranging, for example, from how to meet the daily stresses of coping with a phobia to meeting the needs of aging parents.

The self-help movement has helped to generate funding for education and research and has been a powerful voice for the education of professionals in many fields.

Self-Help Techniques

Since the 1990s, American society has been offered self-help in the form of magazine articles, radio call-in shows, television talk shows, speakers, support groups, audio- and videotapes. Self-help can work if the individual is motivated to make it work. In fact, even with psychotherapy under the guidance of a mental-health professional, much of the improvement in a person's mental health actually comes from self-help.

Self-help techniques include MEDITATION and RELAXATION. Both are skills that can be learned and applied to relieve stress, anxiety and phobias.

Gray, Ross E., Vanessa Orr, June C. Carroll, et al., "Self-help groups: Family physician's attitudes, awareness, and practices," *Canadian Family Physician* 44 (October 1998): pp. 2,137–2,142.

"Special Focus on Self-Help," *Anxiety Disorders Association of America* REPORTER 6, no. 3 (summer/fall 1995).

self-hypnosis   See HYPNOSIS.

self-psychology   The psychological system propounded by Heinz Kohut (1913–81), an Austrian-born American psychoanalyst. This theory holds that all behavior can be interpreted in reference to the self, and that many anxieties are interpreted with reference to the self. Kohut proposed that the young child has tendencies toward assertiveness and ambition as well as toward idealization of parents and the beginnings of ideals and values. Both groups of tendencies contribute to strong ties between the infant and parent.

Kohut believed that the real mover of psychic development is the self, rather than sexual and aggressive drives, as Sigmund Freud suggested. Kohut used the term *self-object* to describe an object in an infant's surroundings that the infant regards as part of him- or herself. People with narcissistic personality disorder cannot separate adequately from the self-object and thus cannot perceive or respond to the individuality of others. Kohut believed that lack of empathic response between parent and infant is the cause of later stresses and psychological disorders in the growing child.

Kohut developed his major theories in several publications, including *The Analysis of the Self* (1971),

The Restoration of the Self (1977), and *The Search for the Self* (1978).

See also PSYCHOTHERAPIES.

self-rating scales Measurements of phobic reactions as reported by the phobic individuals themselves. Self-rating scales or questionnaires are used by researchers and therapists, often to assess the extent of the phobia and also to measure the success of therapy after therapy is underway, and perhaps again after therapy has been concluded. Self-rating scales are particularly useful in working with agoraphobic individuals, as such people are fearful of many varied situations. Scales have been devised for individuals to indicate, for example, on a scale from O to 8, "how much" they "would avoid" or "would not avoid" certain situations. Likewise, questionnaires are used to assess fears relating to AGORAPHOBIA, which might include traveling alone by bus or train, walking alone in busy streets, going into crowded stores, going alone far from home, and being in large open places. Although there is some controversy among researchers regarding the usefulness of self-rating scales because of their lack of specificity, most agree that the scales have a place when used in combination with other assessment techniques that sample behavior and physiological reactions directly.

See, also SELF-HELP.

self-talk Positive affirmations or statements to oneself about overcoming phobias, fears, and anxieties. When positive self-talk replaces negative talk or catastrophizing, projecting the worst case scenarios, the individual moves toward self-confidence and self-esteem. An example of positive self-talk is "I can do this. I can cross the bridge. I am no longer afraid."

semen, fear of Fear of semen is known as spermophobia or spermatophobia. This reaction is usually a variation of "germ" or contamination fears of obsessive-compulsive individuals.

See also PSYCHOSEXUAL ANXIETIES; SEXUAL FEARS.

sense of humor See LAUGHTER.

sensory deprivation Being cut off from usual external stimuli without opportunity for perception through the senses. This may occur accidentally or experimentally. For example, there is sensory deprivation with the loss of hearing or eyesight, or with physical isolation, such as when one is lost in a snowstorm. In some psychological experiments, such as sleep research, subjects are placed in rooms in which day and night are indistinguishable. Sensory deprivation can lead to ANXIETY, PANIC, DELUSIONS, DEPRESSION, and HALLUCINATIONS.

sensory integration disorder Also known as sensory integrative dysfunction. Sensory integration disorder refers to an individual's inability to take in information through the senses (smell, taste, touch, movement, vision, and hearing) and to combine this sensory information with previously known information, memories, and knowledge in order to make meaningful responses. Many parents experience anxiety when their young children appear lazy, stubborn, shy, or headstrong to others. Understanding why this behavior occurs and taking steps to help the child change the behavior can relieve tension between the parent and child.

Sensory integration occurs in the central nervous system and is generally thought to take place throughout complex interactions between the portions of the brain that are responsible for coordination, attention, arousal levels, autonomic functioning, emotions, memory, and higher level cognitive functions.

Sensory integration disorder was first researched and described in *Sensory Integration and the Child*, by A. Jean Ayres in 1994. Said Ayres, "Good sensory processing enables all the impulses to flow easily and reach their destination quickly. Sensory integrative dysfunction is a sort of 'traffic jam' in the brain. Some bits of sensory information get tied up in traffic, and certain parts of the brain do not get the sensory information they need to do their jobs."

According to Linda C. Stephens in the *AAHBEI News Exchange* in 1997, parents and professionals should look at patterns of behaviors and the overall situation of how problems interfere with the child's functioning in his or her play, physical and emotional development, and ability to develop independence. A child suspected of having a sensory integrative disorder should be evaluated by a health care professional who has had additional training in sensory integration evaluation and treatment.

Children with sensory dysfunctions may become discouraged or develop poor self-esteem, especially when they are aware of their differences in functioning compared to those of their peers. If a child has difficulty with motor skills and play activities, it may be hard for him to become part of a group. Some children with the disorder exhibit aggressive behaviors that may cause the child to be shunned by other children.

Symptoms and Diagnostic Path

Sensory integration disorder is usually identified by specialized psychologists, although pediatricians and family practitioners may note the symptoms and make a referral to an appropriate expert. Young children with sensory integration disorder may seem distracted, hyperactive, or uninhibited because they cannot screen out nonessential sensory or visual information. They may constantly ask about or orient to sensory input that others ignore, such as a heater fan or a distant airplane. Other children with the disorder fail to respond to certain stimuli, such as when their name is called. Children with regulatory disorders may have difficulty establishing appropriate sleeping and eating patterns. They may have unusual difficulty with transitioning from one activity to another, such as leaving one place to go to another place.

While young children's attention span is generally short, a child with sensory integration dysfunction shows even more distractibility. In addition, the child does not play, climb, or swing in an organized way. Some children with this disorder are very repetitive in playing with their toys. They may learn one way to play with a toy or playground equipment without adding any variations or playing creatively. Others may have poor balance and trip easily, bumping their heads, because they lack protective responses such as reaching out with the arms when they begin to fall.

Children with ATTENTION-DEFICIT/HYPERACTIVITY DISORDER (ADHD) are also distractible; however, they generally do not have the poor balance and lack of coordination of the child with a sensory dysfunction. In addition, children with ADHD who engage in vigorous sensory input, such as with spinning or swinging, will experience dizziness, while the child with a sensory dysfunction often will not feel dizzy.

Some children have difficulty calming themselves after exciting physical activity. Tantrums may occur and the child may seem inconsolable. Other children with the disorder seek excessive amounts of vigorous sensory input.

Parents should look at behavior patterns and how the problems interfere with the child's functioning in play, physical and emotional development, interaction with other children and adults, and the ability to develop independence.

The child is diagnosed on the basis of behavior as well as with the use of tests, such as the Sensory Integration and Praxis Tests (SOPT). The results of the tests will enable therapists to create recommendations to parents.

Treatment Options and Outlook

Occupational therapists and physical therapists are the key experts who work with children with sensory integration disorder. Young children may be referred to early intervention programs available in most communities through the school system.

Risk Factors and Preventive Measures

According to *The Encyclopedia of Adoption,* children adopted from other countries who have been institutionalized may be at risk for sensory integration disorder, particularly after long stays in orphanages, possibly because of the extreme deprivation they experienced well before the ADOPTION occurred. In addition, children who were exposed prenatally to alcohol or illegal drugs may be at risk for sensory integration disorder.

Adamec, Christine, and Laurie C. Miller, MD, *The Encyclopedia of Adoption* (New York: Facts On File, Inc., 2007).

Ayres, A. Jean, *Sensory Integration and the Child* (Los Angeles: Western Psychological Services, 1994).

Biel, Lindsey, and Nancy Peske, *Raising a Sensory Smart Child: The Definitive Handbook for Helping Your Child with Sensory Integration Issues* (New York: Penguin Books, 2005).

Smith, Karen A., and Karen R. Gouze, *The Sensory-Sensitive Child: Practical Solutions for Out-of-Bounds Behavior* (New York: Harper Resource, 2004).

Stephens, Linda C., "Sensory Integrative Dysfunction," *AAHEI News Exchange* 12, no. 1 (Winter 1997).

separation anxiety   A fear experienced when an individual contemplates being taken or is actually taken from someone to whom he or she has an attachment. Separation fears are evident in school phobias and have been implicated as a factor in AGORAPHOBIA. Freud discussed separation anxieties in his work and noted this fear as a causative factor in many forms of neuroses. Freud himself had separation anxieties.

Separation anxiety is normal for infants who show fear and apprehension when they are removed from their mother or surrogate mother, or when approached by strangers. Separation is seen as the first step toward individuation, personal responsibility, and psychological maturity.

Prolonged separation often is followed by reactions of protest, detachment, and despair. First the child cries, screams, and struggles to find its caregiver, then seems oblivious to the separation, and finally becomes inactive and perhaps depressed. The sequence is similar to what occurs in acute mourning after bereavement, except that grief tends to start with numbness.

Upon reunion following separation, infants are often angry with their caregivers and may avoid or even attack them; when picked up, the infant may be unresponsive at first.

Adolescents and adults show signs of separation anxiety in times of disaster. People search for one another and cling together, as companionship reduces fear. For example, children sometimes want to cling to parents and sleep with them after a tornado hits. The fact that adult phobics' fears are greatly reduced by the presence of companions is a remnant of infant separation anxiety.

See also BIRTH TRAUMA; CHILDHOOD ANXIETIES, FEARS, AND PHOBIAS; LITTLE HANS; SCHOOL PHOBIA; SOTERIA.

Marks, Isaac M., *Fears, Phobias and Rituals* (New York: Oxford University Press), pp. 140–141.

seplophobia   Fear of decaying matter.
See also DECAYING MATTER, FEAR OF.

septophobia   Fear of decaying matter.

serotonin   A NEUROTRANSMITTER substance found in the central nervous system, blood, nerve cells, and other tissues. The substance was identified during the 1950s as 5-hydroxytryptamine (5-HT); it is also known as hydroxytryptamine. Serotonin is derived from tryptophan, an essential amino acid widely distributed through the body and in the brain. Serotonin functions as a smooth-muscle stimulator and constrictor of blood vessels. Serotonin is involved in circuits that influence sleep and emotional arousal and is indirectly involved in the psychobiology of DEPRESSION. One theory suggests low levels of serotonin as a factor in causing depression. Some ANTIDEPRESSANT drugs increase the levels of serotonin and norepinephrine, other neurotransmitters.

See also DRUGS.

serum prolactin   See LACTATE-INDUCED ANXIETY.

sesquipedalophobia   Fear of long words.

Sex Anxiety Inventory (SAI)   A specific-fear questionnaire developed by R. Klorman et al. in 1974. The respondent selects one of two response alternatives on the 25-item questionnaire indicating his or her view concerning sex. Researchers reported that scores on the SAI were related to respondents' actual sexual experiences; those with less sex anxiety reported more sexual activity. See chart on page 437.

See also PYSCHOSEXUAL ANXIETIES; SEX THERAPY; SEXUAL FEARS.

SAMPLE ITEMS FROM THE SEX ANXIETY INVENTORY

Sex:
  a. Can cause as much anxiety as pleasure.
  b. On the whole is good and enjoyable.
I feel nervous:
  a. About initiating sexual relations.
  b. About nothing when it comes to members of the opposite sex.
When I awake from sexual dreams:
  a. I feel pleasant and relaxed.
  b. I feel tense.
When I meet someone I'm attached to:
  a. I get to know him or her.
  b. I feel nervous.

Ronald A. Kleinknecht, *The Anxious Self* (New York: Human Sciences Press, 1986), p. 103.

sex appeal   Attractiveness to others, possibly including some arousal of sexual interest and desire. Healthy, good-looking faces, attractive hair, and an attractive body shape are generally the attributes of sex appeal in the United States today. Many individuals with these characteristics are pictured in advertisements and in films. Many men and women find these advertisements a source of anxiety, as they feel these illustrations are a threat to their SELF-ESTEEM. Many develop negative feelings about their bodies. Some resort to EATING DISORDERS.

A person who has sex appeal may be said to be "sexy" based on cultural patterns and personal tastes. In Western society, standards of what constitutes sex appeal are often established by film and media. Many Americans find men who are muscular and athletic sexy, and relatively slim women attractive. At other periods in history, plumper women were considered attractive, for example, as shown in the paintings of Peter Paul Rubens, a Flemish painter (1577–1640) whose nudes gave our vocabulary the term *Rubenesque*, to refer to the well-developed and heavier body shape.

See also BODY IMAGE.

sex drive   The desire to have sexual activity. Sex drive or sexual desire varies in strength in different women and men and at different ages and stages of life in the same individual. Differences may be due to anxieties, fears, or inhibitions about sexual activity produced by parental attitudes to sex and those of peer groups.

There are differences in sexual desire between persons. How much is too much and how little is too little is a personal choice. However, if one feels that he or she would like to have more sexual desire, medical consultation may be helpful.

One's expression of sexual desire may differ also, according to whether or not one has a partner. For example, sex researchers have found that some widowed postmenopausal women who have no partner do not believe that their sex drive is very strong, while women in the same peer group who have regular, attractive male companions feel a strong sex drive.

While some researchers believe that sex drive decreases with age, many senior adults will attest to the fact that sex drive can persist throughout all stages of life. Good health, freedom from chronic disease, and companionship with others of the opposite sex stimulate the sex drive to continue until older age.

See also SEX THERAPY; SEXUAL DIFFICULTIES.

sexism   An attitude or belief that one sex is superior to the other in certain circumstances. The attitude seems to cause anxieties for all concerned. The term often refers to male attitudes about women. To a large extent, the women's liberation movement during the latter half of the 20th century fought and overcame sexism to some degree.

See also SEXUAL HARASSMENT; WOMEN'S LIBERATION MOVEMENT.

sexophobia   Fear of the opposite sex.

See also OPPOSITE SEX, FEAR OF.

sex therapy   Counseling and treatment of sexual difficulties that are not due to medical or physical causes. Many people encounter sexual difficulties because of anxieties, and at the same time, their sexual difficulties are a cause of anxieties. Many are helped by a combination of sex therapy and marital counseling. The purpose of sex therapy is to reduce anxieties the couple has about sexual activity and increase their enjoyment of their relationship.

In sex therapy, couples learn about normal sexual behavior and learn to reduce their feelings of anxiety about sex by gradually engaging in increasingly intimate activities. Couples learn to communicate better with each other regarding sexual matters and preferences and to retrain their approaches and response patterns.

Sex therapists use several techniques. One is sensate focus therapy, in which the couple explores pleasurable activities in a relaxed manner without sexual sensations. The couple might start with massage of non-erogenous areas of the body. Gradually, as anxieties diminish, the couple progresses to stimulation of sexual areas, and finally to sexual intercourse.

Other techniques sex therapists use are directed toward reducing premature ejaculation, relieving vaginismus (muscle spasm of the vagina), and helping both partners reach orgasm.

For sexual problems related to physical causes or illness, individuals should consult a physician, particularly specialists in gynecology or urology.

See also ANORGASMIA; DYSPAREUNIA; EJACULATION; ORGASM; SEXUAL DIFFICULTIES; SEXUAL RESPONSE CYCLE.

sexual abuse, fear of   Fear of sexual abuse is known as agraphobia or contrectophobia.

See also SEXUAL FEARS.

sexual anxiety   See PSYCHOSEXUAL ANXIETIES; SEX THERAPY; SEXUAL FEARS.

sexual fears   Fears in human love life impair sexual responding so that erotic responses to partners are weakened. Common fears of women include fearing that their vaginas are too tight for insertion of their partners' penises, that they will experience pain during intercourse, and that they will not experience orgasm as often as they desire. Common fears of men include that they will not have an erection, that they cannot maintain an erection long enough during intercourse to achieve orgasm, that they maintain an erection but do not ejaculate, and that they ejaculate sooner than desired.

There are many causes for sexual fears and anxieties. In males, inadequate sexual performance is often due to fear of the same (either through self-judgment—"observer" effect—or perceived rejection or criticism of the partner). Anxiety may either prevent or weaken erection or, more commonly, lead to premature ejaculation. Thus a vicious cycle of fear, failure, and then more fear develops. Fear has these effects only if it is stronger than the sexual excitation. In females, sexual fear may be caused by many things, ranging from the sight of a penis to fear of penetration, to the belief that she will be punished for indulging in sexual pleasure; some men share this last fear. The term frigidity is often applied to women's sexual inadequacies. Frigidity, in actuality, covers situations from a complete inability to be aroused to a failure to reach a climax even when sexual excitement is very high. When a woman has a general inhibition of sexual response, it is often caused by anxiety. Some sexual fears may have origins in relatively trivial situations, such as having been frightened in the act of masturbation, or more serious ones, such as a history of sexual molestation.

Treatment of sexual fears depends on the severity of the fear, the extent to which it interferes with one's functioning, and the perceived cause of the fear. Sexual anxieties are treated with many therapies, including BEHAVIOR THERAPY, in which techniques including DESENSITIZATION are used.

Paraphilias are various sexual deviations that involve sexual arousal by uncommon or bizarre stimuli. FETISHES are one form of paraphilia. A fetishist is almost always a male, and he derives sexual arousal from some inanimate object—such as women's shoes, underwear, etc.—or some specific nongenital part of a person, such as locks of hair, feet, ankles, fingers, etc. Transvestism (cross-sex dressing), incest, pedophilia (sexual gratification through physical and sexual contact with prepubertal children), voyeurism (peeping), and exhibitionism (exposure of genitals) are common forms of paraphilias.

Psychoanalytic theory generally considers the paraphilias as defensive functions that ward off castration anxiety about normal sexual behavior. These views have been challenged by learning theorists, who prefer a theory of stimulus association as explanatory.

See also CLASSICAL CONDITIONING; DYSPAREUNIA, FEAR OF; PSYCHOSEXUAL ANXIETIES; SEX THERAPY.

sexual harassment Sexual harassment is unwelcome sexual attention, usually on the job. It produces anxiety for women and men as well as employers and the families of the people experiencing harassment. Sexual attention is "unwelcome" when it is not initiated or solicited and when it is unwanted. It occurs by men toward women, women toward men, or toward same-sex individuals. Such attentions may include jokes and remarks, questions about the other's sexual behavior, "accidental" touching, and repeated and unwanted invitations for a date or for a sexual relationship. It can be verbal, visual, physical, or written.

Sexual harassment is a source of anxiety to an individual because it is defined in terms of its effect on the recipient. This means behavior that is meant to be humorous or well-intentioned is sexual harassment if it is offensive to another individual. It is not the intent of the sender of the behavior that counts; it is the impact on the recipient. What one may view as harmless may be objectionable to others.

A U.S. Supreme Court decision (*Meritor* v. *Vinson*) in 1980 declared that sexual harassment is a form of sex discrimination and, therefore, a violation of Title VII of the 1964 Civil Rights Act. During the

---

EXAMPLES OF SEXUAL HARASSMENT

- Dirty jokes or sexually oriented language
- Nude or seminude photos, posters, calendars, or cartoons
- Obscene gestures, lewd actions, or leering
- Introduction of sexual topics into business conversations
- Requests for dates or sexual favors that are not mutually acceptable
- Unwelcome hugging, patting, or touching

SEXUAL HARASSMENT: WHAT TO DO

- Tell the offender promptly and clearly that the conduct is unwelcome and unacceptable. Do this verbally, in writing, or both.
- Document in writing every incident, with specific details of the offensive behavior and your response.
- Do not feel guilty. Sexual harassment is not your fault. By clearly voicing your expectations, you force the offender to choose whether to change the unwelcome behavior, or to purposely continue it.
- If the problem continues, tell your supervisor. If your supervisor is the harasser, talk to another executive or report it to the department of human resources.

1980s, American society became increasingly aware of sexual harassment. For example, in the study by the U.S. Merit Systems Protection Board reported in 1988, federal workers were more inclined to define certain types of behavior as sexual harassment than in 1980. In 1987, 42 percent of women and 14 percent of men employed by the federal government said they experienced some form of uninvited and unwanted sexual attention. Federal workers in the survey believed that sexual harassment was not worse in the federal government than in the private sector. In 1991, sexual harassment received national attention when law professor Anita Hill accused nominee to the U.S. Supreme Court Clarence Thomas of sexual harassment and the federal hearing was nationally televised.

Federal workers reported that the most frequently experienced type of uninvited sexual attention was "unwanted sexual teasing, jokes, remarks, or questions." The least frequently experienced type of harassment, "actual or attempted rape or assault," is also arguably the most severe. When victims of sexual harassment took positive action in response to unwanted sexual attention, it was largely informal action, and in many cases, was judged to be effective. For both sexes, simply asking or telling the offender to stop improved the situation most frequently. Threatening to tell others or telling others was the second most effective action for women, while avoiding the person(s) was the second most effective action for men.

Fitzgerald, Louise F., Fritz Drasgow, Charles L. Hulin, et al., "Antecedents and consequences of sexual harrassment in organizations: A test of an integrated model." *Journal of Applied Psychology* 82, no. 4 (August 1997): pp. 578–589.

Karpeles, Michael D., "Risk of sexual harassment on the rise?" *The Rotarian,* (March 1999): p. 8.

sexual intercourse, fear of   Fear of sexual intercourse is known as coitophobia, erotophobia, and genophobia.

See also PSYCHOSEXUAL ANXIETIES; SEXUAL FEARS; SEXUALLY TRANSMITTED DISEASES, FEAR OF.

sexual intercourse, fear of painful   Fear of painful vaginal sexual intercourse is known as dyspareunia.

See also DYSPAREUNIA, FEAR OF; MENOPAUSE, FEAR OF; PSYCHOSEXUAL ANXIETIES; SEXUAL FEARS.

sexual love, fear of   Fear of sexual love is known as erotophobia.

See also PSYCHOSEXUAL ANXIETIES; SEXUAL FEARS.

sexually transmitted diseases (STDs), fear of   Many people fear sexually transmitted diseases (STDs) because such diseases cause discomfort, may lead to infertility, and may be life-threatening. Sexually transmitted disease is the term given to a group of diseases that affect both men and women and are generally transmitted during sexual intercourse. Historically, SYPHILIS and gonorrhea have been wellknown; they were referred to as VENEREAL DISEASES long before the term STD was coined during the latter part of the 20th century. There are several STDs that are feared because they have become notably widespread during the 1980s. These include herpes, chlamydia, and hepatitis B, as well as pubic lice, genital warts, and other vaginal infections. Syphilis and gonorrhea are still prevalent and, some sources say, on the increase due to the upswing in other concurrent STDs.

Fears of acquiring an STD have led many formerly sexually active individuals to seek fewer sexual partners. Fears of STD are prevalent among individuals who are widowed or divorced and who begin seeking new partners after their loss, as well as among never-married individuals. Such fears have also increased the use of condoms, as condoms are thought to reduce the likelihood of spreading most STDs.

Herpes

Herpes (technically known as herpes simplex or herpes virus hominus) is feared because one cannot tell if a partner has herpes, and there is no known cure (as of 2007) for herpes, although there are treatments to decrease the risk of transmitting the disease to others. Herpes is more common in women than in men. Herpes outbreaks cause either single or multiple blisters that occur on mucous membranes such as lips or vagina. Herpes simplex I causes most oral "cold sores." Herpes simplex II causes most vaginal herpes. Transmission can occur when a herpes blister comes in contact with any mucous membrane or open cut or sore. Herpes is most often transmitted through sexual intercourse and can also be transmitted during mouth-genital contact, or with manual contact during heterosexual or homosexual relations.

In its active stage, herpes can be debilitating. Herpes recurs, and often attacks occur when the previously infected individual is under stress, fatigued, or has another illness. Women who know that they have the herpes infection are fearful of giving birth to a baby who may also have herpes, as the infection can be transmitted to the baby during the birth process. Women who have active vaginal herpes blisters are routinely given Caesarean sections.

Many individuals who have herpes take drugs to relieve the pain of the blisters and prophylactically (as a preventive) to reduce the severity of future attacks.

Chlamydia

Chlamydia is two or three times more common than gonorrhea (see below) but less well-known. It is only in the last quarter of the 20th century that information about this disease has appeared in the medical and popular press. Chlamydia is feared because untreated symptoms in women can lead to infections in the fallopian tubes and uterus (pelvic inflammatory disease). The disease affects men and women, but women are less likely to notice symptoms in early stages. The signs in women are unusual vaginal discharge, irregular bleeding, bleeding after intercourse, or deep pain during and after intercourse. Men may notice clear, mucuslike discharge from the penis and burning during urination. Chlamydia is treated with antibiotics, and sexual partners must be treated to avoid a ping-pong effect of reinfection. Thus when one individual discovers that he or she has it, anxieties arise regarding informing the partner(s) and urging treatment.

Hepatitis B

This infection may develop about two months after sexual activity. It usually is acquired during sexual intercourse with an individual from a part of the world in which sanitation is poor and the disease has a high prevalence. People who are fearful of acquiring hepatitis B can receive an immunization against it.

Pubic Lice

Some individuals who fear germs or bugs may also fear pubic lice. These are tiny bugs, also known as "crab lice" or "crabs," that burrow into the skin and suck blood. They thrive on hairy parts of the body, including the pubic mound, outer lips of the vulva, underarms, the head, and even eyebrows and eyelashes. Eggs take from seven to nine days to hatch; persons infected may notice itching in one to three weeks after exposure. The most direct way of acquiring pubic lice is through sexual or close physical contact with an infected person's body. However, pubic lice can also be transmitted by shared towels or bedsheets. Some people fear sleeping in the bedding in which another person has slept for this reason. Pubic lice is commonly treated with a standard pesticide (known in the United States as Kwell) that is also a standard treatment for head lice. Those who have pubic lice (or live in the same household with someone who has them) fear reinfection or unknowingly infecting others, and they often become zealous about washing towels and bedding with disinfectant, such as household bleach, in boiling water, and drying the items in a hot dryer to be sure of killing off the unhatched eggs of the lice.

Genital Warts

Warts, or small bumps on the mucous membrane of the vulva, the clitoral hood, in the perineum, inside the vagina, in the anus, on the penis, or in the urinary tract may be genital warts. They cause discomfort and anxiety to the sufferer and may be particularly painful during sexual intercourse or when the sufferer wears tight clothing. Genital warts are caused by a sexually transmitted virus and can be removed by a physician. Genital warts are particularly feared by women because certain strains of the wart virus have been implicated as a cause of cervical cancer. To reduce anxieties regarding transmission of the wart virus, if either partner has a history of genital warts, a condom should be used during sexual intercourse.

Gonorrhea and Syphilis

Gonorrhea, while treatable, is feared by many people because complications include pelvic inflammatory disease, joint pains, heart disease, liver disease, meningitis, and blindness. Gonorrhea has been referred to as the "dose," "clap," or "drip." Gonorrhea is treated with large doses of penicillin, usually injected, often with follow-up doses of oral antibiotics. During the latter part of the 20th century, many cases of penicillin-resistant gonorrhea have appeared, making the disease more fearsome than during the years when penicillin was hailed as the "magic bullet" against the disease. Because there are fewer symptoms in women than men, usually gonorrhea is detected later in women. In a woman, the gonorrhea germs travel to the uterus, fallopian tubes, and ovaries. As the disease advances she may notice abdominal pain. Males may notice painful urination and pus discharge from the penis.

Detection of gonorrhea historically has caused anxieties for many people because anyone diagnosed with gonorrhea should inform recent partners so that they can obtain treatment.

Syphilis, though less common than gonorrhea, is feared because of serious complications that occur when untreated. Syphilis has been known as "syph," "pox," and "bad blood." Treatment with penicillin or other antibiotics is usually effective during the early stages of the disease and will prevent complications. Treatment is difficult in the later stages of the disease.

Other Diseases

Many women fear acquiring vaginal infections because the vagina becomes red, swollen, and very tender. Women fear the intense itching that accompanies infections and the pain that occurs with any friction, such as during sexual intercourse. One commonly known infection is trichomonas, which is caused by microscopic, parasitic organisms that live in small numbers in the vagina. The organisms, known as trichomonads, also live under the foreskin of a man's penis or in the urethra, usually without producing any symptoms. Medications are available to combat this infection. However, a treated individual must inform his or her sexual partner so that the partner can also be treated. Imparting such information may cause anxiety on the part of the treated person who must inform the other partner as well as the one who hears about the need for treatment.

Yeast infections (monilia) are not necessarily sexually transmitted diseases, but the organisms also live in the vagina and under the foreskin of the penis and can be transmitted during sexual intercourse. Many women, however, have yeast infections without having had sexual intercourse. In fact, some women fear taking certain antibiotic drugs because a fairly well-known side effect of such drugs is the onset of a monilia infection.

Bacterial infections can also be transmitted during sexual intercourse; these are treatable with sulfa creams or oral antibiotics.

Acquired Immunodeficiency Syndrome

AIDS became a widely known and feared sexually transmitted disease during the latter part of the 20th century. The AIDS virus is known to be transmitted by direct exchange of body fluid, such as semen or blood.

Reducing Fears of Acquiring an STD

While some STDs seem to be increasing in prevalence, individuals can reduce their fears of these diseases by taking certain precautions:

1. Have a monogamous relationship. Have sexual contact with only one partner who limits contact to you only.
2. Look your partner over. Ask about any suspicious-looking discharges, sores, or rashes.
3. Be clean. Partners should bathe before and after sexual intercourse. Wash with soap and water.

4. Use condoms. Condoms provide some (though not complete) protection against STDs. However, the condom must be put on before sexual activity begins and not removed until the end of the activity.
5. Use foam, a diaphragm with spermicides, or sponge spermicides, which kill many infectious agents; these should be used in addition to the condom.
6. Avoid the "ping-pong" effect of infection. If one partner has an STD, the other partner must be informed and treated at the same time to avoid reinfection.

sexual perversions, fear of   Fear of sexual perversions is known as paraphobia.

See also SEXUAL FEARS.

sexual revolution   A term that generally covers changes in sexual attitudes and behaviors during the 1960s, 1970s, and early 1980s. With the changes came increased anxieties for many people. Generally, there were more liberal attitudes toward premarital sexual activity, changes in the sexual double standard in which sexual activity is seen as more acceptable for men than for women, and more open discussion of women's sexual needs. Changes in the double standard and increases in premarital activity evolved in part as a result of development of better and easier means of birth control, including oral contraceptives during the late 1950s.

For many young people, dating habits during the sexual revolution included sexual intercourse early in the relationship. However, with the recognition of the increase of SEXUALLY TRANSMITTED DISEASES and acquired immunodeficiency syndrome (AIDS) in the heterosexual population in the 1980s, many people became more cautious and selective about their choice of sexual partners and monogamy regained favor.

The sexual revolution was closely tied with the WOMEN'S LIBERATION MOVEMENT. Many college dormitories became coeducational, offering women more options regarding housing. There was wider acceptance of unmarried adults "living together."

While this arrangement was acceptable to many, for others it was a source of anxiety.

See also ACQUIRED IMMUNODEFICIENCY SYNDROME (AIDS); WOMEN'S LIBERATION MOVEMENT.

shadows, fear of   Fear of shadows is known as sciaphobia or sciophobia. This fear may be related to the fear of LIGHT AND SHADOWS, or of twilight.

shaking, fear of   Because they fear shaking in front of other people, some phobic individuals will not eat in front of others, walk past a line of people, or sit facing another passenger in a bus or train. Some fear public speaking or appearing in front of an audience out of a fear of shaking. Some fear that their hands will shake when they write and so avoid writing anything in front of others. Those who have this fear usually fear going into banks, because they are often asked to sign their name in the course of a transaction. As a practical matter, many who have a fear of shaking rarely do shake in public. Fear of shaking is a SOCIAL PHOBIA and is often overcome with behavior-modification techniques involving exposure therapy.

See also PHOBIA.

sharp objects, fear of   Fear of sharp objects, such as knives, is known as belonophobia.

See also KNIVES, FEAR OF.

sheets of water, fear of   Fear of sheets of water is known as potamophobia. This fear may be related to fear of very heavy rain, rivers, or lakes.

See also LAKES, FEAR OF; RAIN, FEAR OF; WATER, FEAR OF.

shellfish, fear of   Fear of shellfish is known as ostraconophobia. This fear may relate to eating shellfish, getting a disease from them, or to seeing them, thinking of them, or even seeing a picture of them.

See also CONTAMINATION, FEAR OF.

shell shock   A term used during World War I to denote many mental disorders presumed due to experience in battle. The term "combat fatigue" was applied to the same syndrome of effects. More recently, the group of battle-related disorders is referred to as POST-TRAUMATIC STRESS DISORDER.

shiatsu   A specific method for manipulating *tsubos*, (points along the meridians where the flow of energy may become blocked). The manipulation may occur through pressing with the fingers and hands, or through the use of elbows, knees and feet.

Shiatsu is considered a complementary therapy and may be useful for some individuals to prevent or relieve the effects of anxieties. The points that are manipulated are known as acupressure or acupuncture points. Manipulation of the body's approximately 360 *tsubos* is thought to release the flow of energy (*ché*). There are many forms of shiatsu.

See also BODY THERAPIES; COMPLEMENTARY THERAPIES.

shift work   Usually refers to working a series of hours earlier or later in the day than the more usual 9-to-5 routine. Some work an afternoon shift, from 4 to 11 P.M.; others work the night shift, from 11 P.M. to 7 A.M. People who do shift work experience many unique anxieties. Many psychological factors relate to adaptation to night-shift work are based upon how well the individual handles the interruption of the body's CIRCADIAN RHYTHMS. The break in circadian rhythms can affect mental ability, alertness, and temperament. Thus some night-shift workers experience anxiety and lapses in memory as a result of sleep deprivation.

Individuals who do shift work also suffer social anxieties. For example, the rest of the world operates on a 9-to-5 schedule, with most socialization occurring after work and on weekends. For people who work at night to have a family or social life, they must schedule creatively. There may be stresses on the spouse and children of a shift worker because of differences in schedules.

How Night-Shift Workers Can Avoid Anxieties
Workers should move their shifts forward rather than backward whenever possible, says a Stanford

University emergency medicine physician who studies what happens when people's sleep habits change. "The best strategy is to stay on one shift as long as possible," suggests Dr. Rebecca Smith-Coggins, assistant professor of surgery (emergency medicine). "You'll have the best chance of getting restful sleep that way, so you'll be more alert—and potentially safer."

A study of 79,000 nurses published in the December 1, 1995, issue of the journal *Circulation* showed those who worked irregular shifts for more than six years had a moderately higher risk of suffering a heart attack than coworkers.

For people who must change their shifts, the healthiest approach seems to be to start the new shift later in the day. For example, it is easier on your sleep and rest patterns to change from an eight-hour shift starting at 6 A.M. to one starting at 3 P.M. rather than the reverse.

New night workers can help themselves adjust by recognizing that they won't immediately get a full six–eight hours' sleep in one stretch. To help make the change, it is recommended that new night workers take a three-hour nap before starting work, then sleep again after they finish their shift.

Eventually most shift workers will find themselves sleeping longer after they get home and napping less before they start work. For many, a full "night's" sleep is ultimately possible in the morning after work, she says.

Understanding why moving forward is better is a bit complicated, but it is basically because most humans operate on a 25-hour sleep-wake cycle. In other words, our body temperature and other natural functions rotate as if the day were 25 hours long.

Some other ways for night workers to get more efficient rest include darkening the bedroom as much as possible or using a sleep mask. Ear plugs or so-called white noise, such as a humming sound from a fan or air conditioner, can help too. It is also helpful to maintain the same bedtime rituals, such as relaxing with a book or television show, particularly if the material is not unsettling.

See also SLEEP

Smith-Coggins, Rebecca, "Night Shifts Can Be Easier," *Circulation,* December 1, 1995.

Hurley, Margaret, and Elizabeth A. Neidlinger, *Schumpert Medical Quarterly* 9 no. 2 (October 1991).

shock, fear of   Fear of shock is known as hormephobia. This fear relates both to electrical shock and the shock one receives, for example, at hearing extremely bad news.

See also ELECTRICITY, FEAR OF.

shock treatment   See ELECTROCONVULSIVE THERAPY.

shopping, fear of   Fear of shopping may be associated with AGORAPHOBIA as well as a fear of being seen in public. Fear of shopping may also be related to a more underlying fear of spending money or fear of POVERTY. Individuals who fear shopping may lack confidence to make correct purchases or correctly count out money and change or fear coming in contact with STRANGERS. Individuals who have a low sense of self-esteem and a negative body image may fear or avoid shopping for clothes because doing so forces them to confront their appearance, which in turn may make them feel anxious.

Shopaholism

Some individuals resort to shopaholism to relieve anxiety; this can lead to a compulsive syndrome.

AVOIDING ANXIETIES OF SHOPPING ADDICTION

- Learn alternatives to dealing with anxiety; shopping may be your coping technique. Most people with addictive illnesses do not know how to cope with anxieties and stress.
- Cultivate groups of friends with whom you can share activities as a healthful alternative to shopping. Develop new social outlets.
- Physical exercise is a good anxiety reliever and will clear your mind for better concentration later on.
- Shop with a list and buy only what is on the list.
- Shop with a partner who will help you resist.
- Avoid browsing and avoid sales. The excitement can trigger a shopping spree.
- Avoid use of credit cards. Use them only for business, if you need to.

Excessive shopping shares some characteristics with OBSESSIVE-COMPULSIVE DISORDER, in which people perform certain rituals to relieve tension. In this way, compulsive shopping is similar to the problems of alcoholics or compulsive gamblers.

Compulsive shoppers buy things in order to make themselves forget the anxieties of their lives and make themselves feel good. However, what happens is that it takes more and more spending and buying to improve their moods.

Support Group for Shopaholics

Debtors Anonymous is a Chicago area support group for overspenders based on the 12-step recovery program of Alcoholics Anonymous. DA members work toward financial solvency the way AA members work toward abstinence. Experienced DA members review new members' finances and help them formulate an action plan for resolving debts and a spending plan for the future. DA members look to one another for support, hope, and strength in dealing with the stresses of indebtedness.

See also BODY IMAGE, FEAR OF; SOCIAL PHOBIA; STRANGERS, FEAR OF.

Kahn, Ada P., *Stress A–Z: A Sourcebook for Facing Everyday Challenges* (New York: Facts On File, Inc., 1998).

shot, fear of being Fear of being shot involves a fear of violence, injury, and death. The fear has existed since man invented firearms. However, fears of being shot in the latter part of the twentieth century, particularly in the United States, have become more realistic in many places. In 1986, firearms were used in three out of five murders and in 21 percent of all aggravated assault cases. Guns are more frequently used in killings between individuals unknown to each other than in cases involving acquaintances. Homicides involving guns are more frequent in the South than in the North. Victims of fatal shootings are most likely to be male, specifically men in their twenties.

Individuals who fear being the victim of criminal or accidental gunshot wounds have formed a strong gun-control movement in the United States, although there are many opponents to it. Assassinations of prominent figures and random irrational killings have caused fearful speculation that the American inner city will begin to resemble the Wild West, where owning and carrying a gun was standard behavior.

shyness Shyness is a symptom of social anxiety, related to a fear of being unfavorably evaluated by others. Shyness can be observed in several ways. Physically, the shy person may blush and perspire. Emotionally, he or she may feel anxious and insecure. The shy person may think that no one wants to talk to him or her, or that no one likes him or her. A shy person's behavior may actually help to discourage social intercourse, because shy people tend to keep their heads down and even avoid eye contact with others. Shyness may bring on a lack of social relationships, or a distorted view of social relationships, causing the shy person to feel the anxieties of loneliness and emotional unfulfillment.

Shyness may be related to social phobia; social phobia involves fear of scrutiny from other people and leads to gaze aversion and avoidance of eating, drinking, blushing, speaking, writing, or eliminating in their presence.

Almost everyone experiences shyness at some time, especially "situational shyness," which arises in such uncomfortable social situations as meeting

SHYNESS REACTIONS		
Physiological Reactions	**Overt Behaviors**	**Thoughts and Feelings**
Blushing	Silence	Self-consciousness
Perspiration	Avoidance of others	Concerns about impression on others
Increased pulse	No eye contact	
Heart pounding	Avoidance of action	Concern for social evaluation
Butterflies in stomach	Low speaking voice	Unpleasantness of situation

new people or going for a job interview. The term "dispositional shyness" describes a pervasive personality trait, which can be long-lasting or correlated to a particular stage of life, especially adolescence.

Shyness may be handled in different ways, depending on the individual's personal system of DEFENSE MECHANISMS. While it may cause some persons to withdraw and become quiet in social situations (introversion), shyness may encourage others to behave more aggressively in public, trying to cover up their shyness by being "the life of the party" (extroversion).

It is not uncommon for extroverted shy people to become performers or public figures, handling their shyness by keeping themselves in controlled, structured situations, performing well-rehearsed roles in familiar situations. (See chart on bottom of page 445.)

See also BLUSHING, FEAR OF; PERFORMANCE ANXIETY; STAGE FRIGHT.

Jackson, Todd, Shelagh Towson, Karen Narduzzi, "Predictors of shyness: A test of variables associated with self-presentational models." *Social Behavior and Personality* 25 no. 2 (1997): pp. 149–154.

Marks, Isaac M., *Fears, Phobias and Rituals* (New York: Oxford University Press, 1987).

Zimbardo, Phillip, *Psychology and Life* (Glenview, IL: Scott, Foresman, 1985).

sibling relationships   Sibling relationships often include the anxieties caused by competition between brothers and/or sisters. Sibling relationships can also lead to physical, psychological, or sexual abuse, often unknown to the parents. This, in turn, can produce anxiety, POST-TRAUMATIC STRESS DISORDER and repressed memories.

The situation first occurs after the birth of a new baby, when an older sibling feels "displaced" and constantly seeks to command the parents' attention. Feelings of rivalry may persist throughout life. One child may be continuously compared to another in the family, and the parents may influence the feeling of rivalry by showing one child favoritism. Throughout school, brothers and sisters may compete with each other to gain more affection from their parents.

Personality differences may account for sibling rivalry. For example, while one child may have an outgoing personality and make friends easily, another child in the family may be more introspective and find it difficult to mingle. The quieter child may be jealous of the other child, even though he or she excels academically, while the child with many friends may be jealous of his sibling's academic achievements.

Sibling rivalry may persist even after the death of parents, when brothers and sisters become jealous over uneven distribution of their parents' possessions.

See also JEALOUSY.

sick building syndrome   A contemporary personal and societal source of anxiety for many is known as *sick building syndrome;* it was once known as *building-related illness*. People who work in office buildings may experience symptoms such as headaches; itchy eyes, nose and throat; dry cough; diminished mental acuity; sensitivity to odor; and tiredness. These symptoms may be caused by air-conditioning systems, fluorescent lighting systems, and insufficient ventilation. Modern buildings frequently depend on air circulators, as opposed to outside air, for ventilation.

Additionally, the sources of anxiety-related symptoms may be caused by the frustration of feeling closed in and not being able to control the amount of heat or light in the immediate environment. Thus the stress of the syndrome is also related to feelings of lack of personal control.

A ripple effect sometimes occurs when one employee in such a building starts complaining. Soon others believe that they too have headaches as a result of the workplace. The notion of becoming ill from the building in which one works is not entirely far-fetched when one considers the outbreak of Legionnaire's disease, a form of pneumonia, which was first identified among American Legion conventioneers infected from bacteria in the air-conditioning system of a Philadelphia hotel during the 1970s. Outbreaks have occurred as recently as 1995. Tests identified the organisms responsible for the disease as a contaminant of water systems that had been responsible for earlier epidemics of pneumonia, although the cause had not been understood earlier.

Relieving Anxieties Caused by Sick Building Syndrome

Individuals who believe they are being made ill by their workplace should consult their company psychologist, if there is one, or in the human resources department. Reports should be filed in a timely way so that investigations can be made. Removal of the pollutant, if possible, is essential. There may be possibilities for improvement of air balance and adjustment, including percentage of outside air being circulated. All humidifiers, filters, and drip pans must be checked. Overall maintenance of the building should be evaluated and care should be taken regarding selection of cleaning materials, air fresheners, and moth repellents. New carpeting should be installed on a Friday, allowing ventilation of the building over the weekend.

Additionally, individuals should determine if there are any possible steps they can take to relieve their personal anxieties. These may include requesting being moved to another part of the building or bringing a small electric fan or heater to work with them. If necessary, a short vacation away from the pollutants may be helpful.

See also ENVIRONMENT.

sick role The protected position an individual who is anxious, phobic, or considered not well assumes or is put in by family and friends. The sick role may give the individual so labeled the advantages of attention and support, emotional and financial, that he or she might not otherwise have. The individual in the sick role may not be motivated to improve because he or she fears removal of attention (a powerful reinforcer). Some individuals who have AGORAPHOBIA are encouraged in the sick role because their families do chores and errands for them, enabling the phobic individuals to perpetuate their agoraphobic (avoidance) tendencies. The sick role may have positive effects on a family, in that it causes family members to become more cohesive.

See also FAMILY MYTH; PRIMARY GAIN; SECONDARY GAIN.

side effects Reactions or results that follow administration of a drug that are not related to the particular and desired effect of the drug. For example, side effects (such as dizziness, warmth on parts of the body, paradoxical anxiety) can occur after an individual takes an antianxiety or antidepressant drug. Side effects occur for many reasons, including as a result of interaction between drugs and opposing or additive effects; of an individual's allergy to certain substances; or of a drug's interaction with food.

See also ADVERSE DRUG REACTIONS.

siderodromophobia Fear of railroads, trains, or traveling by train. The word is derived from the Greek word *sideros,* meaning "iron," and *dromos,* meaning "course" or "running."

See also MOTION, FEAR OF; RAILROADS, FEAR OF; TRAINS, FEAR OF.

siderophobia Fear of the stars or evil that might come from stars.

See also HEAVEN, FEAR OF; STARS, FEAR OF.

SIDS See SUDDEN INFANT DEATH SYNDROME.

sign An indication of the existence of a disorder. A sign is usually objective evidence and is observed by the examiner or another person rather than reported by the individual. For example, a sign of a panic attack might be visible rapid breathing. A sign should be contrasted with a SYMPTOM, which is a phenomenon reported by the individual himself or herself. The term behavior sign is often used.

See also DIAGNOSIS.

signal anxiety A form of ANXIETY that functions as an early warning system. Signal anxiety, a concept from psychoanalytic theory, comes from the normal ability to anticipate a potentially threatening situation, either from internal or external sources, and to deploy emergency defenses against it before the anxiety intensifies. Such defenses might be fight, flight, or giving in. Signal anxiety may progress to a full ANXIETY ATTACK or even to a PANIC attack if the individual does not pay attention to the early warning or if available defenses are insufficient.

simple phobia   A simple PHOBIA (more recently known as a specific phobia) is a persistent irrational, intense fear of and compelling desire to avoid specific objects or situations.

Almost any object or situation can be phobic for a given individual. All fears that do not fit into other phobic groups are generally categorized as specificphobias. Examples of common specific phobias include driving across bridges, flying, harmless animals such as dogs and cats, heights, darkness, and thunderstorms.

See also DIAGNOSTIC CRITERIA; PHOBIC ANXIETY; PHOBIC DISORDERS.

sin, fear of   Fear of sin is known as hamartophobia, harmatophobia, enissophobia, enosiophobia, peccatiphobia, and peccatophobia.

See also SINNING, FEAR OF.

single, fear of staying   Fear of staying single is known as anuptaphobia. Many people fear remaining single because they view the world as being populated by couples. They find themselves feeling like a "fifth wheel" when they are in the company of couples. The fear of being single is a fear of being considered socially somewhat different from most other people. The fear also includes a fear of growing old and being alone.

sinistrophobia   Fear of things to the left or left-handedness.

See also LEFT, THINGS TO THE, FEAR OF.

sinning, fear of   Fear of sinning is known as peccatiphobia. Fear of sinning has been a strong disciplinary force in religious history. In the church of the middle ages through the 17th century, sinful acts were expected to bring direct retribution from God in the form of illness or natural disaster. Scientific explanations for these phenomena and a more

sophisticated sense of the forces of history lessened but did not eliminate this belief in a cause-and-effect relationship between sinful acts and direct punishment.

Although 20th-century people are concerned with feelings of GUILT (which is the internal form of punishment), the consciousness of specific acts as being sinful seems greatly reduced. Society has become less God-fearing, more secular, and more inclined to depend on law enforcement of a behavioral code than religious discipline.

See also CONSCIENCE.

Sinophobia   Fear of CHINA, the Chinese language, and things relating to the Chinese culture.

sitophobia   Fear of eating or fear of food.

See also EATING, FEAR OF; FOOD, FEAR OF.

sitting, fear of   Fear of sitting is known as cathisophobia, kathisophobia, and thaasophobia. Some individuals who are very anxious and very restless are fearful of sitting or of sitting for very long periods of time. This fear may relate to a fear of one's lap or holding something on one's lap.

skin cancer, fear of   Many individuals fear skin cancer because it can be painful and disfiguring. Skin cancer often occurs on the face and is visible to others, causing the victim anxieties and self-consciousness as well as discomfort. Out of fear of skin cancer, many individuals now avoid suntanning and even being in the sun. Some fearful people cover themselves from head to toe while outdoors on a sunny day. Many people use cream or lotion sunscreens on exposed portions of their skin to avoid any sunburn.

There are three types of skin cancer: basal-cell carcinoma, squamous-cell carcinoma, and malignant melanoma. Basal-cell carcinoma is the most common. Cells just below the surface of the skin become cancerous. Cell damage usually seems to be caused by long-term exposure to strong sunlight, and many years may pass before skin cancer develops. Unlike other malignant growths, basal-cell carcinoma does not spread to other parts of the body until it has been present a long time.

In squamous-cell carcinoma, underlying skin cells are damaged, leading to the development of a malignant or life-threatening tumor. Years of exposure to strong sunlight seems to be the main cause. If this type of cancer is allowed to develop, it may spread to other parts of the body. But good results have been obtained with early detection and treatment.

Malignant melanoma, the most serious of the types of skin cancer, often spreads through the body.

Anxieties about skin cancer, and the suspicion that any skin defect is a symptom of skin cancer, can usually be alleviated by an examination by a dermatologist. With early detection and early treatment, most skin cancers can be successfully controlled.

See also CANCER, FEAR OF; PAIN AND ANXIETIES; SKIN DISEASE AND SKIN LESION, FEAR OF.

skin conductance Certain anxiety-inducing, stressful, or pleasant stimuli change the electrical resistance of the skin, particularly the skin on the palms or other areas without hair. The response is produced by unconscious activity of the sweat glands. This effect is known as GALVANIC SKIN RESPONSE (GSR), electrodermal response (EDR), and psychogalvanic reflex (PGR).

skin disease and skin lesion, fear of Fear of skin disease and skin lesions or injury is known as dermatopathophobia, dermatophobia, and dermatosiophobia. Some individuals who fear skin disease also have fears of contamination and germs. Out of fear they avoid touching items that others have touched. Many individuals fear skin diseases and skin injury or skin lesions because such conditions may be uncomfortable as well as disfiguring. Some individuals who have skin diseases are anxious and self-conscious about their appearance and tend to avoid social situations where others may look at them, criticize them, or ask questions. For example, acne in teenagers causes considerable anxiety because the lesions come and go with relative unpredictability, and often a young person will have a flare-up of acne on a socially or academically important and stressful day.

Fears of skin diseases are related to overall fears of injury and illness, to fear of doctors and hospitals, and to fear of needing medical attention.

Skin conditions such as hives and eczema are themselves symptoms of anxiety disorder, and some skin conditions become worse when an individual is in a state of anxiety.

Among the many specific skin disorders different individuals fear are acne, boils and carbuncles, warts, impetigo, cellulitis, eczema, psoriasis, hives, ichthyosis, keloids, lichen planus, abnormal skin pigmentation, vitiligo, pityriasis, chloasma, and moles.

Individuals who become anxious about any symptoms of skin disease should consult their dermatologist before trying commercial preparations. Many prescription drugs are available to relieve skin problems; seeking treatment usually is the first step toward reducing anxieties about a skin problem.

See also ALLERGIC REACTIONS; BUGS, FEAR OF; CONTAMINATION, FEAR OF; FLYING THINGS, FEAR OF; GERMS, FEAR OF; ILLNESS, FEAR OF; INSECTS, FEAR OF; ITCH, FEAR OF; PAIN, ANXIETY AND DEPRESSION IN; PAIN, FEAR OF.

skin of animals, fear of Fear of the skin of animals is known as dorophobia. This may be related to a fear of textures and a fear of fuzz, or fuzz aversion. It may also be related to a fear of the animals themselves. The classical case of dorophobia was that of Little Albert, who was classically conditioned by John B. Watson and R. Raynor during the 1920s to fear rabbits. The fear quickly generalized to fur, furry objects, beards, and hair.

See ALBERT B.

sleep Fear of sleep is known as hypnophobia. Fear of sleep may be common in individuals suffering from sleep disorders such as NIGHTMARES, sleeptalking, sleepwalking, and especially narcolepsy. Fear of sleep may be related to the individual's feelings of a loss of control of his actions if he falls asleep.

The fear may also be related to a fear of death, as the person may fear NOT WAKING UP.

See also SLEEPTALKING, FEAR OF; SLEEPWALKING, FEAR OF.

Function of Sleep

Sleep is an activity that causes many people anxieties as well as fears. Some individuals become anxious if they do not sleep enough, while others become anxious that they sleep too much. Some have difficulty getting to sleep, and some have difficulty staying asleep. Others have difficulty waking up. Sleep disorders are common in many individuals who have anxiety disorders. Those who have depression may have difficulty sleeping or may sleep too much. For many individuals, physical conditions that make them uncomfortable or anxious also interfere with adequate and satisfying sleep. In some people, sleep may be used as an escape from problems and tensions present during waking hours. Lack of adequate sleep may make one feel nervous and jumpy, affect judgment and decision-making abilities, and slow reaction times.

Sleep is a necessary activity that provides a restorative function. During sleep, daily bodily functions such as digestion and waste removal have a chance to rest and recharge. An evolutionary theory regarding sleep suggests that sleep originally allowed humans and animals to conserve energy during the dark hours when it was less practical to hunt for food and harder to escape from danger.

The average adult needs about eight hours of sleep per 24 hours; the need for sleep seems to decrease as the person ages. Individual sleep patterns vary, however, and may be affected by anxiety. An average person may go through his or her sleep cycle about four to six times each night. A sleep cycle consists of stages (known as Stages I, II, III, and IV) in a cycle lasting about 90 minutes followed by a period of rapid eye movement (REM) sleep for about ten

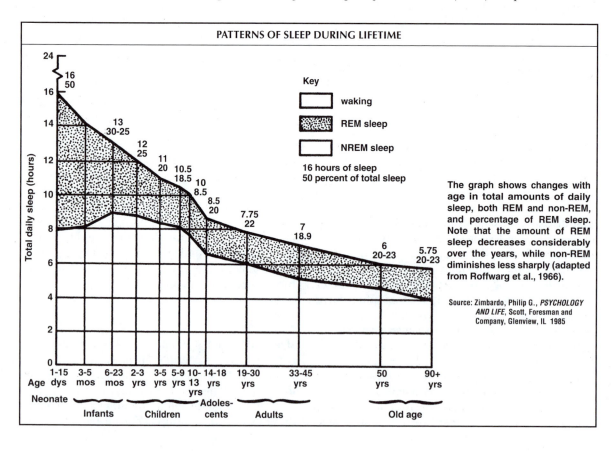

PATTERNS OF SLEEP DURING LIFETIME

The graph shows changes with age in total amounts of daily sleep, both REM and non-REM, and percentage of REM sleep. Note that the amount of REM sleep decreases considerably over the years, while non-REM diminishes less sharply (adapted from Roffwarg et al., 1966).

Source: Zimbardo, Philip G., *PSYCHOLOGY AND LIFE*, Scott, Foresman and Company, Glenview, IL 1985

minutes. With each cycle, REM periods lengthen. During the last cycle, REM sleep may last for 30 to 60 minutes. Dreaming is most likely to occur during REM sleep. This period is characterized by extensive muscular inhibition; most of the voluntary muscles in the body take on a paralyzed state, and there are bursts of rapid movements of the eye, under the closed eyelid, as if the person were watching something occurring in front of him or her.

See also BEDWETTING; DREAM SYMBOLS; DREAMS, FEAR OF; INSOMNIA; NARCOLEPSY; WET DREAMS.

Fear of Sleeptalking

Talking during sleep most often occurs during the early and dreamless stages of an individual's sleep cycle. Persons who have a fear of sleeptalking may be anxious that they might reveal personal secrets or feelings to listeners. In actuality, most sleeptalking is related to unemotional subjects. The habit of sleeptalking has not been related to any specific personality traits or disorders.

See also SLEEP, FEAR OF; SLEEP, FUNCTION OF; SLEEPWALKING, FEAR OF.

Fear of Sleepwalking

Sleepwalking (somnambulism) episodes occur most often in children between ages nine and twelve, although they may happen at any age in a child's or adult's life. Estimates are that as many as 20 percent of the population has experienced sleepwalking at least once. Individuals who walk during sleep will usually perform some familiar or ritualistic activities such as getting dressed, going to the kitchen for something to eat, or getting into their car. In very unusual cases, persons have been known to board trains and wake up hundreds of miles away from home.

Sleepwalking may run in families and may also be related to other sleep disturbances such as sleeptalking and NIGHT TERRORS. If any individual has had an unpleasant or dangerous experience while sleepwalking, this may lead to a fear of the disorder and may also cause increased anxiety concerning sleeping in general.

See also NIGHTMARES; SLEEP, FEAR OF; SLEEP, FUNCTION OF.

Green, Phillip M., and Michael J. Stillman, "Narcolepsy: Signs, Symptoms, Differential Diagnosis, and Management." *Archives of Family Medicine* 7 (September/October 1998): pp. 472–478.

sleep terror disorder   See NIGHT TERRORS.

sliding down the drain, fear of   Many young children view their bathwater going down the drain and worry that they, too, might be caught up in the swirling water and disappear down the water pipe. Commonly, children who have this fear accept the explanation that they are too big to fit in the drain. This fear usually disappears by age five.

See also CHILDHOOD ANXIETIES, FEARS, AND PHOBIAS.

slime, fear of   Fear of slime is known as blennophobia or myxophobia. Individuals who have this fear may fear eating certain foods, such as oysters, or touching or even looking at certain animals, such as frogs and snakes. The fear may also be related to a fear of contamination by dirt or filth.

See also CONTAMINATION, FEAR OF; DIRT, FEAR OF; FILTH, FEAR OF.

slips of the tongue, fear of   Many individuals fear slips of the tongue, or saying one thing when they mean to say something else. Fear of making such slips is based on the interpretation given to these remarks by Sigmund Freud, and they are known as "Freudian slips." It was through the study of slips of the tongue and dreams that Freud formulated his theory of psychic functioning. The Freudian view is that the speaker said exactly what he or she really meant to say. These slips may be the emergence of an unconscious wish or a failure to repress the unconscious desire. Everyone interchanges words frequently, usually without any meaning, but for some social phobics, who fear being heard talking or fear talking with others, this fear is enough to keep them away from social situations. Slips of the tongue often happen when a person is distracted or preoccupied with some stressful situation.

See also SHYNESS; SOCIAL PHOBIA; SPEAKING, FEAR OF.

slowness, compulsive A symptom of OBSESSIVE-COMPULSIVE DISORDER in which individuals take a very long time to do everyday actions. It may take them several hours to bathe, get dressed, and eat their breakfast. When they go out, it may take a long time for them to cross a street because they check and recheck traffic in all directions before setting forth.

small objects Fear of small objects is known as microphobia or tapinophobia. Individuals who fear small objects may fear particular objects, such as figurines, rocks, marbles, and other objects.

smells, fear of Fear of smells is known as osmophobia. Because the sense of smell is closely related to emotions and motivation, the fear of smells may cause anxieties for many individuals.

Unpleasant odors are often precursors to certain anxiety attacks and epileptic seizures. Certain cases of mass hysteria have supposedly been triggered by peculiar smells or other changes in the environment that frightened many people at the same time.

The fear of a particular smell may be related to an individual's previous unpleasant experience with it. Individuals may fear smelling cooking odors or body odors (their own or those of others). Some may fear smelling smoke. Several primary categories of smells have been identified, including musky, floral, peppermint, ether (dry-cleaning fluid), pungent (vinegar), and putrid (rotten eggs). Most smells experienced in daily life are a combination of two or more of these categories.

See also BODY ODOR, FEAR OF.

smoking, fear of Smoking cigarettes, pipes, and cigars is most often feared because of its negative health effects on the smoker. Negative health effects have also been attributed to "secondhand smoke," or the sidestream smoke from the smoker's materials that others unwillingly inhale. In 1987, statistics from the Coalition on Smoking and Health indicated that 350,000 Americans die yearly from cigarette smoking-related diseases.

Although smoking oneself or being near another who is smoking may cause anxiety, many individuals use smoking itself as a means of relieving tension. Smokers often cite the act as a "nervous habit," providing oral gratification and giving them "something to do with their hands." Smokers addicted to the nicotine in tobacco need to smoke to relieve the anxiety caused by their withdrawal between cigarettes. At one time, smoking was looked upon as a sign of maturity and was considered chic, relieving anxiety by raising the smoker's level of confidence and self-esteem. As smoking has become less socially acceptable, however, this has changed, and the more negative image now associated with smoking may actually add to the smoker's anxiety level. Fear of becoming addicted to smoking may keep some individuals from ever starting to smoke.

See also DRUG DEPENDENCE; TOBACCO, FEAR OF.

smothering, fear of Fear of smothering is known as pnigophobia. Smothering to phobic individuals may mean having their air supply cut off in a closed, crowded space, such as an elevator, in which they fear that there may not be enough air for everyone to breathe. Also, such individuals may fear having their faces covered with blankets, masks for anesthesia, or other items that may interfere with their breathing.

See also CHOKING, FEAR OF; SUFFOCATION, FEAR OF.

Snake Questionnaire (SNAQ) A questionnaire devised by R. Klorman et al. in 1974 to measure fear of snakes. The questionnaire is composed of 30 statements concerning snakes to which the respondents answer "true" or "false." Statements concern

SAMPLE ITEMS FROM SNAQ		
	True	False
I avoid going to parks or on camping trips because there may be snakes about.	____	____
I shudder when I think of snakes.	____	____
Some snakes are very attractive to look at.	____	____
I enjoy watching snakes at the zoo.	____	____

Ronald A. Kleinknecht, *The Anxious Self* (New York: Human Sciences Press, 1986), p. 102.

the areas of avoidance of situations where snakes might be present, physical responses felt while in the presence of a snake, and thoughts one might have about snakes. See chart on previous page.

See also SNAKES, FEAR OF.

snakes, fear of Fear of snakes is known as ophidiophobia, ophiophobia, ophiciophobia, and herpetophobia. Fear of snakes is a nearly universal fear among humans as well as animals. Many people fear snakes because of their fangs and the possibility of receiving a fatal snakebite. Many people cannot tell a poisonous snake from a nonpoisonous one and hence fear any snakebite. Also, many people consider snakes slimy and hence disgusting. Some fears of snakes are realistic. In the U.S. and Europe, poisonous snakes include the Eastern diamondback rattlesnake, the Western diamondback rattlesnake, and the European viper (adder).

There is evidence that the vast majority of people who fear snakes have had no direct contact with them. This would suggest a genetic trigger or possibly cultural attitudes conditioning the reaction.

Fear of snakes usually comes with age because small children evidence less fear. In 1928, two American psychologists, H. E. Jones and M. C. Jones, conducted an experiment in which they placed children of various ages in an enclosure with a large, harmless snake and observed their reactions. Children up to the age of two did not show fearful reactions, but those who were three and four years old looked cautious and hesitant. Those over age four showed definite signs of fear. In 1933, Ernest Holmes reported that fear of snakes was shown more frequently by children between the ages of two and four than before or after that age.

In 1965, two British psychologists, Morris and Morris, found that dislike of snakes increases from age four to age six, at which stage it was present in one-third of British children, and then declines to the age of 14. Isaac Marks, in *Fears and Phobias* (1969), commented: "This prevalence is striking when one considers how small the actual danger is from snakes in the British Isles." Children may learn that snakes are dangerous from reading or from their parents. It may be that individuals exposed to a snake for the first time are not frightened by the snake itself, but rather by the writhing movements of the snake.

Researchers have considered the effects of viewing distance on fear of snakes. In a Northampton, Massachusetts, study, phobic subjects made magnitude estimations of the intensity of fear felt when viewing a snake at distances from 2.5 to 15.0 feet. Heart rate, skin conductance, and respiration were also measured throughout each 20-second viewing period. A control group of nonphobic subjects made magnitude estimates of perceived nearness for the empty snake box at the same test distances. Judged fear was inversely proportional to distance. Heart rate and skin conductance decreased significantly for phobics as viewing distance increased.

In psychoanalysis, the snake is a symbol for the penis and is identified with sexual energies. The snake symbol appears frequently in dreams and in primitive rites and art productions, in which it may represent life.

In psychologic, symbolic terms, snakes represent life energy itself. For this reason, snakes carry multivalencies—guardians of life, health, wisdom, immortality, and mystery as well as destruction, illness, temptation, and the principle of will (potentially) inherent in all worldly things. Furthermore, the snake is seen as a symbol of transformation. For example, the ancient Mayan myth tells of the snake (nature principle) climbing the tree, leaping and catching the bird (spirit principle) to become transformed into a "winged serpent."

Probably, the best SYMBOLISM of the serpent is that of the Kundalini, a progressive movement of the life energy through movement of the six Chakras (energy centers of the body in eastern Indian tradition).

The serpent in the Garden of Eden is seen as the life force bringing man into consciousness from unconsciousness. In consciousness, there is fear because man develops awareness of relationships.

In the caduceus, the design of the rod and serpent traditionally used as a medical emblem, there is recognition of illness and health as coexisting in the individual. Of all medical symbols, the serpent is among the most outstanding and widely used. According to mythological tales and records found in excavations and shown by artifacts, the ancients actually used serpents in their healing arts. Before man began recording, he observed the serpent periodically shedding his skin, gliding gracefully along the ground, disappearing into the earth, and then reappearing. These actions fascinated early man, and gradually the powers of wisdom, rejuvenation, convalescence, and long life were attributed to the serpent.

See also PHOBIA; SIMPLE PHOBIAS.

snow, fear of   Fear of snow is known as chionophobia. Because snow is associated with the harshness and sterility of winter, it has come to symbolize death, poverty, and suffering. In the myths of some cultures, the end of the world is predicted to occur in winter, preceded by a barrage of snow. In folk tales, snow has been personified as a beautiful, alluring woman who leads her victims to their doom.

There are realistic reasons for fear of snow. Snow causes falls, traffic accidents, and collapsing roofs. Blizzards can create drifts as high as 30 feet. Victims of a whiteout during a snowstorm suffer from loss of balance and sense of direction because snow blurs the horizon and landscape and cancels shadows. Avalanches, which may travel at speeds of 50 miles per hour, cause death and destruction not only because of the actual weight and force of the snow, but also because of sudden air-pressure changes preceding and following. The sudden melting of large amounts of snow may create destructive floods.

soceraphobia   See FATHER-IN-LAW, FEAR OF; MOTHER-IN-LAW, FEAR OF; RELATIVES, FEAR OF.

social anxiety   Social anxieties involve relationships with other people and one's feelings about them. This concept was once referred to as "interpersonal anxiety." Most people have some social anxieties, such as wanting to be liked and accepted, to avoid criticism, to conform when conformity is desirable, and to be deemed competent. Social anxieties include a wide range of feelings, including worrying about what to wear for an occasion, apprehension upon entering a roomful of strangers, or worries about eating in front of other people.

When these situations become so difficult for an individual that he or she begins to avoid them, they are considered phobias.

See also BLUSHING; PHOBIA; SHYNESS; SOCIAL PHOBIA.

social phobia   The extreme fear of being evaluated, criticized, censured, embarrassed and humiliated, or in some way punished in social settings by the reactions of others. Social phobia is also known as social anxiety disorder. Social phobias affect about 15 million adults in the United States, according to the National Institute for Mental Health (NIMH). Many people with social phobia also suffer from other types of anxiety disorders as well as DEPRESSION. Some turn to substance abuse to self-medicate their anxiety.

Social phobics fear acting or looking stupid and thus avoid engaging in many common activities of daily life that occur when and where they can be seen by others. Social phobias may be limited to one area of life; for example, one person may find it impossible to write on a blackboard in front of other people but is capable of performing other social tasks. Others are severely socially phobic, and they find it difficult to talk to anyone outside of their immediate family. Sometimes, signing one's name in public or urinating in public restrooms are avoided activities.

Symptoms and Diagnostic Path

Social phobia is often accompanied by physical symptoms when the individual is in a social situation that he or she finds distressing, including extreme perspiration, trembling, nausea, blushing, and difficulty speaking.

Social phobics often fear their own responses, fearing that their hands will tremble or shake as they eat or write, and, as a result, they tend to avoid restaurants, banks, and other public places. They will often avert their eyes when talking to another person. Some social phobics have been known to cross the street to avoid greeting someone they know and risk a dismaying response. Social phobics are fearful of attending parties, particularly those that are attended by people they do not know.

Many social phobics have had lifelong shyness and introverted habits. Many agoraphobics have social phobias, and many social phobics have minor agoraphobic symptoms. The social phobic is diagnosed by a mental health professional, based on symptoms and behaviors.

Treatment Options and Outlook

Behavior therapy may be effective among those with social phobia, particularly cognitive-behavioral psychotherapy. In addition, medication may be useful, including antidepressants. Selective serotonin reuptake inhibitors (SSRIs), a form of antidepressant, are often used to treat social phobia. BENZODIAZEPINE drugs may be effective, particularly clonazepam (Klonopin). Some individuals are treated with beta blockers, particularly propranolol (Inderal).

Risk Factors and Preventive Measures

Social phobia appears to have a possible genetic link. Women and men are equally at risk for the development of this disorder, which usually has its onset in adolescence. There is no known way to prevent the development of social phobia.

See also AGORAPHOBIA; PHOBIA.

social support system   A social support system includes significant others—family, people on the job, in the community, and church groups—as well as material resources on which a person can depend for emotional comfort. An individual with a concern about anxieties may have inadequate social support because family members do not understand the individual's circumstances and thus may not offer the assistance or encouragement that would be helpful.

See also SUPPORT GROUPS.

social workers   Trained professionals who can provide counseling for people with concerns about anxieties. Additionally, social workers are familiar with available community resources that offer various types of support and therapy.

Social workers are employed in the public and private sector. Many work in publicly funded health and mental-health clinics, public schools, family agencies, clinics, hospitals, and in private practice. Some work in EMPLOYEE ASSISTANCE PRO-GRAMS (EAP), alcohol and chemical dependency programs, and in religious settings.

Historically, in the 1960s and 1970s, with the establishment of comprehensive community mental health centers, clinical social workers were heavily utilized and provided a major proportion of outpatient mental-health treatment services. In the 1980s, an increasing number of clinical social workers moved into full- or part-time private practice. In the 1990s, private practice is the fastest growing setting for clinical social workers.

There are more than 130,000 members of the National Association of Social Workers (NASW), an organization limited to those persons who have a bachelor's, master's, or doctoral degree from a university program accredited by the Council on Social Work Education.

See also PSYCHOTHERAPIES.

society, fear of   Fear of society in general is known as sociophobia. This fear may be related to AGORAPHOBIA. Many individuals who have several SOCIAL PHOBIAS may also be categorized as sociophobics.

See also PHOBIA.

sodium lactate infusions   See LACTATE-INDUCED ANXIETY.

solitude, fear of   Fear of solitude is known as autophobia, eremophobia, eremiophobia, ermitophobia, and isolophobia.

See also ALONE, FEAR OF BEING; OLD, FEAR OF GROWING.

solo phobia   See ALONE, FEAR OF BEING.

somatization   Experiencing physical symptoms in the absence of disease or out of proportion to a given ailment. Many people experience physical symptoms such as fatigue, shortness of breath, or even pain, as a response to anxiety.

From a public health point of view, somatization is significant. According to the *Harvard Health Letter*,

April 1992, in any given week, almost 80 percent of basically healthy people have symptoms that are not caused by physical disease. About one in five healthcare dollars is spent on patients with somatization. Nearly half of the patients seen in physicians' offices are the "worried well."

Many people who have ongoing complaints may undergo uncomfortable invasive procedures that may cause complications. For example, it is possible that a person who repeatedly reports chest pains could eventually undergo coronary angiography to rule out serious arterial narrowing. Also, these individuals may be taking many medications needlessly, some with serious side effects.

Individuals who "somatize" are said to have *somatoform disorders.*

See also GENERAL ADAPTATION SYNDROME.

somniphobia   Fear of SLEEP.

sophophobia   Fear of learning.

See also LEARNING, FEAR OF; SCHOOL PHOBIA.

soteria   A term that describes the disproportionate comfort some individuals get from the presence of certain objects or situations. The word comes from the Greek *soteria,* which refers to festive entertainment given on a person's recovery from illness or escape from danger. Examples of soterias are the toys and stuffed animals young children carry around with them and the talismans and charms many adults wear. Phobic individuals often develop a soterial attachment to an object that reduces their fear. For example, some get comfort from carrying a bottle of smelling salts with them; some are comforted by the knowledge that they have a supply of sedative drugs in their pocket, even if they don't actually take the drug.

The best known contemporary soteria is the "Linus blanket," the security blanket named for the cartoon-strip character in Charles Schultz's "Peanuts." A soteria has also been called a transitional object. Loss of a soteria usually produces grief.

soteriophobia   Fear of dependence on others.

sounds, fear of   Fear of sounds is known as acousticophobia. This may relate to specific sounds, sound in general, or noise. Parents become anxious when they hear cries of fear or pain from their infants. Many people become fearful when they hear others screaming in agony or panic (for example, hearing other children crying after receiving shots or hearing women in labor). The sound of buzzing bees arouses fear in many people.

See also NOISE, FEAR OF.

Marks, Isaac M., *Fears, Phobias and Rituals* (New York: Oxford University Press, 1987).

sourness, fear of   Fear of sourness or a sour taste is known as acerophobia or acerbophobia. This fear may relate to a fear of taste in general.

See also TASTE, FEAR OF.

space phobia   Fear of falling when one perceives space without nearby support, often occurring with increased age and decreased mobility and flexibility. Space phobics need visual boundaries rather than physical support to walk or drive across open spaces. Space phobia affects more women than men. Although there are many overlapping characteristics of space phobia and AGORAPHOBIA, there are characteristics that distinguish the two. Usually space phobia begins after age 40 and agoraphobia in early adulthood. In space phobia, the individual has intense fears of falling; this usually does not occur in agoraphobia. Space phobics, unlike agoraphobics, rarely have accompanying depression, nonsituational anxiety or panic, or personality difficulties. Space phobics often have diverse cardiovascular or neurological disorders; some progress until the individuals are confined to a wheelchair.

Space phobics respond less well to treatment by exposure in vivo than do agoraphobics.

See also FALLING, FEAR OF.

spacephobia   Fear of outer space.

See also OUTER SPACE, FEAR OF; SPACE TRAVEL, FEAR OF.

space travel, fear of   Fear of traveling in space is a fear of the unknown. Outer space seems dark, still, and mysterious. Modern man realizes that a highly organized system of technology is necessary to sustain life in outer space and also fears that our current system may not be adequate. The classic film of the late 1960s, *2001, A Space Odyssey,* explored the fears of relying on fallible technology in space as well as other frightening aspects of space travel, including isolation, keeping physically and mentally stimulated in a limited environment, and the possibility of encountering the unknown.

The explosion of the space shuttle *Challenger* in 1986 created a new realization of the risks of space travel and a rethinking of the U.S. manned space flight program.

See also OUTER SPACE, FEAR OF; UNKNOWN, FEAR OF.

speaking, fear of   Fear of speaking, a social phobia, is known as laliophobia. This fear may be related to a fear of speaking out loud or speaking over the telephone or fear that one may use the wrong words, have an ineffective tone of voice, or sound powerless. Other fears related to speaking include hearing the sound of one's own voice and stuttering. Public speaking is one of the most prevalent fears among adults.

See also PUBLIC SPEAKING, FEAR OF; SHYNESS; SLIPS OF THE TONGUE, FEAR OF; SPEAKING ALOUD, FEAR OF; STUTTERING, FEAR OF.

speaking aloud, fear of   Fear of speaking out loud is known as phonophobia. This fear may be related to the fear of hearing one's own voice, of stuttering, or of having a poor voice quality. Muteness and aphonia (inability to speak louder than a whisper) may result as traces of avoidance.

See also PUBLIC SPEAKING, FEAR OF; SHYNESS; SLIPS OF THE TONGUE, FEAR OF; SOCIAL PHOBIA; STUTTERING, FEAR OF.

speaking in public, fear of   See PUBLIC SPEAKING, FEAR OF.

specific phobias   Specific phobias are phobias that are restricted to only one situation or object, such as darkness, heights, elevators, closed spaces, or animals. Agoraphobics often have fears of closed places, but that does not mean that all persons who fear closed places are agoraphobic. The gender incidence of specific phobias is approximately equal, except animal phobics are largely women. Onset of specific phobias varies from early childhood to old age. The exceptions are animal and blood phobias, which tend to begin in early childhood.

Most specific phobias are treated successfully by exposure therapy.

See also ANIMAL PHOBIAS; BLOOD AND BLOOD-INJURY PHOBIAS; PHOBIA; SIMPLE PHOBIAS; SOCIAL PHOBIA.

specters, fear of   Some individuals fear specters, or ghosts, because they are supernatural phenomena and involve a fear of the unknown. A specter may be the appearance of a living person at a time or place where he or she could not logically be or the ghost of someone who has died.

See also GHOSTS, FEAR OF.

spectrophobia   Fear of specters or fear of ghosts.

See also GHOSTS, FEAR OF; SPECTERS, FEAR OF.

speed, fear of   Fear of speed is known as tacophobia. This fear may relate to fear of driving fast, walking fast, or doing any sport activity fast, such as skating or bicycling. The fear may be related to a fear of motion.

See also MOTION, FEAR OF.

sperm, fear of   See SPERMATOPHOBIA.

spermatophobia, spermophobia   Fear of semen or sperm is known as spermatophobia.

See also GERMS, FEAR OF; SEXUAL FEARS.

spheksophobia   See WASPS, FEAR OF.

spiders, fear of   A phobic preoccupation or fear of spiders is also known as ARACHNOPHOBIA or arachnephobia. It is unknown how many people have spider phobia but it is believed to be a common phobia, and it is one of what are called *prepared fears* that are indigenous to humans, Experts say that less than 1 percent of all species of spiders can actually be harmful to humans. Spider phobia, like other insect phobias, tends to be stimulus-specific in that the frightened person will usually respond to particular characteristics over others.

Many people dislike spiders and avoid them when possible, but most individuals are not phobic. Among those who are phobic, common stimulus properties that trigger anxiety are the size, color, and texture of the spider, although it should be noted that those who are truly phobic will fear the tiniest and seemingly least threatening of spiders. Individuals who have severe spider phobia are often compelled to fumigate their homes regularly, wash all fruits and vegetables completely, and check incoming bags and other receptacles where spiders might hide. Even the sight of a spider on television or in a magazine can fill the phobic person with extreme revulsion and fear.

Some individuals with spider phobia exhibit symptoms of OBSESSIVE-COMPULSIVE DISORDER, in that they are constantly checking for the feared item and seeking to avoid it, while at the same time fully aware that their behavior is irrational—but they feel compelled to perform illogical behaviors anyway.

Some individuals with severe spider phobia will refuse to enter a room until they first visually scan the room for the presence of spiders. They are usually unable to go on picnics or to stay in strange hotels or houses, and they generally maintain a strong vigilance when they are outside or at particular times of the years, such as the spring and summer. Others have spider phobia that is so severe that it may develop into a refusal to leave the home.

Some experts believe that a fear of spiders may be almost instinctive, a case of what scientists call *prepared learning*. For example, the sight of a spider triggers a rapid heartbeat and the FIGHT OR FLIGHT response. In response to this fear most people's brains manufacture and release natural tranquilizers called endorphins into the bloodstream. These natural painkillers temper the fear and allow the majority of people to react calmly to the sight of the spider.

In a 2006 article in *Body & Society* on the feelings that spiders and other feared objects engender among phobics, authors Smith and Davidson wrote about their experience with patients who were phobic. They noted that many individuals are phobic about items in nature, such as spiders and other insects, snakes, and so forth. The authors hypothesized that it is both an intense feeling of disgust and a strong fear of being touched by a spider or other feared object that are the key factors in the phobic's reactions. The idea of their own personal boundaries being encroached and violated by the spider is extremely distressing to those with spider phobia. In fact, the spider-phobic person anticipates a feeling of disgust and "skin crawling" at the thought of the touch of the spider.

British researchers have used fear of spiders to demonstrate that the meaning of a word associated with a feared situation can interfere with one's ability to name the color in which the word is printed. In one study, 75 spider phobics and 18 nonphobics were asked to name colors of words written on cards. One set of cards contained spider-related words, such as "spider," "creepy," "hairy," "legs," and "crawl."

Researchers also included unrelated words such as "cars" and "effort." Both the phobics and the nonphobics averaged about 78 seconds to name the color of 200 comparison words. However, when the phobics viewed the "spider words," their recall performance rate slowed down to 92 seconds per 100 words, compared with the nonphobics' rate of 76 seconds per 100. Later, the researchers wanted to know if the spider phobics could name the color of the words faster after several SYSTEMATIC DESENSITIZATION sessions.

In their sessions, the phobics began by examining dead spiders or spider fragments. They gradually worked up to live specimens of spiders, and eventually the phobics even handled the spiders. Fourteen of the original phobics had four treatment sessions and 14 were not desensitized. Researchers found that the desensitized phobics improved much more over their original learning performance than did the comparison group of phobics, indicating that their former fear was no longer inhibiting them from learning.

Johann Christoph Friedrich von Schiller (1759–1805), German dramatist, editor, and writer, is said to have feared and hated spiders so much that his fear made him physically sick.

Young children may be encouraged to fear spiders as they repeat the well-known nursery rhyme:

Little Miss Muffet
Sat on a tuffet
Eating her curds and whey.
There came a big spider
Who sat down beside her
And frightened Miss Muffet away.

See also BEHAVIOR THERAPY.

Smith, Mick, and Joyce Davidson, "'It Makes My Skin Crawl . . .': The Embodiment of Disgust in Phobias of 'Nature" *Body & Society* 12, no. 1 (2006): pp. 43–67.

spirits, fear of Those who fear spirits may fear evil spirits, such as the EVIL EYE, demons, or the spirits of deceased persons. Those who believe that the spirits of the dead can communicate with living persons are called spiritualists. Scientists and others have challenged the claims of spiritualists. Some who have attended seances, or meetings in which a dead person's spirit supposedly returns and makes known its presence, say that people are tricked into believing in the return of spirits. According to one explanation, the table in a seance room moves not by any action of the spirit of the deceased, but by the unconscious hand pressure of living persons sitting around it. Nevertheless, there are individuals who fear the spirits of deceased persons and fear the spirits will return in some way to harm them.

See also DEMONS, FEAR OF; EVIL EYE, FEAR OF; GHOSTS, FEAR OF.

spirituality Spirituality has been expressed as experiencing the close presence of a power, a force, energy, or what was perceived of as God. This definition is from the writings of Herbert Benson, M.D., president of The Mind/Body Medical Institute and chief, Division of Behavioral Medicine, Deaconess Hospital, Boston.

Work at the Harvard Medical School involved consideration of the healing effects of spirituality; research later established that people experienced increased spirituality as a result of relaxation therapy whether or not they used religious repetitive focus. This notion came about because for more than 25 years, researchers at Harvard have systematically studied the benefits of mind/body interactions. The research established that when a person engages in a repetitive prayer, word, sound, or phrase and when intrusive thoughts are passively disregarded, a specific set of physiological changes ensue. There is decreased metabolism, heart rate, rate of breathing, and distinctive slower brain waves. These changes are the opposite of those induced by stress and are an effective therapy in a number of diseases that include high blood pressure, cardiac rhythm irregularities, many forms of chonic pain, insomnia, symptoms of cancer and AIDS, premenstrual syndrome, anxiety and mild and moderate depression. To the extent that any disease is caused or made worse by stress; to that extent this physiological state is an effective therapy.

Spirituality, for many, is directly connected to prayer, faith, and religion, and belief systems help many individuals relieve stress.

See also FAITH; MIND/BODY CONNECTION; RELIGION; RELAXATION.

sport anxiety While sports and athletic games give many people satisfaction and relief from stress, for many others, sports lead to anxieties, fears, and avoidance. An example is a young child involved in a highly organized team sport (often known in the United States as "Little League") in which his parents have much interest invested, almost to the point of vicariously playing on the field while watching their children. Such a child may become fearful of losing the game and not pleasing the parents, being ridiculed, or being rejected. Fears developed in this way may remain with a person into adult life.

Adults who wish to excel in their chosen sport but do not may suffer frustration and anxiety because of lack of ability and fear or embarrassment when they are watched by others. Some who fear losing may avoid the sport, even though it was once a source of great personal satisfaction.

Some sports participants have the same feelings of anxiety before a game or a match as speakers and performers; physical symptoms include "butterflies" in the stomach, gastrointestinal upset, vomiting, headache, lightheadedness, and dizziness. Usually these symptoms subside entirely as soon as the participant begins his or her activity. For some, this "nervous anticipation" becomes part of the routine of getting ready for the sport.

Practical anxieties relating to sports include fears of injury, such as fear of injuring a limb and not being able to play, or fear of injury during a game, such as football, in which the risks of being thrown to the ground and trampled are great. There are specific fears within every sport; for example, in tennis, a player may fear being hit in the eye with a ball; in hockey, there may be a fear of being hit with a puck. When the fear leads to avoidance of the sport, the fear becomes a phobia. Mild fear may actually be helpful and may encourage the player to use caution and to react quickly and effectively.

Other fears associated with sports include fear of crowds, fear of noise, and fear of motion.

See also PERFORMANCE ANXIETY; STAGE FRIGHT.

spying, fear of   See BUGGING, FEAR OF.

stage fright   A fear of speaking or performing to an audience is a common ANXIETY. Stage fright is also known as topophobia, or PERFORMANCE ANXIETY. This is a type of panic that affects people in many kinds of situations where they are being evaluated, such as making a speech, playing a musical instrument, or even attending a social affair. Stage fright is related to a fear of making a mistake in front of others, looking foolish or uncertain, etc. Actors, politicians, executives, and others who regularly are in the spotlight often are afflicted. Some anxiety is natural and may even enhance performance, because anxiety pumps more adrenaline into the body's system, making one more alert and motivated. However, when the pressure becomes

extreme, the effects on physical and emotional well-being can be destructive. Migraine headaches, skin and gastrointestinal problems, hot and cold flashes, and hypertension can be typical reactions. As anxiety mounts the individual may become increasingly involved with overcoming it, which depletes energy needed to think, concentrate, and be creative. When the anxiety becomes worse, it can become a phobia. The phobic person may then avoid any situation that might provoke fears.

A typical treatment program gradually reintroduces phobics to stressful situations to help them gain confidence and develop skills one step at a time as they learn to deal with the situation. The starting point is wherever each individual feels comfortable.

See also PHOBIA; SOCIAL PHOBIA.

stages of development   See DEVELOPMENTAL STAGES.

stairs, climbing, fear of   Fear of stairs is known as climacophobia. This fear may be related to fears of falling, injury, heights, high places.

stammering   See STUTTERING; SOCIAL PHOBIA.

Standardized Behavioral Avoidance Tests (SBATs)   Tests used by researchers in AGORAPHOBIA. Researchers have used several different SBATs in assessing the behavioral component of agoraphobia. Examples include driving a car along a progressively more difficult route and assessment of behavior in various areas of functioning, including shopping, driving, crowds, and restaurants.

One useful SBAT for agoraphobics involves the "behavioral walk." This involves a walking course divided into approximately equidistant units. For example, the course might be 1.2 km long and divided into 20 stations that present feared stimulus elements. Individuals are instructed to walk along the course and return when they either complete the course or are unable to proceed further. The major dependent variable from this measure is the number of stations completed. Subjective anxiety ratings and heart rate can be monitored at each station with a portable unit.

See also INDIVIDUALIZED BEHAVIOR AVOIDANCE TESTS.

standing, fear of   Fear of standing is known as stasiphobia or stasophobia. The fear may be related to a fear of falling or of injury.

See also BLOCQ'S SYNDROME; FALLING, FEAR OF; INJURY, FEAR OF.

stared at, fear of being   Fear of being stared at is known as scopophobia, scoptophobia, and ophthalmophobia.

See also BEING LOOKED AT, FEAR OF.

stars, fear of   Fear of stars is known as siderophobia. The fear that man's fate is written in the stars is ancient. Primitive man thought that gods made their home in the stars. The science of astrology, which began in Mesopotamia in the 5th century B.C. gave rise to the fear that human destiny was controlled by the heavenly bodies. In the Egyptian Hellenistic period, a complex set of writings described man's subjection to the demonic powers of stars. An Egyptian scriptural text, *Poimandres*, described how the soul could be saved and ascend to the highest heaven. These beliefs turned into the doctrine of Gnosticism, which portrayed Christ as the deliverer from the power of the stars and the star announcing his birth as the herald of a new order. Astrology continues to attract adherents.

See also ASTROLOGY, FEAR OF.

stasiphobia   Also known as stasibasiphobia.

See STANDING, FEAR OF.

state anxiety   A term used to differentiate types of ANXIETY. State anxiety, also called A-state, is a temporary and changing emotional state involving feelings of tension and apprehension and increased autonomic nervous system activity. It is a response to a specific situation that the individual perceives as threatening, but the response changes as the situation changes. Examples of state anxiety are the unpleasant feelings one experiences when taking an examination or facing a new and strange situation. When the situation is over or one becomes accustomed to it, the anxiety disappears. State anxiety may be contrasted with TRAIT ANXIETY, an integral part of a personality that causes consistent anxiety. The concept of state anxiety was first expressed in 1961 by Raymond B. Cattell, an American psychometrician, and subsequently researched by Charles Spielberger, an American clinical psychologist, and colleagues in 1970.

See also FEAR; PHOBIA.

Catell, R. B., and I. H. Scheirer, *The Meaning and Measurement of Neuroticism and Anxiety* (New York: Ronald Press, 1961).

State-Trait Anxiety Inventory (STAI)   A psychological test developed about 1970 to research anxiety. Use of the test has led to advances in understanding of anxiety. The test differentiates between STATE ANXIETY, also known as A-state, in which the ANXIETY is a temporary and changing response to a situation, and trait anxiety, which is an ongoing personality trait.

The STAI A-Trait portion includes 20 statements relating to anxiety and tension and their opposites. Respondents indicate on a scale ranging from 1 to 4 how often each statement generally pertains to them. The STAI A-Trait is considered reliable and valid. There is also a version of the STAI for children known as the STAIC.

See also EYSENCK PERSONALITY INVENTORY; FEAR; TAYLOR MANIFEST ANXIETY SCALE; TRAIT ANXIETY.

Kleinknecht, Ronald A., *The Anxious Self* (New York: Human Sciences Press, 1986).
Spielberger, C. D., et al., *The State-Trait Anxiety Inventory* (Riverside, Calif.: Consulting Psychologists Press, 1970).

staurophobia   See CRUCIFIX, FEAR OF.

stealing, fear of   Fear of stealing is known as cleptophobia or kleptophobia. Some fear that they will steal something themselves and be caught and punished. Fear of stealing may be related to a fear of punishment, fear of sin, or fear of GUILT. Some fear that others will steal from them; some fear robbers.

See also PUNISHMENT, FEAR OF; ROBBERS, FEAR OF; SINNING, FEAR OF.

steep places, fear of   Fear of steep places or cliffs is known as cremnophobia. This fear may be related to fears of falling, injury, heights, or looking at high places.

See also FALLING, FEAR OF; HEIGHTS, FEAR OF.

stenophobia   Fear of narrow things or places.

See AGORAPHOBIA; CLAUSTROPHOBIA.

stepfamilies   Families formed when a divorced or widowed parent remarries. Anxieties in stepfamilies are far more complex than in traditional nuclear families. Anxieties and challenges arise partly from the fact that society does not define the role of the stepparent as well as that of the natural parent. As a result, everyone may have a different set of ideas regarding how stepparent and stepchild get along. Frequently, a stepparent may feel that he or she should assume the role of an actual parent, but this may be very uncomfortable and objectionable to the child, especially as he or she may continue to have a strong relationship with his or her own natural parent. Children who live with a single parent may have had a partial sense of being the center of attention in the household and may have difficulty giving up that role with the arrival of a stepparent.

The living arrangements that are set up when two families merge may cause anxieties for all involved. For example, some children may be in residence, some may visit. A child who had been living with the other parent may suddenly decide he/she wishes to leave that parent, possibly because of a stepparent in that household. If conflicts erupt between stepsiblings, parents usually side with their own child, rather than being peacemakers, as in traditional families. In cases involving older

couples and adult children, children may also feel that their inheritance rights are threatened by the arrival of a stepfather or mother.

Anxieties may also arise in the stepparented household because there may be a highly charged sexual atmosphere in the home, the stepparents being newlyweds. This may arouse real or potential relationships between stepsiblings, which are technically, although not biologically, incestuous. There is also a potential for technical incest between stepparent and stepchild, particularly if the stepparent is young, even close to the age of the child. In an attempt to be warm and friendly, some stepparents sometimes unwittingly encourage these feelings in children.

Many people help relieve the anxieties brought about by the formation of a stepfamily with family counseling services and support groups for parents and children.

See also DIVORCE; REMARRIAGE; SUPPORT GROUPS.

stepfather, fear of   Fear of a stepfather, or of stepfathers in general, is known as vitricophobia. Some stepchildren experience frightening or unpleasant behavior from their stepfathers because of the tension and guilt he may feel about the breakup of his previous marriage and responsibilities to his own children. A stepfather may seem to favor his own children because they live elsewhere and he puts time aside to visit and entertain them while his stepchildren are taken for granted as part of his everyday life.

A stepfather may exhibit jealousy toward his stepchildren because he would prefer to have their mother to himself. Because of his own insecurity, he may encourage stepchildren to say negative things about their real father.

Some stepchildren fear that a stepfather will try to replace their real father. On the other hand, some children who have lost their father or have a poor relationship with him may have such high expectations of the stepfather that they become hostile when he is unable to meet them. Stepfathers who have no children of their own may be uncomfortable with their new family responsibilities and may set standards, such as of household neatness and quiet, that are impossible to maintain in a home with children.

Stepchildren may also feel fear and resentment toward their stepfather because his relationship with their mother reveals her sexual nature, something most children prefer to ignore.

Studies show that some stepchildren have reason to fear mistreatment from stepfathers. Sexual abuse of stepdaughters is a frequent problem. The stepfather surrogate, the live-in boyfriend, is also the culprit in some cases of physical child abuse.

See also CHILD ABUSE, FEAR OF; RELATIVES, FEAR OF.

stepmother, fear of   Fear of stepmother, or of stepmothers in general, is known as novercaphobia. The cruel fairytale stepmother may be a healthy projection of a child's negative feelings about his or her real mother that are more easily handled as fantasy at a certain stage in the child's development. However, the stepmother image may interfere when stepmother and stepchild meet in real life. Stepmothers may become so anxious to avoid the cruel stepmother image that they discipline their own children but are lenient with their stepchildren, thus ultimately disrupting the household. At the other extreme, some stepmothers favor their own children and are harsh or negligent with their stepchildren. Some negative behavior toward stepchildren may arise from the stepmother's wish to have perfect children to prove that she is the ideal mother. The new stepmother may also feel anxious and pressured to love her stepchildren immediately and, finding that she does not, may convince herself that they are not lovable at all.

When a stepmother takes over, stepchildren may experience anxiety caused by a different household routine, different cooking, and a different value system being applied to homework, neatness, clothing, and other domestic matters. Competition for the father's time and attention and a feeling that the stepmother is trying to replace their real mother may lead to resentment. Stepmothers who have no children of their own may be disturbing to their stepchildren because of their lack of skill and familiarity with domestic problems.

See also RELATIVES, FEAR OF.

Bettelheim, Bruno, *The Uses of Enchantment, The Meaning and Importance of Fairy Tales* (New York: Knopf, 1976).

sticks, fear of   Fear of sticks is known as rhabdophobia. This fear may be related to fears of being beaten or to sexual fears, since to some a stick or rod may be a phallic symbol.

See also BEATING, FEAR OF; SEXUAL FEARS; SYMBOLS, FEAR OF.

stigiophobia   See STYGIOPHOBIA.

stillness, fear of   Fear of stillness is known as eremiophobia. This is related to fears of solitude and of being alone.

See also ALONE, FEAR OF BEING; SOLITUDE, FEAR OF.

stimulus properties   In differentiating between FEAR and ANXIETY, some therapists describe fear and anxiety in terms of stimulus properties, which include *identifiability, specificity,* and *predictability* of the source that brings on a response. Fear is considered a response to a clearly identifiable and circumscribed stimulus, whereas with anxiety, although it is a similar response, the stimulus to which the individual is responding is unclear, ambiguous, and/or pervasive. If a response occurs to a stimulus that is a *realistic* threat and therefore useful, it is said to be fear. Conversely, if a response is elicited by a stimulus that is not seen as a realistic or consensual threat and is therefore irrational and

SIMILARITY AND DIFFERENCE BETWEEN FEAR AND ANXIETY

Stimulus Properties	Fear	Anxiety
Identifiability	Clear	Unclear/ Ambiguous
Specificity	Discrete/ Circumscribed	Pervasive
Predictability	Predictable	Unpredictable
Rationality of Threat	Rational	Irrational

not useful, it is called anxiety. Another factor that differentiates fear from anxiety is the predictability of the source of the threat to which the individual responds. When an object or situation provides a signal of danger or threat and is therefore predictable, the state experienced is called fear. For example, the response of a person in the middle of a thunderstorm who worries about being struck by a lightning bolt would be considered fear because the stimulus is clearly identifiable and predictable and the threat is realistic.

See also PHOBIA; RESPONSE PROPERTIES.

stings, fear of Fear of stings is known as cnidophobia. This fear involves being stung by any type of insect, such as a mosquito, bee, or wasp. Some individuals with severe allergies to stings of particular insects have realistic fears of their reactions to stings. When there is no such justification and when the fear becomes so extreme that it disrupts normal daily life, it has become a phobia. Manifestations of this phobia would involve avoidance of areas, time of day, and weather that is associated with stinging insects. For example, one would not picnic or walk out of doors in warm, balmy weather when bees are likely to be active.

See also BEES, FEAR OF; WASPS, FEAR OF.

stooping, fear of Fear of stooping is known as kyphophobia. This fear may be related to fears of falling, of injury, such as to the back, or of dizziness, which may be brought on by change of posture.

See also FALLING, FEAR OF; INJURY, FEAR OF.

stories, fear of See MYTHOPHOBIA.

storms, fear of Many people fear storms, which may involve lightning, thunder, rain, hail, or snow. While most people do not fear personal injury from the storm, they do fear the unknown causes of the storm, and the unknown consequences. Being near or in a storm leaves one feeling out of control. The power of the storm may overwhelm some people and thus make them fearful. While some individuals become fearful during a storm, others have phobic reactions just at the suggestion of a storm, or at the sight of a little rain, or a little snow. Some avoid going outdoors when any kind of storm is predicted. Some will pull down their window shades or close the shutters on their house when they expect any kind of storm. Some fear hurricanes or tornadoes and do not venture outdoors even in seasons in which hurricanes or tornadoes never occur. Some individuals only fear storms when they have to be traveling through them, such as driving through a blizzard or riding on a train during a rainstorm. Some fear only one type of storm, while others fear all types of storms.

Fears of lightning, thunder, rain, snow, or storms in general are classified as simple phobias or specific phobias.

See also CLIMATE, FEAR OF; LIGHTNING, FEAR OF; RAIN, FEAR OF; SNOW, FEAR OF; THUNDER, FEAR OF.

strangers, fear of The fear of unknown persons is known as xenophobia or zenophobia. The term refers to individuals as well as entire groups of people, such as those from another country.

Fear of strangers is normal in infants between six and 12 months old. The infant learns to recognize a familiar combination of forehead, eyes, and nose that elicits the smile response, and this in turn elicits parental care. An unfamiliar face will frighten the infant and probably make him or her cry.

Other mammals and birds also fear strangers. Chimpanzees, for example, begin fearing strangers at about the same time in life as the human infant.

Stranger fear in human infants may be an evolutionary remnant reflecting widespread abuse and even infanticide by strangers during prehistoric times.

See also SEPARATION ANXIETY.

streets, crossing Fear of crossing streets is known as dromophobia.

See also AGORAPHOBIA; STREETS, FEAR OF.

streets, fear of Fear of streets is known as agyiophobia. Individuals who are fearful of streets may be afraid of getting hit by a vehicle or afraid of crowds. Many agoraphobics are afraid of streets because they will be seen by others there.

See also AGORAPHOBIA; STREETS, CROSSING.

stress The response of the body and mind to strains or burdens that demand adaptation. These may be any hindrance that disturbs an individual's mental and physical well-being. These interferences may range from random nuisances to life-threatening situations. From a scientific perspective, stress causes an imbalance in an individual's equilibrium (HOMEOSTASIS) and produces "wear and tear" in the body (Selye). Controlling stress is important for wellness because extreme effects of stress can lead to mild symptoms, such as a slight headache, to life-threatening conditions, such as high blood pressure and depression.

Stress is an internal response to circumstances known as *stressors*. Stress is the effect of stressors on one's body. Stressors may be external events, such as bad news at work, or internal events, such as personal illness. Stressors include difficulty in getting along with people, feeling trapped or inadequate, finding little pleasure in life, and feeling distrustful. Stress can be caused by good news and happy events too. There are good stressors as well as unpleasant ones. Many normally happy professional and personal events cause stress. "Happy" stressors may include starting a desirable new job, getting married, having a baby, moving to a new area or a new house. HANS SELYE, pioneer in stress research, and author of *Stress Without Distress* and *The Stress of Life,* termed the good events that cause stress as *eustress* and those that caused unpleasant effects as *dis-stress*. The stress reaction depends on how the individual views or interprets a stressor.

When an individual feels stressed, chemical changes take place in the body. The adrenaline starts flowing and the nervous system is activated. The FIGHT OR FLIGHT RESPONSE is activated. During extreme stress, some people notice that they have a faster heartbeat and a sick feeling in their stomach; it is difficult to work or function efficiently at such times. Research has shown that stress also affects the immune system and causes it to be less effective in fighting off diseases. Negative stress also leads to organ damage with time.

Stress and Adaptation

Stressors represent significant changes. How one accommodates to change influences the extent of stress one feels. Hans Selye used the term *General Adaptation Syndrome* to explain how individuals cope with the stressors in their lives. Individuals experience events in different ways. What results in emotional strain and anxiety for one person may not bring about those reactions in others.

Stress affects all aspects of life. Some individuals find that stress actually raises their energy level and helps them focus their mind better on their work or on a sports activity. Some thrive on many kinds of stressors. People who do are often attracted to high-stress occupations and professions.

Stress that starts at work can affect home life, and the reverse is also true for many people. Stress within a family causes tension and difficulty in communicating with each other. In some cases, interpersonal stresses develop when an individual has two feelings at the same time, such as wanting to be an independent adolescent and yet feeling dependent on parents. As life is a series of progressions through emotional stages, it is helpful to remember that change and growth always involve some degree of stress. In a family, several people are trying to cope with their own stress and the stress of others about whom they care. Usually, the closer the relationships the more important the others' stress is for one.

Death of a close relative or friend, divorce or remarriage, marital difficulties, sexual problems, or illness of one's own or one's family are common. Financial problems, such as facing a large mortgage or accumulated bills, can happen to anyone. Individuals faced with serious life stressors may constantly feel out of control and that their world is caving in around them.

Chronic stress results in ongoing wear and tear on the body's organs and systems, making them more susceptible to illness. When symptoms show up, many individuals begin to seek medical or psychological help. "Physicians are aware of stress as a factor in diagnosing and treating many common health concerns. For example, many people seek help for gastrointestinal symptoms, an inability to sleep well, headaches, depression, and chronic fatigue. They may have high blood pressure. The best treatment is to get at the cause of the stress," says Catherine Landers, M.D., a member of the Department of Medicine at Rush North Shore Medical Center, Skokie, Illinois. "Physical problems can interfere with the quality of one's work and ability to meet the needs of family members. Medications won't provide any long-lasting results. There is a strong connection between mental outlook and physical health. Helping the individual change his or her coping styles usually works better than anything we can prescribe as medication."

Managing Stress

"Stressors cannot be eliminated, so our goals should be to control and manage stress," says Elaine Shepp, LCSW, a psychotherapist in private practice on the staff at Rush North Shore Medical Center, Skokie, IL. "It is possible to 'neutralize' the toxic effects of unrelenting stress," says Elaine Shepp. "People I know who win the battle against stress put their personal and professional lives into perspective. They may experience a constantly high level of pressure and unrealistic performance objectives at work. However, they have enough moral courage to become somewhat 'inner directed.' They develop their own ideals of conduct and objectives and test themselves by their own standards," says Shepp. "Some report that they have made a conscious decision not to continue having a 'non-life life.' They are able to prioritize their work and enjoy some diversions."

There are times when individuals find that their mental outlook detracts from the energy required for productive work and effective personal functioning. At these times, talking to a friend just isn't enough. Psychological help is available to help deal with stress. "People who seek professional help to overcome extreme stress should not consider themselves 'weak' or 'losers,'" says Shepp. "Seeking psychological help is an intelligent way of using tools that are available to increase one's level of functioning. Counseling can help prevent 'burn-out' or to assist in dealing with life situations which require the input of a non-involved, knowledgeable person," adds Shepp.

If you find yourself in a position of feeling totally overwhelmed by your stressors and decide to get professional help, how should you choose a psychotherapist? You may want to talk with someone close to you who has experienced psychotherapy. However, the issue of confidentiality is just as important as the need to find a mental-health professional who is nonjudgmental. The psychotherapist should

---

TIPS TO REDUCE STRESS

- Develop a sense of humor and increase your ability to see humor in sometimes intolerable situations.
- Learn to recognize your own signs of stress
    Increased irritability with "difficult" clients or family members
    Headaches
    Overeating
    Increased alcohol consumption
    Sleeplessness
    Depression
    Chronic fatigue
- Identify external stress-producing factors over which you have little or no control. Internal factors include perfectionism and unrealistic expectations.
- Be realistic in your daily outlook. Don't expect too much of yourself or others.
- Prioritize your responsibilities. Learn to occasionally say "no" to requests you consider unreasonable or undoable.
- Focus your energy in other needed areas.
- Pay attention to the basics of living, such as eating a well-balanced diet.
- If you consume a large quantity of caffeinated beverages, cut down. Coffee, tea, and cola can increase your heart rate and your irritability level.
- Develop a regular habit of exercising. A 20-minute walk each day can be effective in fighting muscle tension.
- Keep your job stress separate from stress related to your home life.
- Learn some relaxation techniques that work for you, such as deep breathing, or listening to music you like.
- Recognize that you may need professional help if you feel so overwhelmed that you just cannot cope.
- Understand that getting professional help to deal with major stressful events, such as death, divorce, illness or job loss is a sign of good self-care, not of weakness.

MANAGING STRESS

Learn to recognize your own signs of stress, common stressors, and ineffective coping methods. If you experience any of the symptoms below, consider that stress may be a possible cause of your anxieties.

Stress Signals

Nervous tic
Muscular aches
Inability to sleep
Increased sweating
Stuttering
Nausea of stomach pain
Grinding teeth
Headache, dizziness
Low-grade infections
Rash or acne
Desire to cry or crying
Constipation or diarrhea
Frigidity or impotence
High blood pressure
Dry mouth or throat
Irritability or bad temper
Lethargy or inability to work
Cold, clammy or clenched hands
Sudden bursts of energy
Finger-tapping
Depression
Fear, panic, or anxiety
Hives
Coughing
Nagging
Fatigue
Pacing
Frowning
Restlessness
Accident prone

Common Thoughts and Feelings

Impulsive
Freeze up
Become rigid
Falling apart
Thoughts "jumble up"
Feeling tense
Constant worrying
Feeling time pressure
World is caving in

Stressors (in your family)

Holidays, vacations
Marital difficulties
Injury or illness
Problems with children
Giving a party
Child leaving home
Spouse has new job
Not enough time
Sexual difficulties

Stressors (as an individual)

Aging
Pressure on the job
Feeling unattractive
New job
Great achievement
Change in habits
Success problems

Finances

Inability to pay bills
Mortgage
Major purchase

As a Member of Society

Leading a group
Starting a relationship
Lack of freedom
Feeling insecure
Being popular

As a Family Member

Problems with others
Lack of privacy
Leaving home
Death in family
Divorce or remarriage

Ineffective Coping Methods

Increased smoking
Overeating
Increased consumption of any drug
Denial
Sedentary life
Sleeping all the time

Adapted with permission from The Good Health Program, Rush North Shore Medical Center, Skokie, IL be one with whom you have a sense of comfort, who also understands your particular stressors, and who can suggest practical ways for you to handle these stressors. Find a therapist who is multifaceted in his or her approach to problems and knowledgeable about many options available to treat particular problems. Look for one who is open to consulting with other professionals who have additional expertise.

Finding Relief from Stress

Sources of relaxation are very individual matters. Many people find that regular physical workouts involving running, walking, in a gym, health club, or on exercise equipment at home helps them relieve stress and get ready to effectively face challenges of the day ahead. Using muscles is a way to use up some of the "fight or flight" readiness in the body.

Some people use massage or soothing music as stress relievers. What allows one person to relax may actually cause stress for another. An example is noise level in the workplace or at home. Each individual should try to create an environment in which to work and live that is the least stressful and concentrate on reaching peak performance and a feeling of well-being.

Many so-called alternative therapies are used by many people to relieve stress. These range from acupuncture to biofeedback, guided imagery and hypnosis, meditation, progressive muscle relaxation, and yoga. Also, hobbies help many people relieve stress. When individuals participate in an activity they pursue simply for enjoyment, their stress level goes down. Such hobbies may include dancing, art and painting, sewing, building model trains or plane, bird watching, or playing a musical instrument. Choices of hobbies are as diverse as human nature.

Diet and exercise are basics of wellness and can also help relieve stress. Normal eating of three meals a day reduces effects of stress for some people. "Crash diets" and "fad diets" can lead to anxiety, depression, and an inability to maintain a good weight. Well-balanced meals provide a slow release of necessary nutrients throughout the day. For some people, too much CAFFEINE causes additional stress by bringing on symptoms of anxiety.

See also ANXIETIES; BEHAVIOR THERAPIES; COMPLEMENTARY THERAPIES; GENERAL ADAPTATION SYNDROME; HEADACHES; HOBBIES; MEDITATION; MIND-BODY CONNECTIONS; RELAXATION.

Selye, Hans, *Stress Without Distress* (Philadelphia: J. B Lippincott, 1974).
———, *The Stress of Life,* Rev. ed. (New York: McGraw Hill, 1978).

stress inoculation   This is a concept and therapeutic strategy to prevent anxiety developed by American psychologist Donald Meichenbaum (1940–) that represents an analogue at the psychological/behavioral level to immunization on the biological level. Individuals are given practice with mild stress to modify beliefs and self-statements in order to be more successful and less resistive. The stress situations are then gradually increased in difficulty. Training involves an educational phase (to observe and learn to modify self-statements), rehearsal phase (direct action and cognitive coping), and the application phase (cognitive/somatic skills and strategies are developed).

stressors   See STRESS.

string, fear of   Fear of string is known as linonophobia.

stroke   A term that, when used alone, refers to a cerebrovascular accident, or accident in the brain and blood vessels. Many individuals fear having a stroke when they have any form of chest pain or breathlessness. Some individuals wrongfully consider strokes synonymous with heart attacks. Some individuals fear that their anxieties will bring on a stroke. Many individuals fear having a stroke themselves or fear seeing another individual who has had a stroke because a stroke can cause some permanent impairment of the muscles, limbs, ability to speak, or perceptual abilities. Fear of seeing a stroke victim may be related to a fear of body deformities. The fear of viewing a person who has had a stroke may come from a fear of contagion.

Strokes occur when the blood flow to the brain is interrupted, either by blocking of large or small arteries or veins or by bleeding from a blood vessel into brain tissue. A stroke can also be provoked by an aneurysm, a bulging out of a weakened part of a wall of a blood vessel. An aneurysm may cause mental and physical disturbances of the nervous system by pressing against nearby brain cells, or the bulge may break open and bleed into tissues. In older persons, minor aneurysms or narrowing of blood vessels in the brain may cause "little strokes," particularly in individuals whose circulatory system is already impaired. During these attacks, the individual may have symptoms of anxiety, mental confusion, forgetfulness, irritability, irrational behavior, or headaches.

Strokes come on suddenly, usually reaching a peak within seconds or minutes or a few hours. The stroke victim may collapse, lapse into a coma, or remain conscious with little or no pain or discomfort. Among the many signs of stroke are blindness in one or both eyes or in half of one eye, loss of an ability to smell, dizziness, or reduction of feeling in various parts of the body, a stiff neck, and difficulty in swallowing. When an individual appears to be having a stroke, he should be kept quiet and not moved until a physician arrives.

See also HEART ATTACK, ANXIETY FOLLOWING; HEART ATTACK, FEAR OF.

stuttering, fear of Fear of stuttering is known as psellismophobia and laliophobia. The word stammering is used interchangeably with stuttering and refers to a nonfluency of speech. An individual who stutters has an interrupted flow of words or an inability to articulate certain sounds or repetitions of certain sounds. The speech pattern may be explosive or there may be occasional hesitations. An individual's speech difficulty may be aggravated by situations that arouse anxieties or fears of self-consciousness. Some individuals who have difficulties with speech may avoid certain situations, such as speaking aloud in a community meeting or going to social occasions, because they are fearful that they will stutter when they speak to others. Many forms of speech therapy help individuals overcome their stutters and their fears of stuttering. Also, behavior therapy can help individuals overcome anxieties and phobias about specific situations that bring on stuttering.

See also BEHAVIOR THERAPY; SPEAKING, FEAR OF; SPEAKING ALOUD, FEAR OF.

stygiophobia, styiophobia Fear of hell. The word is derived from the Latin *stygius*, pertaining to the river Styx, the river that surrounds Hades, the underworld of Greek mythology.

See also HELL, FEAR OF.

subconscious An obsolete term for the unconscious as well as the preconscious, which meant remembrances that could be recalled with effort.

See also UNCONSCIOUS.

Subjective Units of Distress (SUDS scale) A standard ANXIETY scale used in BEHAVIOR THERAPY. The scale is a way of quantifying people's feelings of fear and thus provides a way to monitor or assess an individual's responses and make comparisons among people. The individual is asked to think of the worst anxiety and call it the maximum anxiety, or a rating of 100. Being absolutely calm is given a rating of 0. All other fears are ranked in between. The same scale is used later on during therapy to determine the strengths of the person's reactions during desensitization and after treatment. Following are some descriptions of anxiety that an individual may use to equate with the various levels on the scale:

0	No anxiety at all; complete calmness
1–10	Very slight anxiety
10–20	Slight anxiety
20–40	Moderate anxiety; definitely unpleasant feeling
40–60	Severe anxiety; considerable distress
60–80	Severe anxiety; becoming intolerable
80–100	Very severe anxiety; approaching panic

See also BEHAVIOR MODIFICATION.

Wolpe, Joseph, *Our Useless Fears* (Boston: Houghton Mifflin, 1981).

sublimation A defense mechanism. Individuals use sublimation unconsciously by diverting instinctual drives, such as sexual or agressive drives, which may be unacceptable, into personally and socially acceptable channels. Such channeling of energy may protect the individual from the anxiety the original drive might produce and also usually brings the individual satisfactions, such as acceptance and recognition from others. An example of an individual who uses sublimation constructively is one who has exhibitionistic tendencies who becomes a choreographer. While this term is used in PSYCHOANALYSIS, it is also common in psychological vocabularies. The broader use of the term refers to the focusing of one's energy, frustration, anxiety, etc. on an activity that comes to dominate one's life. For example, an active, achievement-oriented person might sublimate his or her energies into sports and fitness, working out or competing on a regular basis.

success, fear of   Some individuals have a fear of success that causes them anxieties while they are striving for an objective and after they achieve it. Fear of success is closely related to fear of failure. The individual who fears achieving success fears being a failure at another plateau, or that he will not be able to fulfill expectations at the higher level. Some find that striving for success, but not quite reaching it, is tolerable; but when an anxious individual imagines himself successful, the level of stress becomes intolerable and turns into fear. Some who fear success fear that success will put them in another academic, social, or athletic class and that they will lose the friendship and comradeship of their peers. Some fear that they will not be conforming to their group if they are successful. Fear of success is related to a fear of RISK TAKING and a fear of CRITICISM.

See also FAILURE, FEAR OF.

succubus   A female demon, evil spirit, or devil who seduces men while they sleep and causes nocturnal seminal emissions. Historically, succubi were thought to cause abnormal behavior. Individuals feared the succubus because she brought on nightmares and a feeling that something heavy was on one's chest during the night, causing suffocation

and exhaustion; the dreamer usually remembered the episode with anxiety and fear upon awakening.

See also DEMONS, FEAR OF; INCUBUS; WITCHES AND WITCHCRAFT, FEAR OF.

Sudden Infant Death Syndrome (SIDS), fear of   Parents of infants fear Sudden Infant Death Syndrome (SIDS) because of its mysteriousness and unpredictability. The exact cause of SIDS, which ends the lives of sleeping infants between the ages of two and four months without warning, is unknown. Physicians believe that each case may be a product of a variety of causes, such as viruses, abnormally small air passages, or momentary interruptions of breathing during sleep. Premature infants and black infants are more likely to be affected, but perfectly healthy babies of affluent white families are also victims. Parents of SIDS babies have at times been treated with suspicion of abuse or neglect by health and law-enforcement professionals. Having a baby taken by Sudden Infant Death may make parents neurotic and overprotective toward surviving children.

suffocation, fear of   Fear of suffocation or smothering is known as pnigophobia. Suffocation means an inability of the body tissues to receive oxygen due to primary failure of the respiratory system to draw adequate amounts of air and oxygen into the lungs. Fears of suffocation may be related to many other fears, such as being buried alive, being in a crowded room, being in an elevator, being in a small, enclosed space, or even being in a bus, train, or airplane. Individuals who fear suffocation may actually have symptoms of suffocation, even though they are breathing in adequate air and oxygen. Symptoms of suffocation are dizziness, along with lethargy and drowsiness, and finally unconsciousness. If no oxygen is administered, there will first be brain damage and then death.

See also BURIED ALIVE, FEAR OF BEING; CHOKING, FEAR OF.

suggestion   The influence a therapist exercises over an individual in a therapeutic setting to accept an attitude or belief. Suggestion may be given to the individual who is anxious or phobic during a conscious state or may be given during a state of HYPNOSIS. Suggestion is used during many forms of BEHAVIOR THERAPY.

suicide, fear of   Taking one's own life. Some individuals who have anxieties and phobias fear that they will kill themselves. Some fear heights because they are afraid that they will feel compelled to jump from a high place. The same may be true of some bridge phobics and even some who fear flying in an airplane. Some individuals whose parent or other relative committed suicide may fear that they will feel compelled to do so, too. However, suicide does not run in the family; it is an individual pattern.

Many who contemplate suicide have an overwhelming feeling of rejection and lack of love and affection in their lives. Individuals who commit suicide often suffer from depression and have deep feelings of hopelessness or helplessness. The attempt at suicide may be brought on by a wish for revenge against the world, for being reunited with an individual who has died, or for instilling guilt in a person who has rejected him or her. Some individuals make threats of suicide in an attempt to dominate and control a spouse or parent or to force favorable treatment. Studies reveal that the suicidal person gives many clues and warnings of his or her contemplated intentions. Such individuals are often confused, alienated, and self-condemning.

Suicide is the eighth leading cause of death in the United States and the second most frequent cause of death for young people in the 15–25 age bracket. About 12 percent of those who threaten or attempt suicide actually kill themselves. Current statistics may understate the actual occurrence of suicide. Many automobile and other accidents may have suicidal intention. Because of social stigma, insurance coverage issues, and legal criteria for classifying cause of death, suicide may not be recorded as the cause in many cases.

Preventing Suicide
Suicide should be understood as a manifestation of DEPRESSION, which can be successfully treated. Friends or loved ones who show signs of depres-

sion or express hopelessness or suicidal impulses should be assisted to get immediate professional help before a suicidal crisis develops. In an acute suicidal crisis, the family should be instructed to remove all weapons and all lethal means from the home, including prescription drugs. They should be told not to leave the individual alone at any time.

One of the most difficult challenges clinicians face is the prevention of suicide by their patients. Such psychiatric clinicians routinely deal with patients whose diagnoses are associated with a high risk for suicide. The problem of suicide risk assessment and intervention is always a high priority. The physician, psychotherapist, or mental-health worker is sometimes the only person with the opportunity to recognize suicidal intent. Studies have shown that from 40 to 75 percent of suicidal individuals will see a physician within six months to a year preceding their self-destructive acts. A number of studies have pointed out that even while receiving psychiatric treatment, psychiatric hospitalization, or treatment with psychotropic drugs, patients do commit suicide.

Although suicide rarely can be a logical, rational decision based on an individual's situation, evidence seems to support the contention that most suicides occur in the context of psychiatric illness. However, the absence of psychiatric treatment at the time of suicide does not necessarily preclude the existence of a serious mental disturbance. It has been observed that severely depressed patients may appear symptom-free just prior to suicide. This may lead to an erroneous assumption that the individual is "normal" at the time of suicide. While suicidal behavior may manifest itself in patients fitting any psychiatric diagnostic category, it has been found most prevalent in depression, especially manic-depression and psychotic depression, as well as in alcoholism, substance abuse, and in schizophrenia, especially in younger age groups.

Relationship Between Suicide and Depression
Often the individual with symptoms of a serious depressive syndrome with such signs as sleep disturbance, weight loss, dry mouth, loss of sexual drive, gastrointestinal discomfort, complete loss of interest, impairment of function, delusional guilt, neglect of personal appearance and cleanliness,

inability to make decisions, a feeling of emptiness, psychomotor retardation or agitation in a depressed mood, characterized by feelings of hopelessness and helplessness, especially with severe anxiety or panic attacks, is a high suicide risk. Generally, the risk of suicide appears to be greatest in the early course of depressive illness (first three episodes) and decreases as drive and affect is "burned out" and where life becomes a kind of partial death, without ambition and seemingly without purpose.

The most commonly understood instances of increased suicidal risk in depressed individuals are situations associated with separation or loss. The loss does not necessarily have to be the final loss or death of a loved one, as Freud emphasized, but may be simply a temporary loss to the individual who is in a depressive crisis. For example, losses may be spouse, home, job, hospital discharge, temporary separation from therapist, money, love, etc.

The "failure situation" ranks high as a precursor of suicide. This situation may occur after a hospital discharge when a patient is trying to regain or attain higher levels of function, such as successful commencement of a job or return to college. Also,

this factor ranks high when individuals try to meet higher expectations of themselves or others.

Additionally, the presence of real or perceived physical illness may be significant in the assessment of suicidal risk. In malignant or incurable illness, two critical suicidal periods seem to be those of: a) uncertainty while diagnosis and prognosis are still at issue and, b) shock following the first realization of the upheavals and suffering, actual or fantasized, that are to follow.

Signs of Chronic Suicide Intentions

A characteristic of the chronically suicidal person is repeated communication of a wish to die or of

---

CHARACTERISTICS OF SUICIDAL INDIVIDUALS

- Ambivalence
- Withdrawn, isolative behavior
- Impaired concentration
- Constricted thought processes; tunnel vision
- Psychomotor agitation
- Psychomotor retardation
- Anxious
- Attentive to internal stimuli
- Verbalizes suicidal thoughts, feelings, plan
- Verbalizes references to death, dying
- Gives away possessions
- Anger, hostility
- Impulsive behaviors
- Depressed mood
- Appetite disturbances
- Hopeless-helpless
- Disturbed sleep patterns

(Adapted with permission from *Encyclopedia of Mental Health.*)

RISK FACTORS AND CHARACTERISTICS OF SUICIDE POTENTIAL

Suicide potential refers to the possibility that an individual will kill himself or herself voluntarily and intentionally.

Risk Factors

- Depression
- Other mood disorders
- Schizophrenia
- Other psychoses
- Neurologic disorders
- Delirium
- Use or withdrawal of alcohol or other substances
- Organic brain disorders
- Hallucinations, delusions
- Stress, acute or chronic
- Isolation
- Loss of significant other
- Loss of self-esteem
- Loss of physical health, function
- Cultural factors
- Spiritual anxiety
- Personality disorders
- Impulse control disorders
- Internal conflicts, guilt
- Family dysfunction, crisis
- Loss of resources, social and economic
- Unmet needs

(Adapted with permission from *Encyclopedia of Mental Health.*)

suicidal thoughts. However, this in itself is not sufficient to distinguish the high- from the low-risk individual, since it has also been observed that the majority of the much larger group of patients who attempt but do not complete suicide also convey intent in advance.

A suicidal individual often shows intense dependency as an underlying lifestyle dynamic. This dependency has been observed throughout all spheres of the suicidal individual's lifestyle where inordinately excessive demands are made on others for constant attention, affection, and approval, and where the individual feels unable to cope for him/herself, thereby needing continual supervision and guidance.

Personalities of many suicidal individuals have shown tendencies toward rigid thinking, which does not allow for alternatives in a crisis, and thinking in opposites. Perfectionism as a personality trait is carried to a pathological state and finds expression in an anxious striving toward perfection in all undertakings.

Suicide in Youth: Guns at Home

There are some clues to predict suicide among youngsters or adolescents. They are more likely to communicate with those in their peer group than their parents. They may give away a prized possession with the comment that they will not be needing it any more. They may be more morose and isolated than usual. Although there may be signs of insomnia, worry, and anorexia, the youngster may not have all the classical signs of depression.

One study listed symptoms occurring in 25 college-age suicides in order of their frequency: despondency, futility, lack of interest in schoolwork, a feeling of tenseness around people, insomnia, suicidal communications, fatigue and malaise without apparent organic cause, feelings of inadequacy or unworthiness, and brooding over the death of a loved one.

Having a gun at home may increase the risk that a psychologically troubled teen will commit suicide, according to an article published in December 1991 in the *Journal of the American Medical Association.* David A. Brent, M.D., Western Psychiatric Institute and Clinic, Pittsburgh, Pennsylvania, and colleagues, noted that the odds that potentially suicidal

adolescents will kill themselves increase 75-fold when a gun is kept in the house. They commented on the differences between teen suicides and that of adults. For teens, they said, a suicide attempt may be an attempt to communicate that they are in great pain, although they may be ambivalent about wanting to die. For such adolescents, ready access to a firearm may guarantee that their plea for help will not be heard.

Researchers found that guns were twice as likely to be found in the homes of suicide victims as in the homes of those who attempted suicide or were under psychiatric control. Handguns were not associated with suicide to any statistically significantly greater extent than long guns. There was no difference in the methods of storage of firearms among the three groups, so that even guns stored, locked, or separated from ammunition were associated with suicide by firearms.

The authors commented that it is clear that firearms have no place in the homes of psychiatrically troubled youngsters . . . Physicians who care for psychiatrically disturbed adolescents with any indicators of suicidal risk, such as depression, conduct problems, substance abuse, or suicidal thoughts have a responsibility to make clear and firm recommendations that firearms be removed from the homes of these at-risk youth. In an accompanying editorial, Mark L. Rosenberg, M.D., Division of Injury Control, National Center for Environmental Health and Injury Control, Centers for Disease Control, Atlanta, Georgia, commented that today the question of whether an adolescent at risk of committing suicide has access to a gun is all but ignored.

Suicide and the Aging Population

A federal study published during 1991 showed that from 1980 to 1986, suicides by Americans aged 65 and older jumped 23 percent for men, and 42 percent for African-American men. The rate for white women rose 17 percent; there were too few suicides among black women to show a meaningful trend. A study in Illinois using a grant from the American Association of Retired People Andrus Foundation showed that the great majority of the elderly who committed suicide were physically healthy. However, 79 percent had shown symptoms of a major

THE SOCIAL READJUSTMENT RATING SCALE

Major life changes can be predictive of physiological or psychological disturbances within two years of the change. The Social Readjustment Rating Scale quantifies the probability of having a disturbance within two years. A score of more than 150 is predictive.

Events	Scale of Impact	Events	Scale of Impact
Death of spouse	100	Son or daughter leaving home	29
Divorce	73	Trouble with in-laws	29
Marital separation	65	Outstanding personal achievement	28
Jail term	63	Spouse begins or stops work	26
Death of close family member	63	Begin or end school	26
Personal injury or illness	53	Change in living conditions	25
Marriage	50	Revision of personal habits	24
Fired at work	47	Trouble with boss	23
Marital reconciliation	45	Change in work hours or conditions	20
Retirement	45	Change in residence	20
Change in health of family member	44	Change in schools	20
Pregnancy	40	Change in recreation	19
Sex difficulties	39	Change in church activities	19
Gain in new family member	39	Change in social activities	18
Business readjustment	39	Taking out a mortgage or loan for a lesser purchase	17
Change in financial state	38		
Death of close friend	37	Change in sleeping habits	16
Change to different line of work	36	Change in number of family get-togethers	15
Change in number of arguments with spouse	35	Vacation	13
Taking out a mortgage or loan for a major purchase	31	Change in eating habits	15
Foreclosure of mortgage or loan	30	Christmas	12
Change in responsibilities at work	29	Violations of the law	11

Note: Scores of 200 or more are associated with stress reactions at a much higher incidence than scores below 200.

treatable psychiatric illness, usually depression or alcoholism.

See also ALCOHOLISM; DEPRESSION.

Fawcett, Jan, and Paul Susman, "A Clinical Assessment of Acute Suicidal Potential: A Review," *Rush-Presbyterian-St. Luke's Medical Bulletin* 14, no. 2 (April 1975).

Fawcett, Jan, William A. Scheftner, Louis Fogg, et al., "Time-Related Predictors of Suicide in Major Affective Disorder," *American Journal of Psychiatry* 147, no. 9 (September 1990).

Kahn, Ada P., and Jan Fawcett, *The Encyclopedia of Mental Health,* 2nd ed. (New York: Facts On File, 2001).

Katz, Marvin, "Critics Fear Misuse of Suicide Books," *Bulletin, American Association of Retired Persons* 32, no. 11 (December 1991).

sun and sunlight, fear of   Fear of sun and sunlight is known as heliophobia and phengophobia. Early men feared the sun because they recognized it as a source of life and worshiped it as the supreme deity. Men paid homage and brought offerings to the sun. They watched the sun and its daily movement across the sky with awe, puzzlement, and terror. They were frightened by the sun's decrease of power in winter; they feared that the sun might die and cause them to freeze to death. A solar eclipse caused the fear that the end of the world had come.

In modern times, the sun is feared as a cause of cancer. Dermatologists and oncologists have repeatedly warned that excessive exposure to sunlight without appropriate covering or use of sunscreen puts people at great risk for developing skin cancers, some of which can be disfiguring or even fatal.

See also AGORAPHOBIA; DEPRESSION; ILLNESS, FEAR OF; SEASONAL AFFECTIVE DISORDER.

superego and superego anxiety In psychoanalysis, superego is the part of the personality representing society's standards, and it determines one's own standards of right and wrong as well as our aims and aspirations. The superego is popularly referred to as the conscience.

Superego anxiety is anxiety that occurs from the anticipation of feeling guilty. An individual is aware that if he violates his own moral standards, his SUPEREGO, or conscience, will let him know by imposing (usually uncomfortable) feelings of guilt or shame. In thinking about the unpleasant guilt that he will experience after committing the transgression, the person may feel tense and anxious, possibly enough to prevent him from carrying out his planned actions.

superiority complex An unrealistic and exaggerated belief that one is better than others. Such a complex can be a source of anxiety for the individual. In some people, this develops as a way to compensate for unconscious feelings of low self-esteem or inadequacy. For example, bullies who push other children around act like they are stronger and smarter than others their age. The reality is that they have low self-esteem. In adults, even business executives may put on a tough facade and try to make others think well of them while inside feeling stressed and inadequate.

See also INFERIORITY COMPLEX; SELF-ESTEEM.

supernatural, fear of Belief in the supernatural with the accompanying fears and sense of terror has been common in many societies. Fears of the supernatural start in the child's vivid imagination and continue into later life; such fears are often associated with and prompted by religions, which use them as methods of discipline and social control. Natural disaster and misfortune, the behavior of wild animals, and the attempt to explain the fate of the soul after death contribute to fears of the supernatural.

As society becomes more scientific and rational and beliefs in the supernatural decrease, stories of the supernatural have become more popular; the supernatural has become a popular subject for novels and films. Supernatural themes allow an escape from the relative security of modern life. Continuing interest in horror stories indicates that people have a capacity to enjoy being frightened. There is a communal quality about the horror story, because a sense of shared terror brings people together, and children may fear the dark, monsters, and other frightening beings less when they are organized into plots.

Interest in the supernatural has heightened in modern times around concerns of death. For example, the dying are isolated in hospitals and cared for by professionals at the time of death. In becoming less a part of life, death has become more remote and mysterious. In spite of modern skepticism, superstitions and half beliefs linger. Frightening stories about the supernatural may be an acceptable way to express and contain these fears. Stories about supernatural, frightening situations may be a type of catharsis and drugless hallucinogen.

The study of death (thanatology) has become a legitimate area of science.

superstition A belief that is not based on scientific or rational evidence. Many people who still hold superstitions become anxious about certain events and situations. Many superstitious notions and customs persist: some are odd or amusing; some are harmless; and some are harmful. Superstitious beliefs are more common among people with little education, but there is a tendency, even among sophisticated, educated persons, to cling to superstitious beliefs. For example, many avoid using the number 13 for fear of it being unlucky.

Stressful interactions may arise between family members or friends when one clings to an old superstition and another counters it with a more practical or scientific explanation.

support groups Groups made up of individuals who have the same anxieties or specific health or social concerns who join together to help each other by sharing experiences, advice, and providing mutual emotional support.

Support groups exist for patients themselves, as well as spouses and family members. For example, individuals with manic-depressive disorder began an organization that now has become nationwide, with chapters in many cities. Individuals with chronic fatigue syndrome (CFS) have done the same, with the result that sufferers no longer need feel alone and that they are the only individuals with the problems. There are support groups for parents of children with specific mental health concerns, as well as groups for middle-age people who care for aging parents.

Many physicians recommend that patients join support groups because they realize that help with the anger and confusion can augment any therapies provided by medical means.

An additional benefit of belonging to a support group for a particular concern is that one can stay up-to-date on research on cures and better treatments. Many groups circulate articles from popular and scientific publications and bring in experts to discuss their latest findings.

According to Karyn Feiden, author of *Hope and Help for Chronic Fatigue Syndrome,* the work of support groups generally falls into three interlinked areas:

- Informing and educating the general public, and particularly patients, their families, and the medical community
- Counseling and consoling those who have been diagnosed with the particular disorder
- Organizing and advocating for the cause at both the local and the national level

See also BEHAVIORAL THERAPY; DEPRESSION.

Kahn, Ada P., *Stress A–Z: A Sourcebook for Facing Everyday Challenges* (New York: Facts On File, 1998).

supportive psychotherapy Psychotherapy that reinforces the individual's defenses and helps the individual suppress disturbing ideas. Supportive PSYCHOTHERAPY may utilize such techniques as suggestion, reeducation, and reassurance to help an individual face his fears, phobias, or anxieties. Unlike PSYCHOANALYSIS, this type of therapy does not look into the historical antecedents to an individual's emotional conflicts.

suppression Conscious efforts to control and conceal experiences, impulses, thoughts, feelings, or acts that are unacceptable to the individual. Some individuals who have specific phobias have suppressed experiences that surface later in life as phobias of situations or objects. Also, these suppressed experiences lead to the development of patterns (e.g., chronic emotional expression) that can trigger anxiety and panic disorders.

See also REPRESSION.

surgical operations (or surgical incisions), fear of Fear of surgical operations is known as ergasiophobia or tomophobia. This fear may extend to any medical procedure that uses operations, instruments, and manipulation, especially cutting and suturing. An individual may be phobic about having an operation himself or herself or of hearing about someone else's operation. A fear of surgical operations may be related to fears of doctors, hospitals, or death. Some individuals have grown up with a fear of surgical operations because they are aware that an older member of their family or someone they knew died during surgery, and they equate surgery with death from an early age. In recent years, knowledge about hospital-induced infections has caused many individuals to fear having anything to do with hospitals and surgery. Some individuals may fear particular types of surgery, such as hysterectomy.

See also DEATH, FEAR OF; DISEASE, FEAR OF; DOCTORS, FEAR OF; HOSPITALS, FEAR OF; ILLNESS, FEAR OF.

suriphobia See MICE, FEAR OF.

surveillance, fear of See BUGGING, FEAR OF; SPYING, FEAR OF.

swallowing, fear of Fear of swallowing is known as phagophobia. Some individuals feel that they have a lump in their throat and find it difficult to swallow when they are very anxious. Muscles of the throat may actually go into spasm, and the individual may make some choking sounds. Fear of swallowing is a SOCIAL PHOBIA and may cause phobic individuals to avoid being seen while they are eating. The fear of swallowing is also related to the feeling of having a "lump in the throat" (globus hystericus).

See also EATING, FEAR OF; FOOD, FEAR OF; GLOBUS HYSTERICUS.

swastika, fear of The swastika causes fear and terror in modern societies because of its association with Hitler and the horrors of the Holocaust preceding and during World War II. Hitler adopted the emblem in 1920, taking it from a badge on the helmets of the German Baltic Corps, which in turn had copied it from the distinguishing mark of the Finnish air force.

The swastika is one of man's earliest and most universal symbols, representing the wheel of the sun as it rolls across the skies, advancing by its feet, or short protrusions at the four ends of its spikes. The term swastika is of Sanskrit derivation, and the sign may have originated in India. The word—derived from two words, *su* meaning good, and *asti*, meaning being—was meant to express and promote good fortune. Throughout history, there have been a variety of meanings attributed to the symbol. For example, some cultures interpreted the emblem sexually, claiming that the joining of two bent lines at their center symbolized the sexual union of the male and female. Thus the emblem became a magic symbol in the promotion of fertility. In Scandinavian countries, the swastika represented the hammer of Thor, the god of thunder and lightning. A similar symbol is also seen in American Indian art.

sweating, fear of Fear of sweating is a SOCIAL PHOBIA. Some individuals avoid crowds, being in close contact with others in elevators, and even eating in restaurants because they fear that they will sweat and look ridiculous. They may also worry about giving off an offensive odor and staining their clothing. They fear attracting attention to themselves. Some women who suffer from HOT FLASHES fear that others will notice while they are having a hot flash. Many individuals who have a low sense of self-esteem worry that others will hold them in even less regard if they sweat at an unpredictable time. Social phobias, such as fear of sweating, are often treated successfully with BEHAVIOR MODIFICATION techniques and exposure therapy.

See also PHOBIA.

swimming, fear of Fear of swimming may be a SOCIAL PHOBIA in that many who fear swimming fear being seen in their bathing suits by others, fear criticism about their body shape, and fear that they may look ridiculous while swimming or approaching the pool or body of water. Fear of swimming may also come from a fear of water or a fear of drowning. Some fear being out of control if a wave or the undertow overtakes them while swimming in an ocean or large lake. Some individuals are comfortable standing in a pool or body of water but fear swimming; some can float or swim but fear putting their face in the water while they do so. For many, a fear of swimming can be overcome by taking lessons and learning to use appropriate breathing techniques while in the water. For others, behavior modification techniques may be effective.

See also PHOBIA; WATER, FEAR OF.

symbolism, fear of Fear of symbolism is known as symbolophobia. Many personal fears can be produced by phobic stimuli. Individuals may fear the symbols themselves with or without understanding their unconscious representation. For example, water has been viewed symbolically as a representation of the mind. Going underwater—the "deep dive," for example, in *Moby Dick*—is symbolic of going into the unconscious or going into the "dark side."

Jung, to a greater degree than Freud, explored the enduring and universal evolutionary aspects of symbols. Jung used the word "archetype" to designate universal symbols that possess constancy and efficiency and can force the way to psychic evolution. These ready-made systems of images are inherited, powerful, instinctive guides to creative action and growth. The deeper significance of these archetypes are secret and require an opening to the beyond or unknown. Some archetypes are the mother, father, wise man, warrior, magician, etc.

Freud viewed symbolism in dreams as important in understanding concealed unconscious wishes or conflicts. In the English school of psychoanalysis, also known as the Kleinian school, symbol formation was viewed as an essential prerequisite of early normal development. Investigations by Melanie Klein (1882–1960), an Austrian psychoanalyst, led to an understanding of how symbolism helps the child construct his internal world at an early age. The infant's transference of interest from his subjective world to the outside world of external reality begins with symbols. For example, the baby regards objects as symbolizing others, if there is some resemblance between them. The baby's fingers symbolize the breast when the breast is not available, and the symbol serves as a bridge to the actual object.

Behavior therapists acknowledge that symbolism distinguishes between radical objective theorists who are not interested in mediating processes and those who view cognitions and imagery as mediating between the stimulus and response in the behavioral sequence that governs human behavior. The development of language presupposes an ability to utilize symbols and symbolization.

See also COLLECTIVE UNCONSCIOUS.

symbolophobia   Fear of symbolism.
See also SYMBOLISM.

symmetry   Fear of symmetry is known as symmetrophobia. Symmetry is a relationship of characteristic equivalence or balance. It is an exact correspondence of form and configuration on opposite sides of a dividing line or plane or about a center or axis. An example of fear of symmetry is an individual's compulsion to rearrange furniture so that end tables are not exactly the same distance from a couch, or so that identical lamps are not placed equidistant from a chair. A compulsion to rearrange pictures on a wall in a random fashion

rather than in a row or equidistant from each other is another example of fear of symmetry.

sympathetic nervous system   One of two major divisions of the AUTONOMIC NERVOUS SYSTEM, and the one that prepares an individual for fighting, fleeing, action, or sexual climax. During a PHOBIC REACTION, the sympathetic nervous system becomes quickly activated. The sympathetic nervous system tends to excite or arouse one by speeding up the contractions of the blood vessels, slowing those of the intestines, and increasing the heartbeat to prepare the body for exertion, emotional stress, and extreme cold, while the parasympathetic nervous system tends to depress many bodily functions. These two divisions of the autonomic nervous system coordinate to control bodily activities and respond appropriately to physical and psychological challenges. When an individual wants to be aroused (such as when fleeing from fear) the sympathetic system speeds up and the parasympathetic system slows down. When one wants to relax, the parasympathetic system increases its activities and the sympathetic system slows down.

The sympathetic nervous system consists of a group of 22 neural centers on or close to the spinal cord. From these 22 centers fibers connect to all parts of the body, including the sweat glands and tiny blood vessels near the surface of the skin. When one is suddenly afraid, the sympathetic nervous system activates the following physiological responses:

- Heart pumps more blood to the brain and muscles and to the surface of the skin
- Breathing becomes faster and harder
- Blood-sugar level becomes elevated
- Digestion slows down
- Skin perspires to remove waste products created by exertion and to keep one cool
- Pupils in the eyes open up to let in more light
- Controls orgasm and ejaculation during sexual arousal

See also HYPERVENTILATION.

symptom Evidence of a disorder as noticed personally by the individual afflicted with it. For example, phobic individuals report that they experience rapid heartbeat and a tight feeling in their chest when they view their feared object. A symptom is usually distinguished from a SIGN, which is a manifestation of a disorder that is noticed on an objective, observable basis by another person, such as a therapist or physician. However, in common usage, the word symptom often includes objective signs of disordered conditions as well.

See also DIAGNOSIS; SYNDROME.

Symptom Substitution

Development of a SYMPTOM to replace one that has been removed after therapy. An example of symptom substitution is replacement of one phobia with another. Some therapists, including dynamic therapists, who oppose behavioral therapy techniques, argue that such therapy's removal of a symptom, such as a phobia, without addressing the "underlying cause" will result in the emergence of a new substitute symptom. Behaviorists have found no evidence for this hypothesis and have successfully treated phobias without adverse effects. Since symptom substitution is a major corollary of the medical or dynamic model of behavioral pathology, the lack of evidence for the occurrence of symptom substitution calls into question the medical model.

See also BEHAVIOR THERAPY; HYPNOSIS; MEDICAL MODEL; SUGGESTION.

syndrome A group of symptoms that occur together that constitute a recognizable condition, either physical or mental. Syndrome is also called symptom complex or disease entity. For example, the group of symptoms exhibited by agoraphobics is known as the agoraphobic syndrome. "Syndrome" is less specific than "disorder" or "disease," which generally implies a specific cause or disease process. In the American Psychiatric Association's DIAGNOSTIC AND STATISTICAL MANUAL OF MENTAL DISORDERS, most disorders are considered syndromes.

American Psychiatric Association, *Diagnostic and Statistical Manual of Mental Disorders* (Washington, DC: American Psychiatric Association, 1987).

syngenesophobia Fear of relatives.
See also RELATIVES, FEAR OF.

syphilis, fear of See SEXUALLY TRANSMITTED DISEASES.

syphilophobia Fear of syphilis. Also known as syphilidophobia.
See also SEXUALLY TRANSMITTED DISEASES; VENEREAL DISEASE, FEAR OF.

systematic desensitization A behavioral therapy procedure that is highly effective in the treatment of excessive emotional states such as anxiety and anger. It originated with Joseph Wolpe, who used in vivo and imaginal desensitization with his patients and reported over 80 percent recovery rates for a variety of anxiety, phobic, and emotional reactions. The essence of systematic desensitization is the

---

DIFFICULTIES SOME INDIVIDUALS EXPERIENCE DURING SYSTEMATIC DESENSITIZATION

Following are some of the difficulties phobic individuals learn to overcome during systematic desensitization.

- *Difficulties during relaxation:*
    Sleepiness
    Poor concentration
    Fear of losing control
    Muscular relaxation without mental relaxation
    Severe anxiety and depression
- *Problems of imagery:*
    Inability to obtain images
    Dissociation of anxiety
    Dilution of image to more protective setting
    Intensification of image to panic proportions
- *Misleading hierarchies:*
    Irrelevant hierarchies
    Fluctuating hierarchies
- *Relapse of desensitized phobias*
- *Lack of cooperation*
- *Life situation influences outside treatment*

gradual exposure of an individual to components of a feared situation while he or she is relaxed. Systematic desensitization is the major treatment procedure for phobias and agoraphobia. Exposure may occur in imagination or self-visualization or in actuality (in vivo). Systematic desensitization is best applied with the help of a skilled therapist. Once relaxation skills are mastered (which takes five to six weeks), a hierarchy involving gradually more intimate (and reactive) triggering stimuli is developed, and imaginal or in vivo exposure is started. Systematic desensitization is a highly effective treatment method for simple phobias. The cure rate for simple phobias is about 80 percent to 85 percent with 12 to 15 sessions. Social phobias, agoraphobia, and panic require more patience, time, and skill in using systematic desensitization. These reactions also usually require in vivo exposure rather than imaginal to be effective. See chart on preceding page.

See also AGORAPHOBIA; BEHAVIOR THERAPY.

tabophobia Fear of a wasting sickness.

tachycardia Rapid, intensive heartbeat, often associated with a fearsome situation or high levels of ANXIETY that occur during phobic attacks and PANIC ATTACKS. Tachycardia is not dangerous to the person's health but, if persistent, should be checked by a physician.

See also PANIC; PANIC DISORDER; SYMPATHETIC NERVOUS SYSTEM.

tacophobia (tachophobia) Fear of speed.

See also SPEED, FEAR OF.

taeniophobia See TAPEWORMS, FEAR OF.

tai chi chuan A Chinese martial art and form of stylized, meditative exercise, characterized by methodically slow circular and stretching movements planned to rebalance bodily energy. Practitioners of tai chi chuan usually perform their routines early in the morning to keep themselves anxiety-free during the day.

Chen, W. William, and Wei Yue Sun, "Tai Chi Chuan, an alternative form of exercise for health promotion and disease prevention for older adults in the community," *International Quarterly of Community Health Education* 16, no. 4 (1997): pp. 333–339.

taijin kyofusho See CROSS-CULTURAL INFLUENCES.

talking, fear of Fear of talking is known as glossophobia, laliophobia, lalophobia, and phonophobia.

Fear of talking may be a SOCIAL PHOBIA in that the individual is afraid to speak up in a crowd, fears embarrassment, or fears saying something ridiculous or inappropriate. Also, fear of talking may relate to fear of hearing the sound of one's own voice or a fear of stuttering.

See also ONE'S OWN VOICE, FEAR OF; STUTTERING, FEAR OF; TELEPHONES, FEAR OF.

tapeworms, fear of Fear of tapeworms is known as taeniophobia or teniophobia. Some individuals fear tapeworms because they can cause disease and discomfort. Tapeworms, a member of the class Cestoda, are a parasite of man and other vertebrates. If a human or animal eats improperly cooked pork or beef containing worm larvae, the digestive juices of the consumer free the larvae; the young parasites then attach themselves to the new host's intestinal lining and develop into adults. Treatment is either by surgery or drugs. Reinfection is possible unless the victim practices proper hygiene. Thoroughly cooking all meat and fish products will also eliminate the possibility of infection.

See also WORMS, FEAR OF.

taphophobia (taphephobia) Fear of being buried alive is known as taphophobia. These terms also refer to fears of graves and tombs.

See BURIED ALIVE, FEAR OF BEING; GRAVES, FEAR OF; TOMBS, FEAR OF.

tapinophobia See SMALL OBJECTS.

tardive dyskinesia A severe and permanent side effect caused by the use of some older antipsychotic drugs that causes a noticeable and uncontrollable impairment of the individual's voluntary movement. This side effect may present after years of taking certain types of antipsychotic medications that block the transmissiong at the dopamine synapses. Some examples of such drugs that may cause tardive dyskinesia include haloperidol (Haldol), chlorpromazine (Thorazine), or trifluoperazine (Stelazine).

These medications were often used in the past to treat patients with SCHIZOPHRENIA, and they were also sometimes used with patients with other forms of PSYCHOSIS, such as BIPOLAR DISORDER or DEPRESSION with psychotic features. In some cases, such drugs were used in the short term for patients with ANXIETY DISORDERS. They were also sometimes used with combative children or with elderly patients with dementia.

Typical symptoms of tardive dyskinesia include tremors and involuntary movements of the mouth and tongue, as well as drooling. The patient is often aware of these behaviors but cannot regain physical control. It is an irreversible condition. This condition persists long after drug withdrawal and sometimes worsens even after treatment is suspended altogether. It is believed that the blocked dopamine synapses become hypersensitive to any dopamine that does reach them, leading to these uncontrollable behaviors.

More recently developed antipsychotic drugs are much *less* likely to cause tardive dyskinesia because they affect the brain in a different manner. Some examples of more recent drugs are aripiprazole (Abilify) and risperidone (Risperdal).

Stahl, Stephen, *Essential Psychopharmacology: The Prescriber's Guide* (Cambridge: Cambridge University Press, 2005).

taste, fear of Fear of taste is known as geumaphobia, geumophobia, or geumatophobia. Individuals may fear certain tastes because of their associations with past experiences or situations that caused anxieties. The fear also may be generalized to other foods in the particular taste category. For example, a child who becomes nauseous after eating a lemon for the first time, or who is always given lemons to eat by a feared authority figure, may grow to associate lemon with discomfort and begin to fear not only this taste but any sour-tasting food.

There is a disorder known as gustatory agnosia, in which food becomes tasteless or even has a disgusting taste. Individuals who have this condition may also lose their ability to smell or may find that formerly pleasant odors are offensive. With an inability to smell, they may fear that they are unaware that they are eating or drinking something that formerly caused them anxieties.

See also EATING, FEAR OF; FOOD, FEAR OF; SWALLOWING, FEAR OF.

tattoos, fear of Many individuals who fear tattoos do so because ornamental tattooing can produce tumors, or individuals may develop allergic skin reactions to some of the color pigments used. Those who fear contamination or infection may fear those problems from needles used in tattooing. The most common infections from needles are hepatitis and AIDS (acquired immunodeficiency syndrome).

Some fear tattooing because it seems to be a permanent coloration of the skin. Because the pigment in a tattoo extends deep into the skin, its removal, by any method, is likely to leave a scar. Small tattoos can be removed by excision, leaving a small, minimal scar. Dermabrasion (skin planing) is also used to make the tattoo fainter.

Others may fear tattoos because the tattoos depict their phobic object, such as butterflies, lips, or the word "mother."

See also CONTAMINATION, FEAR OF; NEEDLES, FEAR OF.

taurophobia Fear of bulls.

Taylor Manifest Anxiety Scale (TMAS) A scale used by therapists to assess trait ANXIETY and useful in helping individuals who have phobias understand themselves better and deal with their phobias. The TMAS was one of the first self-report ("paper and pencil") scales designed specifically to measure anxiety. The scale was adapted by Janet Taylor in the early 1950s from the Minnesota Multiphasic

Personality Inventory, a multifactorial personality scale.

The test is a reliable, valid, and economical means to determine levels of anxiety; it has been used to test effects of anxiety on learning and conditioning and in hundreds of clinical and experimental studies of anxiety. Janet Taylor believed that anxiety was a drive or motivating force and that persons with high drive, or high anxiety, would develop conditioned responses more rapidly than low-anxiety or low-drive subjects.

See also EYSENCK PERSONALITY INVENTORY; STATE-TRAIT ANXIETY INVENTORY.

Taylor, J. A., "A Personality Scale of Manifest Anxiety," *The Journal of Abnormal and Social Psychology* 48 (1953): pp. 285–290.

technology, fear of   Fear of technology is known as technophobia. Many individuals fear technological devices in modern society. For example, some individuals look with fear upon computers, highly technical telephone answering systems, and even videocassette recorders. Some individuals become very anxious when faced with a set of instructions that are supposed to be easy for the average individual to follow. Another aspect of technophobia is the fear that machines will be able to do what people do now. Fear of robots is part of this fear.

See also COMPUTER PHOBIA.

teeth, fear of   Fear of teeth is known as odonophobia.

See also DENTAL ANXIETY.

teeth grinding   Known medically as *bruxism*, teeth grinding is a habit many people practice when they feel anxious or fearful. Some people grind their teeth during the day and some only do it at night.

For about 5 percent of the population, teeth grinding causes serious consequences. For example, it is possible to grind the enamel off the teeth, making them more susceptible to cavities and very sensitive to heat and cold. Years of grinding can cause facial and jaw pain from fatigued muscles. Grinding also may damage the joint between the jaw and the cranium (temporomandibular joint). When a person eats, the muscles responsible for chewing exert just enough pressure to hold in place the disk of cartilage that cushions the joint. When the person grinds his or her teeth, this disk gradually becomes displaced, causing soreness, inflammation, and even arthritis.

Dentists can prepare plastic retainer-like appliances, called mouth guards or night guards, that prevent grinding. Many people find that RELAXATION THERAPY, GUIDED IMAGERY, HYPNOSIS, and BIOFEEDBACK also help to relieve this unwanted habit.

See also TEMPOROMANDIBULAR JOINT SYNDROME.

teleology   In psychology and psychiatry, teleology is the concept that mental processes have purposes and are directed toward goals. Within this concept, behavior, including phobic or avoidant behavior, can be explained in terms of purposes as contrasted with causes. Alfred ADLER's emphasis on ideals and goals that the individual chooses for self-fulfillment is a teleological approach, as is Carl JUNG's concentration on religious and moral values and on development of individual purposes.

telephone, fear of the   Known as telephonophobia, there are many variations of the fearful syndrome. Some individuals fear talking on the telephone. Others fear the ringing of a telephone, perhaps because they fear hearing bad news. Some are afraid to pick up the phone and answer it because they fear that they will say something that will be criticized by the listener. Some experience a great deal of anxiety if they have to pick up the telephone to inquire about a job, place an order, or make any kind of an inquiry. Some individuals feel that they are powerless when speaking to another person by telephone, because when deprived of visual clues, such as body language, they feel they cannot control the response they will get. Some express anxiety that they are intruding on the person they are calling and can never seem to find a "good" time to place their call. Others are fearful of using the telephone because doing so reminds them of overhearing conversations their parents had, of listening when they should not have been, or of hearing something specifically traumatic. Individuals who have telephone phobia experience symptoms of nervous stomach and sweaty palms, which are typical anxiety reactions. Many telephone phobics are motivated to overcome their phobia because they realize that the telephone can be a bridge between themselves and someone about whom they care and between themselves and necessary services. Individuals who have overcome this phobia have suggested rehearsing the conversation before making the call, writing down what they want to say when they call, or standing up while speaking into the telephone. Behavior therapy techniques can be helpful for telephone phobics.

See also BEHAVIOR THERAPY.

teletophobia   Fear of religious ceremonies.

See also RELIGIOUS CEREMONIES, FEAR OF; CHURCHES, FEAR OF.

television, role of in phobias   Television can be a powerful source of observational learning for both children and adults. Children observe models of fearful behavior on television, such as people who are afraid of the dark and of harmless animals. Television presents many unrealistic and exaggerated situations in cartoon form that can frighten children, such as goblins, dragons, and vampires. Children may later think about these situations, dream about them, and even develop night terrors because of what they have seen. Crime programs make children as well as adults fearful of criminal attack, and news programs that report murders, arson, and robberies reinforce the notion that these events are more frequent than they actually are.

See also CHILDHOOD ANXIETIES, FEARS, AND PHOBIAS.

temporomandibular joint syndrome (TMJ)   A condition that occurs when the ligaments and muscles that control and support the jaw, face, and head do not work together properly. The disorder can be brought on by a spasm of the chewing muscles, teeth grinding (bruxism), or clenching the teeth as a response to anxiety and tension.

Symptoms of TMJ may include tenderness of the jaw; HEADACHES and dull, aching, facial pain; jaws that lock; pain brought on by chewing or yawning; and a clicking or popping noise when opening the jaw.

Psychological counseling sometimes helps individuals overcome the underlying anxieties and helps them to cope better with the stresses in their lives. Some people try GUIDED IMAGERY and RELAXATION exercises.

Treatment may include relieving pain by applying moist heat to the face, taking muscle-relaxant drugs, and using a bite splint at night to prevent teeth clenching and grinding. Some individuals undergo orthodontia to correct their bite; others undergo surgery on their jaw.

See also MEDITATION; STRESS; TEETH GRINDING.

TENS (transcutaneous nerve stimulation)   See PAIN, ANXIETY AND DEPRESSION IN.

tension headache   See HEADACHES.

teratophobia   Fear of deformed people or of bearing a monster. Some women develop this fear while pregnant. Others fear becoming pregnant because of this fear.

See also BEARING A MONSTER, FEAR OF; DEFORMED PEOPLE, FEAR OF.

terdekaphobia   Also known as triskadekaphobia. Fear of the number 13.

termites, fear of   Fear of termites (also known as white ants) is known as isopterophobia. The word *termites* applies to many antlike insects which feed on wood and are highly destructive to trees and wooden structures. Individuals who fear termites actually may fear being buried alive if the termites cause collapse of the buildings in which they live.

TERRAP   The TERitorrial APprehensiveness Program (TERRAP) is a multifaceted approach to treatment of AGORAPHOBIA and panic attack syndromes. TERRAP was founded in 1965 by Arthur B. Hardy, M.D., of Menlo Park, CA, together with a number of agoraphobic patients. By 1988, there were over 35 TERRAP centers in the United States.

Before acceptance into a TERRAP program, an individual is evaluated and diagnosed during a private consultation with a psychotherapist, at which time decisions about the need for medication are made. However, many people arrive at the program already addicted, for example, to imipramine, alprazolam, or combinations of several drugs. Many individuals who enter the TERRAP program have seen several therapists without result.

Following are the basic principles of TERRAP:

1. A 20-session program. Each session addresses a separate complication regarding phobias. Education is emphasized, because the individuals who have a problem must understand what they have, why they have it, and what they can do to assure the best possible results for recovery.
2. A pre-group. This is preparatory to going into the main therapy group. In the pre-group, individuals ask basic questions, learn about what they will be doing, and prepare for the basic treatment in a group. Pre-group is led by ex-phobics who have recovered using the TERRAP method and offers group support, information, and skill building. Homework is required. Participants then join the regular treatment group, which also serves as an ongoing support group during therapy.
3. Anxiety attacks are considered a response to some noxious stimuli. Participants learn to recognize the stimuli that trigger the anxiety reactions. This is referred to as "stimulus hunting."
4. Participants learn relaxation exercises and calming procedures in order to decrease excessive anxiety and tension. This includes use of progressive muscular relaxation exercises, visual clues such as pictures, colors, decorations, pleasant sights, sounds (such as favorite music), smells (such as perfume), tastes, and tactile sensations (such as hugging, soft fur, or movement such as rocking in a rocking chair)—all of which are natural tranquilizers.

5. Once the fundamentals have been accomplished, participants are ready for DESENSITIZATION. Desensitization procedures include the use of BIOFEEDBACK, pictures of the noxious stimuli (providing an opportunity to face the fear in a safe setting), mental desensitization (bringing to mind anxiety-producing situations, alternating with pleasant thoughts and thus relaxing mentally at the thought of them), and IN VIVO DESENSITIZATION with the entire group, as demonstrated by a trained guide.
6. Fieldwork is available individually with a trained guide who is a recovered phobic. This consists of going out into the natural situation accompanied by a trained field worker who assists in the implementation of the program.
7. Treatment includes spouse participation. Spouses can be particularly helpful with in vivo desensitization. Spouses are educated about the problem, how they can help, and what they may do that makes the problem worse (if that is the case). Marriage counseling is available when necessary. Agoraphobia frequently creates tension between spouses, and help is almost always needed to assist in resolving marital conflicts.
8. Participants learn to chart their progress on graphs during goal-setting sessions, which are highly motivating.
9. Participants learn self-talk to help them develop realistic, logical, positive, and practical thinking and offset their ever-present negative thoughts. Self-talk consists of positive coping statements.
10. Participants learn ASSERTIVENESS TRAINING to correct the tendency to please others and to enable them to speak up for themselves to get what they want.
11. Participants learn the principles of problem solving and apply those principles to conflict resolution.
12. Participants experience emotional breakthroughs about halfway through the program. Breakthroughs are part of recovery, and by understanding and allowing their feelings to emerge, people can learn to accept and understand their feelings better, as well as reduce their intensity.
13. Participants are prepared in advance for the inevitable setbacks that occur to almost all

recovering people. Participants are taught what to do about setbacks, so they do not become panicky when and if they happen.

14. Medication, when and if needed, is available. Medication is always carefully monitored to assure best results and to avoid addiction.

15. Participants return to the support group for continued association with recovered phobics and to allow time to consolidate their gains from the treatment group. This makes recovery as lasting and permanent as possible. The support group utilizes field trips, networking, buddy systems, distance trips, driving practice, lecture sessions, and videotapes.

16. Advanced goal setting and individual and group therapy continue to be available if necessary.

17. Follow-up interviews are used for information and research.

See also PHOBIA.

(Arthur B. Hardy, M.D., Menlo Park, California.)

terrorism   Terrorism is meant to make many people fearful and apprehensive about traveling and trusting others. It increases their levels of anxiety in airports and other public places. The destruction of the Twin Towers at the World Trade Center in New York City on September 11, 2001, killed thousands and shocked Americans and the world and caused greatly increased concern and levels of insecurity in the United States and other countries. The bombing of the Murrah Federal Building in Oklahoma City, Oklahoma, in 1995 killed many people and terrorized countless others, particularly those working in government buildings around the world. Hostage-taking, which had made the headlines many times in the latter 1990s, is an act of terrorism.

Terrorists are individuals who are fanatical about their cause and often have no concern for their victims or for their own lives. Most terrorist groups are supported by governments who find terrorism an effective and inexpensive way to wage war compared to the high costs of a conventional military operation. Terrorism is a way to traumatize a population, create chaos, and demobilize people by fear and inaction.

In 1986, Vice President George Bush's Task Force on Combating Terrorism defined terrorism as: "The unlawful use or threat of violence against persons or property to further political or social objectives. It is usually intended to intimidate or coerce a government, individuals, or groups to modify their behavior or politics." Terrorism aimed at U.S. diplomats has increased dramatically since the Bush report.

While little can be done to protect against most types of terrorism, certain precautions, such as awareness of surroundings and vigilance in public places, should be taken. Thorough security measures to ensure safety should help ease levels of anxiety. Terrorism has become a new form of war.

See also HOSTAGES; POST-TRAUMATIC STRESS DISORDER.

test anxiety   Fear of taking tests is common among individuals of all ages, but it is particularly noticeable in students. Test anxiety may be related to a desire for perfectionism and fear of failure. Outside of academic settings, individuals face many test situations in everyday life, including tests for acquiring a driver's license, medical tests, and tests as part of employment applications. Desensitization programs have been used to treat test anxiety with varying degrees of success.

See also ANXIETY.

testophobia   Fear of taking tests.
See also TEST ANXIETY.

testosterone   A male HORMONE produced by the testes that stimulates development of male reproductive organs, including the prostate, and secondary features, such as the beard and bone and muscle growth. Testosterone stimulates the male sexual drive. Testosterone level usually decreases in men during ANXIETY and stress.

See also STRESS MANAGEMENT.

tetanus, fear of   Fear of tetanus is known as tetanophobia. Tetanus is an acute infectious disease caused by a toxin produced in the body by *Clostridium tetani.* Tetanus is commonly called lockjaw.

See also LOCKJAW, FEAR OF.

Teutophobia   Fear of Germany and German things.

textophobia   Fear of certain fabrics.

See also FABRICS, FEAR OF CERTAIN.

textures, fear of certain   Some people have aversions to fuzzy surfaces, such as certain carpets, tennis balls, peach skins, or the skins of kiwi fruit. Some avoid suede, velvet, corduroy, or other fabrics, or shiny buttons. Usually aversions to textures make the individual uncomfortable but do not elicit phobic reactions.

thaasophobia   Fear of sitting down.

See also SITTING, FEAR OF.

thalassophobia   Fear of the sea, ocean, or other large body of water.

See also SEA, FEAR OF.

thanatophobia   Fear of death.

See also DEATH, FEAR OF.

theaters, fear of   Fear of theaters is known as theatrophobia. Individuals who fear theaters may do so because they feel closed in and unable to get out easily. They may be agoraphobics and may also be afraid of crowds, suffocation, fire, or being far from a bathroom. Some people fear being in the center section of a theater and will not go unless they can be assured of an aisle seat. They may fear contamination from the seat or the back of the seat. Some individuals who fear head lice fear that they will contract them while sitting in a theater seat (as well as in a bus or train).

See also AGORAPHOBIA.

Thematic Apperception Test (TAT)   A personality diagnostic test. The TAT may be useful in giving therapists information about an anxious or phobic individual, because in doing the test, the individual projects attitudes, feelings, conflicts, and personality characteristics. Individuals are asked to make up stories with a beginning, middle, and end about a series of pictures; then the therapist looks for common themes in the stories. Scoring is primarily subjective.

See also PERSONALITY TYPES.

theology, fear of   Fear of theology is known as theologicophobia. Some people fear theology because explanations of theological concepts are often made in specialized and obscure terms. Some believers with a mystical or personal approach to religion resent the scholarly application of theological thinking. Such individuals become anxious when they try to analyze and categorize religious ideas because the structured academic approach interferes with their personal sense of contact with God.

See GOD, FEAR OF; RELIGIOUS CEREMONIES, FEAR OF.

theophobia   Fear of God.

See also GOD, FEAR OF.

therapeutic touch   A nontraditional therapy (alternative or complementary) developed by Dr. Dolores Krieger, professor of nursing at New York University, by which she relieves the pain and distress of illness by passing her hands over the patient. It is also known as *healing touch* and is derived from the laying-on of hands. Her method is described in her book *The Therapeutic Touch, How to Use Your Hands to Help or to Heal.*

Since the mid-1970s, Dr. Krieger has conducted courses in therapeutic touch and taught thousands of people. New York University offers a fully accredited graduate course at the master's level designed to formally teach the process of therapeutic touch and to investigate how and why it works. In addition, more than 50 universities offer formal instruction in therapeutic touch, usually as part of the curriculum for nurses' training.

How the Technique Works

The healer eases into an altered state of consciousness while focusing energy on the patient, then slowly passes his or her hands about four to six inches above the patient's body in an effort to sense a transfer of energy. The healer scans the body for an area of temperature change, indicating the part of the body troubled, then lays hands on the affected area. The patient senses a change in temperature, perhaps a feeling of deep heat, in the area being touched.

According to Dr. Krieger, at the very least, the method produces a relaxation response in the patient and works well for inflammation, musculoskeletal problems, and psychosomatic disorders. Explanation by healers whose patients have been helped say that energy passes between themselves and their patients. Skeptics believe that this healing has a PLACEBO EFFECT, but it seems to work for some individuals.

Historically, physicians touched their patients far more than they do today with the advent of so many highly technical diagnostic machines. Until the invention of the stethoscope in the mid-1800s, physicians pressed their naked ears to the bodies of patients to listen for heartbeats and other internal sounds. This intimate gesture probably had a soothing effect on the patient, much as therapeutic touch has today. As author Lewis Thomas wrote in *The Youngest Science*, "it is hard to imagine a friendlier human gesture, a more intimate signal of personal concern and affection, than the close-bowed head affixed to the skin."

Now, many nurses and other health care practitioners, including body therapists, realize the need for human touch and practice healing touch either knowledgeably or unconsciously along with massage and other techniques.

See also BODY THERAPIES; MASSAGE THERAPY.

thermophobia   Fear of heat or of being too warm.
See also HEAT, FEAR OF.

thieves, fear of   Fear of thieves or burglars is known as cleptophobia, kleptophobia, and harpaxophobia. Because of high crime rates in modern urban areas, many individuals have become excessively fearful of burglars and muggers. Antidotes to this fear seem to include burglar-alarm systems, training in self-defense techniques, and carrying weapons (although the last may be illegal in many places).

things that go bump in the night, fear of   This term has contemporary meaning in referring to fears of strange noises in the dark. There is an anonymous Scottish prayer, presumed to have been used popularly during the 1800s:

> From ghoulies and ghosties and long-leggety
>   beasties
> And things that go bump in the night,
> Good Lord, deliver us!

Bartlett, John, ed., *Bartlett's Familiar Quotations*, 15th ed. (Boston: Little Brown, 1980).

third force   The term given to approaches to psychotherapy that include HUMANISTIC PSYCHOLOGY and existential and experiential therapies. Many individuals who have anxieties and phobias are helped by such techniques. The term is used to contrast these approaches from the "first force" of psychoanalysis and the "second force" of behavior therapy. Leaders of third-force therapy have included Abraham Maslow, Carl Rogers, Gordon Allport, and Kurt Goldstein. In general, third-force therapy emphasizes direct experience, the here-and-now, responsibility for oneself, group interactions, personal growth rather than symptom alleviation or adjustment, and self-exploration and self-discovery.

See also EXISTENTIAL THERAPY; GESTALT THERAPY; REALITY THERAPY.

thirteen, fear of the number   Fear of the number thirteen, or of having thirteen people at a table, is known as tridecaphobia, tredecaphobia, and triskaidekaphobia. Individuals who fear the number 13 may fear any situation or event involving this number, such as a house number, floor of a building, apartment or office number, or the 13th day of the month. Because this is such a common fear, many buildings have omitted labeling the 13th floor as such.

Residents of the 13th floor are less anxious believing that they live on the 14th floor.

thixophobia   Fear of touch.
See also HAPTOPHOBIA; HAPHOPHOBIA.

Thought Field Therapy (TFT)   A form of therapy based on body meridians and restoration of energy balance in the body used to help some people deal with certain anxiety disorders. It is based on a principle in Chinese medicine that energy flows along meridians and can be balanced and released by contact on acupressure points.

The therapy is aimed at breaking up negative emotions and beliefs. Clients learn to press certain pressure points on glands and energy pathways in particular patterns based on the type of energy blockage involved.

The therapy is said to have no adverse side effects. TFT does not require the individual to talk about their problem, something that often causes considerable distress or embarrassment and which discourages many for seeking treatment.

The technique was developed in the 1980s by Roger D. Callahan, Ph.D., an American psychologist.

thought stopping   A cognitive BEHAVIOR THERAPY technique developed by Joseph WOLPE. The therapist asks the phobic or anxious individual to recognize fear-producing thoughts. When the individual begins to verbalize or produce these undesirable thoughts, he is asked to interrupt them with an internal shout of "stop." Eventually the individual learns to control and reduce the incidence of such thoughts. Thought stopping is also useful in treating smoking and sexual deviations.
See also REINFORCEMENT.

thumb sucking, fear of   Some parents fear that their infant's habit of thumb sucking will lead to infection or a malformed mouth. Young infants put anything they can into their mouths, and as they get older they usually grow out of the habit of thumb sucking. However, parents who have fears of contamination or germs may worry that their infant will contract a disease because of something on his or her fingers. Fears about thumb sucking may be related to fears of nail biting.
See also CONTAMINATION, FEAR OF; GERMS, FEAR OF.

thunder, fear of   Fear of thunder is known as brontophobia, ceraunophobia, keraunophobia, and tonitrophobia.
See also THUNDERSTORMS, FEAR OF.

thunderbolt, fear of   Fear of a thunderbolt is known as keraunosophobia.
See also THUNDERSTORMS, FEAR OF.

thunderstorms, fear of   Fear of thunderstorms is known as astraphobia. Individuals who fear thunderstorms listen intently to weather forecasts and may call their local weather bureau with questions. Such individuals will avoid going outdoors when thunderstorms are predicted. Some phobics hide in a closet or under a bed during a thunderstorm, and some become incontinent as a result of their fear. Some fear the noise of the thunder, and others fear injury or death.
See also THUNDER, FEAR OF; THUNDERBOLT, FEAR OF.

tic   A tic is a frequent involuntary muscle spasm. A person with a tic is known as a tiquer. Tics can occur in any muscle group, but the ones most noticeable to others involve the facial muscles, such as the eyelids or the lips. Additionally, tics may also be vocal, involving sudden, uncontrollable, loud sounds. The individual who has a tic may not be aware of it until someone else points it out. On the other hand, once an individual knows that he has a tic, he may become very anxious and embarrassed about it and may even avoid people, becoming a social phobic. Some people associate tics with nervousness and anxiety, and to some extent this is correct. Tics may disappear in time as the individual becomes more relaxed. Tics are treated with therapy to determine the conditions causing the anxiety, then with behavioral methods of relaxation training and SYSTEMATIC DESENSITIZATION. Tics are characteristic of Gilles de la TOURETTE SYNDROME, a disorder of the nervous system; they can also be brought about by certain drugs.

See also BEHAVIOR THERAPY.

tied up, fear of being   Fear of being tied up is known as merinthophobia. This fear may relate to fears of burglars, of violent crime, of being out of control, and of helplessness. It is a close relative of claustrophobia. The fear may also relate to a sexual fear, as being tied up is sometimes involved in certain sadomasochistic sexual practices.

See also BOUND, FEAR OF BEING; BURGLARS, FEAR OF; SEXUAL FEARS.

time, fear of   Fear of time is known as CHRONOPHOBIA. This fear relates to fear of time passing, either too slowly or too rapidly; free time, either too much or too little; or running out of time.

time management   Realistically prioritizing projects and avoiding procrastination. *Time management* was a catch phrase during the 1980s and 1990s as organizations strove to educate employees, particularly middle managers, to avoid the anxiety caused by a growing need to define business priorities and deal with the paper pileup in their in-boxes. Seminars on time management were often sponsored by date book and planning calendar manufacturers who offered products as solutions to the time-management problem. However, it persists and is compounded today by staff reductions that add responsibilities to existing jobs and computerization that has raised the standards for quality and promises to reduce time and effort when in fact the opposite is often true.

Another aspect of time management is the growing anxiety of balancing career and family. While this is applicable to both men and women, it is a particular problem for the working mother (both

---

TIME MANAGEMENT TIPS TO REDUCE ANXIETIES

- Set realistic goals; don't overestimate what you can do.
- Don't procrastinate.
- Establish priorities; make lists.
- Pace yourself; set "time-outs."

---

married and single) who continues to have major responsibility for running the home and caring for the children as she shares the family's financial burden.

See also PERFECTION; PROCRASTINATION; STRESS; WORKPLACE.

timidity   A lasting tendency to show fearful behavior.

See also SHYNESS; SOCIAL PHOBIA.

TM   See MEDITATION; TRANSCENDENTAL MEDITATION.

TMJ   See TEMPOROMANDIBULAR JOINT SYNDROME; TEETH GRINDING.

toads, fear of   The toad has a long history as an object of fear and superstition. It has been viewed as a repulsive, warty creature as well as a favorite item in witchcraft. Ozark Mountain-area residents once feared that killing toads would cause cows to give blood instead of milk. Others feared, erroneously, that they would break out in warts if they touched toads.

See also FROGS, FEAR OF.

tobacco, fear of   Modern fears of tobacco are related to the evidence that smoking is a risk factor in the development of many types of cancer, lung diseases, and heart disease. Historically, in certain parts of Russia the tobacco plant was feared because some individuals believed that it was inhabited by the devil.

See also DEVIL, FEAR OF; SMOKING, FEAR OF.

tocophobia Fear of childbirth.

See also CHILDBIRTH, FEAR OF.

toilet training The process of teaching a child to use the toilet for urination and bowel movements. It can be an exercise in anxiety for both the child and the parent because children generally will become toilet trained when they are ready. There is little to gain in speeding up the toilet-training process at a very early age or holding the child to a rigid, demanding schedule.

Some professionals connect toilet training, if it occurs when a child is too young or is too harsh in its administration, with later behavior that is obedient but resentful. On the other hand, a child whose toilet training was delayed may develop a self-centered personality.

Even when trained, accidents happen, and children can revert to soiling or wetting, particularly when they are anxious or under stress. The best advice for parents is to begin toilet training at a reasonable age; view the training as an educational experience; exhibit a great deal of patience; support performance with praises and rewards; and accept occasional accidents even after training is completed.

Behavior therapists have perfected toilet-training methods to the point where 80–90 percent of interventions are successful in brief periods of training.

See also BED-WETTING; PARENTING.

tombs, fear of The common fear of tombs relates to the fear of being buried alive, of suffocation, and of death.

See also BURIED ALIVE, FEAR OF; SUFFOCATION, FEAR OF.

tombstones, fear of Fear of tombstones is known as placophobia. This fear is related to a fear of cemeteries and, indirectly, to a fear of death.

See also CEMETERIES, FEAR OF; DEATH, FEAR OF.

tomophobia Fear of surgical operations.

See also SURGICAL OPERATIONS, FEAR OF.

tonitrophobia Fear of thunder.

See also THUNDER, FEAR OF; THUNDERBOLT, FEAR OF; THUNDERSTORMS, FEAR OF.

toothache, fear of Having a toothache causes everyone to feel a certain amount of anxiety and uneasiness. However, fear of a toothache extends beyond just the pain in the mouth. Some individuals fear any kind of PAIN. Many people fear having a toothache because they fear going to the DENTIST. Some fear that they will need an INJECTION if the dentist does any drilling as preparation for filling a cavity in a tooth. Some fear the drilling, or even the sound of the drill. Some who have blood or injury phobia fear that they will see blood during the visit to the dentist, or that they may receive further injury in the course of treatment. Some fear having a tooth pulled. Some fear toothaches because going to the dentist means confinement in the dental chair. During treatment for the toothache, they will be covered with a waterproof apron and may have any number of devices working in their mouth at one time. All these prospects make some individuals fearful because there will be no easy escape from the situation once they are in it. Anxiety sometimes arises when the individual is uncertain which tooth is hurting. A visit to the dentist, even if one is fearful of dentists and dentistry, will do much to allay the fear aroused by a toothache. Dentists today have many techniques to help fearful patients relax enough and to treat dental problems with a minimum of pain.

See also DENTAL FEARS; PAIN, ANXIETY AND DEPRESSION IN; PAIN, FEAR OF.

topological vs. functional approach See MEDICAL MODEL.

topophobia Fear of certain places. This term also refers to a fear of being on the stage, or STAGE FRIGHT.

See also PLACES, FEAR OF.

tornadoes, fear of Fear of tornadoes is known as lilapsophobia.

See also HURRICANE, FEAR OF; THUNDER, FEAR OF; THUNDERBOLT, FEAR OF; THUNDERSTORMS, FEAR OF.

touched, fear of being   Fear of being touched is known as haphephobia; haptephobia; hapnophobia; aphephobia, haptophobia; and thixophobia. This fear may relate to a fear of contamination or to a sexual fear.

Tourette's syndrome   Gilles de la Tourette syndrome is a movement disorder characterized by repeated, involuntary, rapid movements of various muscle groups and by vocal tics, such as barks, sniffs, or grunts. It was first described by the French physician Georges Gilles de la Tourette in 1885. The cause of the disorder is unknown. The syndrome is a lifelong disorder that often begins during adolescence with eye spasms. Tourette individuals and members of their families may have an increased incidence of compulsive rituals and agoraphobia, although the role of these disorders in the disease is not understood.

See also AGORAPHOBIA; OBSESSIVE-COMPULSIVE DISORDER.

toxicophobia, toxiphobia, and toxophobia   Fear of poison.

See also POISON, FEAR OF.

trains, fear of   Fear of trains is known as siderodromophobia. Some people fear long waits for trains. Others fear trains for their noise, motion, or speed. Individuals who fear trains may fear being in an enclosed space, feel trapped on a train, or fear becoming ill and being seen by others with no place to take refuge. Some fear trains if there are no toilet facilities available. Fear of trains is fairly common among agoraphobics. However, trains may be less frightening if they stop frequently at stations and have corridors and a toilet. If there are toilets, though, some people may fear being seen entering the toilet booth.

See also ENCLOSED PLACES, FEAR OF; MOTION, FEAR OF; SPEED, FEAR OF; WAITS, FEAR OF LONG.

trait anxiety   A general, persistent pattern of responding with ANXIETY. Trait anxiety resembles timidity and indicates a habitual tendency to be anxious over a long period of time in many situations, also known as A-trait. The person with a high A-trait perceives more situations as threatening than a person who is low in A-trait. Phobic individuals are high in A-trait. The term is used in research projects to differentiate between types of anxieties. For example, American psychologist Charles Spielberger has developed an instrument to measure A-trait vs. A-state anxiety, the latter being more situational and varied over time.

See also STATE ANXIETY; STATE-TRAIT ANXIETY INVENTORY (STAI).

Spielberger, C. D., et al., *The State-Trait Anxiety Inventory* (Riverside, CA: Consulting Psychologists Press, 1970).

trait theorists   See PERSONALITY DISORDERS (chart).

tranquilizers   Tranquilizers are pharmacological agents that act on the emotional state of the individual, quieting or calming the person without affecting clarity of consciousness. As a class of drugs, tranquilizers can be divided into two groups: antianxiety agents (called ANXIOLYTICS or "minor" tranquilizers) and antipsychotic drugs (called neuroleptics or "major" tranquilizers).

Antianxiety Agents (Minor Tranquilizers)

BENZODIAZEPINE compounds such as DIAZEPAM and ALPRAZOLAM are generally favored over SEDATIVES (such as BARBITURATES) for relief of ANXIETY. Phenothiazines (which are antipsychotic drugs) are sometimes used to relieve anxiety, although their side effects are a major drawback. A group of drugs known as BETA-ADRENERGIC BLOCKERS (e.g., PROPRANOLOL) may also have some effectiveness in relieving anxiety.

Antipsychotic Drugs
(Major Tranquilizers; Neuroleptics)

The neuroleptic drugs have gone a long way in advancing psychiatric health care. They are often used to maintain an individual's psychiatric state at a level to allow some enjoyment of life. There are four main subgroups of neuroleptic drugs: the PHENOTHIAZINES, the butyrophenones, the thioxanthenes, and the nearly obsolete rauwolfia alkaloids. Most of these drugs have major side effects and physiological effects with prolonged use.

See also HYPNOTICS; MEPROBAMATE; TARDIVE DYSKINESIA.

transactional analysis (TA) A type of group therapy developed by Eric Berne, a Canadian-born American psychoanalyst (1910–70). TA is based on his theory of personality structure. According to Berne, the personality is made up of three constructs: the parent, the adult, and the child, which correspond in a general way to Freud's superego, ego, and id. The parent ego state can be nurturing or critical ("I love you," "You should . . ."); the adult is practical and evaluative, taking in information and making rational decisions; and the child is primarily made up of feelings, expressing them naturally, as they occur, or adaptively, as they have been socialized.

In TA, group members make determined efforts to change their patterns of communications (or "transactions") with others by engaging in "games" and role-playing scenarios that manipulate the way they choose to use their different ego states. Berne believed that transactions were frequently set up to satisfy only one person's needs, not allowing for mutual fulfillment. This unhealthy pattern can stem from an individual's fear of presenting the true self to another person and risking rejection.

Berne also stressed that each person is responsible for accepting himself and his own feelings (I'm OK), and realizing that other people must do the same (You're OK). He believed that psychological disturbance would occur when the personality was inappropriately dominated by the parent, adult, or child ego state.

The essence of TA therapy is to help the individual develop psychological independence and identity, marked by awareness of self and others and spontaneity and intimacy in his or her lifestyle rather than the more common human coping attributes of manipulation and self-defeating behavior.

TA sees anxiety as the outcome of faulty lifestyle, hence the focus is on modification of lifestyle rather than specific symptoms. For example, Eric Berne, in his book about transactional analysis (*Games People Play*), did not make one reference to anxiety in the subject index.

transcendental meditation (TM) A type of MEDITATION developed in the early 1960s by Maharishi Mahesh Yogi. Some individuals find relief from their anxieties in TM. In TM, the individual sits quietly with eyes closed and focuses his attention solely on the verbal repetition of a special sound or "mantra." The person practicing TM usually spends about twenty minutes, twice a day, engaged in meditation. This process of focused attention should have the effect of taking the person's mind away from his anxieties and worries, helping him to relax. TM claims benefits of reducing anxiety and aggression and possibly changing certain body states by slowing metabolism and heart rate and lowering blood pressure.

transcutaneal nerve stimulation (TENS) See PAIN, ANXIETY AND DEPRESSION IN.

transference A process through which the individual displaces to the therapist feelings, attitudes, and attributes of a significant attachment figure from the past, usually a parent, and then responds to the therapist accordingly. In a general way, transference refers to the tendency to transfer to the current relationship with the therapist feelings and emotions that belonged to a past relationship. An understanding and resolution of transference is a necessary part of all psychoanalytic therapies. FREUD believed that transference was a necessary part of analysis because new forms of the old conflicts could be brought to consciousness, where they could be relieved, understood, and worked through to a more satisfactory resolution. During this process, the sources for anxieties and phobic behaviors are often discovered. Transference thus becomes a major aspect of psychoanalytic work.

See also COUNTERTRANSFERENCE; PSYCHOANALYSIS.

transfusion, fear of blood See BLOOD TRANSFUSION, FEAR OF.

transitional object An object an infant selects because of its anxiety-reducing qualities, such as a "security blanket" or soft doll. The child perceives that the transitional object acts as a defense against outside threats and is especially important at bedtime or during periods of regression to an earlier phase of development. The term was introduced by Donald W. Winnicott, an English pediatrician and psychoanalyst, in the early 1950s.

See also SOTERIA.

trauma Real or imaginary incidents that occur and affect the individual's later life and ability to cope with anxieties. Freud believed that all neurotic illnesses were the result of early psychological trauma. The term *trauma* comes from the Greek word meaning "wound." In medicine, the word trauma refers to a violent shock or severe wound. Traumatic stress is associated with phobia onset in about 3 percent of cases, with panic disorder in about 4 percent of cases, and with OBSESSIVE-COMPULSIVE DISORDER in more than 10 percent of cases.

traumatophobia Fear of injury.

See also INJURY, FEAR OF.

travel, fear of Fear of travel is known as hedonophobia or hodophobia. Individuals who are afraid to travel are likely to be fearful of new things and new places. They may also have a fear of moving. Generally, agoraphobics fear traveling. Also, some individuals who fear airplanes, trains, or moving vehicles fear traveling.

See also FLYING, FEAR OF; TRAINS, FEAR OF.

trees, fear of Fear of trees is known as dendrophobia. Individuals who fear trees may fear certain landscapes, may fear being hit on the head with apples, acorns or other falling objects, or may fear blossoms or fruit from the trees. Some individuals fear seeing trees with leaves turning brown; this may represent a fear of death to them. In mythology and legends, trees were considered special, mysterious places because they gave shade and shelter; wood from trees enabled man to build fires, homes, and bridges, and the fruit of trees fed man and animals. Trees were a link from earth to heaven, and tree worship was an early form of religion. The common practice to "touch wood" for luck is a carryover from tree worship. Early believers tried to summon friendly spirits by knocking on the trunks of the tree.

See also SUPERNATURAL, FEARS OF.

trembling, fear of/tremophobia Fear of trembling is known as tremophobia. Individuals who fear trembling in themselves are afraid that others will notice and be critical or frightened. Some people who have trembling hands due to disease, such as Parkinson's, fear that if they are seen trembling they will appear helpless. Some who fear trembling in others are afraid that the other individual may have a contagious disease or may act violently.

See also SOCIAL PHOBIA.

trichinosis, fear of Fear of trichinosis is known as trichinophobia. Trichinosis is caused by eating undercooked pork containing *Trichinella spiralis*. In the early stages, symptoms of trichinosis are diarrhea, nausea, colic, and fever, and later, stiffness, pain, swelling of the muscles, fever, sweating, and insomnia. Some individuals avoid eating certain foods because of this fear.

See also EATING, FEAR OF; FOOD, FEAR OF.

trichopathophobia Fear of hair disease is known as trichopathophobia.

See also HAIR, FEAR OF; HAIR DISEASE, FEAR OF.

trichophobia Fear of hair is known as trichophobia.

See also HAIR, FEAR OF.

trichotillomania See HABITS; HAIR FEARS.

tricyclic antidepressants One of a group of ANTIDEPRESSANTS whose molecular structure is characterized by three fused rings. Tricyclic DRUGS are effective primarily in alleviating ENDOGENOUS DEPRESSION. Imipramine, one of the tricyclic antidepressive drugs, has been used extensively for treatment of panic disorder. While results are mixed, it does seem to be effective in the short run with a small percentage of people who have panic reactions.

triskaidekaphobia   Fear of the number thirteen also known as terdekaphobia.

See also THIRTEEN, FEAR OF THE NUMBER.

tropophobia   Fear of moving or of making changes.

See also CHANGE, FEAR OF; MOVING, FEAR OF; NEWNESS, FEAR OF.

trypanophobia   Fear of injections.

See also INJECTIONS, FEAR OF; NEEDLES, FEAR OF.

tuberculosis, fear of   Fear of tuberculosis is known as tuberculophobia, or phthisiophobia. Tuberculosis is an infectious disease caused by *Mycobacterium tuberculosis,* or the tubercle bacillus. The disease is characterized by formation of tubercles, or pockets of infection, in the tissues throughout the body. Persons who have tuberculosis tend to cough, spreading moist particles of the TB germ into the air. Some of these particles continue floating in the air until they enter the respiratory passages of another person and find their way down to the lungs to cause common tuberculosis. The germ may remain dormant for many years before making the individual ill. The bacillus responsible for tuberculosis was identified in 1882, but it was not until 1944 that the drug streptomycin was found, which was effective against tuberculosis. Now that most forms of tuberculosis are treatable, the disease is not as feared as it once was. During the 19th and the early part of the 20th century, tuberculosis was feared by many. Individuals who had tuberculosis were often isolated or sent to sanitariums where they could be outdoors; even before the discovery of streptomycin, it was known that the tubercle bacillus is killed by exposure to sunlight. Tuberculosis was always

more common among families subject to poor housing, overcrowding and generally substandard health conditions, although it has affected all socio-economic groups because of contagion.

The word tuberculosis, used alone, has come to mean pulmonary, or lung, tuberculosis. However, the infection may take hold elsewhere in the body. When it does, the problem is identified by the area it affects: tuberculosis of the bones, intestinal tuberculosis, tuberculous meningitis (in the brain), tuberculous peritonitis (in the membrane surrounding the abdomen), or tuberculosis of the urinary tract.

See also DISEASE, FEAR OF; HEALTH ANXIETY; ILLNESS PHOBIA.

twins, fear and phobias in   Studies of panic disorders in families and among twins suggest that such disorders may have a genetic basis. Individuals who have relatives with panic attacks are more likely to suffer similar attacks than are those with no such family history. Identical twins, who have exactly the same genetic makeup, are more likely to both suffer from panic attacks than are fraternal twins, who share the same environment and are genetically no more similar than other siblings.

Through studying twins, researchers have determined that some fears and phobias may have genetic contributions. In a study of 15 pairs of identical twins reared apart, University of Minnesota researchers found three sets of twins with multiple phobias. Two siblings were afraid of water and heights and had claustrophobia. Three other pairs of twins shared a single phobia. One of these pairs, although separated soon after birth, worked out the same solution to their water phobia: they waded into the ocean backward, averting their eyes from the surf. Researchers speculate that evolution selected genes for such fears because they conferred a survival advantage on early man. For example, avoiding heights and water helped them avoid falling off cliffs and drowning.

Genes may make individuals more sensitive to their environment. At the Medical College of Virginia, where 3,798 pairs of identical and fraternal twins were examined, identical twins were found to have a higher concordance than fraternal twins for anxiety and depression. While these results are interesting and suggestive, scientifically acceptable twin studies are rare and usually consist of too few subjects to allow one to generalize the results.

Type A behavior pattern   See CORONARY-PRONE TYPE-A BEHAVIOR.

tyramine   A substance found in some foods that may contribute to causing HEADACHES and may interfere with the effectiveness of certain ANTIDEPRESSANT medications. Tyramine affects the constriction or expansion of blood vessels. This reaction to certain foods occurs only in about 30 percent of people who have migraine headaches. Since there is no way to know whether an individual is in this sensitive group, physicians generally recommend that all migraine sufferers and individuals who take MAO (MONOAMINE OXIDASE) INHIBITORS as mood elevators for depression avoid ripened cheeses, including cheddar, Emmentaler, Gruyère, Stilton, Brie, and Camembert (cottage, cream, and some processed cheeses are permitted), herring, chocolate, vinegar (except white vinegar), anything fermented, pickled, or marinated, sour cream, yogurt, nuts, peanut butter, seeds, pods of broad beans (lima, navy, pinto, garbanzo, and pea), any foods containing large amounts of monosodium glutamate (some Asian foods), onions, and canned figs.

tyrants, fear of   Fear of tyrants is known as tyrannophobia. Many individuals who have survived such an oppressive environment develop this fear.

UFOs, fear of Individuals and groups of people often become anxious when they think they see unidentified flying objects (UFOs). Anxieties about sightings of UFOs are related to the times. For example, in the 20th century, when space travel became a reality, there was increased speculation about life on other planets, and some came to fear invasion by alien beings. However, in the Middle Ages, when dragon shapes were seen in the clouds or a fiery cross was sighted in the sky, people feared divine retribution. Fear of UFOs is an example of fear of the unknown, because no one is sure where the UFOs are from or exactly what they are.

See also FLYING THINGS, FEAR OF; UNKNOWN, FEAR OF.

ulcers A peptic ulcer is a sore on the lining of the stomach or duodenum (the first part of the small intestine). In the recent past (until the late 20th century), most doctors believed that severe stress and spicy foods caused the development of ulcers, but physicians now know that these theories were wrong. However, once an ulcer develops, stress and anxiety can exacerbate the existing pain, as stress and anxiety can also do with headaches and many other pain syndromes.

Most ulcers have one of two primary causes. First, the common bacteria, *Helicobacter pylori,* are responsible for 60–90 percent of all ulcers. Australian physicians Marshall and Warren discovered that *H. pylori* was responsible for most ulcers in 1982, however, they were ridiculed for years until their theory was finally tested and found to be a sound one. It is now believed that in the United States, 20 percent of those under age 40 harbor *H. pylori* in their gastrointestinal system, as do about 50 percent of those over age 60. Most people with *H. pylori* in their systems do not develop ulcers, but some do. It is unknown why some individuals with the bacteria develop ulcers and others do not.

The second primary cause of ulcers is the use of nonsteroidal antiiflammatory medications (NSAIDs), whether they are prescribed NSAID drugs or over-the-counter drugs such as aspirin, ibuprofen, naproxen sodium, and ketoprofen. These NSAIDs are responsible for nearly all remaining ulcers. In addition, among elderly individuals who take NSAIDs, these drugs may be responsible for the majority of ulcers.

Symptoms and Diagnostic Path

Some patients have no symptoms. When there are symptoms, the outstanding symptom of peptic ulcers is stomach pain, which usually occurs at certain regular times and is relieved by eating. The pain may be a gnawing and dull ache, and it may come and go over a period of days or weeks. Constipation, nausea, vomiting, loss of appetite, and even anemia may also be symptoms of ulcers. Other symptoms include poor appetite, weight loss, and a bloated feeling, as well as frequent burping. Symptoms may be severe or mild.

Many people suffer with symptoms of ulcers for five years or longer before seeking medical advice.

Physicians who suspect an ulcer generally order tests, such as an upper gastrointestinal study or endoscopy. The upper gastrointestinal study is an X-ray of the esophagus (the food tube that connects to the stomach), the stomach, and the duodenum. Barium is administered so it will highlight the organs and show the presence of an ulcer clearly. An *endoscopy* is an examination of the esophagus, stomach, and duodenum through the insertion of a tiny tube (endoscope) down the throat and into the esophagus and other organs while the patient is under a mild anesthesia.

If the patient may have *H. pylori,* the physician can test for the presence of these bacteria, either through taking a tissue sample during an endoscopy or through analyzing the blood or stool of the patient. In addition, there is a breath test for *H. pylori.*

Emergency symptoms.   According to the National Digestive Diseases Information Clearinghouse, individuals with any of the following symptoms should immediately contact their doctor because they could be signs of a perforated ulcer, a bleeding ulcer, or an ulcer that is obstructing food on its path outside the stomach. These symptoms include

- sharp, sudden, persistent stomach pain
- bloody or black stools
- bloody vomit or vomit that looks like coffee grounds

Treatment Options and Outlook

A variety of drugs are available to alleviate ulcer symptoms and bring them under control. Acid-suppressing drugs such as histamine 2 blockers as well as drugs known as proton pump inhibitors are often part of the treatment. These drugs cause the stomach to release less acid and give the stomach lining a chance to heal. A stomach-lining protector drug such as bismuth subsalicylate (Pepto Bismol or other brand names) may be given. However, if *H. pylori* is the cause of the ulcer, antibiotics are administered to kill the bacteria. Treatment to eradicate *H. pylori* takes at least two to three weeks.

If the cause of the ulcer is the use of NSAIDs, these drugs are usually discontinued, and H2 blockers and proton pump inhibitors are used to allow the lining of the stomach or duodenum a chance to heal. However, in some cases, individuals need to continue to take NSAIDs, and in such cases, the physician may prescribe drugs such as misoprostol (Cytotec) to reduce the amount of stomach acid and prevent gastric ulcers in those individuals.

Whatever the cause of the ulcer, some behaviors should be avoided by the person with an ulcer; for example, smoking and the use of alcohol may aggravate ulcers and delay healing. As a result, individuals who have ulcers are usually advised to abstain from both tobacco and alcohol.

If the individual is also very anxious, which can worsen an existing ulcer, psychotherapy is recommended to help reduce anxiety, tension, and anger.

Some individuals require surgery for their ulcers.

Risk Factors and Preventive Measures

Individuals who have had ulcers in the past are at risk for developing them again. Patients who have chronic pain for which they take an NSAID medication are also at risk for developing an ulcer. Alcohol can increase the risk for the development of ulcers, because alcohol irritates the stomach lining. In addition, if patients take NSAIDs in combination with corticosteroids, such as prednisone, the risk of the development of an ulcer is increased seven times. Patients who take a combination of NSAIDs and anticoagulants such as warfarin (Coumodin) have a 12 times greater risk of developing an ulcer. In such cases, physicians and patients themselves should be aware of ulcer symptoms so they can be reported if they occur and any ulcer that develops can be treated.

It is best to always wash the hands after using the bathroom and before eating to avoid the transmission of *H. pylori.*

See also STRESS MANAGEMENT.

Minocha, Anil, MD, and Christine Adamec, *The Encyclopedia of the Digestive System and Digestive Disorders* (New York: Facts On File, Inc., 2004).

unconditional positive regard   A term used by client-centered therapists to denote the worth of the individual under treatment. Unconditional positive regard is used interchangeably with the words "ACCEPTANCE" and "prizing" and is viewed as necessary to promote effective psychotherapy. If a person is raised in a situation without unconditional positive regard, he or she is more likely to develop anxieties. For example, phobic individuals often come from families in which they received criticism (the opposite of unconditional positive regard).

See also CLIENT-CENTERED THERAPY; FAMILY THERAPY.

unconditioned response   Behavior that is elicited reliably following an UNCONDITIONED STIMULUS and not based upon learning. Classical CONDITIONING theory views the unconditioned response as automatic and resulting from innate sensory processes not governed by experience. With conditioning (the association of a new stimulus with the unconditioned stimulus) new learning occurs. For example, the sight and smell of food is an unconditioned stimulus for hunger and salivation. With learning by association, words and images (conditioned stimuli) can come to elicit hunger and salivation (conditioned response). Many anxieties are thought to be acquired in this manner so that an apparently neutral stimulus (such a seeing the brake lights on an automobile) may come to elicit anxiety (part of the unconditioned response) because of its association with the trauma and suffering of an automobile accident.

unconditioned stimulus   A signal that provokes a response not based on learning. For example, experiments have shown that a child's fear of loud noises could be generalized (transferred) to a white rat. This is done by pairing the presentation of loud noises with the white rat. For effective conditioning, the conditioned stimulus (white rat) must be presented slightly before the onset of the unconditioned stimulus. With repetition, the conditioned stimulus will come to elicit a portion of the unconditioned response. The loud noise was the unconditioned stimulus because it existed before the experiment. Loud noise, falling, certain animals, being out of control, suffocation, and perhaps a few other fears are unconditioned stimuli that elicit the unconditioned response of fear.

See also CONDITIONING; UNCONDITIONED RESPONSE.

unconscious, the   The designation given by Sigmund Freud to a region of the psyche comprising all mental functions and products of which the individual is unaware and which he or she cannot recognize or remember at will. The unconscious in its most simplistic form refers to the availability (or unavailability) of psychic material. Some individuals develop phobias because of unconscious memories.

See also PSYCHOANALYSIS.

undressing (in front of someone), fear of   Fear of undressing in front of someone is known as dishabillophobia. The term also includes the fear of being seen in a less than fully clothed state, or being seen in a state of disarray. There may be some sexual connotations to this fear, insofar as the individual fears being seen in the nude. There also may be an obsession with wanting to be seen only at one's best.

unknown, fear of the   Fear of the unknown is a common thread among many phobias and anxieties. For example, fears of death and darkness represent fears of the unknown, as do fears of outer space and the future. Many anxieties in illness conditions are fears of the unknown, as the individual does not know whether medications will work or what complications might occur. Some who fear traveling or doing new activities have these fears because of their fears of the unknown.

See also CANCER, FEAR OF; NEWNESS, FEAR OF; OUTER SPACE, FEAR OF.

uranophobia   Fear of heaven.

See also HEAVEN, FEAR OF.

urinary incontinence   The inability to control the evacuation of liquids from the body. Urinary incontinence affects people of all age groups; an overwhelming number are women. Incontinence is a cause of extreme anxiety for the individual who must cope with a problem that can mean personal FRUSTRATION, emotional devastation, social isolation, and physical discomfort.

Incontinence in Women

According to a study by the National Institutes of Health in 1996, 26 percent of women age 30–59 have experienced episodes of urinary incontinence. The most common form, *stress* incontinence, occurs when the pelvic floor muscles become weak and no longer support the bladder. Without support, such everyday events as laughing, coughing, or lifting a heavy object apply stress or pressure to the bladder. In younger women, childbirth often causes the weakening of the pelvic floor muscles; estrogen deficiency brought on by menopause is often a cause of this weakness in older women.

Urge incontinence usually occurs during involuntary bladder contractions, which may be caused by a variety of problems, including urinary infections. Help is available from urogynecologists (gynecologists who are specially trained in problems of the urinary tract). Surgical techniques for correcting the problem have advanced dramatically in the latter part of the 20th century. Exercises are also sometimes prescribed (Kegel exercises) by gynecologists to help restore muscle strength, particularly in milder cases. These exercises involve tightening the urinary muscles (as if to stop urination) repeatedly for five to 10 minutes at a time, with repetitions several times a day.

Urinary incontinence is sometimes a symptom of nervousness. In many cases, anxiety can affect one's control over urinating, either causing one to feel the urge very frequently or not being able to void even though the urge seems present.

Understanding the mechanisms for the problem can help one cope with its attendant anxieties. A thorough examination by a physician is essential to determine possible physical causes.

Male Incontinence

In males, the cause of incontinence is frequently an enlarged prostate gland that presses on and blocks the duct through which urine leaves the body. As more urine accumulates in the bladder and dilates it, the bladder cannot hold any more and it dribbles out. After surgical removal of the prostate, nerves controlling the urinary sphincter may be damaged, leaving a man incontinent. Radiation treatment for cancer also sometimes contributes to male incontinence.

Symptoms of a prostate problem in a man include having trouble emptying the bladder; getting up several times a night to urinate; taking longer than usual to start urination and after starting, noticing a very slow stream; dribbling after finishing urination and having the urge to void again just after voiding; or rectal pain. Any man experiencing these symptoms should consult a physician.

Elderly people sometimes develop urinary incontinence because of neurological reasons, such as

---

RELIEVING ANXIETIES OF INCONTINENCE

- Keep a diary for a week or so noting how often you urinate, how often you leak, and what you are doing at the time of the incontinent episode. You may notice a pattern, either in the length of time you are able to wait between episodes or in the circumstances surrounding these episodes.

- If you find that you are wet every hour or two, empty your bladder as completely as you can every 30 to 60 minutes.

- Try to stop the urge to void at unscheduled times by relaxing or distracting yourself. For example, if you are at home, do a small household task until the urge to urinate passes; then void according to your planned schedule.

- If you become too uncomfortable to wait until the scheduled time, go and use the toilet, but void again at the next scheduled time.

- Reward yourself for staying on schedule. It takes effort, practice and patience.

- Keep a daily log to track your progress. If you are aware of fewer incontinent episodes and have been able to void on schedule for about a week, extend the times between voiding periods by 30 minutes or so each week.

- Extend the intervals until you reach a comfortable schedule, such as two-and-a-half to three hours between voidings.

---

after a stroke or a spinal-cord injury. In some cases, a diuretic prescribed for high blood pressure or heart failure may increase the output of urine and lead to incontinence.

In the late 1990s, advertisements for "adult diapers" and products to hide the problem of incontinence attest to the fact that urinary incontinence is a common problem and, as the elderly population increases, its prevalence will increase. According to the *Harvard Health Letter,* many people resign themselves to wearing adult diapers or pads because they mistakenly believe that urinary incontinence is a normal part of aging. Others are too embarrassed to bring it to their doctor's attention or fear that invasive tests and surgery might result. Those who have the condition can benefit from discussing the problem with a caring and knowledgeable physician.

See also BED-WETTING; HORMONE REPLACEMENT THERAPY; MENOPAUSE.

urinating, fear of   Fear of urinating is called urophobia. This can be a very embarrassing and debilitating fear and is a form of SOCIAL ANXIETY. It occurs more frequently in men than in women. Fear of urinating usually occurs when others are present when the person wants to or is actually urinating. Some men may be unable to urinate in front of any other person, and many waste time waiting at work and other places until the men's room becomes empty. Some women cannot urinate in any toilet except in their own home. In its extreme form, the fear of urinating with another person nearby necessitates holding in urine through the working day until the home bathroom can be used. The victim often avoids parties, restaurants, and social gatherings that might involve long commitments of time. The fear usually develops as a form of social anxiety and is often traced to adolescent fears of public exposure and possible criticism, which are common in youth.

Some individuals fear that they might urinate when far from a toilet, wet themselves, and be seen by others. Such individuals may visit public toilets frequently and try to urinate so that they will not feel the urge far from a toilet. They may avoid social gatherings where no toilets are readily available. Individuals who become incontinent, or unable to control the flow of their urine, due to illness or injury fear odor and offending others. Urinary incontinence due to physical causes can be treated with medication, surgery, or commercially available adult diapers. Other fears relating to urination can be treated with psychotherapy and/or behavioral therapy quite effectively. DESENSITIZATION, RELAXATION THERAPY, and EXPOSURE THERAPY are generally helpful.

See also DEFECATION, FEAR OF.

vaccination, fear of Fear of vaccination is known as vacciniophobia. Some people fear vaccination because they fear INJECTION. Some fear NEEDLES or devices that pierce the skin. Some fear unwanted side effects from vaccination. Those who have ILLNESS PHOBIA or fear of CONTAMINATION may fear contamination from the inoculation device. Many people worldwide fear being vaccinated and taking their infants for vaccination because they do not understand what vaccination means.

Valium An antianxiety drug. Chemically known as DIAZEPAM, Valium is in a class of drugs called BENZODIAZEPINES. It has been used more extensively and for more conditions than any of the other benzodiazepines.

See also ANTIANXIETY DRUGS.

vampire A fearsome creature that sucks blood, usually at night. There is a deep, archetypal fear of images that can transform from humans to animals and back to human form. Vampires seem to fall into this category of creatures. During the Middle Ages, vampires, like werewolves, were highly feared. The fear that the vampires would come after one during the NIGHT in quest of blood, the only food on which he could survive, brings with it all of the psychological associations with human BLOOD. To be drained of blood is to be drained of strength and one's soul. Offering blood was associated with sacrifice in many cultures; primitive gods demanded blood. Blood, symbolized by wine, plays a part in the Christian communion service. Blood, particularly the blood of a virgin, was considered to have healing properties during the Middle Ages. Warriors drank the blood of their fallen victims.

Blood is also a sexual symbol, directly associated with MENSTRUATION and less directly with SEMEN. The vampire's bite of a sleeper, usually of the opposite sex, is linked closely with a kiss. In *The Vampire Myth*, James Twitchell described this aspect of the vampire as a symbol: "The myth is loaded with sexual excitement; yet there is no mention of sexuality. It is sex without genitalia, sex without confusion, sex without responsibility, sex without guilt, sex without love—better yet, sex without mention." This quality of the legend created an eager Victorian audience for *Dracula*, since they could read it as an exciting and superficially proper story that both expressed and suppressed their sexual desire, GUILT, and ANXIETY.

The hero of Bram Stoker's *Dracula* described the tension between attraction and revulsion that has made the vampire a significant psychological symbol: "There was something about them that made me uneasy, some longing and at the same time some deadly fear. I felt in my heart a wicked burning desire that they would kiss me with those red lips."

Because of this unique combination of qualities, the vampire has been referred to as a "psychic sponge" and "a kind of incestuous, necrophilous, oral-anal-sadistic-all-in-wrestling match." The historical inspiration for Stoker's Count Dracula was Vlad the Impaler, a 15th-century ruler of Wallachia, who was a cruel and violent man, but not a vampire. The concept of a bloodsucking evil spirit goes back to antiquity, but the vampire as thought of today emerged in 16th-century eastern Europe, where the Magyar term *vampir* came into use. The vampire legend spread throughout Europe and was taken up by literary figures such as Goethe, Baudelaire, Byron, and Dumas. *Dracula* was published in 1897 and subsequently adapted for the stage and then the screen, with Bela Lugosi playing the evil count. Over 200 vampire films have been produced throughout the world. An upsurge of interest in vampires in the 1970s produced still more vampire-related plays, films, books, and music.

Centuries ago, certain practical situations involving DEATH and BURIAL may have contributed to fears about vampires. As premature burial was a possibility before the days of modern technology to confirm death, live bodies were sometimes actually interred. Incidents of multiple deaths from the PLAGUE and less-than-formal burials added to these fears. Actual cases of body snatching in eras when corpses were not available for medical research also contributed to the belief that some dead bodies did not stay in their proper places.

Unusual cases of deviant individuals who desire human blood further reinforced vampire fears. Elizabeth Bathory, a Hungarian countess, tortured and killed over 600 young women, partly for her own perverse enjoyment and partly from the belief that their blood would prolong her youth and beauty. More common psychological deviations that endorsed a belief and fear of vampires were necrophagia (eating dead bodies), necrosadism (mutilation of dead bodies), and necrophilia (sexual intercourse with a corpse).

Historically, superstitions have led many people to believe in and fear vampires. Many cultures follow rituals resulting from beliefs that CORPSES will wander freely from their GRAVES with ill intentions toward the living, particularly relatives, unless proper precautions are taken. Suicides, excommunicants, and criminals were thought to be assured of this fate after death.

Fear of vampires may also symbolize a type of human relationship that is both attractive and frightening. A particularly magnetic individual can influence and hold others in his power, draining away talent, energy, and individuality for his own purposes.

The vampire's superhuman strength, capacity to live forever, and ability to create other vampires at will appeal to the basic human fear of death and desire for eternal life. However, those who fear vampires also believe that the vampire is vulnerable. They believe that silver, a CRUCIFIX, or garlic can ward off a vampire, and that one can end the eternal existence of a vampire by driving a stake through his heart, if he can be found sleeping in his coffin.

See also SUPERNATURAL, FEAR OF; WEREWOLVES, FEAR OF; WITCHES AND WITCHCRAFT, FEAR OF.

vasovagal response   See BLOOD AND BLOOD-INJURY PHOBIA; FAINTING.

vegetables, fear of   Fear of vegetables is known as lachanophobia. This fear may be related to fears of certain foods or fear of eating things that have grown in the ground. Some individuals who fear pollution in the air or water may fear eating vegetables.

See also FOODS, FEAR OF; POLLUTION, FEAR OF.

vehicles, fear of   Fear of vehicles is known as amaxophobia or ochophobia. This fear may relate to driving a car or riding in a car or other form of transportation such as trains, boats, buses, and airplanes. This phobia may be part of a fear of motion or a fear of being in an enclosed place. Sometimes the fear relates to being away from a safe place (such as home) or a fear of losing emotional or psychological control in front of others.

See also AUTOMOBILES, FEAR OF; FLYING, FEAR OF; MOTION, FEAR OF; TRAINS, FEAR OF.

venereal disease, fear of   Fear of venereal disease is known as cypridophobia, cypriphobia, and venereophobia. A venereal disease is a SEXUALLY TRANSMITTED DISEASE (STD). Individuals who have a phobia of venereal disease may also fear prostitutes and sexual activity. The outbreak of acquired immunodeficiency syndrome (AIDS) in the 1980s has increased many persons' fears of sexually transmitted diseases and has caused them to take measures to prevent their spread.

See also PROSTITUTES, FEAR OF; SEXUAL INTERCOURSE, FEAR OF; SEXUALLY TRANSMITTED DISEASES, FEAR OF; SYPHILLIS, FEAR OF.

venustaphobia   Fear of beautiful women.

See also WOMEN, FEAR OF.

verbal slips   See SLIPS OF THE TONGUE, FEAR OF.

verbophobia   See WORDS, FEAR OF.

vermiphobia   See WORMS, FEAR OF.

vertigo, fear of   Fear of vertigo is known as illyngophobia. Vertigo is an anxiety response to a situation and also the medical term that refers to dizziness. Dizziness is a common symptom of many phobics, such as those who fear heights, looking over cliffs, bridges, elevators, and riding in automobiles. Many agoraphobics experience dizziness when venturing out alone or to places they fear. Fear of dizziness is known as dinophobia.

Individuals who experience vertigo because of phobias should sit, lie down, or brace themselves. Sitting with one's head between one's legs is a good precaution if one thinks he or she may lose consciousness, but it may not stop the dizziness. Behavior therapies sometimes help individuals who experience dizziness because of phobic reactions.

See also ACROPHOBIA; AGORAPHOBIA; DIZZINESS, FEAR OF; HEIGHTS, FEAR OF.

vestiphobia   Fear of clothing, either one's own or that of another. Some individuals fear particular items of clothing, such as textured items, silk or velvet garments, undergarments, or a particular style of clothing.

See also CLOTHING, FEAR OF.

virginity, fear of losing   Fear of losing one's virginity is known as esodophobia or primeisodophobia. Attitudes toward retaining virginity until marriage have changed with the new morality of the 1960s and 1970s, but the experience of defloration may still be frightening for many reasons. Women's fears are in part a product and reflection of male anxiety. In many cultures, men have wanted to marry virgins as insurance that children from the union will be their own. A male attitude that inexperience is synonymous with purity of mind encourages the feeling that a virgin bride will more truly belong to her husband. Male fear of defloration has arisen from the feeling that sexual intercourse, particularly with a virgin, will rob a man of his strength and put him in the woman's power. Loss of virginity may be more directly frightening to a woman because of the threat of pain and pregnancy and also the fear of appearing inexperienced or awkward. Defloration also represents a sudden, radical change, a break with the past that is the end of girlhood.

virgins, fear of   Fear of virgins is known as parthenophobia.

See also YOUNG GIRLS, FEAR OF.

virgivitiphobia   Fear of rape.

See also RAPE, FEAR OF.

vitricophobia   Fear of a stepfather.

See also STEPFATHER, FEAR OF.

vomiting, fear of   Fear of vomiting is known as emetophobia. Fear of vomiting is considered a social phobia. Some individuals fear that they might vomit in public or that they may see others vomiting. Some individuals who have this phobia avoid any situation that is remotely likely to provoke vomiting in themselves or in others, such as going on a boat or riding in a car.

See also FOOD, FEAR OF; NAUSEA; SWALLOWING, FEAR OF.

voodoo, fears in   Voodoo is a religion and set of related superstitions that include many different magical figures and frightening beliefs. Witches, sorcerers, medicine men, and priests all have their places in voodoo. At night, believers fear bloodsucking spirits call loupgarous. Noon is frightening, too, because the human shadow, which believers equate with the soul, disappears. The soul, called the *gros bon ange*, or "large good angel," is a fragile, easily disturbed link between the body and the conscience, the *ti bon ange* or "good little angel." Magical spells aim at the soul in the culture of Haiti, where voodoo was transplanted from African tribal beliefs. Any sort of enmity may be a source for possession by evil spirits resulting in violent mental and physical symptoms.

Believers undertake initiation into voodoo, a type of purified intentional form of possession, as a safeguard against calamity, a way to please ancestral spirits, and a way to get the powerful voodoo spirits known as *loa* on one's side. The initiation procedure is essentially a ritual death, a giving up of the soul, which is imagined to leave the body to be captured in a sacred vessel where it will be protected by the gods and safe from evildoers. The initiate is then considered to be a servant of the *loa*, reborn with a new name. The ceremony, during which the initiate learns the secrets and rites of voodoo, is long and complex, lasting over a month. At the end of this time the initiate is called a *hounsi canzo*, the initiated spouse of the god. On the death of an initiate, a rite called *dessounin* releases his spirits into the water of death and again captures his soul in a sacred vessel to await resurrection.

A fear associated with voodoo belief is the possibility of becoming a ZOMBIE, a walking corpse in the service of the person who has reanimated him. The initiation and *dessounin* rituals are supposed to give some sort of assurance that the initiate's soul is safe from anyone with the magical powers to create a zombie.

See also ZOMBIE, FEAR OF BECOMING A.

waits, fear of long Fear of long waits is known as macrophobia. Long waits are common in modern society; people are asked to wait on the telephone, in stores, at airports, and for one another. Many individuals become impatient and anxious; some are so fearful of waiting that they will not frequent busy restaurants; they take scheduled transportation so that waits are predictable. This fear may be somewhat related to AGORAPHOBIA, in which individuals do not like to be away from a secure place for very long. Also, some individuals experience a feeling of being trapped while in line, as they cannot leave easily and still maintain their place.

See also TRAINS, FEAR OF.

waking up, fear of not Fear of not waking up may be related to a fear of death. Many individuals who fear going to bed or going to sleep have this fear. Fear of not waking up is somewhat common in physically ill and elderly persons and in individuals who have anxieties about death. This fear is related to fear of going to sleep.

See also BED, FEAR OF; DEATH, FEAR OF; SLEEP, FEAR OF.

walking, fear of Fear of walking and/or standing upright is known as basiphobia, basistasiphobia, stasiphobia, and stasibasiphobia. The fear is often related to fear of falling, collapse, and death.

See also BLOCQ'S SYNDROME; STANDING UPRIGHT, FEAR OF.

war, fear of Fear of war is not a phobia, since it is realistic and quite sane. The fear of war appears to follow an inverse "U" function with age. That is, the fear at very young ages (before age five or so) is low but increases in intensity up to about ages 12 to 14, when it peaks. At late adolescence and young adulthood it declines considerably, and at adulthood it is low relative to economic and health fears.

Studies of junior and senior high school students indicate that fear about nuclear war is intense in about 30 percent of that population. On a worldwide basis, this intensity seems to be steady across countries. If children's fears are ranked, the fear of nuclear war is always second or third. The only item to be ranked consistently higher is the fear of parents dying. The high intensity of this fear together with its pervasive nature would classify fear of nuclear war as a major social stressor to children worldwide. The effects on family life and social and psychological development may become evident soon.

war exposure See POST-TRAUMATIC STRESS DISORDER.

warlock See WITCHES AND WITCHCRAFT, FEAR OF.

war neuroses See POST-TRAUMATIC STRESS DISORDER.

washing, fear of Fear of washing is known as ablutophobia. Usually this refers to fear of washing oneself, or even of thinking of washing oneself. However, it also refers to a fear of viewing another individual washing himself or herself.

wasps, fear of Fear of wasps is known as spheksophobia. Individuals who fear wasps often fear stings, pain, bees, or flying insects in general.

See also BEES, FEAR OF; FLYING THINGS, FEAR OF.

water, fear of Fear of water is known as aquaphobia and hydrophobia. Fear of water is related to a fear of drowning and a fear of death. In some aquaphobes, this fear extends to bathing, swimming, or seeing or imagining bodies of water or running water. Fear of water is a learned fear. By age three, children are ready to learn to swim, unless they become fearful of water, particularly deep water. Some individuals who fear water may have had a traumatic experience in a pool or other body of water. They may have been cautioned not to go near the water. Some children of water phobics are taught at an early age to also be afraid of the water and consequently grow up fearful. Many individuals are phobic about going into water that is over their head, even though they know how to swim. Some fear putting their faces in the water and getting water up their nose; when this happens, they have a rapid heartbeat and breathe faster, often inhaling water, which further increases their anxiety. Some individuals avoid boat rides because they are afraid of falling out into deep water. Some panic when flying in an airplane over water. For still others, fear of water may be related to a fear of landscape that includes a body of water. Former aquaphobics advise persons afraid of water to take swimming lessons to become more comfortable in water and to learn to relax and breathe correctly.

The word for fear of water, hydrophobia, may have been the first term using the suffix "phobia" to denote a morbid fear. The term was used by Celsus, a Roman medical authority of the first century A.D., who said of hydrophobia, "There is just one remedy, to throw the patient unawares into a water tank which he has not seen beforehand. If he cannot swim, let him sink under and drink, then lift him out; if he can swim, push him under at intervals so that he drinks his fill of water even against his will; for so his thirst and dread of water are removed at the same time."

See also LAKES, FEAR OF; LANDSCAPES, FEAR OF CERTAIN.

waves, fear of Fear of waves is known as cymophobia. This fear may be related to a fear of motion, a fear of water, or a fear of landscapes in which water and leaves are prominent.

See also LANDSCAPE, FEAR OF CERTAIN; MOTION, FEAR OF; WATER, FEAR OF.

weakness, fear of Fear of weakness is known as asthenophobia. Individuals fear weakness because they fear losing physical, emotional, social, or political control.

See also LOSING CONTROL, FEAR OF.

wealth, fear of See MONEY, FEAR OF.

weekend depression A type of DEPRESSION that some individuals experience when away from their work. Particularly for some individuals who live alone, facing solitude creates anxiety.

To overcome the anxiety of being alone, as well as the change in mood from the work week when one is surrounded by people, individuals can schedule pleasurable activities with FRIENDS or like-minded others so that they will not spend the entire weekend alone. Weekend depression should be distinguished from chronic depression, or SEASONAL AFFECTIVE DISORDER, which affects some individuals during dark months of the year.

See also AFFECTIVE DISORDERS.

weight gain, fear of Fear of gaining weight is known as obesophobia or pocrescophobia. Some individuals who fear gaining weight stop eating, or eat very little, a condition known as ANOREXIA NERVOSA, which is found most often among teenage girls. Some individuals who fear gaining weight practice BULIMIA, or bingeing and purging, in which they gorge themselves and then induce vomiting. Fear of weight gain is related to concerns about one's body image and social fears.

See also EATING DISORDERS.

weight loss, fear of Fear of losing weight may be related to a fear of illness or a fear of death. Some individuals fear "losing themselves" or disappearing if they lose too much weight. Fear of losing weight may be related to a fear of being out of control of one's body.

See also ANOREXIA NERVOSA; BULIMIA; EATING DISORDERS; LOSING CONTROL, FEAR OF; WEIGHT GAIN, FEAR OF.

werewolves   Some men fear that they will become werewolves, and some people fear that they will be devoured by werewolves. Like satyrs, centaurs, and mermaids, werewolves are a combination of human being and animal. The word werewolf is derived from the Anglo-Saxon term *wer,* or man. Fear of werewolves in the classical world were recorded by Herodotus, Plato, and Pliny. Fear of werewolves developed out of fear of wolves, which are known to be ferocious, cruel, and howling. Werewolves change back and forth between human and animal form. Legends describe different methods of metamorphosis or change. Methods include removal of a hide of human skin, donning of an animal skin under the power of a full moon, rolling on the ground in the nude, and immersion in water. Some legends say that transformation is complete, while others say that in animal form the werewolf has some human characteristics and vice versa. Reversal occurs at daybreak or if the animal is injured or killed. In their animal form, werewolves murder and devour human flesh.

There are many fears and beliefs about the creation of werewolves. The metamorphosis may be voluntary or involuntary. Ritual may be used to call up an evil spirit; some may use fire, or application of a magic ointment to the skin. Some may urinate in a circle under the full moon; some become werewolves because they were conceived under a new moon. Others say that werewolves are created by contact with a magic flower, drinking from a stream where wolves commonly go, from a wolf paw print, eating wolf meat or brains, or making a pact with the devil. Still other origins of werewolves may be heredity, living an evil life, and self-hypnosis. Some say that a priest or saint can turn a living human being into a werewolf, that witchcraft and sorcery can turn an innocent victim into a werewolf, and that evil individuals may return after death as werewolves.

Once a man becomes a werewolf, he can be cured of his affliction through religious exorcism, shedding blood, being addressed by his human name, and abstaining from eating flesh for years. In some legends werewolves can be killed by ordinary means; other stories say that they must be shot with a consecrated silver bullet.

There have been cases of lycanthropy, a mental disorder more common in the past, in which the victim believes himself to be a wolf and runs wild, eats raw meat, rapes, murders, and eats human flesh.

In one anthropological study of the werewolf, researchers suggested that the werewolf image is a product of the COLLECTIVE UNCONSCIOUS, which has recorded a transition in man's evolution from a pastoral, vegetarian society to a meat-eating, possibly cannibalistic, aggressive culture in which males took females by violence.

See also SUPERNATURAL, FEAR OF; WITCHES AND WITCHCRAFT, FEAR OF.

wet dreams, fear of   Fear of wet dreams is known as oneirogmophobia. Wet dreams are nocturnal emissions from the penis while asleep. Some men fear wet dreams because of embarrassment that others might become aware of the problem. Nocturnal emissions are part of normal adolescent development and are brought about by accumulated normal tensions that find release during sleep.

See also DREAMS, FEAR OF; SEXUAL FEARS.

whirlpools, fear of   Fear of whirlpools is known as dinophobia. This fear may be related to a fear of motion or of water. The swirling action of a whirlpool may make the individual feel that he will be swept away; the fear may also represent a fear of being out of control.

See also MOTION, FEAR OF; WATER, FEAR OF.

whistling, fear of   Those who fear whistling may do so because whistling is associated with unseen dangers, such as the sound of wind or the hiss of a snake. Whistling has been associated with the casting of spells and has been called the devil's music. On the other hand, whistling in the dark or in other frightening situations historically has been thought to work a kind of countermagic to keep away evil.

In some cultures, if a woman whistles, bad luck is thought to follow. In the theater, newspaper offices, mines, and on shipboard, whistling is thought to bring misfortune.

See also SOUNDS, FEAR OF.

white, fear of the color   Fear of the color white is known as leukophobia. To some individuals, paleness may represent ill health. White may also symbolize virginity to some individuals who fear virginity or chastity. White may also represent ghosts to those who fear the supernatural.

See also COLORS, FEAR OF.

"white coat" hypertension   A term referring to high blood pressure caused by anxiety induced by visiting a doctor's office. Some individuals appear to be victims of "white coat" hypertension, a condition in which blood pressure is generally normal but increases when the patient is tested by a doctor. This type of hypertension occurs more frequently among young women than men. Because of this type of anxiety, some patients may be misclassified as hypertensives.

Some individuals' blood pressure may rise in the doctor's office or clinic because they are fearful of doctors or fearful of the surroundings, including laboratories where they might encounter needles or blood-testing devices (particularly if they are phobic about these things).

There may be some aspect of conditioned response involved in "white coat" hypertension, too. When a subject's blood pressure is checked once, it may be high due to anxiety. In a small number of cases, the remembrance that it was high once may lead to anxiety that in turn causes the blood pressure to rise. Some experience a rise in blood pressure just by looking at the blood pressure (sphygmomanometer) cuff.

See also DOCTORS, FEAR OF; HIGH BLOOD PRESSURE, FEAR OF.

Pickering, Thomas G., et al., "How Common Is White Coat Hypertension?" *Journal of the American Medical Association* (January 8, 1988), pp. 225–228.

wiccaphobia   Fear of witches and witchcraft.
See also WITCHES AND WITCHCRAFT, FEAR OF.

wigs, fear of   Individuals who are phobic about wigs may become so frightened that they cannot come close to anyone wearing a wig or other false hairpiece. Wigs may be disturbing because they represent artificiality or disguise or because they resemble severed scalps. For some, hair has deep psychological associations. For example, some associate hair with youth, life, the seat of the soul, and strength; lack of hair represents aging, sacrifice, and punishment. Thus they find anything that covers, confines, or substitutes for hair may be distasteful. Fears of wigs may be closely related to fear of hair in general, or fear of damage to the hair.

See also HAIR, FEAR OF.

will therapy   A form of psychotherapy. Will therapy was introduced by Otto Rank, an Austrian psychoanalyst (1884–1939), in 1936. Rank viewed therapy as a way to free the individual from anxieties and fears and enable him or her to become independent and responsible, take risks, and achieve an ability for self-expression. He viewed life as a struggle to separate oneself psychologically from the mother, just as one is separated physically during birth. Rank viewed human behavior as derived from an innate condition of conflict between patterns of dependence and independence. Fear develops if one pattern predominates. For example, if independence (self-assertion) predominates, fear of isolation, being alone, and losing love develops. Guilt is also a byproduct of independence as individuals perceive themselves rejecting others. Will therapy is also known as Rankian therapy. This viewpoint on therapy has influenced many different approaches to HUMANISTIC PSYCHOLOGY.

See also BIRTH TRAUMA; CHARACTER TRAINING APPROACHES.

wind, fear of   Fear of wind is known as aerophobia or anemophobia. Individuals who fear wind may also fear all movement of air, such as tornadoes and hurricanes. They may fear being out of control and may be afraid that they will be pushed over by a strong wind and not be able to get to safety. They may fear falling or being helpless. Some fear injury from getting particles in their eyes during a windstorm. Some who fear wind also fear all types of inclement weather, such as rain, snow, or sleet.

See also HURRICANE, FEAR OF; TORNADO, FEAR OF.

wine, fear of Fear of wine is known as oenophobia or oinophobia. Some individuals who fear drinking wine fear becoming intoxicated or alcoholic. They may fear being out of control and perhaps doing something to embarrass themselves or others.

See also INTOXICATION, FEAR OF.

winged things, fear of Many people fear winged things, such as birds, bats, and flying insects because their quick, unpredictable movements simulate attack. Phobics react to this fear by keeping their houses closed to the point of discomfort, carrying umbrellas, or avoiding the out-of-doors and enclosed spaces where they might become trapped with a flying animal or insect.

See also BATS, FEAR OF; BEES, FEAR OF; BIRDS, FEAR OF; FLYING THINGS, FEAR OF; INSECTS, FEAR OF; WASPS, FEAR OF.

witches and witchcraft, fear of Historically, many individuals have feared witches and witchcraft because witches appear to be inherently evil and have mystical powers. Witches usually have been women, but male witches, known as warlocks, have also been feared. The term witchcraft derives from the Saxon word *wicca,* a contraction of *witega,* a prophet or wise person. Beliefs that have led to persistent fears include the notions that witches can inflict misfortune and a state of demonic possession on their victims, fly through the air, become invisible, appear in spectral form as seductive women or men, eat human flesh and have a mysterious link with animals. Some have believed that witches possessed the power of the EVIL EYE and that they could change winds to adversely affect sailors, cause the neighbor's wheat to rot, control certain animals, and turn themselves into animals. Witches were

believed to possess the power to make themselves invisible by means of magic given to them by the devil, and of harming others by thrusting nails into a waxen image representing them. Other beliefs include notions that witches can be identified by marks on their bodies and by the use of tests and ordeals.

Witchcraft was at times associated with religious heresy, condemned in the Bible and by religious authorities. In some cultures, witches were thought to be in league with the Devil, and to have had sexual intercourse with the Devil.

Beliefs in witches have persisted in part because such beliefs were a way to handle social strain and competition in primitive societies. Witchcraft provided a fear inducement for social control and promoted conformity within the society. Witchcraft provided an explanation for misfortune, which, unlike other systems of metaphysical belief, provided an opportunity for redress of wrongs. Beliefs in witches have also served a social and political purpose by punishing incompetent behavior and discouraging begging.

See also DELUSIONS; HALLUCINATIONS; INCUBUS; SUCCUBUS; SUPERNATURAL, FEAR OF.

Razali, S. M., "Depression and witchcraft induced psychosomatic symptoms." *European Psychiatry* 12, no. 8 (1997): pp. 420–421.

withdrawal effects of addictive substances Many people fear the effects of withdrawing from an addictive substance, whether they are using drugs on an abusive or therapeutic basis. There is a good basis for this fear because a series of symptoms often appears when a drug on which the user is physically dependent is abruptly stopped or severely reduced. Withdrawal symptoms occur most consistently in cases of addiction to central nervous system depressants or narcotics. Symptoms are usually opposite to the usual effects of the drugs (a rebound effect).

Intensity and duration of withdrawal symptoms usually depends on the susceptibility of the individual, properties of the particular drug, and the degree of addiction. Usually, shorter-acting substances, such as heroin, cause more rapidly developing, shorter, and more severe withdrawal symptoms than longer-lasting, more slowly eliminated drugs, such as methadone. If administered during heroin withdrawal, methadone can ease the intensity of the withdrawal experience.

Many people experience withdrawal symptoms after taking tranquilizers and other sedatives on a prescription basis. Withdrawal symptoms from depressants (barbiturates, SEDATIVES, and tranquilizers) may occur within a few hours after the drug is stopped. Physical weakness, anxiety, nausea and vomiting, dizziness, sleeplessness, hallucinations, delirium, delusions, and convulsions may occur as long as three days to a week following withdrawal and may last for many days. Withdrawal from the minor tranquilizers is similar but may take longer to develop. Not all symptoms that emerge after taking tranquilizers are withdrawal effects. Some may be anxiety that was repressed by the medications.

While certain substances, such as stimulant drugs (AMPHETAMINE and CAFFEINE), are considered more psychologically than physically addictive, sudden abstinence may produce withdrawal effects. These may include headache, stomach cramps, lethargy, chronic fatigue, and possibly severe emotional depression.

Individuals taking tricyclic ANTIDEPRESSANTS or MAO inhibitors should be aware that use of these drugs should be tapered off to avoid withdrawal reactions. If symptoms of withdrawal occur, the drugs may be reinstated temporarily and then tapered off even more gradually. The longer the period of use, the likelier there are to be withdrawal effects.

See also ADDICTION, FEAR OF; DEPRESSION; DRUG DEPENDENCE; LITHIUM; MANIC-DEPRESSIVE DISORDER.

Wolf Man, case of   A well-known case of animal phobia, documented in the writings of SIGMUND FREUD. In the case titled "From the History of an Infantile Neurosis," Freud analyzed the reasons for a young man's childhood animal phobia, religious obsession with conflicting blasphemous thoughts, and sudden change to unruly behavior. A key point in the analysis revealed a dream about wolves with fairy-tale symbolism. Using this dream, Freud attributed the young man's mental instability to early sexual experiences and observations and an erotic attachment to his father.

women, fear of   Fear of women is known as gynophobia, gynephobia, and feminophobia. Some men who fear women may have a fear of heterosexual activity or sexual intercourse. From a psychiatric point of view, they may have an unresolved conflict with their own mothers and hence fear all women. They may fear marriage because they will feel confined or limited in their activities.

See also MARRIAGE, FEAR OF; WOMEN, FEAR OF BEAUTIFUL.

women, fear of beautiful   Fear of beautiful women is known as venustaphobia.

See also WOMEN, FEAR OF.

woods, fear of   Fear of woods is known as hylophobia. Some may fear being lost in the woods or being in the woods after dark. They may feel closed in when they are surrounded by tall trees. This fear may be related to fear of trees or fear of landscape that includes wooded areas.

See also LANDSCAPE, FEAR OF; TREES, FEAR OF.

words, fear of   Fear of words is known as verbophobia or logophobia. This may be a fear of hearing words in general or of specific words. Those who have this fear become anxious even at the thought of certain words. Some individuals fear certain words because they fear that they will stammer or stutter when they try to say them.

See also NAMES, FEAR OF; STUTTERING, FEAR OF; TALKING, FEAR OF.

work, fear of   Fear of work is known as ergasiophobia, ergophobia, and ponophobia. The term ergasiophobia also sometimes refers to fear of surgical operations.

workplace violence   Murders, shootings, knifings, beatings, and other aggressive assaults and attacks that victimize employees, employers, or members of the public who are present in a workplace site. These incidents often result in severe anxiety for management as well as for coworkers. Workers may experience POST-TRAUMATIC STRESS DISORDER as a result of extreme incidents of violence that they have directly suffered from or witnessed.

Anxiety in the workplace is becoming more and more prevalent due to violence, assaults, and deviant behavior in this setting. Future research will assess the degree and extent of such problems and their effect on productivity.

According to the Federal Bureau of Investigation (FBI) in its report on workplace violence, the issue first came to the public's attention in 1986, when part-time letter carrier Patrick H. Sherrill, who thought he was going to be fired, walked into the Edmond, Oklahoma, post office where he worked and shot 14 people to death before killing himself. Other workplace crimes that subsequently held the public's attention were, for example, when four state lottery executives in Connecticut were killed by a lottery accountant in 1998 or when six people were killed by a plant worker at the Lockheed-Martin plant in Meridian, Mississippi, in 2003.

Despite the publicity and concern surrounding multiple homicides that occur in the workplace, homicides represent less than 1 percent of all incidents of workplace violence, while assaults that do not lead to death are far more common. Assaults at work represent about 94 percent of all cases of workplace violence, followed by robbery (4 percent) and rape/sexual assault (2 percent).

The FBI report stated, "According to popular opinion, sensational multiple homicides represent a very *small* number of workplace violent incidents. The majority of incidents that employees/managers have to deal with on a daily basis are lesser cases of assaults, domestic violence, stalking, threats, harassment (to include sexual harassment), and physical and/or emotional abuse that make no headlines."

Homicide. According to the National Institute of Occupational Safety and Health (NIOSH), homicide is the third leading cause of death on the job, and there were 609 homicides of workers in 2002. (The first leading cause of death was motor vehicle crashes of workers, followed by falls at the workplace). Workplace homicides peaked in 1994, at 1,080, and decreased thereafter. It is unknown why the numbers of homicides fell, but the drop may have occurred due to an increased awareness of employers about workplace violence as well as security measures that they began taking.

Researchers report a difference between the circumstances of workplace violence and those of other types of homicides that occur off the job. While most workplace homicides are robbery related, less than 10 percent of the homicides in the general population occur during a robbery. Also, about 50 percent of all murder victims in the general population are related to their assailants, whereas in the majority of workplace homicides, the assailant and the victim do not know each other.

According to the FBI, violence by criminals who are not associated with the workplace accounts for most (80 percent) of workplace homicides. The motive in most of these cases is theft, and the criminal is usually carrying a gun or other weapon. Individuals who are the most at risk for being victimized by this type of violence are taxi drivers (who have the highest risk of murder), followed by late-night retail or gas station clerks. Those who work at night are also at risk for homicide or assaults, as are those who deliver goods or services or who handle money.

Some workplace homicides are driven by an underlying desire for suicide. The perpetrator knows that if he kills others, the police are likely

---

FACTORS LEADING TO AN INCREASED RISK FOR VIOLENCE AT WORK

- interacting with the public
- exchanging money
- having a mobile workplace, such as a taxicab or a police cruiser
- delivering services or goods
- working late at night or during early morning hours
- working alone or among small numbers of people
- working in high crime areas
- guarding valuable goods or property
- dealing with unstable people
- working with volatile persons in healthcare, social services, or criminal justice settings

Source: Rugala, Eugene A., ed., *Workplace Violence: Issues in Response*. Washington, DC: U.S. Federal Bureau of Investigation, 2002.

to kill him. Law enforcement authorities call this "suicide by cop."

Assaults. Violence may lead to injuries on the job, such as when workers are attacked by clients or others. Assaults may be minor or may lead to permanent injuries. Nurses and other health-care workers are at a high risk for assaults, as are police officers, correctional officers and security guards.

Workers may also be assaulted as a result of incidents of domestic violence that then lead to violence against the worker in the workplace, as when the spouse or partner comes to the place of work and attacks the individual.

Predicting Violence at Work. According to Julian Barling in the *Encyclopaedia of Occupational Health and Safety,* Fourth Edition, a profile of a potentially violent or disgruntled employee may be created to predict possible workplace violence. Some potential characteristics of prospective offenders are

- male
- white
- age 20–33 years
- a loner
- an individual fascinated with guns

In addition, alcohol and/or drugs are often factors in precipitating violence in the workplace, when combined with the other risk factors. Some personal characteristics that are exhibited outside the workplace may also be predictive of violence at work. Such factors may include low self-esteem and an overall history of aggression toward one's family.

Other factors that may lead to on-the-job aggression and violence include high levels of STRESS, feelings of job insecurity, and perceptions that management and supervision policies are harsh and unjust. In addition, perceived crowding and extreme noise and heat on the job may lead to violence.

Prevention of Violence. Experts report that while no single strategy is appropriate for preventing violence in all workplaces, all workers and employers should assess the risk of violence in their workplaces and then take appropriate actions to reduce those risks and fears. A number of environmental, administrative, and behavioral strat-

---

INDICTORS OF PROBLEMATIC BEHAVIOR AT WORK THAT MAY LEAD TO VIOLENCE

- increasing belligerence
- ominous, specific threats
- hypersensitivity to criticism
- recent acquisition/fascination with weapons
- apparent obsession with a supervisor or coworker or employee grievance
- preoccupation with violent themes
- interest in recently publicized violent events
- outbursts of anger
- extreme disorganization
- noticeable changes in behavior
- homicidal/suicidal comments or threats

Source: Rugala, Eugene A., ed., *Workplace Violence: Issues in Response.* Washington, DC: U.S. Federal Bureau of Investigation, 2002.

---

egies may reduce the risk of workplace violence. These include good visibility and lighting within and outside the workplace, cash handling policies, the physical separation of customers or clients in some workplaces, the use of security devices and/or escort services, and employee training.

In one case, a company hired an organization to screen employees they were about to fire, so that high-risk employees could be identified and any danger minimized. All employees were told that the facility would be staffed by security officers subsequent to the layoff. The company identified four individuals about to be laid off to be at a high risk for workplace violence and escorted them off the premises prior to removing other employees. No violence occurred.

According to the FBI, there are some behavioral precursors of potentially risky behavior among workers, such as specific threats, noticeable behavioral changes, and a newfound fascination with weapons.

See also AGGRESSION; DOMESTIC VIOLENCE.

Barling, Julian, "Workplace Violence," in *Encyclopaedia of Occupational Health and Safety,* 4th ed. (Geneva, Switzerland: International Labor Organization, 1998).

Kahn, Ada P., *Encyclopedia of Work-Related Injuries, Illnesses, and Health Issues* (New York: Facts On File, Inc., 2004).

National Institute for Occupational Safety and Health, *Worker Health Chartbook, 2004* (Atlanta, GA: Centers for Disease Control and Prevention, September 2004).

Rugala, Eugene A., ed., *Workplace Violence: Issues in Response* (Washington, DC: U.S. Federal Bureau of Investigation, 2002).

worms, fear of   Fear of worms is known as vermiphobia or scoleciphobia. Those who have this fear may avoid going into certain places, such as near rivers, swamps, or even out on rainy days because they fear the presence of worms. Fear of worms may be related to a fear of slimy things, slime, or of other small creatures that thrive in the water or ground, such as frogs, toads, and lizards.

See also FROGS, FEAR OF; SLIME, FEAR OF.

worms, fear of infestation with   Fear of infestation with worms is known as helminthophobia or vermiphobia. Some individuals fear eating certain foods, such as pork, because they fear infestation with worms. This fear is related to a fear of contamination and of disease.

See also CONTAMINATION, FEAR OF; GERMS, FEAR OF; PARASITES, FEAR OF; TRICHINOSIS, FEAR OF.

worrying   Worrying is a common expression or symptom of ANXIETY. Persons troubled about a past, present, or future event may worry. Worrying is characterized by a feeling of uneasiness and mental discomfort. Excessive or highly irrational worry may be a symptom of an anxiety disorder. Individuals who have OBSESSIVE-COMPULSIVE DISORDER worry excessively. It is often worry that leads them to perform certain RITUALS such as repeated handwashing or checking for locked doors. Individuals who have AGORAPHOBIA are commonly worriers, as are social phobics. Agoraphobics may worry that they will not be able to get to a secure place, while social phobics may worry that they will be seen not looking their best or will find themselves in an embarrassing situation. Furthermore, anxiety sufferers almost always worry in anticipation of a situation in which they may experience anxiety.

Phobics and those who have obsessive-compulsive disorder differ in the ways in which they worry. Phobics have persistent worries around one theme, such as their phobic object or situation, whereas obsessive-compulsives have repetitive worries that lead them to actions (such as checking repeatedly to see that the door is locked). Obsessive-compulsives worry about remote, abstract, and future consequences of contact with an evoking stimuli, while phobics worry more about coming into contact with a specifically feared object or situation.

See RUMINATION; SOCIAL PHOBIA.

wrinkles, fear of getting   Fear of wrinkles or of getting wrinkles is known as rhytiphobia. The most feared wrinkles are those on the face, particularly around the eyes and mouth. Wrinkles are feared because they are a sign of AGING. Contemporary society places emphasis on youth as a standard of beauty, and many individuals, particularly women, fear losing their attractiveness because of wrinkles. Some who are so motivated seek reconstructive cosmetic surgery to remove wrinkles.

See also AGING, FEAR OF.

writer's block   Nearly all writers suffer from writer's block at some time, and many people fear that it will happen to them. Writer's block is a seeming inability to get started with a writing project, and, specifically, to set words down on paper. Anxiety about writing generally occurs before one begins to write; the hardest part of writing may be putting the first words down. Writer's block often includes many self-doubts. The writer may worry about the validity of his topic, his ability to communicate on paper, and acceptance by teachers, publishers, or readers.

Writer's block is sometimes difficult to recognize because it may hide behind other activities, such as procrastination. At the beginning of a writing project, one often thinks of many things to do except write. Overresearch is another symptom. One can always collect more information, visit one more library, or do one more interview as an excuse for staying away from the desk, typewriter, word processor, or paper and pencil.

The process of writing includes several steps: incubation, planning, research, organization, first draft, incubation, revision, and final draft. Before one starts, one unconsciously develops ideas and insights for the written material. This is the important incubation process. To bring these ideas out of the mind and onto paper and break writer's block, or overcome writer's anxiety, one must reach a state of relaxed, energized concentration in which one sets aside self-criticism and freely expresses creative thoughts.

There are a number of exercises one can perform to help reach the state of energized relaxation. Physical exercise energizes and is conducive to a relaxed state of mind. Meditation and imagery exercises are also very useful in reducing stress and minimizing the self-doubt that obstructs expression. Proper nutrition and enough sleep are similarly important to the writer.

Too much stress can paralyze the writer, and too little stress can lead to apathy. The ideal state of mind, the one that unblocks, is called "eustress," or good stress, by HANS SELYE, the Canadian author well known for writing about subjects relating to stress. That middle point in the stress spectrum is the state of relaxed concentration accompanied by energy. Because writing is hard work, one must be in the right mental framework to take risks and have confidence and self-esteem regarding one's own talents.

Another useful measure in avoiding writer's block is staying away from people who are critical of one's work or ideas in the early stage of the writing project. While their criticisms may be helpful later, early in the project criticism may be inhibitory.

A writer is usually his or her own best critic, and also a source of writing anxiety. One cannot get rid of the internal critic, but one can negotiate with it. The aim in any project is to express before you become critical and evaluate. The internal critic wants to evaluate before you put the ideas on paper. To overcome writer's block, try to keep the internal critic hidden until the revision stage.

(Adapted with permission from Sloane, Beverly LeBov, *Town Hall of California Reporter* [March–April 1987], pp. 6–7.)

writing, fear of Fear of writing is known as graphophobia. Some fear writing in public and having others observe as they write. They may fear criticism of their handwriting or of their posture while writing. Some fear writing anything at any time, because they do not want to commit their ideas to paper for others to see. Fear of writing is a SOCIAL PHOBIA and can be treated with behavior modification therapy.

See also BEHAVIOR THERAPY.

Xanax An anxiolytic and antidepressant drug. Chemically known as alprazolam, Xanax is a triazolobenzodiazepine belonging to the benzodiazepine class of drugs. It has antianxiety, antidepressant, and antipanic qualities.

See also ALPRAZOLAM; ANXIETY DRUGS; CORONARY BYPASS ANXIETY, POST-OPERATIVE; HEART ATTACK, ANXIETY FOLLOWING.

xanthophobia Fear of the color yellow and even the word *yellow*.

xenophobia Fear of strangers.
See also STRANGERS, FEAR OF.

xerophobia Fear of dryness.
See also DRYNESS, FEAR OF.

X-rays Fear of X-rays is known as radiophobia. Many people refuse to have diagnostic X-rays out of fear of harmful effects of radiation. This fear is becoming more prevalent as more people are aware of the possible effects of radiation. Dental X-rays are part of routine dental examinations, and chest X-rays are often part of routine physical examinations, particularly before admission to a hospital or before a surgical procedure.

See also RADIATION, FEAR OF.

xylophobia Fear of forests.
See also FORESTS, FEAR OF.

yoga Many individuals attempt to reduce anxieties through yoga, a system of beliefs and practices first described comprehensively in the third century B.C. Yoga is a way to balance energy and thus achieve relaxation, absence of anxiety, and better functioning. The most well-known form of yoga in the United States in Hatha yoga, which emphasizes physical well-being and mental concentration through stretching and breath-control exercises.

Yoga proposes that the human ego produces attachments, dependencies, obsessions, and fantasies that in turn produce anxiety. Meditation reduces the effects of these anxiety-producing mental conditions not by fighting them, but by allowing the meditator to observe them in a state of detachment. Like other meditation techniques, yoga focuses on a higher level of consciousness than the ordinary waking state.

Yoga exercises and postures are based on the observation that an individual's mental state is reflected in his physical posture. Thus exercises are intended to promote self-awareness of the condition of the body. Stimulation of the spinal column and glands is thought to create a feeling of well-being. Concentration on breathing is central to yoga practice; breath control helps the individual conserve and focus energy.

See also TRANSCENDENTAL MEDITATION.

young girls, fear of Fear of young girls is known as parthenophobia.

See also GIRLS, FEAR OF.

Z

zelophobia Fear of jealousy.
See also JEALOUSY, FEAR OF.

zemmiphobia Fear of the great mole rat.

Zen therapy Zen is one of many anxiety-reducing meditative techniques. Some individuals who begin Zen meditation are sufferers from depression who have not found help from other self-help techniques or therapy. Zen has been helpful to many individuals who have a strong sense of their own internal control. Meditation may be effective because extreme emotions produce a hypnotic, exclusive state of mind that meditation helps to break down. Also, meditation helps the individual balance arousal, tranquility, and objective observation of behavior and thoughts.

Zen, derived from the Chinese word for meditation, emerged as a Buddhist movement in seventh-century China and evolved further as a Japanese practice. Two central concepts of Zen are the individual's ability to control his mind and the desirability of a state of detachment. An attitude common to the meditative techniques is that man's usual state of awareness is clouded and distorted with fantasies, emotions, and associations that produce many psychological problems and result from the lack of control of thought processes. Zen meditative techniques known as *zazen* are intended to break through this distortion of perception. Zen meditation is practiced with the eyes open, the back upright and unsupported, the whole body in a firmly balanced position. The *zazan* technique may be a controlled method of breathing or concentration on a *koan*, a nonrational problem put to the meditator by a teacher. An example of a *koan* is the question: "While we know the sound of two hands clapping, what is the sound of one hand clapping?" The meditator is to think about the *koan* but not to force himself if his thoughts wander. He should simply observe his own thoughts in a detached state. The goal of this technique is a breakthrough in thought process. A transcendental state of mind called *satori,* which is beyond thought and language, is the ultimate goal. A meditator who reaches this state is capable of accepting daily experience with a clear mind and without dwelling on the past or events over which he has no control.
See also TRANSCENDENTAL MEDITATION.

zombie, fear of becoming a The fear of becoming a zombie results from the belief that a lifeless corpse can be reanimated by magic and continue a robot-like existence under the control of the person who revived it. The belief is founded in the set of superstitions surrounding the Voodoo religion of Haiti, which originated in African tribal tradition. Practitioners of voodoo believe that a voodoo priest can raise a dead corpse from the grave to create a zombie. Thus special burial precautions are taken, such as sewing the mouth of the body closed to prevent the spirit from escaping. Another belief that frightens many people is that a sorcerer can draw out a man's soul, cause his death, and subsequently have him in his power.

A recent expedition to Haiti uncovered a rational explanation for fear of becoming a zombie. Some voodoo experts know the secret of using a certain kind of poison from the puffer fish. The poison creates a condition simulating death. The victim is buried, exhumed, and, because the poison suppresses the activity of certain areas of the brain, the "corpse" continues his existence as a zombie.
See also VOODOO, FEAR OF.

zoophobia Fear of animals.
See also ANIMALS, FEAR OF.

RESOURCES

Acupuncture

See Complementary Therapies

Addictions

American Society of Addiction Medicine
4601 North Park Avenue
Upper Arcade #101
Chevy Chase, MD 20815
(301) 656-3920
http://www.asam.org

Cocaine Anonymous World Services Organization
P.O. Box 2000
Los Angeles, CA 90049
(310) 559-5833
http://www.ca.org

Debtors Anonymous
General Services Office
P.O. Box 920888
Needham, MA 02492
(781) 453-2743
http://www.debtorsanonymous.org

Gamblers Anonymous-International
International Services Office
P.O. Box 17173
Los Angeles, CA 90017
(213) 386-8789
http:/www.gamblersanonymous.org

Marijuana Anonymous World Services
P.O. Box 2912
Van Nuys, CA 91404
(800) 766-6779 (Toll-free)
http://www.marijuana-anonymous.org

Narcotics Anonymous World Services, Inc.
P.O. Box 9999
Van Nuys, CA 91409
(818) 773-9999
http://www.na.org

National Center on Addiction and Substance Abuse at Columbia University
633 Third Avenue
New York, NY 10017
(212) 841-5200
http://www.casacolumbia.org

National Center on Substance Abuse and Child Welfare
4940 Irvine Boulevard
Suite 202
Irvine, CA 92620
(714) 505-3525
http://www.ncsacw.samhsa.gov

National Clearinghouse for Alcohol and Drug Information (NCADI)
11426-28 Rockville Pike
Rockville, MD 20852
(800) 729-6686 (Toll-free)
http://www.health.org

National Council on Problem Gambling
216 G Street NE
Suite 200
Washington, DC 20002
(202) 547-9204
http://www.ncpgambling.org

National Institute on Drug Abuse
National Institutes of Health
6001 Executive Boulevard
Room 5213

Bethesda, MD 20892
(301) 443-1124
http://www.nida.nih.gov

**Substance Abuse and Mental Health Services
    Administration (SAMHSA)**
Department of Health and Human Services
1 Choke Cherry Road
Rockville, MD 20857
(240) 276-2000
http://www.samhsa.gov

Aging and Elder Care

AARP
601 E Street NW
Washington, DC 20049
(888) 687-2277
http://www.aarp.org

Administration on Aging
Department of Health and Human Services
200 Independence Avenue SW
Washington, DC 20201
(202) 619-0724
http://www.aoa.gov

Alliance for Aging Research
2021 K Street NW
Suite 305
Washington, DC 20006
(202) 293-2856
http://www.agingresearch.org

**National Association of State Units on
    Aging**
1201 15th Street NW
Suite 350
Washington, DC 20005
(202) 898-2578
http://www.nasua.org

National Institute on Aging
Building 31, Room 5C27
31 Center Drive, MSC 2292
Bethesda, MD 20892
(301) 496-1752
http://www.nia.nih.gov

Agoraphobia

**Agoraphobics Building Independent Lives
    (ABIL)**
2501 Fox Harbor Court
Richmond, VA 23235
(804) 353-3964
http://www.anxietysupport.org

Anxiety Disorders Association of America
8730 Georgia Avenue
Suite 600
Silver Spring, MD 20910
(240) 485-1001
http://www.adaa.org

AIDS (Acquired Immunodeficiency Syndrome)

AIDS Health Project
1930 Market Street
San Francisco, CA 94102
(415) 476-3902

AIDS Info
P.O. Box 6303
Rockville, MD 20849
(800) 448-0440 (Toll-free)
http://aidsinfo.nih.gov

Alcoholism

**Al-Anon/Alateen World Service
    Headquarters**
1600 Corporate Landing Parkway
Virginia Beach, VA 23454
(888) 425-2666 (Toll-free)
http://www.al-anon.alateen.org

Alcoholics Anonymous World Services, Inc.
Grand Central Station
P.O. Box 459
New York, NY 10163
(212) 870-3400
http://www.alcoholics-anonymous.org

**National Council on Alcoholism and Drug
    Dependence (NCADD)**
22 Cortlandt Street
Suite 801

New York, NY 10007
(212) 269-7797
http://www.ncadd.org

National Institute on Alcohol Abuse and Alcoholism
5635 Fishers Lane, MSC 9304
Bethesda, MD 20892
(301) 443-0595
http://www.niaaa.nih.gov

Allergies and Asthma

American Academy of Allergy, Asthma and Immunology
555 East Wells Street
Suite 1100
Milwaukee, WI 53202
(414) 272-6071
http://www.aaaai.org

American College of Allergy, Asthma and Immunology
85 Algonquin Road
Suite 550
Arlington Heights, IL 60005
(847) 427-1200
http://www.acoai.org

Asthma and Allergy Foundation of America
1233 20th Street
Suite 402
Washington, DC 20036
(202) 466-7643
http://www.aaia.org

National Institute of Allergy and Infectious Diseases
6610 Rockledge Drive
MSC 6612
Bethesda, MD 20892
(301) 402-3573
http://www3.niaid.nih.gov

Alzheimer's Disease

Alzheimer's Association
225 North Michigan Avenue
Floor 17
Chicago, IL 60601

(800) 272-3900 (Toll-free)
http://www.alz.org

Alzheimer's Disease Education and Referral Center
P.O. Box 8250
Silver Spring, MD 20907
(800) 438-4380 (Toll-free)
http://www.nia.nih.gov/alzheimers

Anxiety Disorders

Anxiety Disorders Association of America
8730 Georgia Avenue
Suite 600
Silver Spring, MD 20910
(240) 485-1001
http://www.adaa.org

Mood and Anxiety Disorder Programs (MAP)
National Institute of Mental Health
9000 Rockville Pike
Bethesda, MD 20892
(866) 627-6464 (Toll-free)
http://intramural.nimh.nih.gov/mood

Attention-Deficit/Hyperactivity Disorder

Attention Deficit Disorder Association
P.O. Box 543
Pottstown, PA 19464
(484) 945-2101
http://www.add.org

Children and Adults with Attention Deficit Disorder (CHADD)
8181 Professional Place
Suite 150
Landover, MD 20785
(800) 233-4050 (Toll-free)
http://www.chadd.org

Body Therapies

American Society for the Alexander Technique
P.O. Box 60008
Florence, MA 01062
(800) 473-0620 (Toll-free)

Feldenkrais Educational Foundation of North America
3611 Southwest Hood Avenue
Suite 100
Portland, OR 97239
(866) 221-6612 (Toll-free)
http://www.feldenkrais.com

Feldenkrais Movement Institute
721 The Alameda
Berkeley, CA 94707
(510) 527-2634
http://www.feldenkraisinstitute.org

The Rolf Institute of Structural Integration
5055 Chaparral Court
Suite 103
Boulder, CO 80301
(800) 530-8875
http://www.rolf.org

Cancer

American Cancer Society
1599 Clifton Road NE
Atlanta, GA 30329
(800) ACS-2345
http://www.cancer.org

National Cancer Institute
6166 Executive Boulevard
Room 3936A
Bethesda, MD 20892
(800)-4-CANCER
http://www.cancer.gov

Sloan Kettering Institute for Cancer Research
1275 York Avenue
New York, NY 10021
(212) 639-2000
http://www.mskcc.org/mskcc.html/5804.cfm

Susan G. Komen Breast Cancer Foundation
5055 LBJ Freeway
Suite 250
Dallas, TX 75244
(972) 855-1600
http://www.komen.org

Us TOO Interactive, Inc. (prostate cancer organization)
5003 Faireview Avenue
Downers Grove, IL 60515
(630) 795-1002
http://www.ustoo.com

Y-Me National Breast Cancer Organization
212 West Van Buren
Suite 1000
Chicago, IL 60607-3903
(312) 986-8338
http://www.y-me.org

Chronic Fatigue Syndrome

The CFIDS Association of America
P.O. Box 220398
Charlotte, NC 28222
(704) 365-2343
http://www.cfids.org

National Chronic Fatigue Syndrome and Fibromyalgia Association
P.O. Box 18426
Kansas City, MO 64133
(816) 313-2000
http://www.ndfsfa.org

Complementary Therapies

The Academy for Guided Imagery
30765 Pacific Coast Highway
Suite 369
Malibu, CA 90265
(800) 726-2070 (Toll-free)
http://www.academyforguidedimagery.com

Acupuncture and Oriental Medicine Alliance
6405 43rd Avenue Court NW
Suite A
Gig Harbor, WA 98335
(253) 851-6896
http://actuall.org

American Alliance for Health, Physical Education, Recreation and Dance
1900 Association Drive
Reston, VA 20191
(703) 476-3400
http://www.aahperd.org

American Art Therapy Association
5999 Stevenson Avenue
Alexandria, VA 22304
(888) 290-0878 (Toll-free)
http://www.artherapy.org

American Association of Naturopathic Physicians
4435 Wisconsin Avenue NW
Suite 403
Washington, DC 20016
(866) 538-2267 (Toll-free)
http://www.naturopathic.org

American Association of Oriental Medicine
P.O. Box 162340
Sacramento, CA 95816
(916) 443-4770
http://www.aaom.org

American Chiropractic Association
1701 Clarendon Boulevard
Arlington, VA 22209
(703) 276-8800
http://www.amerchiro.org

Association of Applied Psychophysiology and Biofeedback
10200 West 44th Avenue
Suite 304
Wheat Ridge, CO 80033
(800) 477-8892 (Toll-free)
http://www.aapb.org

Ayurvedic Institute
P.O. Box 23445
Albuquerque, NM 87192
(505) 291-9698
http://www.ayurveda.com

The Herb Research Foundation
4140 15th Street
Boulder, CO 80304
(303) 449-2265
http://www.herbsorg

Mind-body Medical Institute
824 Boylston Street
Chestnut Hill, MA 02467
(617) 941-0102
http://www.mbmi.org

National Center for Complementary and Alternative Medicine
National Institutes of Health
9000 Rockville Pike
Bethesda, MD 20892
(888) 644-6226 (Toll-free)
http://nccam.nih.gov

National Center for Homeopathy
801 North Fairfax Street
Suite 306
Alexandria, VA 22314
(877) 624-0613 (Toll-free)
http://www.homeopathic.org

Cults

Cult Hotline and Clinic
120 West 57th Street
New York, NY 10019
(212) 632-4640
http://cultclinic.org

Task Force on Missionaries & Cults
70 West 36th Street
Suite 700
New York, NY 10018
(212) 983-4800, extension 155
http://www.tfmc.us

Dental Fears

American Dental Association
211 East Chicago Avenue
Chicago, IL 60611
(312) 440-2500
http://www.ada.org

Depression

Depression and Bipolar Support Alliance
730 North Franklin
Suite 501
Chicago, IL 60610
(800) 826-3632 (Toll-free)
http://dbsalliance.org

Depression and Related Affective Disorders Association
8201 Greensboro Drive
Suite 300
McLean, VA 22102
(703) 610-9026
http://www.drada.org

International Foundation for Research & Education on Depression
7040 Bembe Beach Road
Suite 100
Annapolis, MD 21403
(404) 268-0044
http://www.ifred.org

National Institute for Mental Illness
6001 Executive Boulevard
Room 8184
MSC 9663
Bethesda, MD 20892
(866) 615-6464 (Toll-free)
http://www.nimh.nih.gov

Developmental Delays

National Down Syndrome Society
666 Broadway
New York, NY 10012
(212) 460-9330
http://www.ndss.org

National Organization on Fetal Alcohol Syndrome (NOFAS)
900 17th Street NW
Suite 910
Washington, DC 20006
(202) 785-4585
www.nofas.org

Domestic Violence

National Coalition Against Domestic Violence
1120 Lincoln Street
Suite 1603
Denver, CO 80203
(303) 839-1852
http://www.ncadv.org

National Council on Child Abuse and Family Violence
1025 Connecticut Avenue NW
Suite 1000
Washington, DC 20036
(202) 429-6695
http://www.nccafv.org

Dreams

International Association for the Study of Dreams
1672 University Avenue
Berkeley, CA 94703
(209) 724-0889
http://www.asdreams.org

Eating Disorders

National Association of Anorexia Nervosa and Related Disorders
P.O. Box 7
Highland Park, IL 60035
(847) 831-3438
http://www.anad.org

National Eating Disorders Association
603 Stewart Street
Suite 803
Seattle, WA 98101
(206) 382-3587
http://www.edap.org

Eye Movement Desensitization and Reprocessing (EMDR)

Eye Movement Desensitization and Reprocessing International Association
5806 Mesa Drive
Suite 360
Austin, TX 78731
(512) 451-5200
http://emdria.org

Flying, Fear of

The Institute for Psychology of Air Travel
551 Boylston Street
Suite 202

Boston, MA 02116
(617) 437-1811
http://fearlessflying.net

Grief

Caring Connections
National Hospice and Palliative Care Organization
1700 Diagonal Road
Suite 625
Alexandria, VA 22314
(800) 658-8896 (Toll-free)
http://www.caringinfo.com

Parents of Murdered Children
100 East Eighth Street
Suite B-41
Cincinnati, OH 45202
(513) 721-5683
http://pomc.org

Headaches

American Association for Headache Education
19 Mantua Road
Mt. Royal, NJ 08061
(856) 423-0258
http://www.achenet.org

National Headache Foundation
820 North Orleans
Suite 217
Chicago, IL 60610
(888) NHF-5552 (Toll-free)
http://www.headaches.org

Heart Disease

American Heart Association
7272 Greenville Avenue
Dallas, TX 75231
(800) 242-8721 (Toll-free)
http://www.americanheart.org

National Heart, Lung, and Blood Institute
P.O. Box 30105
Bethesda, MD 20824
(301) 592-8573
http://www.nhlbi.nih.gov

Hypnosis

American Society of Clinical Hypnosis
140 North Bloomingdale Road
Bloomingdale, IL 60108
(630) 980-4740
http://www.asch.net

Learning Disabilities

Learning Disabilities Association of America
4156 Library Road
Pittsburgh, PA 15234
(412) 341-1515
http://www.ldaamerica.org

Marriage and Family

American Association for Marriage and Family Therapy
112 South Alfred Street
Alexandria, VA 22314
(703) 838-9808
http://www.aamft.org

Mental Health

American Psychiatric Association
1000 Wilson Boulevard
Suite 1825
Arlington, VA 22209
(703) 907-7300
http://www.psych.org

American Psychological Association
750 First Street NE
Washington, DC 20002
(800) 374-2721 (Toll-free)
http://www.apa.org

National Alliance for the Mentally Ill
Colonial Place Three
2107 Wilson Boulevard
Suite 300
Arlington, VA 22201
(703) 524-7600
http://www.nami.org

National Institute of Mental Health
9000 Rockville Pike
Bethesda, MD 20892

(866) 627-6464 (Toll-free)
http://intramural.nimh.nih.gov

National Mental Health Association
2000 North Beauregard Street
Sixth Floor
Alexandria, VA 22311
(703) 684-7722
http://www.nmha.org

Mental Health: Children and Adolescents

American Academy of Child and Adolescent Psychiatry
3615 Wisconsin Avenue NW
Washington, DC 20016
(202) 966-7300
http://www.aacap.org

American Academy of Pediatrics
141 Northwest Point Boulevard
Elk Grove Village, IL 60007
(847) 434-4000
http://www.aap.org

Obsessive-Compulsive Disorder

Obsessive-Compulsive Foundation
676 State Street
New Haven, CT 06511
(203) 401-2070
http://www.foundation.org

Parkinson's Disease

American Parkinson's Disease Association
135 Parkinson Avenue
Staten Island, NY 10305
(800) 223-2732 (Toll-free)
http://www.apdaparkinson.org

National Parkinson Foundation, Inc.
1501 NW 9th Avenue/Bob Hope Road
Miami, FL 33136
(800) 327-4545 (Toll-free)
http://www.parkinson.org

Phobias

Anxiety Disorders of America
8730 Georgia Avenue
Suite 600
Silver Spring, MD 20910
(240) 485-1001
http://www.adaa.org

National Mental Health Association
2000 North Beauregard Street
Sixth Floor
Alexandria, VA 22311
(703) 684-7722
http://www.nmha.org

Post-traumatic Stress Disorder

Anxiety Disorders Association of America
8730 Georgia Avenue
Suite 600
Silver Spring, MD 20910
(240) 485-1001
http://www.adaa.org

Sexually Transmitted Diseases

American Social Health Association
P.O. Box 13827
Research Triangle Park, NC 27709
(919) 361-8400
http://www.ashastd.org

Sexuality Information and Education Council of the United States (SIECUS)
1706 R Street NW
Washington, DC 20009
(202) 265-2405
http://www.siecus.org

Skin and Hair

American Academy of Dermatology
P.O. Box 4014
Schaumburgh, IL 60618
(866) 503-SKIN
http://www.add.org

National Alopecia Areata Foundation
P.O. Box 150760
San Rafael, CA 94915

(415) 472-3780
http://www.naaf.org

Sleep

American Academy of Sleep Medicine
One Westbrook Corporate Center
Suite 920
Westchester, IL 60514
(708) 492-0930
http://www.aasmnet.org

American Sleep Apnea Association
1424 K Street NW
Suite 302
Washington, DC 20005
(202) 293-3650
http://www.sleepapnea.org

Narcolepsy Network
79 Main Street
North Kingstown, RI 92852
(888) 292-6522 (Toll-free)
http://www.narcolepsynetwork.org

National Sleep Foundation
1522 K Street NW
Suite 500

Washington, DC 20005
(202) 347-3471
http://www.sleepfoundation.org

Suicide

American Association of Suicidology
5221 Wisconsin Avenue NW
Washington, DC 20015
(202) 237-2280
http://www.suicidology.org

American Foundation for Suicide Prevention
120 Wall Street
22nd Floor
New York, NY 10005
(888) 333-AFSP (Toll-free)
http://www.asfsp.org

Volunteerism

Volunteer Management Associates
320 South Cedar Brook Road
Boulder, CO 80304
(720) 304-3637
http://www.volunteermanagement.com

BIBLIOGRAPHY

ACQUIRED IMMUNODEFICIENCY SYNDROME (AIDS)

Andre, Pierre. *People, Sex, HIV & AIDS: Social, Political, Philosophical and Moral Implications.* Huntington, WV: University Press, 1995.

Centers for Disease Control and Prevention. "Basic Statistics." Centers for Disease Control and Prevention. Available online. URL: http://www.cdc.govfhiv/topics/surveillancelbasic.htm. Downloaded May 11, 2006.

Greenwald, Jeffrey L., MD, et al. "A Rapid Review of Rapid HIV Antibody Tests." *Current Infectious Disease Reports* 8 (2006): pp. 125–131.

Joint United Nations Programme on HIV/AIDS, 25 Years of AIDS, 2006. Available online. URL:http://data.unaids.org/pub/FactSheet/2006/20060428_FS_25yearsofAIDS_en.pdf. Downloaded May 19, 2006.

United Nations General Assembly, Declaration of Commitment on HIV/AIDS: Five Years Later. Report of the Secretary General. March 26, 2006. Available online. URL: http://data.unaids.org/ pub/Report/2006/20060324_SGReport_GA-A60737_en.pdf. Downloaded May 19, 2006.

ADDICTIONS
(See also ALCOHOLISM; SMOKING)

Chopra, Deepak. *Overcoming Addictions: The Spiritual Solution.* New York: Harmony Books, 1997.

Gwinnell, Esther, MD, and Christine Adamec. *The Encyclopedia of Drug Abuse.* New York: Facts On File, Inc., 2007.

Johnston, Lloyd D., et al. *Monitoring the Future: National Survey Results on Drug Use, 1975–2004. Volume II: College Students & Adults Ages 19–45.* Bethesda, Md.: National Institute on Drug Abuse, National Institutes of Health, 2005.

Substance Abuse and Mental Health Services Administration. *Overview of Findings from the 2004 National Survey on Drug Use and Health.* Washington, DC: Department of Health and Human Services, September 2005.

Thombs, Dennis L. *Introduction to Addictive Behaviors.* 2nd ed. New York: The Guilford Press, 1999.

ADOPTION

Adamec, Christine, and Laurie C. Miller, MD, *The Encyclopedia of Adoption.* 3rd ed. New York: Facts On File, Inc., 2006.

AGORAPHOBIA
(See also ANXIETY AND ANXIETY DISORDERS)

Ballenger, James C., ed. *Biology of Agoraphobia.* Washington, DC: American Psychiatric Press, 1984.

Goldstein, Alan J. *Overcoming Agoraphobia: Conquering Fear of the Outside World.* New York: Viking, 1987.

Scrignar, Chester H. *From Panic to Peace of Mind: Overcoming Panic and Agoraphobia.* New Orleans, La.: Brunn Press, 1991.

Seagrave, Ann, and Faison Covington. *Free From Fears: A New Help For Anxiety, Panic and Agoraphobia.* New York: Poseidon Press, 1987.

ALCOHOLISM

Berger, Gilda. *Alcoholism and the Family.* New York: Franklin Watts, 1993.

Gwinnell, Esther, MD, and Christine Adamec. *The Encyclopedia of Drug Abuse.* New York: Facts On File, Inc., 2007.

Miller, Laurie, MD, and Christine Adamec. *The Encyclopedia of Adoption.* New York: Facts On File, Inc., 2006.

Petrakis, Ismene L., MD, et al. "Comorbidity of Alcoholism and Psychiatric Disorders." *Alcohol Research & Health* 26, no. 2 (2002): pp. 81–89.

Varley, Chris. *Alcoholism.* New York: M. Cavendish, 1994.

ALTERNATIVE THERAPIES
(See COMPLEMENTARY THERAPIES; MIND/BODY CONNECTIONS)

ALZHEIMER'S DISEASE

Davies, Helen D. *Alzheimer's: The Answers You Need.* Forest Knolls, Calif.: Elder Books, 1998.

Medina, John. *What You Need to Know About Alzheimer's.* Oakland, Calif.: New Harbinger, 1999.

Reekum, Robert van, Martine Simard, and Karl Farcnik. "Diagnosis of dementia and treatment of Alzheimer's disease." *Canadian Family Physician* 45 (April 1999): pp. 945–952.

Warner, Mark L. *The Complete Guide to Alzheimer Proofing Your Home.* West Lafayette, Ind.: Purdue University Press, 1998.

ANIMALS, FEAR OF

Freud, Sigmund. *Totem and Taboo.* London: Routledge & Kegan Paul, 1950.

ANOREXIA NERVOSA
(See EATING DISORDERS)

ANXIETY AND ANXIETY DISORDERS
(See also OBSESSIVE-COMPULSIVE DISORDER; PHOBIAS; POST-TRAUMATIC STRESS DISORDER.)

Agras, M. W. *Panic: Facing Fears, Phobias, and Anxiety.* New York: W. H. Freeman, 1985.

Barlow, D. H., and Michael Craske. *Mastery of Your Anxiety and Panic II.* Albany, N.Y.: Graywind Publications, 1994.

Bassett, Lucinda. *From Panic to Power.* New York: Harper-Collins, 1995.

Beck Aaron T., MD, and Gary Emery. *Anxiety Disorders and Phobias: A Cognitive Perspective.* New York: Basic Books, 2005.

Bloomfield, Harold H. *Healing Anxiety with Herbs.* New York: HarperCollins, 1998.

Feniger, Mani. *Journey From Anxiety to Freedom: Moving Beyond Panic and Phobias and Learning to Trust Yourself.* Rocklin, Calif.: Prima Pub., 1997.

Gold, Mark S. *The Good News About Panic, Anxiety & Phobias.* New York: Bantam Books, 1990.

Marks, Isaac. *Living with Fear.* New York: McGraw-Hill, 1980.

———. *Fears, Phobias, and Rituals: Panic, Anxiety, and Their Disorders.* New York: Oxford University Press, 1987.

Ross, Jerilyn. *Triumph over Fear: A Book of Help and Hope for People with Anxiety, Panic Attacks, and Phobias.* New York: Bantam Books, 1994.

Swedo, Susan, and H. L. Leonard. *It's Not All in Your Head.* New York: HarperCollins, 1996.

Warneke, Lorne. "Anxiety Disorders: Focus on Obsessive-Compulsive Disorder." *Canadian Family Physician* 39 (July 1993).

ARTHRITIS

Cook, Allan R. *Arthritis Sourcebook.* Detroit, MI: Omni-graphics, 1999.

Rados, Carol. "Helpful Treatments Keep People with Arthritis Moving." *FDA Consumer Magazine* (March–April 2005). Available online. URL: http://www.fda.gov/fdac/features/2005/205_pain.html. Downloaded June 16, 2006.

Trien, Susan F., and David Piseisky. *The Duke University Medical Center Book of Arthritis.* New York: Fawcett, 1992.

ASTHMA

Adams, Francis V. *The Asthma Sourcebook: Everything You Need to Know.* Los Angeles, Calif.: Lowell House, Contemporary Books, 1998.

Astor, Stephen. *What's New in Allergy and Asthma: New Developments and How They Help You Overcome Allergy and Asthma.* Mountain View, Calif.: Two A's Industries, 1996.

Firshein, Richard. *Reversing Asthma: Reduce Your Medications with This Revolutionary New Program.* New York: Warner Books, 1996.

Freedman, Michael R. *Living Well With Asthma.* New York: Guilford Press, 1998.

Stalmaiski, Alexander. *Freedom from Asthma: The Revolutionary 5-Day Treatment for Healing Asthma With the Breath Connection Program.* New York: Three Rivers Press, 1999.

ATTENTION-DEFICIT/HYPERACTIVITY DISORDER

Biederman, J., et al. "Is ADHD a Risk Factor for Psychoactive Substance Use Disorders: Findings from a Four-Year Prospective Follow-up Study." *Journal of the American Academy of Child & Adolescent Psychiatry* 36, no. 1 (1997): pp. 21–29.

Connelly, Elizabeth Russell. *Conduct Unbecoming: Hyperactivity. Attention Deficit, and Disruptive Behavior Disorders.* Philadelphia: Chelsea House Publishers, 1999.

Hallowell, Edward M., and J. J. Ratey. *Driven to Distraction.* New York: Pantheon, 1994.

———. *Answers to Distraction.* New York: Pantheon, 1995.

Ingersoll, Barbara D. *Daredevils and Daydreamers: New Perspectives on Attention Deficit/Hyperactivity Disorder.* New York: Doubleday, 1998.

Silver, Larry B. *Dr. Larry Silver's Advice to Parents on Attention Deficit Hyperactivity Disorder.* New York: Times Books, 1999.

Wilens, T. E., et al. "Characteristics of Adolescents and Young Adults with ADHD Who Divert or Misuse their Prescribed Medications." *Journal of the American Academy of Child & Adolescent Psychiatry* 45, no. 4, pp. 408–414.

BINGE DRINKING

Brewer, Robert D., MD, and Monica H. Swahn. "Binge Drinking and Violence." *Journal qf the American Medical Association* 294, no. 5 (August 2005): pp. 616–618.

National Institute on Alcohol Abuse and Alcoholism. *Alcohol Use and Alcohol Use Disorders in the United States: Main Findings from the 2001–2002 National Epidemiologic Survey on Alcohol and Related Conditions (NESARC).* U.S. Alcohol Epidemiologic Data Reference Manual 8, 1 (January 2006).

Weitzman, Elise R., et al. "Reducing Drinking and Related Harms in College: Evaluation of the 'A Matter of Degree' Program." *American Journal of Preventive Medicine* 27 (October 2004): pp. 196–197.

BIOFEEDBACK

Basmajian, John V., ed. *Biofeedback: Principles and Practice for Clinician.* Baltimore: Williams & Wilkins, 1983.

Brown, Barbara. *Stress and the Art of Biofeedback.* New York: Harper & Row, 1977.

Olton, D. S., and A. R. Noonbeng. *Biofeedback: Clinical Applications in Behavioral Medicine.* Englewood Cliffs, N.J.: Prentice Hall, 1980.

Soroka, George F. *Twelve Steps to Biofeedback.* Demarest, NJ: Ariel Starr Productions, 1998.

BLOOD AND NEEDLE PHOBIA

Hamilton, James G. "Needle Phobia: A Neglected Diagnosis." *The Journal of Family Practice* 41, no. 2 (August 1995): pp. 169–175.

Hellstrom, Kerstin, Jan Fellenius, and Lars-Goran Ost. "One Versus Five Sessions of Applied Tension in the Treatment of Blood Phobia." *Behav. Res. Ther* 34, no. 2: (1996): pp. 101–112.

Kleinknecht, Ronald A., Robert M. Thorndike, and Marilyn M. Walls. "Factorial Dimensions and Correlates of Blood, Injury, Injection and Related Medical Fears: Cross Validation of the Medical Fear Survey." *Behav. Res. Ther* 34, no. 4 (1996): pp. 323–331.

Mavissakalina, Matig R., and Robert F. Prien, eds. "Blood Phobia." In *Long-Term Treatments of Anxiety Disorders.* Washington, DC: American Psychiatric Press, Inc., 1996.

CAFFEINE

Gwinnell, Esther, MD, and Christine Adamec. *The Encyclopedia of Addictions and Addictive Disorders.* New York: Facts On File., Inc., 2005.

Hering-Hanit, R., and N. Gadoth. "Caffeine-Induced Headache in Children and Adolescents." *Cephalgia* 23, no. 4 (2003): p. 332.

National Institutes of Health. "Caffeine." NIH. Available online. URL: http://www.nlm.nih.gov/ medlineplus/druginfo/uspdi/202105.html. Downloaded May 26, 2006.

Ross, G. Webster, MD, "Association of Coffee and Caffeine Intake with the Risk of Parkinson Disease." *Journal of the American Medical Association* 283, no. 20 (March 24/31, 2000): pp. 2674–2679.

Tuomilehto, Jaako, M.D. "Coffee Consumption and Risk of Type 2 Diabetes Mellitus Among Middle-aged Finnish Men and Women." *Journal of the American Medical Association* 291, no. 10 (March 2004): pp. 1213–1219.

CANCER

Anderson, Greg. *Cancer: 50 Essential Things to Do.* New York: Plume, 1999.

Hersh, Stephen P. *Beyond Miracles: Living with Cancer: Inspirational and Practical Advice for Patients and Their Families.* Lincolnwood, IL: Contemporary Books, 2000.

National Cancer Institute. "What You Need to Know About Breast Cancer." Available online. URL: http://www.caner.gov/pdf/WYNTKIWYNTK_breast.pdf. Accessed April 25, 2006.

Terkel, Susan Neiburg, and Marlene Lupiloff-Bnass. *Understanding Cancer.* New York: Franklin Watts, 1993.

CHILD ABUSE

Administration on Children and Families. *Child Maltreatment.* Washington, DC: U.S. Department of Health and Human Services, 2006.

Clark, Robin E., and Judith Freeman Clark, with Christine Adamec. *The Encyclopedia of Child Abuse.* 3rd ed. New York: Facts On File, Inc., 2007.

Dube, Shanta R., et al. "Long-Term Consequences of Childhood Sexual Abuse by Gender of Victim." *American Journal of Preventive Medicine* 28, no. 5 (2005): pp. 430–438.

Office of Justice Programs. *Full Report of the Prevalence, Incidence and Consequences of Violence Against Women: Findings from the National Violence Against Women Study.* Washington, DC: United States Department of Justice, November 2000. Available online. URL: http://www.ncjrs.org/pdffiles1/nij/183781.pdf. Downloaded April 22, 2006.

CHILDHOOD ANXIETIES, FEARS, AND PHOBIAS

Eisen, Andrew R., Christopher A. Kearney, and Charles E. Schaefer. *Clinical Handbook of Anxiety Disorders in Children and Adolescents.* Northvale, NJ: Jason Aronson Inc., 1994.

Husain, Syed Arshad, Jythsna Nair, William Holcomb, et al. "Stress Reactions of Children and Adolescents in War and Siege Conditions." *Am J Psychiatry* (December 1998): pp. 155–612.

King, Nevil!e J., Viv Clowes-Hollins, and Thomas H. Ollendick. "The Etiology of Childhood Dog Phobia." *Behav. Res. Ther* 35, no. 1 (1997): p. 77.

Last, C. G., and C. C. Straus. "School Refusal and Anxiety-Disordered Children and Adolescence." *Journal of the American Academy of Childhood and Adolescent Psychology* 29 (1990): pp. 31–35.

Muris, Peter, Harald Merckelbach, and Ron Collaris. "Common Childhood Fears and Their Origins." *Behav. Res. Ther* 35, no. 10 (1997): pp. 929–937.

Turecki, Stanley. *The Emotional Problems of Normal Children.* New York: Bantam, 1994.

COMPLEMENTARY THERAPIES
(See also MIND/BODY CONNECTIONS)

Bensky, Dan, and Andres Gamble. *Chinese Herbal Medicine, Materia Medica.* Seattle, Wash.: Eastland, 1986.

Butt, Gary, and Frena B!oomfield. *Harmony Rules.* London: Arrow Books, 1985.

Christi, Hakim. *The Traditional Healer: Handbook: A Classic Guide to the Medicine of Avicenna.* Rochester, Vt.: Healing Arts Press, 1991.

Eisenberg, David. *Encounters with Qi.times.* New York: Norton, 1985.

———, et al. "Unconventional Medicine in the United States: Prevalence, Costs, and Patterns of Use." *New England Journal of Medicine* 328 (1993): pp. 246–252.

Facklam, Howard. *Alternative Medicine: Cures or Myths?* New York: Twenty-first Century Books, 1996.

Feldenkrais, Moshe. *Awareness Through Movement.* New York: Harper & Row, 1977.

Fradet, Brian. *Stress, Anxiety and Depression: The Natural Medicine Collective.* New York: Dell Publishing, 1995.

Frawley, David, and Vasant Lad. *The Yoga of Herbs: An Ayurvedic Guide to Herbal Medicine.* Santa Fe, N. Mex.: Lotus Press, 1986.

Gordon, James S. *Manifesto for a New Medicine: Your Guide to Healing Partnerships and Wise Use of Alternative Therapies.* Reading, Mass.: Addison-Wesley Publishing Company, 1996.

Heyn, Birgit. *Ayurveda: The Indian Art of Natural Medicine to Life Extension.* Rochester, Vt.: Healing Arts Press, 1990.

Kaminski, Patricia, and Richard Katz. *Flower Essence Repertory: A Comprehensive Guide to North American and English Flower Essences for Emotional and Spiritual Well-Being.* Nevada City, Calif.: The Flower Essence Society, 1994.

Krieger, D. *Therapeutic Touch: How to Use Your Hands to Help or to Heal.* Englewood Cliffs, N.J.: Prentice Hall, 1979.

Lad, Vasant. *Ayurveda: The Science of Self-Healing—A Practical Guide.* Santa Fe, NM: Lotus Press, 1984.

McGill, Leonard. *The Chiropractor's Health Book: Simple Natural Exercises for Relieving Headaches, Tension and Back Pain.* New York: Crown, 1995.

Morrison, Judith M. *The Book of Ayurveda.* New York: Fireside, 1995.

Morton, Mary, and Michael Morton. *5 Steps to Selecting the Best Alternative Medicine.* Novato, Calif.: New World Library, 1996.

Reid, Daniel. *The Complete Book of Chinese Health and Healing.* Boston: Shambhala, 1994.

Rondberg, Terry A. *Chiropractic First: The Fastest Growing Healthcare First Before Drugs or Surgery.* Chandler, AZ: The Chiropractic Journal, 1996.

Ryman, Danielle. *Aromatherapy: The Complete Guide to Plant and Flower Essences for Health and Beauty.* New York: Bantam Books, 1991.

Sachs, Judith. *Nature's Prozac: Natural Therapies and Techniques to Rid Yourself of Anxiety, Depression, Panic Attacks & Stress.* Englewood Cliffs, N.J.: Prentice Hall, 1997.

COMPUTERS

Kenwright, Mark, Isaac M. Marks, Lina Gega, and David Mataix-Cols. "Computer-Aided Self-Help for Phobia/Panic via Internet at Home: A Pilot Study." *British Journal of Psychiatry* 184 (2004): pp. 448–449.

COSMETIC SURGERY

Gwinnell, Esther, MD, and Christine Adamec. *The Encyclopedia of Addictions and Addictive Disorders.* New York: Facts On File, Inc., 2005.

CROSS-CULTURAL INFLUENCES ON PHOBIAS, FEARS, AND ANXIETIES

Friedman, Steven. *Cultural Issues in the Treatment of Anxiety.* New York: Guilford Press, 1997.

Pachter, Lee M. "Culture and Clinical Care: Folk Illness Beliefs and Behaviors and Their Implications for Health Care Delivery." *JAMA* 271, no. 9 (March 2, 1994): pp. 690–694.

DENTAL FEARS

Getka, Eric J., and Carol R. Glass. "Behavioral and Cognitive-Behavioral Approaches to the Reduction of Dental Anxiety." *Behavior Therapy* 23 (1992): pp. 433–448.

Jongh, Ad De, Peter Muris, Guusje Ter Horst, et al. "One-session Cognitive Treatment of Dental Phobia: Preparing Dental Phobics for Treatment by Restructuring

Negative Cognitions." *Behav. Res. Ther* 33, no. 8 (1995): pp. 947–954.

Walker, Edward A., Peter M. Milgrom, Philip Weinstein, et al. "Assessing Abuse and Neglect and Dental Fear in Women." *JADA* 127 (April 1998): pp. 485–490.

DEPRESSION AND BIPOLAR DISORDER (MANIC-DEPRESSIVE DISORDER)

Baskin, Valerie D. *When Words Are Not Enough: The Women's Prescription for Depression and Anxiety.* New York: Broadway Books, 1997.

Bloomfield, Harold H., and Peter McWilliams. *How to Heal Depression.* Los Angeles: Prelude Press, 1994.

Bohn, John, and James W. Jefferson. *Lithium and Manic Depression: A Guide.* Rev. ed. Madison: Lithium Information Center, University of Wisconsin, 1990.

Greist, John H., and James W. Jefferson. *Depression and Its Treatment: Help for the Nation's #1 Mental Problem.* Rev. ed. New York: Warner Books, 1992.

Healy, David. *The Anti-Depressant Era.* Cambridge, MA: Harvard University Press, 1997.

Kim, Henny H., ed. *Depression.* San Diego: Greenhaven Press, 1999.

Lewy, Alfred J., Bryan J. Lefler, Jonathan S. Emens, and Vance K. Bauer. "The Circadian Basis of Winter Depression." *Proceedings of the National Academy of Sciences* 103 (2006): pp. 7414–7419.

Martin, Philip. *The Zen Path Through Depression.* San Francisco: HarperSanFrancisco, 1999.

Quinn, Brian. *The Depression Sourcebook.* Los Angeles: Lowell House, 1997.

Reichenberg-Ullman, Judyth. *Prozac-free: Homeopathic Medications for Depression, Anxiety and Other Mental and Emotional Problems.* Rocklin, Calif.: Prima Health, 1999.

Robbins, Paul R. *Understanding Depression.* Jefferson, NC: McFarland & Co., 1993.

Rosen, David H. *Transforming Depression.* New York: G. P. Putnam's Sons, 1993.

Sanders, Pete. *Depression and Mental Health.* Brookfield, CT: Copper Beech Books, 1998.

Stahl, Stephen M. *Essential Psychopharmacology: The Prescriber's Guide.* Cambridge: Cambridge University Press, 2005.

Turkington, Carol. *Making the Prozac Decision: A Guide to Antidepressants.* Los Angeles: Contemporary Books, 1997.

Warneke, Lorne. "Management of Resistant Depression." *Canadian Family Physician* 42, (October 1996): p. 1973.

Whybrow, Peter C. *A Mood Apart: Depression, Mania and Other Afflictions of the Self* New York: Basic Books, 1997.

DIVORCE (See MARRIAGE AND DIVORCE)

DRIVING PHOBIA

Ehlers, Anke, Stefan G. Hofmann, Christoph A. Herda, et al. "Clinical Characteristics of Driving Phobia." *Journal of Anxiety Disorders* 8, no. 4 (1994): pp. 323–339.

EATING DISORDERS

Cassell, Dana K., and Donald H. Gleaves. *Encyclopedia of Obesity and Eating Disorders,* 2nd ed. New York: Facts On File, 2000.

Kinoy, Barbara P., ed. *Eating Disorders: New Directions in Treatment and Recovery.* New York: Columbia University Press, 1994.

Sonder, Ben. *Eating Disorders: When Food Turns Against You.* New York: Franklin Watts, 1993.

EXERCISE COMPULSION

Garman, J. G., et al. "Occurrence of Exercise Dependence in a College-Aged Population." *Journal of American College Health 52,* no. 5 (March–April 2004): pp. 221–228.

Gwinnell, Esther, MD, and Christine Adamec. *The Encyclopedia of Addictions and Addictive Disorders.* New York: Facts On File, Inc., 2005.

Hausenbias, Heather, and Danielle Symons Downs. "Exercise Dependence: A Systematic Review." *Psychology of Sport and Exercise* 3 (2002): pp. 89–123.

FERTILITY/INFERTILITY (See also PREGNANCY)

Conkling, Winifred. *Getting Pregnant Naturally: Healthy Choices to Boost Your Chances of Conceiving Without Fertility Drugs.* New York: Avon Books, 1999.

Indichova, Julia. *Inconceivable: Winning the Fertility Game.* New York: Adell Press, 1997.

Lauerson, Niels H. *Getting Pregnant: What Couples Need to Know.* New York: Rawson Associates, 1991.

Domar, A, D., M. M. Seihel, and H. Benson. "The Mind/Body Program for Infertility: A New Behavioral Treatment Approach for Women with Infertility." *Fertility and Sterility* 53 (1990): pp. 246–249.

Mahlstedt, P. "The Psychological Component of Infertility." *Fertility and Sterility* 43 (1985): pp. 335–346.

Seibel. M. M., ed. *Infertility: A Comprehensive Test.* Norwalk, CT: Appleton & Lange, 1990.

FLYING, FEAR OF

Beckham, Jean C., Scott R. Vrana, Jack G. May, et al. "Emotional Processing and Fear Measurement Synchrony as Indicators of Treatment Outcome in Fear of

Flying." *J. Behav. Tlzer & Exp. Psychiat.* 21, no. 3 (1990): pp. 153–162.

Brown, Duane. *Flying Without Fear.* Oakland, CA: New Harbinger Publications, 1996.

Hartman, Cherry. *The Fearless Flyer: How to Fly in Comfort and Without Trepidation.* Portland, Oreg.: Eighth Mountain Press, 1995.

McCarthy, Geoffrey W., and Kenneth D. Craig. "Flying Therapy for Flying Phobia." *Aviation, Space, and Environmental Medicine* 66, no. 12 (December 1995).

McNally, Richard J., and Christine E. Louro. "Fear of Flying in Agoraphobia and Simple Phobia: Distinguishing Features." *Journal of Anxiety Disorders* 6 (1992): pp. 319–324.

Ost, Lars Goran, Mats Brandberg, and Tomas Aim. "One Versus Five Sessions of Exposure in the Treatment of Flying Phobia." *Behavior Res. Ther* 35, no. 11 (1997): pp. 987–996.

Remington, John. *How Avioanxiely Becomes Controlled: Now Fly Without Fear.* St. Louis, Mo.: Inner Marker to Growth, 1992.

Wilhelm, Frank H., and Walton T. Roth. "Clinical Characteristics of Flight Phobia." *Journal of Anxiety Disorders* 11, no. 3 (1997): pp. 241–261.

GUIDED IMAGERY
(See also COMPLEMENTARY THERAPIES; MIND/ BODY CONNECTIONS.)

Achterberg, Jeanne. *Imagery in Healing: Shamanism and Modern Medicine.* San Francisco: Shambhala Publications, 1985.

Burns, David. *Feeling Good: The New Mood Therapy.* New York: Avon Books, 1992.

Epstein, Gerald. *Healing Visualizations, Creating Healing Through Imagery.* New York: Bantam Books, 1989.

Samuels, Michael. *Healing with the Mind's Eve.* New York: Random House, 1992.

Siegel, Bernie. *Love, Medicine and Miracles.* New York: Harper & Row, 1986.

———. *Peace, Love and Healing.* New York: Harper & Row, 1986.

HEADACHES

Blanchard, E. B., K. A. Appelbaum, et al. "Placebo-controlled Evaluation of Abbreviated Progressive Muscle Relaxation and of Relaxation Combined with Cognitive Therapy in the Treatment of Tension Headache," *Journal of Consulting and Clinical Psychology* 58 (1990): pp. 210–215.

Blanchard, E. B., N. L. Nicholson, et al. "The Role of Regular Home Practice in the Relaxation Treatment of Tension Headache." *Journal of Consulting and Clinical Psychology* 59 (1991): pp. 467–470.

Diamond, Seymour. *The Hormone Headache: New Ways to Prevent, Manage, and Treat Migraines and Other Headaches.* New York: Macmillan, 1995.

Finnigan, Jeffry. *Life Beyond Headaches.* Olympia, WA: Finnigan Clinic, 1999.

Hartnell, Agnes. *Migraine Headaches and the Foods You Eat: 200 Recipes for Relief.* Minneapolis: Chronimed, 1997.

Inlander, Charles B., and Porter Shimer. *Headaches: 47 Ways to Stop the Pain.* New York: Walker & Company, 1995.

Maas, Paula, and Deborah Mitchell. *The Natural Health Guide to Headache Relief: The Definitive Handbook of Natural Remedies for Treating Every Kind of Headache Pain.* New York: Pocket Books, 1997.

Minirth, Frank B., with Sandy Dengler. *The Headache Book.* Nashville, TN: Nelson Publishers, 1994.

Solomon, Seymour, and Steven Fraccaro. *The Headache Book.* Yonkers, N.Y.: Consumer Reports Books, 1991.

HEALTH, WELLNESS, AND STRESS

Benson, Herbert. *The Wellness Book: The Complete Guide to Maintaining Health and Treating Stress-Related Illness.* Secaucus, NJ: Carol Publishing Group, 1992.

Bohm, David. *Wholeness and the Implicate Order.* London: Ark, 1980.

Campbell, Joseph. *The Inner Reaches of Outer Space.* New York: Alfred Van Der Marck, 1985.

Capra, Fritjof. *The Turning Point.* New York: Bantam, 1982.

Castenada, Carlos. *The Art of Dreaming.* New York Harper-Collins, 1993.

Dubos, Rene. *Mirage of Health.* New York: Anchor Books, 1959.

Hoffer, Eric. *The True Believer.* New York: Harper & Row, 1951.

Illich, Ivan. *Medical Nemesis: The Expropriation of Health.* New York: Pantheon, 1982.

Ornstein, Robert, and David Sobel. *The Healing Brain: Breakthrough Discoveries About How the Brain Keeps Us Healthy.* New York: Simon & Schuster, 1987.

Pelletier, Kenneth R. *Sound Mind, Sound Body: A Model for Lifelong Health.* New York: Simon & Schuster, 1994.

Peterson, Christopher, and Lisa M. Bossio. *Health and Optimism.* New York: Macmillan, 1991.

Strasburg, Kate, et al. *The Quest for Wholeness: An Annotated Bibliography in Patient-Centered Medicine.* Bolinas, CA: Commonweal, 1991.

Stutz, David, and Bernard Feder. *The Savvy Patient: How to Be an Active Participant in Your Medical Care.* Yonkers, NY: Consumer Reports Books, 1990.

Weil, Andrew. *Eight Weeks to Optimum Health: Proven Program for Taking Full Advantage of Your Body's Healing Power.* New York: Knopf, 1997.

Williams, R. W., and V. Williams. *Anger Kills: 17 Strategies for Controlling the Hostility that Can Harm Your Health.* New York: Times Books, 1993.

Wolinsky, Stephen. *Quantum Consciousness: The Guide to Experiencing Quantum Psychology.* Norfolk, Conn.: Bramble Books, 1993.

HEART DISEASE

Dembroski, T. M., et al. "Components of Hostility as Predictors of Sudden Death and Myocardial Infarction in the Multiple Risk Factor Intervention Trial." *Psychosomatic Medicine* 51 (1989): pp. 514–522.

Kerman, D. Ariel, and Richard Trubo. *The Hart Program: Lower Your Blood Pressure Without Drugs.* New York: HarperCollins, 1992.

McGowan, Mary P. *Heart Fitness for Life: The Essential Guide to Preventing and Reversing Heart Disease.* New York: Oxford University Press, 1997.

Ornish, Dean. *Dr. Dean Onrnish's Program for Reversing Heart Disease.* New York: Ballantine, 1992.

Sachs, Judith. *Natural Medicine for Heart Disease.* New York: Dell Publishing, 1997.

Skerritt, Paul W. "Anxiety and the Heart—a Historical Review." *Psychological Medicine* 13 (1983): pp. 17–25.

HIV
(See ACQUIRED IMMUNODEFICIENCY SYNDROME)

HOLISTIC MEDICINE
(See COMPLEMENTARY THERAPIES; MIND/BODY CONNECTIONS)

HYPNOSIS

Caprio, Frank Samuel. *Healing Yourself With Self-Hypnosis.* Paramus, N.J.: Prentice Hall, 1998.

Erickson, M. H., and E. L. Rossi. *Hypnotherapy: An Exploratory Casebook.* New York: Irvington, 1979.

Hadley, Josie, and Carol Staudacher. *Hypnosis for Change.* Oakland, Calif.: New Harbinger Publications, Inc., 1996.

Haley, J. *Advanced Techniques of Hypnosis and Therapy: Selected Papers of Milton H. Erickson, M.D.* New York: Grune & Stratton, 1967.

Lankton, S. R., ed. *Ericksonian Hypnosis: Application, Preparation, and Research.* New York: Brunner/Mazel, 1989.

Rhue, J. W., Lynn, S. J. and Kirsch, I., eds. *Handbook of Clinical Hypnosis.* Washington, DC: American Psychological Association, 1993.

Rossi, E. L. *The Psychology of Mind-Body Healing: New Concepts of Therapeutic Hypnosis.* New York: Norton, 1993.

Stockwell, Shelley Lessin. *Hypnosis: How to Put a Smile on Your Face and Money in Your Pocket: The Stockwell System.* Rancho Palos Verdes, Calif.: Creatively Unlimited Press, 1998.

IMMUNE SYSTEM
(See also PSYCHONEUROIMMUNOLOGY)

Borysenko, M. "The Immune System: An Overview." *Annals of Behavioral Medicine* 9 (1987): pp. 3–10.

Cohen, S., D. A. J. Tyrrel, and A. P Smith. "Psychological Stress and Susceptibility to the Common Cold." *New England Journal of Medicine* 325 (1991): pp. 606–612.

Herbert, Tracy B. "Stress and the immune system." *World Health*, March–April 1994.

Locke, Steven, and Douglas Colligan. *The Healer Within.* New York: New American Library, 1986.

MARRIAGE AND DIVORCE

Bray, James H. *Stepfamilies: Love, Marriage and Parenting in the First Decade.* New York: Broadway Books, 1998.

Briscoe, D. Stuart. *Marriage Matters! Growing Through the Differences and Surprises of Life Together.* Wheaton, IL: H. Shaw Publishers, 1994.

Conover, Kris. *Marriage Made Simple: Fifty Hints for Building Long-Lasting Love.* New York: Plume, 1999.

Gottman, John Mordechai. *Why Marriages Succeed or Fail: What You Can Learn from the Breakthrough Research to Make Your Marriage Last.* New York: Simon & Schuster, 1994.

Heyn, Dalma. *Marriage Shock: The Transformation of Women Into Wives.* New York: Villard, 1997.

Roleff, Tamara L., and Mary B. Williams, ed. *Marriage and Divorce.* San Diego: Greenhaven Press, 1997.

Simpson, Eileen B. *Late Love: A Celebration of Marriage After Fifty.* Boston: Houghton Mifflin, 1994.

MEDITATION
(See also MINDFULNESS MEDITATION)

Benson, Herbert. *The Relaxation Response.* New York: Avon Books, 1975.

———. *Beyond the Relaxation Response.* New York: Berkeley Press, 1985.

Borysenko, Joan, and Duscher, J. *On Wings of Light: Meditations for Awakening to the Source.* New York: Warner, 1992.

Chopra, Deepak. *Quantum Healing.* New York: Bantam, 1989.

———. *Creating Health: How to Wake Up the Body's Intelligence.* Boston: Houghton Mifflin, 1991.

———. *Unconditional Life.* New York: Bantam, 1992.

———. *Ageless Body, Timeless Mind.* New York: Crown, 1993.

———. *Creating Affluence: Wealth Consciousness in the Field of All Possibilities.* San Rafael, Calif.: New World Library, 1993.

Connor, Danny, with Michael Tse. *Qigong. Chinese Movement & Meditation for Health.* York Beach, ME: Samuel Weiser, 1992.

Cousins, Norman. *The Healing Heart.* New York: Norton, 1983.

Denniston, Denish, and Peter McWilliams. *The TM Book: Transcendental Meditation, How to Enjoy the Rest of Your Life.* Allen Park, Mich.: Versemonger Press, 1975.

Dossey, L. *Space, Time and Medicine.* Boston, MA: Shambhala, 1982.

———. *Meaning and Medicine: A Doctor's Tales of Breakthrough and Healing.* New York: Bantam, 1991.

———. *Recovering the Soul.* New York: Bantam, 1989.

Dychtwald, K. *Bodymind.* Los Angeles: Tarcher, 1986.

Goleman, Daniel. *The Meditative Mind.* Los Angeles: Tarcher, 1988.

Levey, Daniel. *The Fine Arts of Relaxation, Concentration and Meditation.* London: Wisdom Publications, 1987.

Mahesh Yogi, Maharishi. *Science of Being and Art of Living: Transcendental Meditation.* New York: Meridian, 1995.

Nuernberger, Phil. *Freedom from Stress.* Honesdale, PA: The Himalayan International Institute of Yoga Science and Philosophy, 1985.

Trungpa, Chogyam. *Shambhala: The Sacred Path of the Warrior.* Boston: Shambhala, 1984.

MENTAL ILLNESS (See also ANXIETY AND ANXIETY DISORDERS; DEPRESSION.)

P. Lowing, et al. "The Inheritance of Schizophrenia Disorder: A Reanalysis of the Danish Adoption Study Data." *American Journal of Psychiatry* 1400 (1983): pp. 1,167–1,171.

MINDFULNESS MEDITATION (INSIGHT MEDITATION)

Goldstein, Joseph, and Jack Komfield. *Seeking the Heart of Wisdom: The Path of Insight Meditation.* Boston: Shambhala, 1987.

Hanh, Thich Nhat. *Being Peace.* Berkeley: Parallax Press, 1987.

———. *The Miracle of Mindfulness: A Manual of Meditation.* Boston: Beacon Press, 1976.

———. *The Sun My Heart.* Berkeley: Parallax Press, 1988.

Kabat-Zinn, Jon. *Full Catastrophe Living: Using the Wisdom of Your Body and Mind to Face Stress, Pain and Illness.* New York: Delacorte Press, 1991.

———. *Wherever You Go, There You Are.* New York: Hyperion, 1994.

Levine, Stephen. *A Gradual Awakening.* Garden City, N.Y.: Anchor/Doubleday, 1979.

Suzuki, Shunryu. *Zen Mind, Beginner's Mind.* New York: Weatherhill, 1986.

MIND/BODY CONNECTIONS
(See also COMPLEMENTARY THERAPIES; PSYCHONEUROIMMUNOLOGY)

Benson, Herbert. *The Relaxation Response.* New York: Avon Books, 1975.

———. *Beyond the Relaxation Response.* New York: Berkeley Press, 1985.

Borysenko, Joan. *Minding the Body. Mending the Mind.* New York: Bantam, 1988.

———. *Guilt Is the Teacher, Love Is the Lesson.* New York: Warner, 1991.

Cannon, Walter. *The Wisdom of the Body.* New York: Norton, 1939.

Chopra, Deepak. *Perfect Health.* New York: Harmony Books. 1990.

———. *Quantum Healing: Exploring the Frontiers of Mind/Body Medicine.* New York: Bantam Books, 1989.

Cousins, Norman. *Head First: The Biology of Hope and the Healing Power of the Human Spirit.* New York: Viking Penguin, 1990.

———. *Anatomy of an Illness as Perceived by the Patient.* New York: Norton, 1979.

———. *The Healing Heart.* New York: Norton, 1983.

Dienstfrey, Harris. *Where the Mind Meets the Body.* New York: HarperCollins, 1991.

Dossey, Larry. *Space, Time and Medicine.* Boston: Shambhala, 1982.

Goleman, Daniel, and Joel Gurin, eds. *Mind Body Medicine: How to Use Your Mind for Better Health.* Yonkers, N.Y.: Consumer Reports Books, 1993.

Gordon, James S., et al. *Mind, Body and Health: Toward an Integral Medicine.* New York: Human Sciences Press, 1984.

Locke, Steven E., and Douglas Colligan. *The Healer Within: The New Medicine of Mind and Body.* New York: Dutton, 1986.

Moyers, B. *Healing and the Mind.* New York: Doubleday, 1993.

Omstein, Robert, and David Sobel. *The Healing Brain.* New York: Simon & Schuster, 1988.

Pelletier, Kenneth R. *Mind as Healer Mind as Slayer.* Rev. ed. New York: Delacorte, 1992.

———. *Sound Mind, Sound Body: A New Model for Lifelong Health.* New York: Simon & Schuster, 1994.

———. *Holistic Medicine: Front Stress to Optimum Health.* Magnolia, Mass.: Peter Smith, 1984.

Siegel, Bernie. *Love, Medicine and Miracles.* New York: Harper & Row, 1986.

———. *Peace. Love and Healing.* New York: Harper & Row, 1989.

NUTRITION

Brody, Jane. *Jane Brody's Nutrition Book.* New York: W. W. Norton, 1981.

Brown, Judith B. *Everywoman's Guide to Nutrition.* Minneapolis: University of Minnesota Press, 1991.

Finn, Susan Calvert, and Linda Stern. *The Real Life Nutrition Book: Making the Right Food Choices Without Changing Your Life-Style.* New York: Penguin Books, 1992.

Haas, Robert. *Eat Smart, Think Smart: How to Use Nutrients and Supplements to Achieve Maximum Mental and Physical Performance.* New York: HarperCollins, 1994.

Kotsanis, Frank N., and Maureen A. Mackey, eds. *Nutrition in the '90s: Current Controversies and Analysis.* Vol. 2. New York: M. Dekker, 1994.

Quillan, Patrick. *Beating Cancer with Nutrition.* Tulsa, OK: Nutrition Times Press, 1994.

Werhach, Melvyn. *Healing Through Nutrition: A Natural Approach to Treating 50 Common Illnesses with Diet and Nutrients.* New York: HarperCollins, 1993.

OBSESSIVE-COMPULSIVE DISORDER
(See also ANXIETY AND ANXIETY DISORDERS)

Alper, Gerald. *The Puppeteers: Studies of Obsessive Control.* New York: Fromm International Publishing Corporation, 1994.

Bejerot, S., and M. Humble. "Low Prevalence of Smoking among Patients with Obsessive-Compulsive Disorder." *Comprehensive Psychiatry* 40, no. 4 (July–August 1999): pp. 268–272.

De Silva, Padmal. *Obsessive-Compulsive Disorder: The Facts.* New York: Oxford University Press, 1998.

Gravitz, Herbert L. *Overcoming Obsessive-Compulsive Disorder: New Help for the Family.* Santa Barbara, Calif.: Healing Visions Press, 1998.

Hanna, Gregory L., et al. "Genome-Wide Linkage Analysis of Families with Obsessive-Compulsive Disorder Ascertained through Pediatric Probands." *American Journal of Medical Genetics* 114 (2002): pp. 541–552.

Marks, Isaac. *Fears and Phobias.* New York: Academic Press, 1969.

National Institute of Mental Health. "The Numbers Count: Mental Disorders in America." Available online. URL: http://www.nimh.nih.gov/publicat/numbers.cfm. Downloaded November 14, 2006.

Rappaport, Judith. *The Boy Who Couldn't Stop Washing: The Experience and Treatment of Obsessive-Compulsive Disorder.* New York: Dutton, 1989.

PAIN

Corey, David, with Stan Solomon. *Pain: Free Yourself for Life.* New York: NAL-Dutton, 1989.

Hardy, Paul A. J. *Chronic Pain Management: The Essentials.* London: Greenwich Medical Media, 1997.

Singh Khalsa, Dharma. *The Pain Cure: The Proven Medical Program That Helps End Your Chronic Pain.* New York: Warner Books, 1999.

Stacy, Charles B., et al. *The Fight Against Pain.* Yonkers, NY: Consumer Reports Books, 1992.

PANIC ATTACKS AND PANIC DISORDER
(See ANXIETY AND ANXIETY DISORDERS)

PERFORMANCE ANXIETY

Dunkel, Stuart Edward. *The Audition Process: Anxiety Management and Coping Strategies.* Stuyvesant, N.Y.: Pendragon Press, 1989.

Moss, Robert. "Stage Fright Is Actors' Eternal Nemesis." *New York Times,* January 6, 1992.

Salmon, Paul. *Notes from the Green Room: Coping with Stress and Anxiety in Musical Performance.* New York: Lexington Books, 1992.

Steptoe, A., and H. Fidler. "Stage Fright and Orchestral Musicians: A Study of Cognitive Behavioral Strategies and Performance Anxiety." *British Journal of Psychology* 78 (1987): pp. 241–249.

Wesner, R. B., R. Noyes Jr., and L. L. Davis. "The Occurrence of Performance Anxiety Among Musicians." *Journal of Affective Disorders* 18 (1990): pp. 177–185.

PHARMACOLOGICAL APPROACH
(DEPRESSION, PHOBIAS, ANXIETIES)

Appleton, William S. *Prozac and the New Antidepressants: What You Need to Know About Prozac, Zoloft, Paxil, Luvox, Wellbutrin, Effexor, Serzone, and More.* New York: Plume, 1997.

Davidson, J. R. T., S. M. Ford, R. D. Smith, and N. L. S. Potts. "Long-term Treatment of Social Phobia Clonazapam." *Journal of Clinical Psychiatry* 52, no. 11 (1991, suppl.): pp. 16–20.

Fieve, Ronald R. *Prozac.* New York: Avon, 1994.

Liebowitz, M. R., F. R. Schneier, and B. Hollander, et al. "Treatment of Social Phobia with Drugs Other Than Benzodiazepines." *Journal of Clinical Psychiatry* 52 (1991, suppl.): pp. 10–15.

Monroe, Judy. *Antidepressants.* Springfield, NJ: Enslow Publishers, 1997.

Stahl, Stephen M. *Essential Psychopharmacology: The Prescriber's Guide.* Cambridge: Cambridge University Press, 2005.

Turkington, Carol. *Making the Prozac Decision: A Guide to Antidepressants.* Los Angeles: Lowell House, 1997.

Wilkinson, Beth. *Drugs and Depression.* New York: Rosen Publishing Group, 1994.

PHOBIAS
(See also ANXIETY AND ANXIETY DISORDERS)

Bourne, Edmund J. *The Anxiety & Phobia Workbook.* Oakland, Calif.: New Harbinger Publications, 1995.

Cheek, J. *Conquering Shyness.* New York: Dell Publishing, 1989.

DuPont, Robert L. *Phobia: A Comprehensive Summary of Modern Treatments.* New York: Brunner/Mazel, 1982.

Jampolsky, Gerald. *Love Is Letting Go of Fear.* New York: Bantam Books, 1979.

Marks, Isaac M. *Living with Fear* New York: McGraw-Hill, 1980.

———. *Fears, Phobias, and Rituals.* New York: Oxford University Press, 1987.

Markway, B. G., et al. *Dying of Embarrassment: Help for Social Anxiety and Phobias.* Oakland, Calif.: New Harbinger, 1992.

Marshall, John R. *Social Phobia: From Shyness to Stage Fright.* New York: Basic Books, 1994.

Monroe, Judy. *Phobias: Everything You Wanted to Know, But Were Afraid to Ask.* Springfield, N.J.: Enslow Publishers, 1996.

Nardo, Don. *Anxiety and Phobias.* New York: Chelsea House, 1992.

Uhde, T. W., M. B. Tancer, B. Black, and T. M. Brown. "Phenomenology and Neurobiology of Social Phobias: Comparison with Panic Disorder." *Journal of Clinical Psychology* 52 (November 1991): pp. 31–40.

Zane, Manuel D., and Harry Milt. *Your Phobia.* Washington, DC: American Psychiatric Press, Inc., 1984.

POST-TRAUMATIC STRESS DISORDER
(PTSD) (See also ANXIETY AND ANXIETY DISORDERS)

Catherall, Donald Roy. *Back from the Brink: A Family Guide to Overcoming Traumatic Stress.* New York: Bantam Books, 1992.

Egendorf, A. *Healing from the War: Trauma and Transformation After Vietnam.* New York: Houghton Mifflin, 1985.

Eitinger, Leo, and Robert Krell, with Miriam Rieck. *The Psychological and Medical Effects of Concentration Camps and Related Persecutions on Survivors of the Holocaust.* Vancouver: University of British Columbia Press, 1985.

Eth, S., and R. S. Pynoos. *Post-Traumatic Stress Disorder in Children.* Washington, DC: American Psychiatric Press, Inc., 1985.

Herman, Judith. *Trauma and Recovery.* New York: Basic Books, 1992.

Lindy, Jacob D. *Vietnam: A Casebook.* New York: Brunner/Mazel, 1987.

Peterson, Kirtland C., Maurice F. Prou, and Robert A. Schwarz. *Post-Traumatic Stress Disorder: A Clinician's Guide.* New York: Plenum Press, 1991.

Porterfield, Kay Marie. *Straight Talk About Post-traumatic Stress Disorder: Coping with the Aftermath of Trauma.* New York: Facts On File, 1996.

Sonnenberg, S. M., A. S. Blank, and J. A. Talbott, eds. *The Trauma of War: Stress and Recovery in Vietnam Veterans.* Washington, DC: American Psychiatric Press, 1985.

Van der Kolk, B. A., ed. *Post-Traumatic Stress Disorder: Psychological and Biological Sequelae.* Washington, DC: American Psychiatric Press, Inc. 1996.

PREGNANCY
(See also FERTILITY/INFERTILITY)

Kitzinger, Sheila. *The Complete Book of Pregnancy and Childbirth.* Mississauga, Ontario: Random House of Canada, Ltd., 1996.

Stoppard, Miriam. *Healthy Pregnancy.* New York: DK Publishing, 1998.

Stone, Joanne. *Pregnancy for Dummies.* Foster City, Calif.: IDG Books worldwide, 1999.

Westheimer, Ruth K. *Dr. Ruth's Pregnancy Guide for Couples: Love, Sex, and Medical Facts.* New York: Routledge, 1999.

PSYCHOLOGY, CONTEMPORARY (See also COMPLEMENTARY THERAPIES; MIND/BODY CONNECTIONS; PSYCHONEUROIMMUNOLOGY)

Berne, Eric. *Games People Play.* New York: Grove Press, 1964.

Borysenko, Joan. *Guilt Is The Teacher; Love Is The Lesson.* New York: Warner Books, 1990.

Bradshaw, John. *Bradshaw On: The Family.* Deerfield Beach, Fla.: Health Communications, Inc., 1988.

———. *Healing the Shame That Binds You.* Deerfield Beach, Fla.: Health Communications, Inc., 1988.

Cousins, Norman. *The Healing Heart.* New York: Avon Books, 1984.

Csikszentmihalyi, Mihaly. *Flow: The Psychology of Optimal Experience.* New York: HarperCollins Perennial, 1991.

Peck, M. Scott. *The Road Less Traveled.* New York: Simon & Schuster, 1978.

Wolinsky, Stephen H. *Trances People Live: Healing Approaches in Quantum Psychology.* Norfolk, Conn.: Bramble Co., 1991.

PSYCHONEUROIMMUNOLOGY

Ader, Robert, D. Felton, and N. Cohen, eds. *Psychoneuroimmunology.* 2nd ed. San Diego: Academic Press, 1990.

Bohin, David. *Wholeness and the Implicate Order.* London: Routledge & Kegan Paul, 1980.

Cousins, Norman. *Anatomy of an Illness.* New York: Bantam Books, 1981.

Kiecolt-Glaser, J. K., and R. Glaser. "Psychoneuroimmunology: Can Psychological Interventions Modulate Immunity?" *Journal of Consulting and Clinical Psychology* 60 (1992): pp. 569–575.

RELAXATION

Agras, W. S., C. B. Taylor, H. C. Kraemer, M. A. Southam, and J. A. Schneider. "Relaxation Training for Essential Hypertension at the Worksite: II. The Poorly Controlled Hypertensive." *Psychosomatic Medicine* 49 (1987): pp. 264–273.

Benson, Herbert. *The Relaxation Response.* New York: Avon Books, 1975.

———. *Beyond the Relaxation Response.* New York: Berkeley Press, 1985.

———. *Your Maximum Mind.* New York: Times Books, 1987.

———, Eileen M. Stuart, and staff of the Mind/Body Medical Institute. *The Wellness Book: The Comprehensive Guide to Maintaining Health and Treating Stress-Related illness.* New York: Carol, 1992.

Blumenfeld, Larry, ed. *The Big Book of Relaxation: Simple Techniques to Control the Excess Stress in Your Life.* Roslyn, N.Y.: Relaxation Company, 1994.

Davis, Martha, Elizabeth Robbins Eshelman, and Matthew McKay. *The Relaxation and Stress Reduction Workbook.* Oakland, Calif.: New Harbinger Publications, 1995.

SELF-ESTEEM

Dobson, James C. *The New Hide and Seek: Building Self-Esteem in Your Child.* Grand Rapids, Mich.: Fleming H. Revell, 1999.

Hazelton, Deborah M. *Solving the Self-Esteem Puzzle.* Deerfield Beach, Fla.: 1991.

Hiliman, Carolynn. *Recovery of Your Self-Esteem.* New York: Simon & Schuster, 1992.

Johnson, Carol. *Self-Esteem Comes In All Sizes.* New York: Doubleday, 1995.

Kahn, Ada P., and Sheila Kimmel. *Empower Yourself: Every Woman's Guide to Self-Esteem.* New York: Avon Books, 1997.

Lindenfield, Gael. *Self-Esteem.* New York: HarperPaperbacks, 1997.

McKay, Matthew. *The Self-Esteem Companion: Simple Exercises to Help You Challenge Your Inner Critic and Celebrate Your Personal Strengths.* Oakland, Calif.: New Harbinger Publications, 1999.

Minchinton, Jerry. *Maximum Self-Esteem: The Handbook for Reclaiming Your Sense of Self-Worth.* Yanzant, Miss.: Arnford House Publishers, 1993.

Prato, Louis. *Be Your Own Best Friend: How to Achieve Greater Self-Esteem, Health, and Happiness.* New York: Berkley Books, 1994.

Steinem, Gloria. *Revolution from Within: A Book of Self-Esteem.* Boston: Little, Brown and Co., 1992.

SENSORY INTEGRATION DISORDER

Adamec, Christine, and Laurie C. Miller, MD *The Encyclopedia of Adoption.* New York: Facts On File, Inc., 2007.

Ayres, A. Jean. *Sensory Integration and the Child.* Los Angeles: Western Psychological Services, 1994.

Biel, Lindsey, and Nancy Peske. *Raising a Sensory Smart Child: The Definitive Handbook for Helping Your Child with Sensory Integration Issues.* New York: Penguin Books, 2005.

Smith, Karen A., and Karen R. Gouze. *The Sensory-Sensitive Child: Practical Solutions for Out-of-Bounds Behavior.* New York: Harper Resource, 2004.

Stephens, Linda C. "Sensory Integrative Dysfunction." *AAHEI News Exchange* 12, no. 1 (Winter 1997).

SMOKING (See also ADDICTIONS)

Buckley, Christopher. *Thank You for Smoking.* New York: Random House, 1994.

Gwinnell, Esther, MD, and Christine Adamec. *The Encyclopedia of Addictions and Addictive Behaviors.* New York: Facts On File, Inc., 2005.

Hammond, S. Katharine. "Environmental Tobacco Smoke Presents Substantial Risk in Workplaces." *The Journal of the American Medical Association* (September 1995).

Liesges, Robert C., and Margaret Deflon. *How Women Can Finally Stop Smoking.* Alameda, Calif.: Hunter House, 1994.

Mowat, David L., Darlene Mecredy, and Frank Lee, et al. "Family Physicians and Smoking Cessation." *Canadian Family Physician* 42 (October 1996): p. 1946.

Rogers, Jacquelyn. *You Can Stop Smoking.* New York: Pocket Books, 1995.

Sanders, Pete, and Steve Myers. *Smoking.* Brookfield, Conn.: Copper Beech Books, 1996.

Pietrusza, David. *Smoking.* San Diego: Lucent Books, 1997.

SOCIAL PHOBIAS
(See ANXIETY AND ANXIETY DISORDERS; PHOBIAS)

SOCIAL SUPPORT, SUPPORT GROUPS, AND SELF-HELP

Kreiner, Anna. *Everything You Need to Know About Creating Your Own Support System.* New York: The Rosen Publishing Group, 1996.

Pilisuk, Marc, and Susan H. Parks. *The Healing Web: Social Networks and Human Survival.* Hanover, N.H.: University Press of New England, 1986.

Spiegel, David. *Living Beyond Limits.* New York: Times Books, 1993.

White, Barbara J., and Edward J. Madara. *The Self-Help Sourcebook: Finding & Forming Mutual Aid Self-Help-Groups.* Denville, N.J.: American Self-Help Clearinghouse, St. Clare's-Riverside Medical Center, 1992.

SPIDER PHOBIA

Fredrikson, Mats, Peter Annas, and Gustav Wik. "Parental History, Aversive Exposure and the Development of Snake and Spider Phobia in Women." *Behav Res. Ther.* 35, no. 1 (1997): pp. 23–28.

Kindt, Merel, Jos F Brosschot, and Peter Muris. "Spider Phobia Questionnaire for Children (SPQ C): A Pyschometric Study and Normative Data." *Behav. Res. Ther.* 34, no. 3 (1996): pp. 277–282.

Kirkby, Kenneth C., Ross G. Menzies, Brett A. Daniels, et al. "Aetiology of Spider Phobia: Classificatory Differences between Two Origins Instruments." *Behav. Res. Ther.* 33, no. 8 (1995): pp. 955–958.

Ost, Lars-Goran. "One-Session Group Treatment of Spider Phobia." *Behav Res. Ther.* 34, no. 9 (1996): pp. 707–715.

Smith, Mick, and Joyce Davidson. "'It Makes My Skin Crawl . . .': The Embodiment of Disgust in Phobias of 'Nature'" *Body & Society* 12, no. 1 (2006): pp. 43–67.

STRESS AND STRESS MANAGEMENT

Brammer, L. M. *How to Cope with Life Transitions: The Challenge of Personal Change.* New York: Hemisphere Publishing, 1991.

Bridges, W. *Managing Transitions: Making the Most of Change.* Reading, Mass.: Wesley, 1991.

Eliot, Robert S. *From Stress to Strength: How to Lighten Your Load and Save Your Life.* New York: Bantam Books, 1994.

Faelten, Sharon, and David Diamond. *Take Control of Your Life: A Complete Guide to Stress Relief.* Emmaus, Penn.: Rodale Press, 1988.

Gordon. James S. *Stress Management.* New York: Chelsea House Publishers, 1990.

Kahn, Ada P. *Stress A–Z: A Sourcebook for Facing Everyday Challenges.* New York: Facts On File, 1998.

Lark, Susan M. *Anxiety and Stress: A Self Help Program.* Los Altos, Calif.: Westchester Publishing Company, 1993.

Lehrer, Paul M., and Robert L. Woolfolk, eds. *Principles and Practice of Stress Management.* 2nd ed. New York: Guilford Press, 1993.

Maddi, Salvatore, and Suzanne Kobasa. *The Hardy Executive: Health Under Stress.* Homewood, Ill.: Dow Jones-Irwin, 1984.

Miller, Lyle H., and Alma Dell Smith. *The Stress Solution: An Action Plan to Manage the Stress in Your Life.* New York: Pocket Books, 1993.

Ornish, Dean. *Stress, Diet, and Your Heart.* New York: Holt, Rinehart-Winston, 1983.

Padus, Emrika, ed. *The Complete Guide to Your Emotions and Your Health.* Emmaus, PA: Rodale Press, 1992.

Patel, Chandra. *The Complete Guide to Stress Management.* New York: Plenum Press, 1991.

Sapolky, Robert M. *Why Zebras Don't Get Ulcers.* New York: W. H. Freeman & Company, 1994.

Seaward, Brian Luke. *Managing Stress: Principles and Strategies for Health and Wellbeing; Managing Stress: A Creative Journal.* Boston: Jones & Bartless Publishers, 1994.

Selye, Hans. *Stress Without Distress.* New York: Lipincott, 1974.

———. *The Stress of Life.* Rev. ed. New York: McGraw-Hill Book Company, 1978.

Snyder. Solomon H., ed. *Stress Management.* New York: Chelsea House Publishers, 1990.

THYROID DISEASE

Hallowell, Joseph G., et al. "Serum TSH, T_4, and Thyroid Antibodies in the United States Population (1988 to 1994): National Health and Nutrition Examination Survey (NHANES III)." *Journal of Clinical Endocrinology & Metabolism* 87, no. 2 (2002): pp. 489–499.

Petit, William A., MD, and Christine Adamec. *The Encyclopedia of Endocrine Diseases and Disorders.* New York: Facts On File, Inc., 2005.

ULCERS

Minocha, Anil, MD, and Christine Adamec. *The Encyclopedia of the Digestive System and Digestive Disorders.* New York: Facts On File, Inc., 2004

VISUALIZATION (See GUIDED IMAGERY)

WOMEN

Berg, Barbara J. *The Crisis of the Working Mother.* New York: Summit Books, 1986.

Freudenberger, Herbert, and Gail North. *Women's Burnout: How to Spot It, How to Reverse It, and How to Prevent It.* Garden City, N.Y.: Doubleday & Company, Inc., 1985.

Lerner, Harriet Goldhor. *The Dance of Anger.* New York: Harper & Row, 1985.

———. *The Dance of Intimacy.* New York: Harper & Row, 1989.

Long, B. C., and C. J. Haney. "Coping Strategies for Working women: Aerobic Exercise and Relaxation Interventions." *Behavior Therapy* 19 (1988): pp. 75–83.

Powell, J. Robin. *The Working Woman's Guide to Managing Stress.* Englewood Cliffs, N.J.: Prentice Hall, 1994.

Siress, Ruth Hermann. *Working Women's Communications Survival Guide: How to Present Your Ideas With Impact. Clarity, and Power and Get the Recognition You Deserve.* Englewood Cliffs, N.J.: Prentice Hall, 1994.

Weinstock, Lorna, and Eleanor Gilman. *Overcoming Panic Disorder: A Woman's Guide.* Chicago: Contemporary Books, 1998.

Witkin, Georgia. *The Female Stress Syndrome: How to Become Stress-Wise in the '90s.* New York: Newmarket Press, 1991.

WORKPLACE

Adams, Scott. *The Dilbert Principle: A Cubicle's-Eye View of Bosses. Meetings, Management Fads and Other Workplace Afflictions.* New York: HarperBusiness, 1997.

Brown, Stephanie. *The Hand Book: Preventing Computer Injury.* New York: Ergonomne, 1993.

Frankenhaeuser, Marianne. "The Psychophysiology of Workload, Stress, and Health: Comparison Between the Sexes." *Annals of Behavioral Medicine* 13, no. 4: pp. 197–204.

Karasek, Robert, and Tores Theorell. *Health Work: Stress, Productivity, and the Reconstruction of Working Life.* New York: Basic Books, 1990.

Leana, Carrie R., and Daniel C. Feldman. *Coping with Job Loss: How Individuals, Organizations and Communities Respond to Layoffs.* New York: Lexington Books, 1992.

Meyer, G. J. *Executive Blues: Down and Out in Corporate America.* New York: Franklin Square Press, 1997.

Peterson, Michael. "Work, Corporate Culture, and Stress: Implications for Worksite Health Promotion." *American Journal of Health Behavior* 21, no. 4 (1997): pp. 243–252.

Repetti, Rena, Karen Matthews, and Ingrid Waidron. "Employment and Women's Health Effect of Paid Employment on Women's Mental and Physical Health." *American Psychologist* 44, no. 11: pp. 1394–1401.

Schnall, Peter L., Carl Pieper, and Joseph E. Schwartz. "The Relationship between Job Strain, Workplace Diastolic Blood Pressure, and Left Ventricular Mass Index: Results of a Case-Control Study." *Journal of the American Medical Association* 263, no. 7 (April 11, 1990).

Schor, Juliet. *The Overworked American: The Unexpected Decline of Leisure.* New York: Basic Books, 1991.

Snyder, Don J. *The Cliff Walk: A Memoir of a Lost Job and a Found Life.* Boston: Little, Brown, 1997.

Veninga, Robert L., and James P. Spradley. *The Work Stress Connection.* New York: Ballantine Books, 1981.

Wolf, Stewart G. Jr., and Albert J. Finestone. *Occupational Stress.* Littleton, Mass.: PSG Publishing, 1986.

WORKPLACE VIOLENCE

Barling, Julian. "Workplace Violence." In *Encyclopaedia of Occupational Health and Safety.* 4th ed. Geneva, Switzerland: International Labor Organization, 1998.

Kahn, Ada P. *Encyclopedia of Work-Related Injuries, Illnesses and Health Issues.* New York: Facts On File, Inc., 2004.

National Institute for Occupational Safety and Health. *Worker Health Chartbook, 2004.* Atlanta: Centers for Disease Control and Prevention, September 2004.

Rugala, Eugene A., ed. *Workplace Violence: Issues in Response.* Washington, DC: U.S. Federal Bureau of Investigation, 2002.

WORRY

Hallowell, Edward M. *Worry: Controlling It and Using It Wisely.* New York: Random House, 1997.

YOGA

Devananda, Swami Vishnu. *The Swivananda Companion to Yoga.* New York: Fireside, 1983.

Groves, Dawn. *Yoga for Busy People: Increase Energy and Reduce Stress in Minutes a Day.* Emeryville, Calif.: New World Library, 1995.

Iyengar, Geeta S. *Yoga: A Gem for Women.* Palo Alto, Calif.: Timeless Books, 1990.

Lad, Vasant, and David Frawley. *The Yoga of Herbs,* Santa Fe, N. Mex.: Lotus Press, 1986.

Taylor, Louise. *A Woman's Book of Yoga: A Journal for Health and Self-Discovery.* Boston: Charles F. Tuttle Company, 1993.

Terkel, Susan Neiburg. *Yoga Is for Me.* Minneapolis: Lerner Publications Company, 1987.

Vishnudevananda, Swami. *The Complete Illustrated Book of Yoga.* New York: Pocket, 1981.

INDEX